University of California at Berkeley

THE NEW WELLNESS ENCYCLOPEDIA

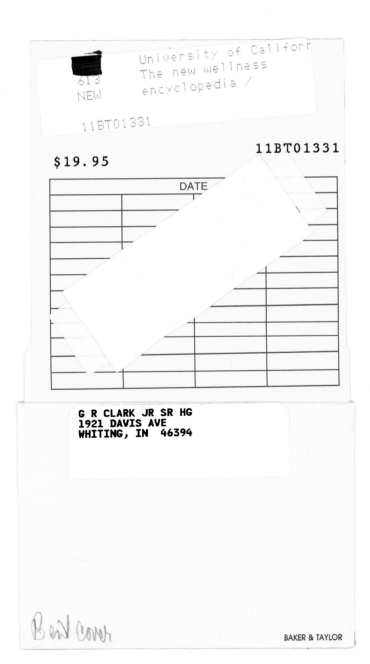

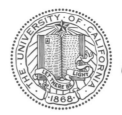

University of California at Berkeley

THE NEW WELLNESS

ENCYCLOPEDIA

From the Editors
of the University of California at Berkeley
WELLNESS LETTER

Houghton Mifflin Company
Boston • New York 1995

THE UNIVERSITY OF CALIFORNIA AT BERKELEY WELLNESS LETTER

The *Wellness Letter* is a monthly eight-page newsletter that delivers brisk, useful
coverage on health, nutrition and exercise topics in language that is clear, engaging and nontechnical. It's a
unique resource that covers fundamental ways to prevent illness.
For information on how to order this award-winning newsletter from the world-famous School of Public Health
at the University of California at Berkeley, write to
Health Letter Associates, Department 1108, 632 Broadway, New York, New York 10012.

Copyright ©1995 by Health Letter Associates
All rights reserved.

This book was created and produced by Rebus, Inc.
New York, New York

For information about permission to reprint selections from
this book, write to Permissions, Houghton Mifflin Company,
215 Park Avenue South, New York, NY 10003

CIP data is available.

ISBN 0-395-73345-6

Printed in the United States of America

DOW 10 9 8 7 6 5 4 3 2 1

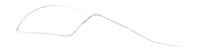

This book is not intended as a substitute for the advice of a
physician. Readers who suspect they may have specific
medical problems should consult a physician about any
suggestions made in this book.

Preventive health is something that can and should be practiced every day by every person. With that conviction, we launched the *University of California at Berkeley Wellness Letter* more than a decade ago with only 20,000 subscribers. We believed that thousands more would be attracted by our wellness concept—the idea that health is your most precious possession, and that nutrition, exercise, good health care, a positive attitude, a healthy environment, and, most of all, knowledge are the crucial factors in maintaining good health and longevity. Our intention was to create a publication that would clarify the often conflicting and superficial health information presented by the popular media. We chose the word "wellness" because it conveys what we consider to be a primary goal: leading a full and productive life. And one of the crucial tenets of wellness is that preventing illness is just as important as treating it—perhaps *more* important because most chronic diseases are incurable.

In 1990, in the spirit of the *Wellness Letter* (which by then had grown to more than 600,000 subscribers in the United States and Canada), we developed the first edition of this encyclopedia—a comprehensive resource that differed from other medical reference books in that it focused on tomorrow's health, rather than today's illness. Since then, there have been more than enough developments to merit a new edition.

This book updates and expands upon most of the topics that appeared in the first edition, and adds a number of new ones as well. Here you'll find authoritative information on the potential protection against heart disease and cancer offered by antioxidants; new cholesterol testing guidelines; optimal calcium intakes for men and women; expanded vitamin and mineral charts; a comprehensive discussion of weight control, with recommendations on how to evaluate diet plans; a new (and more moderate) prescription for exercise that can contribute to a vigorous, long life; how to treat and prevent low-back pain; updates on environmental and safety issues; recent guidelines on mammograms and other screening tests—just to name a few of the hundreds of topics that are covered in the following pages.

As we noted in the first edition, this is not a reference book that should sit on your shelf until something goes wrong. The information here, like that in the *Wellness Letter,* contains positive, practical guidelines you can take advantage of right away.

SHELDON MARGEN, M.D.
Professor Emeritus, School of Public Health
University of California at Berkeley

Contents

Part 5 ENVIRONMENT AND SAFETY

While the past twenty-five years have seen tremendous advances in medicine—in the development of new drugs and new diagnostic and surgical techniques—these discoveries have a downside: drugs are prescribed too readily; an excessive number of X-rays and other diagnostic tests are often ordered; hospitals have grown overcrowded and impersonal; and the cost of health care has soared.

Even when applied effectively, the medical approach to sustaining life is incomplete. Consider this: a major study showing that the mortality rate from heart disease has been dropping since 1963 also found that lifestyle changes in diet and smoking habits—rather than new medical treatments—accounted for over half of the decline. Another large-scale study at the Carter Center at Emory University showed that fourteen primary causes of illness and premature death—causes ranging from drug abuse to cancer and heart disease—were dramatically influenced by risk factors for which preventive action can be taken. (The six factors most frequently cited were tobacco, alcohol, injuries, unintended pregnancy, lack of preventive services, and improper nutrition.) Indeed, the researchers concluded that about two-thirds of the deaths under age sixty-five are potentially preventable.

The clear conclusion of these and other studies cited throughout this book is that we are not dependent on medical breakthroughs to achieve an enormous improvement in our health. Rather, good health depends to a large extent on certain lifestyle choices we make that include what we eat, how active we are, whether or not we smoke, the precautions we take to avoid injuries and accidents, how we deal with tension and anxiety, even how we manage the environments in which we live and work. This book is intended to inform you about these choices and to help you integrate them into your life.

Bear in mind that wellness is not "alternative" medicine—it doesn't promote special diets, regimens that rely on vitamin supplements, herbal medications, or other treatments based on fads or anecdotal evidence. Nor is wellness a substitute for medical care when you are ill. Physicians, nurses, and other well-trained medical providers can diagnose, alleviate, and cure many types of health problems. Your doctor can also perform routine tests and examinations that can greatly increase your chances of avoiding or recovering from an illness. Nevertheless, the medical community by and large is devoted to helping people get well after they have become ill. The premise of wellness is that there are many ways to prevent problems that affect your health, and correct information is essential for you to make the proper choices.

The recommendations in this book

As the idea of taking charge of your own health has gained acceptance, claims about how to do this have proliferated. Newspapers and magazines bombard us with advice on how to eat right, what to do about heart disease, when and how to exercise, and a hundred other health-related matters. Some of this information is straightforward, but much of it is confused, contradictory, or misleading. The information in the following pages is backed by the consensus of researchers and professors at the School of Public Health at the University of California at Berkeley, one of the nation's leading research and teaching institutions. In drawing upon their expertise, the book provides conclusions that have emerged from reviews of hundreds of scientific studies. The intent is to sort out claims and misconceptions, and to supply explanations and guidelines that are clear, practical, and as up-to-date as possible.

Though knowledge in preventive health care is expanding rapidly, we have made an effort to arrive at recommendations that will hold up over time—that are based not on one or two small studies, but on a more substantial body of research. For example, researchers may argue over exactly how much exercise is the optimal amount to lower the risk for heart disease. But several large-scale studies have shown unequivocally that even moderate amounts of physical activity offer a dramatic benefit compared to being sedentary. Clarifying such distinctions is one of the ways that this book serves as a truly authoritative reference source.

How to use this book

The New Wellness Encyclopedia is divided into five major parts: Longevity, Nutrition, Exercise, Self-Care, and—one of the most recent areas of concern—Environment and Safety. Each part contains chapters dealing with major topics; each chapter is organized around subtopics, with guidelines or special topics highlighted in charts, tables, and boxes. Many of the guidelines offer manageable steps on how to change old habits for healthier ones. You will also find tips and interesting facts in the margin of almost every page. The index, which is extensively cross-referenced, simplifies access to information on any topic. The text also contains cross-references to related topics.

In addition, the book features The Wellness Food Guide—a 75-page mini-encyclopedia that offers advice on a wide variety of foods, including shopping and preparation tips. And a glossary at the back of the book provides brief definitions of key terms.

Part 1   LONGEVITY

The first and foremost goal of wellness is preventing illness, in particular illness that can shorten your life or decrease the quality of life, especially as you get older. Today, in Western societies, the health problems that most significantly affect longevity are chronic diseases such as heart disease, stroke, and cancer—the current leading causes of mortality. Researchers have determined that the factors promoting these illnesses are strongly linked to lifestyle, behavior patterns, and complex environmental factors. This part of the book provides practical information on how you can lower your risk of chronic disease. In the following pages, you'll find that many of the recommendations for longevity overlap and work together; for example, a diet that reduces blood cholesterol levels also helps you lose weight and reduces your risk of developing certain kinds of cancer. The opening chapter clarifies the concept of health risk. Subsequent chapters provide a detailed look at the most important risk factors that affect your health and explain what you can do to reduce or control them.

Health Risks: A Perspective

Efforts to identify health risks—and reduce them, if possible—are as old as medicine itself. Hippocrates advised his fellow physicians to "consider the seasons of the year and what effects each of them produces" and to take note of what people drank and ate and how they lived. Scientists today are still looking for the determinants of health, albeit with a little more sophistication and scientific knowledge. Epidemiology (literally, the study of epidemics) is the attempt to identify the factors that cause diseases and injuries in order to determine what the probabilities are that they will cause them, and to determine how to decrease or eliminate the identified risks. This is often referred to as risk hazard appraisal, which is of growing importance in medical science, especially in the effort to prevent disease and promote health. Once the risk factors are known, the next job is to make changes in the environment (for example, to persuade car manufacturers to install seat belts of a certain design) and to persuade people to change their behavior (for example, convince them to fasten the belts).

When media reports talk about risk, they are basically quoting odds. No one can honestly assure you that doing one thing will kill you, while refraining from doing it will keep you safe. For example, on average, one out of ten smokers gets lung cancer, but a nonsmoker also occasionally gets it. If you are an average smoker, your lifetime chances of getting lung cancer are twenty-four times higher than those for a nonsmoker, and the risk increases as the amount of smoking increases.

In the science of risk assessment, there is no such thing as absolute safety; however, you can choose to widen or narrow your safety margins. And though scientists may assess the risks, it's often hard to evaluate what the experts say. The press seldom makes your task simpler. The headline "Alcohol Shown to Cause Breast Cancer" will attract more readers than "Study Suggests Alcohol Intake Slightly Increases Breast Cancer Risk for Some Women." It is always easier to oversimplify than to tell people how complicated things really are.

Examples of risk assessment

How do experts figure your odds against different risks? Here are two examples:

•You are about to plan a thousand-mile journey, and you aren't pressed for time. Rank the following means of transportation from the safest to the riskiest: bus, train, plane, and passenger car.

According to recent statistics from the National Safety Council, in the United States you are safest in a plane or bus—the fatality rates are almost equal—and in greatest danger in a car. About ten people die per billion car and taxi miles, whereas it takes some five billion bus or plane miles to produce one fatality. Trains are thirty times safer than cars, but only about half as safe as buses and planes.

•You're a healthy forty-five-year-old man, slightly overweight. Your father and his brother both died in their fifties of heart disease. Your mother, now sixty-five, has had non–insulin-dependent diabetes (NIDDM, adult-onset or type II diabetes) for several years. Are you likely to get one of these ailments?

Many experts now believe that continual exposure of breast tissue to the hormone estrogen (beginning at puberty) is probably at the root of breast cancer. Additional nonalterable risk factors include the early onset of menstruation, late menopause, a family history of breast cancer, and just growing older. Recently a gene that predisposes people in certain families to breast cancer has been identified, but it is still poorly understood.

Research into the role of dietary factors has led nowhere in particular: there's no conclusive evidence that a high fat intake or any other kind of diet is related to breast cancer, though it's true that women who live in countries with high fat intakes tend to have higher rates of breast cancer. Presumably, a very healthy diet would be as protective against breast cancer as against other cancers—yet even that is uncertain.

Smoking—the chief risk factor for lung cancer—appears to have no connection to breast cancer.

Both heart disease and diabetes have genetic components. If your father died young of a heart attack, you have a good chance of following in his footsteps. Knowing your inherited liabilities, though, gives you an excellent opportunity to alter them. The genetic odds may be lowered significantly if you are not overweight, keep your blood pressure under control, and maintain a low blood cholesterol level. If your mother has diabetes, that's an indication that weight control and exercise are crucially important for you, and that periodically your doctor should measure your blood sugar level.

For many of us, familial tendencies constitute an emotional trap. People whose parents or grandparents died at comparatively young ages of heart disease or cancer, or some other disease with a genetic component, usually realize that this heritage works against them and may falsely conclude that taking care of their own health is irrelevant. On the other hand, if all your relatives were as indestructible as Winston Churchill—who drank brandy, smoked habitually, was overweight, yet lived into his eighties and died peacefully in his sleep—you may have an equally false sense of invulnerability.

Researchers may one day unravel the genetic code and come closer to predicting your chances of getting a disorder such as heart disease or hypertension. But of the hundreds of diseases that have been genetically defined, most are fairly rare. The few that are more common include hemophilia, in which a blood-clotting factor is absent; sickle cell anemia, a blood disorder that occurs most commonly among people of African descent; cystic fibrosis; and certain forms of kidney disease.

In many ailments that show signs of running in families, such as cancer, heart disease, or diabetes, heredity is only one factor in the mix. Your biological and cultural heritage, your lifestyle, and your environment interact, and it's the interaction that counts. Your diet or exercise habits or your environment may foster, or foil, the tendencies with which you were born.

Making sense of "increased risk": the alcohol/breast cancer connection

Reports that warn about doubling or tripling your risk of heart disease or any other specific illness need to be viewed cautiously. You have to know how likely you are to get the disease in the first place. For example, if your chances of developing a certain illness are 1 in 100,000, a doubled risk brings you up to 2 in 100,000 (or 1 in 50,000). Those are still pretty low odds. However, if 1 out of 10 people develops this illness and you do something that doubles your risk, your chances are now 1 in 5. That's a very significant increase.

Let's say, for example, that you're a forty-eight-year-old woman, a good cook, and you enjoy a glass of wine with fine food. You've heard about a report stating that even moderate alcohol consumption—equivalent to one or two glasses of wine per day—may double a woman's risk of getting breast cancer, and that quitting now might not reduce the risk. Nevertheless, you stop drinking wine. Your sister is a teetotaler. Are you twice as likely to get breast cancer as she is?

Consider two figures that have appeared in the press. Several studies of alcohol and breast cancer, most recently a Spanish study and an American one, have showed that even moderate alcohol intake was associated with a 50 percent risk for breast cancer—a figure hard for women to ignore. Along with this 50 percent figure was another statistic issued by the American Cancer Society—namely, that one in nine American women is at risk of developing breast cancer at some time in her life. That's a risk of 11 percent, a figure that is sufficiently intimidating in itself. Is it logical to conclude that women drinkers run a risk closer to 16 percent, a terrifying narrowing of the safety margin?

What one has to understand is that the one-in-nine figure applies to *lifetime* risk, not risk at any given moment; it encompasses all American women indiscriminately, from age one to eighty-five. That is, it's a lifetime average and does not describe the odds for an individual over shorter intervals. The incidence of breast cancer in the population rises with age. A fifty-year-old woman has about a 1 in 50 chance of developing breast cancer, or 2 percent. If she's a moderate drinker, her chances would increase by half—to 1.5 in 50, or 3 percent—if the reported studies are correct. That's a little less horrifying than 16 percent.

Consider this, too. In a review of all population studies to date on alcohol intake and breast cancer, Dr. Lynn Rosenberg, writing in *Epidemiological Review,* observed that while many studies have shown an association, "the associations have been weak and inconsistent," and "confounding cannot be ruled out as an explanation." That is, something in the lifestyle or environment of women who drink might be responsible for any association. The causes of breast cancer remain unknown.

Being realistic

Many people, of course, choose to focus on news that is reassuring rather than alarming. For example, say that you're fifty, female, and a smoker. Your last checkup showed that both your blood pressure and blood cholesterol level were somewhat higher than they should be. You know this means you risk a heart attack or stroke, but you read an article that said that even fifty-year-old male smokers with high blood pressure and elevated cholesterol levels have only a 13 percent chance of getting sick within six years. So you're looking on the bright side: you've got an 87 percent chance of staying healthy for the next six years. Is this a constructive attitude?

A fifty-year-old smoker, male or female, with elevated blood cholesterol and blood pressure is seriously courting cardiovascular disease. You may have only a 13 percent chance of developing it (though neither you nor your doctor has any way of predicting whether you'll fall into the lucky 87 percent who do not develop heart disease or the unlucky 13 percent who do). If these sound like favorable odds, you may decide not to make any changes in your habits. However, a more realistic way for you to consider the odds is as follows: if your risk factors are low (that is, you don't smoke and your blood

When Risk Factors Synergize

If you smoke and drink, you are worse off than if you only smoke or only drink. Alcohol seems to multiply the cancer-causing effects of smoking—a phenomenon called synergism. According to some studies, a person who has one drink per day but doesn't smoke has a somewhat higher risk of oral cancer than a nonsmoking teetotaler. A person who smokes up to a pack of cigarettes a day and doesn't drink has about the same relative risk.

But the risk for a moderate smoker and drinker (a pack or less a day and one drink a day) is four times greater (400 percent) than that for a total abstainer. For a heavy smoker (two packs) and drinker (more than two small drinks a day), the risk is fifteen times greater. No one knows exactly why these risks synergize in this instance. However, if you both smoke and drink and decide you'll give up one of these habits, quit smoking. In terms of risk for potentially fatal cancers as well as heart disease, it's the more harmful of the two.

Genetic screening

Many would-be or expecting parents today face choices based on genetic considerations. An ever-expanding range of disorders can now be diagnosed prior to conception—thus more avenues are open to would-be parents than ever before. If their genetic history and/or the results of such screening suggest problems, the couple may decide to undergo prenatal testing, or else choose not to conceive children.

Once a child is conceived, tests such as amniocentesis and chorionic villus sampling, which examine fetal tissue, may be recommended to determine the presence of certain genetic disorders, such as Down's syndrome, sickle-cell disease, Tay-Sachs disease, and spina bifida. (Many other birth defects still cannot be detected, however.) For more information and referrals, contact your local chapter of the March of Dimes. Many university hospitals have genetic counseling programs.

Words to Watch

The following words are commonly used in reporting scientific studies—and both reporters and lay readers often misinterpret their meaning.

Breakthrough: is so overworked as to be meaningless.

Contributes to, is linked to, is associated with: none of these terms means "causes."

Doubles the risk, triples the risk: may or may not be meaningful. Does the reporter tell you what your risk was in the first place? If your risk is 1 in a million, and you double it, that's still only 1 in 500,000. If your risk is 1 in 100, and increases by 25 percent, that is 1 in 80, which may be cause for concern.

Dramatic proof: probably neither.

Indicates, suggests: do not mean "proves."

In some people: does not mean "in all people."

May: does not mean "will."

Proves: scientific studies gather evidence in a systematic way, but they seldom prove anything. A dubious word.

---

pressure and blood cholesterol levels are low), your chance of having a heart attack between age forty and sixty-four is only 6 percent. But, if you continue to smoke and do nothing about your other risk factors, your chance of having a heart attack during these years is 40 percent—a substantial difference. Giving up cigarettes, controlling your blood pressure, and lowering your cholesterol level would significantly widen your safety margin. Obviously, that's the constructive action to take.

Another example of this kind of reasoning can be seen in the relationship between oral contraceptives and heart attacks. The high-dose oral contraceptives that were introduced in the 1960s—but are rarely used now—increased the risk of heart attack by a factor of 4.7. This sounds like a very large increase. However, for a twenty- to twenty-four-year-old woman, heart attack risk is estimated to be less than 1 in 500,000. Thus a fivefold increase represents only about 5 in 500,000 (or 1 in 100,000). This means that if all the 9.5 million American women in this age group were to take high-dose oral contraceptives, ninety of them (instead of the expected nineteen) would die of heart attacks. This is many fewer deaths than might result from unwanted pregnancies in the same age group. And even this small risk has been markedly reduced by the introduction of low-dose estrogen contraceptives (which are discussed on page 384).

Interpreting health news

Nowadays almost anything can be called a study or be so designated by the press. Major journals in the medical field attempt to limit unproven or overstated claims by carefully reviewing what is submitted to them. However, a phenomenal amount of research is published each year: an average of 240,000 biomedical articles in English alone are indexed each year by the National Library of Medicine. If every study "proved" something, there would be no questions left unanswered. A dose of skepticism is always in order, even when the study comes from an important institution and appears in a respected journal.

Some years ago, for example, the *New England Journal of Medicine* published a study from the Johns Hopkins Medical Institutions showing that heavy coffee drinkers had two to three times the risk of heart disease—a study conducted over many years and using many subjects. From reports in the media, it sounded like proof positive, unless you actually read the complete study. The authors didn't ask participants about important risk factors such as their diet (did they habitually eat a lot of fat and cholesterol?), smoking habits, and exercise levels. It wasn't clear, therefore, whether coffee was at fault, or diet, or other factors altogether. "A need for further investigation" was the final word—though this didn't keep reporters from citing this study as proof of the dangers of caffeine consumption.

Or consider a 1994 Finnish study that made front-page news because of its finding that beta carotene supplements, instead of protecting against cancer, as expected, seemed to increase the risk of the disease among smokers. Scientists were surprised and reporters dumbfounded, but they should have also been skeptical. Any study must be evaluated in the context of other studies, and this study—which flies in the face of all other research on the subject—had problems. For one thing, it was too short—the development of most cancers appears to take decades, but the study only followed the sample of smokers for six years. It also focused on a homogenous group—white, middle-aged male smokers who had smoked for decades. But what is true for smokers may not hold for others. And the men were all Finns, who may, due to some genetic trait, utilize beta carotene differently from other peoples. What is more, even the researchers expressed surprise at their study's results, and acknowledged that an adverse effect of beta carotene was unlikely and might be due to chance.

When you read or listen to health news, keep the following points in mind:

Don't jump to conclusions. Changing your daily habits on the basis of a single study is almost never a good idea. Scientific findings should be duplicated by others for validity, and even then there's an element of uncertainty.

Try to distinguish between promising advances, reported as scientific news, and public health recommendations. If doctors at some medical center have just done the first successful liver transplant, that's interesting. But it doesn't mean there's now a cure for liver disease. On the other hand, if the Surgeon General or the American Cancer Society says "eat less fat" or "don't smoke," you can assume that many studies point in this direction.

Keep your skepticism in working order. Science is an uncertain undertaking. Progress is measured less often by dramatic insights than by the slow accumulation of knowledge. "Astounding" medical advances are rare. "Medical milestone" in a press report is like the word "natural" on a food package: something to arouse rather than allay your suspicions. No matter how enthusiastically a finding is hailed in the press, see what the experts are saying next week and next month.

Notice where the information is coming from. Does the author of the article cite any authorities, appear to rely on scientific evidence—or simply tell a lot of anecdotes? "Thousands of people say..." "It's well known that..." Is any source given for astounding statistics? Even fully sourced statistics can be wrong, of course, but if the author is willing to give sources, that may be a good sign.

Use your own logic and common sense. If the article says that the Japanese are healthier than Americans and claims it's because they eat more fish, stop and think. The Japanese also eat a lot of rice. They also sleep on mats instead of mattresses. How does the writer know it's the fish? The heart attack rate tends to be higher in countries where most households have telephones, but that doesn't mean the telephones are causing heart attacks.

Be wary when studies are cited to sell you a product. Manufacturers and industry groups have been known to stretch the truth.

Health Risks:
A Perspective

Your family's medical tree

One of the best presents you can give your children is a record of your family's medical tree. It should include the age at death and cause of death (as well as other medical problems) of your parents and siblings. Data on your grandparents may be helpful, but harder to uncover. In the past, the cause of death may not have been known, may have been misdiagnosed (a heart attack mistaken for "acute indigestion"), or may have been labeled with a euphemism (since the term "cancer" carried a stigma). You may be able to get medical records from family members' doctors or from the hospitals where relatives died; the state health department can provide a copy of death certificates. Besides cancers, heart disease, and diabetes, you'll want to list high blood pressure, stroke, kidney disease, anemia, miscarriages, arthritis, epilepsy, osteoporosis, peptic ulcer, mental illness, and other major disorders that appear to "run in families."

Heart Disease: Rating the Risks

Since 1960, the mortality rate from heart attack in the U.S. has dropped by half, according to the National Center for Health Statistics—and since 1980 alone, by one-third. This success has been due not only to improved medical treatment of coronary artery disease (CAD), but also to preventive steps people have taken. Heart attack is still our leading killer, however, accounting for about 500,000 deaths every year—45% in people under age 65. Most of these deaths, too, could be avoided or at least postponed if everyone paid attention to the risk factors for CAD and if they took preventive measures to counter them.

Just how far we have to go in preventing this disease can be seen in a new report from the Centers for Disease Control and Prevention that showed that only 18% of adults are free of the six major coronary risk factors. And among those over fifty, only about 10% report that they are free of the major risks. Many people don't even know what these risk factors are, except perhaps high blood cholesterol. The other five proven risks—smoking, obesity, high blood pressure, diabetes, and being sedentary—are as bad, or even worse, for the heart.

The pillars of prevention

Scientists now know far more about the major controllable risk factors for CAD than for most other diseases. A risk factor merely increases the probability that you will develop CAD; it doesn't guarantee that you will, nor does its absence (or even the absence of all risk factors) guarantee that you won't have a heart attack. If you have more than one CAD risk factor, the combined impact is greater than it would be if you added the individual risks together.

Most of the risk factors can be countered by relatively simple preventive measures. In 1992 Dr. JoAnn Manson and colleagues from Harvard reviewed nearly 200 studies on CAD to evaluate the role of the known preventive measures; the results were published in the *New England Journal of Medicine (NEJM)* . Here are some of the details:

1. Quit smoking. This is perhaps the single most effective step you can take. Anywhere from 20 to 40% (100,000 to 200,000 every year) of all CAD deaths are still directly attributable to smoking. It more than doubles your chance of eventually having a heart attack and increases the chance of dying from it by 70%; it is also the leading cause of sudden cardiac death. Smoking low-tar, low-nicotine cigarettes does not significantly reduce coronary risk. Smoking even a few cigarettes a day can endanger your heart. In addition, it's estimated that more than 35,000 non-smoking Americans die each year from heart disease because of long-term exposure to other people's smoke. But quitting smoking markedly reduces your CAD risk: within five to ten years of quitting, your risk declines to a level similar to that of people who never smoked.

2. Reduce cholesterol. For every 1% reduction in blood cholesterol, there's a 2 to 3% decline in the risk of heart attack. Since 1960, the average blood cholesterol level in the U.S. has declined from 220 to 205 mg/dl (a "desirable" level is below 200), a 7% decline, according to the National Center for Health Statistics. That's a significant decline, but still leaves about 20% of American adults who have "high" cholesterol levels (above 240) and another 30% with "borderline-high" levels (200 to 239). For information on the government's new guidelines on how to monitor blood cholesterol and for advice on how to lower total cholesterol and raise protective HDL cholesterol, see pages 47-50.

3. Avoid or control hypertension. About 50 million Americans have high blood pressure, which is a risk factor for stroke and heart attack. For every 1 mm Hg reduction in diastolic blood pressure, there's a 2 to 3% decline in the risk of heart attack. Reducing systolic blood pressure also decreases risk. If you can lower your blood pressure by making lifestyle changes—including limiting intake of sodium, calories, and alcohol—the coronary benefits are likely to be dramatic.

4. Stay active. Dozens of studies have shown that exercise protects against CAD. The *NEJM* report estimated that sedentary people who begin a regular program of exercise reduce their risk of a heart attack by 35 to 55%. And yet an estimated 60 to 80% of Americans are sedentary, with little improvement evident in decades. Even low-

Risk factors you can't change

There are several risk factors for CAD that you can do nothing about. But they should give you even more incentive to address the factors that can be improved.

Heredity. *People with a parent or sibling who had a premature heart attack (before age 55 in a man or 65 in a woman) are at increased risk of CAD. Race is also a factor: African-Americans have an elevated risk of CAD, primarily because they have a higher risk of hypertension and diabetes than whites.*

Increasing age. *About 55% of all heart attacks occur after age 65. More than four out of five who die of such attacks are over 65.*

Sex. *Before age 55, men have a much higher rate of CAD than women. By the time they reach 60, women develop cardiovascular disease at the same rate as men at 50—and this 10-year gap prevails until about the age of 75 or 80, when the differences disappear and the rates become similar. Women who have a heart attack, especially at older ages, are more likely to die from it than are men.*

intensity activities, such as walking, if done regularly and over the long term, can decrease the risk of heart attack. The important thing is to find a type and level of activity you can maintain regularly with pleasure. Exercise helps the heart work more efficiently, reduces blood pressure, boosts HDL cholesterol, decreases the tendency of blood to form clots, moderates stress, helps the body use insulin, and helps people control their weight.

5. Maintain a healthy weight. About one in four American adults is obese (weighing at least 20% above the "suggested" weight for their height), which doubles their risk for CAD at a given age. And the more overweight you are, the greater the effect on CAD. Obesity also increases the risk for diabetes, hypertension, and high blood cholesterol, which further worsen CAD risk. How fat is distributed affects the risk. People who put weight on around the waist (apple-shaped or pot-bellied) have a greater chance of CAD than those who put weight on the hips (pear-shaped).

6. Avoid or control diabetes. Non–insulin-dependent diabetes (also called adult-onset diabetes), which afflicts about 12 million Americans, is an important risk factor for both CAD and hypertension. Diabetic women are three to seven times more likely to have coronary heart disease than those without diabetes, and diabetic men have two to three times the risk. Even people who merely have slightly elevated blood sugar levels but no detectable diabetes are at increased risk. Weight control and exercise can improve the utilization of blood sugar and prevent or slow down the onset of diabetes.

Additional steps
7. Consider hormone therapy after menopause. Estrogen therapy raises HDL cholesterol and also lowers the risk of heart attack in other ways. It also decreases the risk of osteoporosis and perhaps stroke. Today hormone replacement therapy, or HRT, usually includes progestin (a synthetic form of progesterone) along with estrogen. Recent studies suggest that the combined estrogen-progestin therapy also protects against heart disease. HRT is not appropriate for all women, so talk to your doctor.

8. Consider a drink a day. There's a growing consensus that light to moderate alcohol consumption—two drinks or less a day for a man, one drink for a woman (a drink is defined as twelve ounces of beer, four ounces of wine, or 1.5 ounces of 80-proof spirits)—has a minor beneficial effect for the heart. However, drinking more than this can increase the risk of heart attack and stroke, as well as cirrhosis, cancer, and accidents. As the *NEJM* report put it, "the difference between drinking small-to-moderate quantities of alcohol and drinking large amounts may mean the difference between preventing and causing disease."

9. Consider aspirin. Low-dose aspirin—usually half an aspirin a day (160 milligrams)—can lower the risk of heart attack by about one-third by reducing the ability of platelets in the blood to stick together and thus form a clot. It is particularly advisable if you have an elevated risk of CAD. The research has focused mostly on men so far, but at least two encouraging studies have suggested that women benefit, too. Aspirin can have side effects and isn't right for everyone, so don't start aspirin therapy on your own—ask your doctor about it.

What about diet?
Although "eat a healthful, low-fat diet" is not generally considered a separate preventive measure, it clearly plays a role in many of the listed measures, such as controlling cholesterol and body weight. In addition, there has been accumulating evidence that a high intake of antioxidant vitamins (usually supplements of C, E, and beta carotene) helps reduce the risk of CAD.

Mind/body: stress and anger

Until recently, people with so-called Type A personality (aggressive, competitive, tense) were considered coronary-prone. But subsequent studies were contradictory and failed to confirm the link. Many researchers then shifted their focus to various components of Type A—notably anger or hostility. Some studies found a link between anger or hostility and CAD, but other did not. People who suppress their anger appear to be at greatest risk for CAD and other illness, though some studies have found that venting anger isn't necessarily better.

Some of the best research on stress has involved the workplace. A worker's sense of control, or lack thereof, is perhaps the major determinant of how he reacts to stress. Studies in the U.S. and Europe have consistently shown that people in high-strain jobs (heavy pressure to perform but little sense of control), such as bus drivers, have the highest rates of hypertension and heart attacks. Stereotypical "high-stress" jobs such as managers, engineers, and doctors tend to have the lowest rate, because these professionals get to make more of their own decisions. Even when such risk factors as age, race, education, and smoking are statistically eliminated from the equation, people in the bottom 10% of the job echelon turn out to be in the top 10% for illness. Researchers have found that these workers have four to five times the risk of heart attack as those at the top 10% of the ladder, whose jobs give them a high sense of control. (See page 450 for more on stress and its effects on health.)

The Role of Diet and Exercise

The relevance of diet and physical activity to wellness cannot be overstated. The foods you eat and your level of physical activity affect a number of risk factors implicated in longevity, particularly blood cholesterol levels, hypertension, and obesity. Moreover, diet and exercise are the elements of your health care over which you have the most control.

Drawing on hundreds of studies, researchers have compiled considerable evidence showing the extent to which diet and exercise influence the risk of disease. This chapter summarizes the key findings concerning this connection; other benefits that you can derive from changes in diet and exercise, as well as specific recommendations, are covered in the nutrition and exercise sections of this book.

Diet and Longevity

The evidence that a proper diet can help prevent the leading chronic diseases comes from a wide range of sources: large-scale studies of what certain populations eat and the prevalence of various diseases in these groups; studies of humans and animals under experimental conditions showing how specific diets change their chronic disease risk; and laboratory experiments showing how chemicals alter the structure and function of cells and tissues in the test tube.

Based on these studies, scientists now estimate, for example, that 40 percent of all cancer incidence in men and nearly 60 percent in women are related to diet. Diet has also been clearly implicated in two of the three major factors in the development of heart disease—high blood cholesterol levels and hypertension. Furthermore, there is now a consensus among experts as to which dietary elements play a role in the development of disease. The American Cancer Society, the American Heart Association, the National Research Council, the National Cancer Institute, and many other scientific organizations all basically agree on the dietary changes individuals must make to reduce their risks of chronic disease. In addition, a comprehensive review of the available evidence on diet and health, conducted by the Surgeon General and released in 1989, confirmed the findings and recommendations of other organizations, and has been compared in importance to the 1964 Surgeon General's report on the relationship between tobacco use and disease.

What are the foods that play a role in disease prevention or promotion? Actually, it is not foods per se that contribute, but substances contained in foods. These range from fats—which in excessive amounts can contribute to heart disease—to antioxidant compounds, which can protect against cancer and other diseases, and enhance immune system functioning.

The following substances can contribute to health problems when consumed in excess:

Fat. Of all the changes you can make in your diet, cutting back on fat will have the greatest effect on reducing disease risk. A diet high in fat has been strongly linked to an increased risk of heart disease and certain forms of cancer, such as breast, colon, rectum, endometrium, and prostate. While there is no definitive evidence that a high-fat diet is a factor in breast cancer, population studies have suggested a link. A low-fat diet is helpful to those with diabetes, since diabetes accelerates the development of heart disease. In particular, a diet high in saturated fat (the type found in animal products, such as meats and whole-milk dairy products, and in tropical vegetable oils—coconut, palm, and palm kernel) contributes to heart disease by raising levels of total blood cholesterol and low-density lipoprotein (LDL) cholesterol—the type referred to as "bad" cholesterol.

A high-fat diet also contributes to obesity, which is an independent risk factor for heart disease and cancer, and the primary risk factor for developing non–insulin-dependent diabetes mellitus (NIDDM, also called adult-onset or type II diabetes).

Dietary cholesterol. Cholesterol from foods (cholesterol is found only in animal products) contributes to the development of heart disease because it can raise blood

Good sources of vitamin C

Asparagus
Blackberries
Broccoli·
Cantaloupe
Cauliflower
Chinese cabbage
Grapefruit
Grapefruit juice
Kale
Kiwifruit
Kohlrabi
Mangoes
Mustard greens
Oranges
Orange juice
Peas, edible pod
Peppers
Raspberries
Red cabbage
Strawberries
Tangerines
Tomatoes
Tomato juice

Is a Low-Fat Diet Worth the Effort?

In a study published in the *Journal of the American Medical Association* in 1991, researchers calculated that, if the amount of fat in the American diet were reduced from 37 percent of daily calories to 30 percent, the number of deaths from coronary artery disease and various forms of cancer would indeed decline—but that the benefit worked out to what the researchers called a "disappointing" gain of only three months for women and four months for men. The news media picked up on this—you torture yourself on a low-fat diet (actually such a diet is relatively easy) to gain "only a few months of life." Does that mean a low-fat diet isn't worth the effort? No. This type of statistical study is not useful in assessing the impact of modifying particular risk factors for disease or even eliminating certain diseases altogether. Since the gain in life expectancy is an average for the population as a whole, rather than for just people at high risk, it is small. This, however, is not surprising.

For instance, if all deaths from coronary artery disease (the leading killer) could be eliminated in the United States, there would be only a gain of 3.8 years in life expectancy for the entire population, according to research by the National Center for Health Statistics. But for those people who would have died of coronary artery disease, there would be a gain of 12.4 years.

Another dramatic example from NCHS: if breast cancer were eliminated in this country, Americans would live on average only about three more months (for all women, about seven months). That doesn't sound like much, but for those women who would have died of breast cancer, the extension of life would be more than seventeen years. Similarly, a middle-aged man with high blood cholesterol and other coronary risk factors might delay a fatal heart attack for decades by reducing his fat intake.

Thus the three-to-four-month gain in life expectancy for the general population suggested by this study tells you little. Another fundamental problem is that this study looked only at length of life, not at quality of life. By cutting down on fat and delaying disease, you may not only live longer, but also perhaps avoid many years of pain and suffering.

In addition, people who reduce their fat intake also usually cut down on calories and thus lose weight—which reduces their risk of diabetes, high blood pressure, and other diseases. But the researchers assumed that people would continue to consume the same number of calories, which is highly unlikely. And people who cut down on fat typically eat more fruits, vegetables, and grains. Thus they usually consume more fiber and antioxidant nutrients, which may reduce the risk of certain cancers and other diseases. The study did not consider these variables.

If we knew exactly who would die of fat-related coronary heart disease or cancer, of course, a low-fat diet would be recommended only for them. Since we don't know, a low-fat diet remains best for everyone. There's simply too much evidence about the substantial benefits of a low-fat, high-fiber diet in reducing the risk of the most common chronic diseases.

cholesterol levels, but not to as great an extent as saturated fat. Elevations in total cholesterol levels from dietary cholesterol are predominantly in the form of LDL.

Sodium. In populations with a high-sodium intake, there is an increased incidence of hypertension. While not everyone is sodium sensitive—responding to a high-sodium intake with a rise in blood pressure—there is no way to tell who is and who is not. In addition, there is some evidence that high-sodium intake over a lifetime may cause some people to become sodium sensitive.

Alcohol. A moderate intake of alcohol—the amount in one or two drinks per day—has been shown to slightly increase the levels of HDL ("good") cholesterol and offer protection against coronary artery disease. But alcohol consumed to excess can lead to decreased HDL levels, high blood pressure, and heart damage. Heavy drinking also increases the risk of cancer of the mouth, pharynx, esophagus, and larynx. These risks increase dramatically when alcohol is used in conjunction with tobacco. In addition, there is some association between alcohol intake and cancers of the pancreas, rectum, and breast. There is no evidence that alcohol causes these cancers, but once they have developed, alcohol may help promote their spread. Except when combined with smoking, the risk of cancer from alcohol appears to be most commonly linked with heavy alcohol consumption. In addition, drinking alcohol to excess can contribute to a decrease in bone mass, increasing the risk for developing obvious symptoms of osteoporosis, or bone weakening.

Nitrites and nitrates. These chemicals, which are used to preserve cured meats—such as bacon, hot dogs, sausages, and ham—have been found to promote cancers of the stomach and esophagus in laboratory animals, most probably because the chemicals can be converted by stomach acid to nitrosamines, which are carcinogenic. Foods high in vitamin C may block the conversion of nitrites and nitrates to cancer-causing nitrosamines.

Char-broiled foods. Grilling or barbecuing foods can create cancer-causing agents. This is most dangerous when fatty meats are cooked over a heat source because when the fat drips on the coals or hot coils, it forms carcinogenic substances that are then deposited on the food by the rising smoke.

The following substances are positive additions to a healthy diet:

Fiber. Both soluble and insoluble fiber help prevent disease. In combination with a low-fat, low-cholesterol diet, soluble fiber—found in oat and rice bran, legumes, and many fruits and vegetables—has been shown to help control cholesterol in individuals with elevated levels. In those with diabetes, soluble fiber appears to lower blood glucose levels when it makes a substantial contribution to the diet. Insoluble fiber—the type found in wheat bran—has been associated with a lower risk of colon cancer. Researchers theorize that fiber does this by helping to speed the elimination of waste matter and/or possibly by binding carcinogenic matter in the intestine in some way.

Antioxidants. Vitamins C and E, beta carotene (the precursor of vitamin A, which is formed in the body), and the mineral selenium are antioxidant compounds that appear to protect against cancer and possibly other diseases because they neutralize free radicals—unstable molecules created by various normal chemical processes in the body, or by solar or cosmic radiation, cigarette smoke, and other environmental influences. In the human body, the most damaging free radicals are derived from the complex chemical process by which oxygen is utilized inside the cells.

Good sources of beta carotene

Apricots
Asparagus
Broccoli
Cantaloupe
Carrots
Cherries
Cress
Dandelion greens
Kale
Mangoes
Peaches
Peas
Romaine lettuce
Sweet potatoes
Spinach
Tomatoes
Winter squash

The Potential Benefits of Antioxidants

Exactly how the antioxidant vitamins act to prevent or reduce the risk of cancer and other chronic diseases is under active investigation. The evidence, while not yet conclusive or clear, is nevertheless promising:

Cancer. Low intakes of vitamin C are associated with elevated cancer risk: Dr. Gladys Block of the University of California at Berkeley recently cited more than ninety epidemiologic studies examining the effects of vitamin C against cancer. "In about three quarters of the studies, high vitamin C intake was found to significantly reduce the risk of cancer. Evidence of this protective role was particularly strong for cancers of the oral cavity, esophagus, stomach and pancreas. Substantial evidence also suggests that vitamin C has a risk-reducing effect on cervical, rectal, breast, and even lung cancer." In 1993, a Yale University School of Medicine study of non-smoking lung cancer patients concluded that a diet rich in beta carotene reduces lung cancer risk in men and women who don't smoke. Supplements of vitamin E seem to be similarly protective.

Vitamin E first showed promise as an anti-carcinogen in the 1930s, when laboratory experiments showed that it greatly reduced certain cancers in mice. The past decade has seen a number of human studies on this antioxidant vitamin, but the results, unfortunately, are not so clear-cut. However, two recent studies focusing on specific cancers do seem to point to vitamin E as a protective factor. A major study published in 1992 in the *American Journal of Epidemiology* found that people who took vitamin E supplements had half the risk of oral cancers compared to those who didn't take them. A study published in *Nutrition and Cancer* in 1993 found that vitamin E reduced the risk of esophageal as well as oral cancer.

The problem with many of these antioxidant studies is that they involved populations that had very low intakes of these nutrients to begin with. The question remains whether supplementation would have the same effect on people whose antioxidant intakes were not deficient. However, in studies from all over the world, low antioxidant intake and low blood levels of antioxidants have been linked with increased risk for lung, colon, and cervical cancers, among others.

It's still not possible to say that antioxidants—in food or in supplements—prevent cancer, or that either may ever be useful in treating cancer. There may be other factors besides antioxidants in vitamin-rich foods that are protective. Nevertheless, these findings hold great promise.

Heart disease. One theory about how antioxidants may help prevent heart disease is that oxidation of LDL (low-density lipoprotein, or "bad") cholesterol on artery walls is what leads to the buildup of plaque. Thus the antioxidants would act to reduce this buildup. Evidence to support the idea is fast accumulating. In 1993, two large studies from Harvard Medical School suggested that vitamin E may reduce the risk of heart disease by one quarter to one half. One study followed more than 87,000 female nurses age thirty-four to fifty-nine; the other study followed 45,000 male health professionals. The protective effect of vitamin E held even after adjusting for vitamin C and beta carotene intake. The reduced risk of heart disease was seen in people taking more than 100 IU daily for at least two years: that's far more than you could get from food alone.

A study published in the American Heart Association's journal, *Circulation,* showed that high doses of vitamin E have the same positive effects as a combination of antioxidants; it also demonstrated that doses of vitamin E as high as 800 IU produce no side effects.

According to Dr. Charles H. Hennekens of the Harvard Medical School, writing in *Clinical Cardiology,* antioxidant vitamins may one day have a substantial impact on heart disease. Though findings from all studies have not been consistent, some important clinical trials are under way. One of these, the Physicians' Health Study, is testing beta carotene supplements in men, and another, the Women's Health Study, is testing vitamin E and beta carotene supplements in women. And future studies may test whether antioxidant vitamins will help prevent second heart attacks.

Antioxidants, however, are not a substitute for a healthy diet low in saturated fats or for aerobic exercise, and they are unlikely to counteract the heart-damaging effects of smoking. They may be helpful against heart disease and other ailments, but they are not a miracle cure. As a means of decreasing heart disease risk, they are, according to Dr. Hennekens, "promising, but unproven." And there is a persistent problem in all the studies: it may well be that people who have healthy diets and take supplements—and thus have a lower risk of heart disease—also have other good health habits that are more protective than the antioxidants they consume. And the protective factor might turn out to be some as yet unrecognized compound in antioxidant-rich foods.

Cataracts and other eye disorders. Vitamin C may play a role in preventing cataract formation and in fighting macular degeneration, a retinal problem that can lead to blindness. Eye fluids are normally rich in vitamin C (as well as other antioxidants), which may protect against sunlight-induced free-radical formation in the eye. Studies conducted worldwide have suggested that vitamin E might also prevent or delay the development of cataracts. Among others, a recent Finnish study published in the *British Medical Journal* found that low blood levels of vitamin E and beta carotene were associated with a higher risk of cataracts.

Other disorders. Research on other health problems is still in its infancy, and no conclusions can be drawn at this time, although there are some positive indications. For example, vitamin E, in particular, has shown promise in the treatment of Parkinson's disease. The antioxidants are also under investigation as playing some protective role against diabetic retinopathy (which can lead to blindness), AIDS, arthritis, other diseases, and aging.

Chemically incomplete, free radicals may "steal" particles from other molecules, creating abnormal compounds and thus setting off a chain reaction that can damage cells by causing fundamental changes in their genetic material and other important parts of the cell. In simplest terms, the manner in which free radicals damage the body's cells is similar to the process by which oxygen causes paper to turn yellow or butter to turn rancid.

Antioxidant nutrients render free radicals harmless by neutralizing them without becoming free radicals themselves; they are chemical "good guys," potentially conferring a number of health benefits, as outlined in the box on the previous page. Antioxidant nutrients are abundant in fruits, vegetables, and grains. But even if you are eating a very healthy diet, you may not obtain the high levels of antioxidant vitamins that many authorities think you need, and supplements may be recommended. For more information on specific vitamins and guidelines, see the chart on page 126.

Potassium. An adequate potassium intake may lessen the blood-pressure-raising effect of sodium, and independently contribute to a reduced risk of death from stroke. Potassium is abundant in fruits and vegetables. One study found that if you add even one piece of fruit or serving of vegetables or other food high in potassium to your regular diet, you may reduce your risk of fatal stroke by 40 percent.

Calcium. Calcium is the most important dietary factor associated with the risk of developing osteoporosis, the loss of bone mass. An adequate intake of calcium throughout life—and especially from birth to the age of twenty-five—can help build bone density and therefore ward off osteoporosis. Generally, calcium obtained from foods is better absorbed by the body than calcium obtained from supplements (see page 138).

Vitamin D. Vitamin D helps the body to absorb calcium. A number of studies have shown that elderly people are at increased risk for vitamin D deficiency. Milk—an excellent source of calcium—is usually fortified with vitamin D (choose low-fat or skim varieties). In addition, the body produces vitamin D in response to sunlight.

Cruciferous vegetables. These members of the cabbage family—such as broccoli, kale, Brussels sprouts, and cauliflower—not only contain antioxidant vitamins, but are rich in folacin and in lesser-known substances such as indoles and sulforaphane, which may reduce the risk of a variety of cancers and help keep you healthy in other ways.

Can diet cure disease?

Much of the research on diet and health focuses on the prevention—not the treatment—of chronic diseases. But the distinction between "reducing disease risk" and "delaying the onset of further symptoms" is sometimes blurred. Certainly, diet can help control many chronic diseases. For example, if you have diabetes, eating a diet high in complex carbohydrates and maintaining an appropriate weight can help keep the disease in check. Hypertensives may lower their blood pressure by losing weight and eating less sodium. And studies of people with severe heart disease, conducted by Dr. Dean Ornish and his colleagues at the University of California at San Francisco, found that a vegetarian diet extremely low in fat (10 percent calories from fat) and cholesterol (5 milligrams daily) can not only help keep more plaque from building up in the coronary arteries, but also help reduce the plaque already there and thus actually unclog arteries. In addition to changing their diet, the men and women in these studies participated in a moderate exercise program, practiced stress management techniques, and quit smoking. After one year, the participants experienced a significant regression of the plaque that had built up in their arteries plus a reduction in chest pain. On average, total blood cholesterol levels dropped 24 percent, and levels of LDL ("bad" cholesterol) dropped a dramatic 37 percent. However, the study did not determine which, if any, of the lifestyle changes had the greatest effect; thus, diet alone may not be enough to reverse atherosclerosis.

In none of these instances, though, does diet cure chronic disease the way an antibiotic can wipe out an infection. Yet the myths proliferate, especially when it comes to fighting cancer. Claims have been made for a wide variety of dietary cures—everything from aloe vera to carrot and celery juice to vitamin B_{15} (pangamic acid) supplements. One persistent belief is that macrobiotic diets have the ability to cure cancer. These diets consist chiefly of whole grains plus selected vegetables, a few fruits, seaweed, and occasionally some fish. The diet is progressive—that is, you are eventually supposed to cut out all foods except brown rice. This is just one example of how nutrition quackery can be especially harmful. Not only is there no evidence that any kind of macrobiotic diet can cure cancer, but it can actually interfere with the treatment of the disease by contributing to malnutrition and weight loss. Even worse, people might decide to substitute the diet for effective treatment.

Nevertheless, a proper diet—one that is low in fat, high in complex carbohydrates, and supplies an adequate amount of nutrients—can serve as an adjunct to medical intervention and treatment in the management of many diseases.

Exercise and Longevity

Perhaps the most comprehensive research on the effects of exercise on health and longevity is the series of long-term studies conducted by Dr. Ralph S. Paffenbarger, Jr., and his associates. Under way for more than twenty-five years, the studies have produced strong evidence that regular exercise is an important health-promoting factor. One study has examined the lifestyles of 16,936 Harvard alumni who entered college between 1916 and 1950 and ranged in age from thirty-five to seventy-four at the start of the study. Their exercise habits (self-reported) and mortality rates were followed by Dr. Paffenbarger beginning in the mid-1960s, and surviving subgroups are still being followed. The exercises included walking, stair-climbing, and various sports.

The researchers have found that, for the most part, the more a person exercised, the better his chances to outlive his peers. For example, during more than two decades of observation, men who walked nine or more miles a week had a 21 percent lower mortality rate than those who walked three miles or less. In terms of calories burned per week, life expectancy improved steadily, starting at an expenditure of 500 calories per week of exercise (a 150-pound man burns off about 500 calories walking six miles) and continuing upward to 3,500 calories per week (the equivalent of walking six miles daily for a week). No additional benefit occurred above 3,500 calories a week, however. The beneficial effects of exercise were evident in all of the men studied, and the benefits tended to intensify with age.

In a recent report examining data on more than 10,000 of the alumni, the

It is now widely accepted that there is an inverse relationship between the level of physical activity and the incidence of cardiovascular disease—so much so that the American Heart Association has cited being sedentary as one of the important risk factors for cardiovascular disease. While exercise alone is not sufficient to prevent heart disease, it is a critical part of any program.

researchers found that middle-aged and elderly men (forty-five to eighty-four years old) who take up moderately vigorous activities such as tennis, swimming, jogging, or brisk walking have a 23 to 29 percent lower overall death rate than nonexercisers, and up to a 41 percent reduction in the risk of coronary artery disease. In effect, the men who started exercising could expect to live nine or ten months longer, on average, than those who remained sedentary. Even men who waited until they were sixty-five to eighty-four to begin moderate exercise gained two to six months.

Six or even ten months may not sound like a lot, but it is indeed a big gain in life expectancy in this type of population study. For comparison: men who gave up smoking gained about 1.5 years; and those who quit smoking and started exercising gained 2.5 years. These figures are averages, and men who were at highest risk who began to exercise probably gained more time, while others may have gained less. Moreover, this study looked only at length of life; it didn't attempt to measure the improvements in quality of life. People who exercise regularly tend to control their weight and blood pressure, raise their HDL ("good") blood cholesterol, and have fewer chronic diseases like diabetes—thus they also have a better chance of leading vigorous, healthful lives and avoiding years of chronic illness and suffering. And the study also showed that it's never too late to start.

As Dr. Paffenbarger has pointed out, the Harvard alumni in his study were not necessarily typical of the general population. Their mortality rates from every major cause were generally half that of most white males—except for suicides, where their rate was 50 percent higher. Since those studied clearly enjoy a special status (white, male, and well-off economically), Dr. Paffenbarger cautioned against drawing sweeping conclusions for all of society. Moreover, such a study does not prove that exercise by itself makes people live longer, since the exercisers may have been more likely to have other healthful habits (such as following a low-fat diet) that may have been partly responsible for the lowered risk of heart disease and other illnesses. Though all the subjects claimed to be healthy, some may have experienced subtle symptoms of an undiagnosed illness that discouraged or prevented them from exercising. And women weren't included in this study or in most of the other major studies on exercise.

The benefits of moderate activity

Subsequent studies show that other groups in the population have benefited from being active—and that the greatest surge in life expectancy is derived by incorporating a relatively modest amount of activity into what was previously a sedentary lifestyle. Indeed, the weight of evidence overwhelmingly supports the life-extending and life-improving power of regular exercise—and that even moderate exercise, such as walking or gardening, provides a number of significant health benefits.

For example, one study looked at 3,000 railroad workers—all white, male, and middle-aged—over a period of seventeen to twenty years. The subjects who passed their leisure time being sedentary—defined as expending less than 250 calories a week in moderate- or low-intensity exercises like strolling, bowling, gardening, or cycling at an easy pace—had a 30 to 40 percent greater risk of dying from coronary heart disease as well as from all causes than those who expended between 1,000 and 2,000 calories a week in these activities. This was true even after adjust-

Exercise and cancer risk

While it has not been shown that a given level of physical activity per se can reduce overall cancer risk, research suggests that exercise often modifies some of the risk factors associated with certain kinds of cancer. Obesity, for example, has been linked to cancer of the breast and the female reproductive system—and regular exercise helps promote weight loss. Several studies have also found that men who worked at sedentary jobs for most of their lives had a greater incidence of colon cancer (but not rectal cancer) than those in more active jobs. And an ongoing study of Harvard alumni found that those who were highly or even moderately active had a substantially lower risk of both colon and lung cancer than alumni who were less active.

Exercise will not counteract the effects of a high-fat diet or smoking. Still, it can contribute, even indirectly, to a reduced risk, and is recommended by the American Cancer Society as part of its cancer prevention program.

ing for age, blood pressure, smoking, and blood cholesterol levels. The researchers estimated that it takes about thirty minutes of moderate activity every day to expend 1,000 calories in a week.

How much is enough? As other studies have found, this one indicated that going beyond an average of about an hour's worth of moderate leisure activity a day (more than 2,000 calories a week) did not add substantially to the health benefits. This is not to say that high-intensity workouts are a waste of time—a number of studies have shown that while a little exercise is good, more is better—but for the estimated 78 percent of Americans who are either totally or mostly sedentary, just walking briskly for 30 minutes a day is adequate to confer health benefits.

In a more well-rounded and systematic study conducted by researchers at the Institute for Aerobics Research in Dallas, researchers surveyed more than 13,000 healthy men and women for an average of eight years and related their exercise and activity habits to overall mortality. Subjects were evaluated according to objective standards of fitness—the results of treadmill tests. (In contrast, most earlier research relied only on how much people said they exercised; such self-reports, without any evaluative testing, are not as reliable.)

The results are impressive. Of five groups of people, divided according to fitness levels, the least-fit group (who were also the most sedentary) had the highest mortality rates by far. The big surprise was that the death rate dropped most sharply in the second-least-fit group, by 60 percent for men and 48 percent for women. To be in this group, the researchers estimated, all a person would have to do is walk briskly for thirty to sixty minutes every day. The three fittest groups— including people who jogged up to forty miles a week—derived comparatively minor additional benefits.

In addition, the women (more than 3,100 of them) were found to benefit as much from being fit as the men. The few earlier studies of fitness in women were small and had ambiguous results. In this study, being physically fit lowered the risk not only of heart disease among both men and women, but also cancer (for which there is less evidence) as well as all causes of death. The researchers couldn't adjust for the fact that nearly all the participants were white and well-to-do. But they did adjust their data statistically to be sure that the higher mortality rate was due to lack of fitness and not other important risk factors, such as age, smoking, high cholesterol or blood pressure levels, and family history of heart disease.

Fitness and aging

Our bodies change as we age. For example, aerobic capacity (the ability of the cardiovascular system to deliver oxygen to working muscles) declines slightly every year after age thirty. Heart muscle contractibility slowly declines, as does general muscle strength. Percentage of body fat, as opposed to lean muscle tissue, tends to increase with age.

Yet some people stay vigorous and active much longer than others. Most gerontologists now believe age-associated declines can be explained in terms of lifestyle, habits, diet, and other factors not directly part of the aging process. Thus exercise may certainly be a factor in slowing the hands of time. Consider the following evidence:

•As reported in the *Journal of Gerontology,* a study of walkers in three age groups (nineteen to twenty-nine, thirty-nine to forty-nine, and fifty-five to sixty years old)

Impressive evidence

One of the most surprising findings about the potential of benefitting from exercise came from a study conducted at Tufts University in which ten very frail ninety-year-olds, already institutionalized, participated in a nine-week program of high-intensity weight training. They began slowly, lifting only 50 percent of their maximum weight in a sitting position (eight repetitions three times a week), then moving up to 80 percent of their maximum capacity, and increasing their exercises in number and intensity each week (under careful supervision). The nonagenarians were able to build muscle mass and become, as the researchers pointed out, more mobile and self-sufficient.

showed that aerobic capacity is not necessarily correlated with age. That is, some fast walkers in the older group were as fit as those in the younger groups.

•A study conducted at Washington University School of Medicine in St. Louis showed that heart function in men and women in their sixties improved by 25 to 30 percent after a year of endurance exercise. And men in their seventies showed increased muscle strength after just eight weeks of strength training.

•Women in their sixties and beyond have been to shown to benefit from strength training. In one study reported in the *Journal of the American Geriatric Society,* thirty-six women over sixty who were already engaging in some form of regular aerobic exercise were given training sessions on heavy-resistance weight-training machines. After six months, the women experienced significant decreases in body fat and increases in lean muscle mass. And there were no injuries.

•Burning extra calories through exercise protects against the slow but steady weight gain that is a common pattern among Americans as they grow older.

•Exercise increases bone density in women over forty, many of whom are at high risk for menopausal bone loss.

•Comparisons of the mental agility of younger people and healthy older individuals who exercise at about the same level show that the elders react about as fast as their juniors and significantly faster than their sedentary peers. Regular aerobic exercise seems not only to help preserve neurological functioning into old age, but also potentially to enhance it in older people who have been sedentary.

If maintaining a healthy heart, strong muscles, and flexible joints is part of staying young, then exercise is part of the answer. Americans spend millions on potions that "guarantee" the glow of youth but accomplish nothing. Exercise, which can truly maintain your body's youthful functions, usually costs nothing.

Controlling Your Weight

For most people, "overweight" and "obese" are not scientific terms, but loaded words that trigger anxiety and frustration. Like gender and ethnicity, weight is an essential part of every person's self-image, and when pounds go haywire, the result is distress. Our culture is, to put it mildly, preoccupied with weight. Weight gain is always noticed and generally perceived as an important change—in an adult, usually for the worse. Bathroom scales are almost as common as bathrooms; millions of people weigh themselves daily as part of their morning routine.

In our culture, the ideal human body is lean and trim with an abdomen taut as an army cot—an image depicted everywhere and a model to which few conform. Some surveys show that as many as 90 percent of Americans believe they weigh too much—indeed, more than a third of American women and nearly a quarter of men are following some weight-loss program at any given moment—and even small children worry about diets. The young are always extremely susceptible to whatever ideal standards of beauty are being purveyed—no matter how unreachable—and many studies have shown that among teenage girls, in particular, poor body image is a factor in depression as well as in poor health habits, resulting in self-starvation or compulsive exercising. Though little is known about how adult women feel about their bodies and how they are affected by the "thin" ideal, discontent about body image certainly does not vanish at age twenty-one or even thirty-five.

Lurking in the back of our minds is the notion that fat is the visible evidence of self-indulgence and a weak will. And according to the National Institutes of Health, of all the health risks of being overweight or obese, probably none has a more adverse effect than the psychological suffering and social ostracism. Fortunately, medical discoveries of the past few years have begun to offer new ways of thinking about overweight and obesity.

What is obesity?

Although often used interchangeably, "overweight" and "obese" do not mean the same thing. Obesity is a medical term meaning the storage of excess fat in the body. Often referred to as a "disease," obesity is actually a sign of what may well be a spectrum of different kinds of disorders—genetic or environmental. In fact, there is no single definition of obesity. It may be simply an extreme degree of overweight, but a person can be overweight without being obese: a 250-pound six-foot linebacker, for example, may be overweight according to ordinary standards, but may actually have a below-average amount of body fat. In contrast, a person in a normal-weight range but with very sedentary habits could have a small muscle mass and be storing excess fat and thus be classifiable as obese.

During the 1980s, the obesity rate in the United States rose by nearly one-third. Between 1976 and 1980, about 26 percent of adults were classified as "overweight," which made us one of the most overweight nations in the world. As reported in the journal *Obesity & Health* and confirmed by the National Center for

Health Statistics, the percentage rose to 34 percent in 1988-91, according to data from the Third National Health and Nutrition Examination Survey (NHANES III), an important large-scale study.

The increase in overweight has affected all groups—men and women, young and old, and various ethnic groups. Among American men, being overweight increased over the decade from 24 percent to 32 percent; among women, from 27 percent to 35 percent. The survey uses the body mass index (BMI) to define overweight, and most experts consider this to be the best method (the formula for calculating BMI is given in the box on the next page). Being overweight according to the BMI definition used in this survey is roughly equivalent to weighing more than the range for a given height listed in the government's chart of suggested "healthy" weights (see above).

Healthy Weights

Check your height on the chart below, now used as the government's guidelines for healthy weight. The two sexes are combined in this one table. The higher weights generally apply to men, the lower to women. Allowance has been made for some weight gain with age. Don't forget, though, that healthy and attractive people come in many shapes and sizes.

SUGGESTED WEIGHT (without clothes or shoes)

Height	Age 19 to 34	35 and over
5'0"	97-128	108-138
5'1"	101-132	111-143
5'2"	104-137	115-148
5'3"	107-141	119-152
5'4"	111-146	122-157
5'5"	114-150	126-162
5'6"	118-155	130-167
5'7"	121-160	134-172
5'8"	125-164	138-178
5'9"	129-169	142-183
5'10"	132-174	146-188
5'11"	136-179	151-194
6'0"	140-184	155-199
6'1"	144-189	159-205
6'2"	148-195	164-210
6'3"	152-200	168-216
6'4"	156-205	173-222

It's important to remember, however, that the line between desirable weight and overweight, and between overweight and obese, is not clear-cut, even for the experts. Both "overweight" and "obesity" must be measured against some arbitrary standard, and the definition must take into account the the amount of muscle mass a person has (someone who is very muscular may be categorized as overweight) and where the fat is distributed on the body (excess abdominal fat is more of a health risk than fat on the hips). Nevertheless, by virtually any definition, Americans have been getting fatter.

Risks of too much poundage

Doctors have observed for many years that overweight and obesity are associated with greater risk for some diseases, and the evidence continues to accumulate. (The risks are greatest for the very overweight and the obese; if you're only a few pounds—less than 10 to 15 percent—over your desirable weight, your increased risks are small.)

Hypertension. High blood pressure, or hypertension, is 5.6 times higher in overweight people aged twenty to forty-four and twice as high for those forty-five to seventy-four. An Australian study of young overweight hypertensives, published in *The New England Journal of Medicine,* showed them all to be prone to the kind of heart enlargement usually associated with high blood pressure. One group was placed on a weight-reduction regimen, and although they lost an average of only eighteen pounds, their systolic and diastolic blood pressure dropped significantly. Moreover, their heart size decreased somewhat, providing additional evidence of the connection between being overweight and cardiovascular disease.

Coronary artery disease (CAD). Numerous other studies have shown the relationship between being overweight and high blood cholesterol levels as well as heart attacks. Obesity is associated with an increased risk of developing, and dying from, CAD because it may raise LDL (low-density lipoprotein, or "bad") cholesterol and lower HDL (high-density lipoprotein, or "good") cholesterol. Hypertension and diabetes, also associated with obesity, are themselves contributing factors to heart disease mortality.

In addition, obesity puts women in particular at increased risk of heart disease. A study conducted at Harvard Medical School of 115,000 women aged thirty to fifty-five found that of all the women in the study who developed heart disease during an eight-year period, 40 percent of them had no other risk factors (diabetes, family history, smoking, or high cholesterol, for example) except being 20 percent or more over their ideal weight. And of this group, 70 percent were women in the very obese category (they were at least 30 percent over their ideal weight). Women who had been slim at age eighteen and gained weight in adulthood seemed to be at increased risk.

Diabetes. Although diabetes is probably an inherited disease, non–insulin-dependent diabetes mellitus (NIDDM, also called adult-onset or type II diabetes) can be delayed or averted by weight control. Diabetes is three times as frequent in overweight people as in those who are not overweight.

Smoking appears to cause a dangerous redistribution of fat to the abdomen, even though smokers tend to weigh less than nonsmokers. On the other hand, when smokers quit and then gain weight, it tends to accumulate around the hips.

How Much Should You Weigh?

How to determine your "desirable" weight is still a matter of controversy. The fastest, though not the most accurate, way to determine what you should weigh is to consult a standard height/weight table. According to an analysis in the *Annals of Internal Medicine,* one trouble with these tables is that they take no account of many factors that affect weight—family history, race, or age, for instance. At age fifty, even the trim and muscular weigh more than they did at twenty-five, and there is some evidence that modest weight gain between age twenty-five and sixty-five is healthy.

A better way to define overweight is to measure the proportion of fat in the body, but this is a difficult task to do accurately, even with professional training. Therefore, the preferred way to figure out your healthy weight is to calculate your body mass index—the figure you get by dividing your weight in kilograms by the square of your height in meters. This is the most useful figure because it minimizes the effect of height and provides reasonable guidelines for defining overweight. You can calculate your body mass index by following the steps below. (A calculator, while not a necessity, will help.)

1. To convert your weight to kilograms, divide the pounds (without clothes) by 2.2: _____.

2. To convert to meters, divide your height in inches (without shoes) by 39.4 (_____), then square it:_____.

3. Divide (**1**) by (**2**):_____. This figure is your body mass index.

For men, desirable body mass index is 22 to 24. Above about 28.5 is overweight. Body mass index above 33 is seriously overweight.

For women, desirable body mass index is 21 to 23, overweight begins at about 27.5, and seriously overweight is above 31.5.

Cancer. Studies conducted by the American Cancer Society have shown that certain cancers (of the colon and prostate in men, of the uterus in women, and of the breast in postmenopausal women) are more prevalent in the obese than in the nonobese. One large, long-term study conducted by the Society revealed that the overall cancer risk was 55 percent higher for women who were 40 percent over average weight than for normal-weight women; for obese men, the cancer risk was about one third higher than for normal-weight men.

Clearly, then, weight has a serious and direct effect on longevity and seems to take its greatest toll in those under fifty. Leading health professionals have already stated that younger overweight people stand to gain even more by reducing than do the middle-aged and elderly.

Does body shape matter?

People with "apple" shapes (fattest in the abdomen area) have a greater risk of coronary artery disease, stroke, hypertension, and diabetes than those with "pear" shapes (fattest in the hips, buttocks, and thighs). In addition, researchers have found that fat distribution may also affect the risk of breast cancer in postmenopausal women. It's long been known that increased body weight is a risk factor for various cancers, but several studies have indicated that women who tend to store fat in the midsection and upper body are at even greater risk.

Men are more likely than women to store excess fat in the midsection and develop a "beer belly" whether they drink alcohol or not. Women typically store fat lower on the body. Because of these gender differences, researchers suggest that sex hormones determine where body fat is deposited. Still, women can be "apple-shaped," too, with all the risks that entails. Heredity and physical activity level are other major factors affecting your body shape.

While fat in the hip and thigh region is mainly stored just under the skin, fat in the midsection is stored deeper inside the body. Scientists theorize that abdominal fat also releases more fatty acids, leading to a rise in triglycerides and some forms of cholesterol in the bloodstream, and interfering with the action of insulin in the body (thus increasing the risk of diabetes). The elevated risk of breast cancer, the researchers theorize, may be due to increases in the availability and activity of estrogen associated with abdominal obesity.

The role of fat

Fat cells are not mere storage tanks for excess calories; they cushion organs and insulate against the cold. Even more important, the ability to store excess

The eye-mouth gap

Numerous studies have shown that perhaps 80 percent of us underestimate our food intake—lean and athletic people as well as the obese. One national survey found that adults underestimate their daily diet, on average, by about 800 calories. In one study, researchers found that obese people ate twice as much as they reported.

This discrepancy has been called the "eye-mouth gap." One reason for it: people don't know how much food they put on their plates. So if you are trying to lose weight, don't trust your eyes. Weigh or measure the food you eat, at least for a while, to get a sense of what a "serving" is. A kitchen scale is a wise investment. Use it when you cook, especially for such calorie-dense foods as meat, fish, or cheese. The scale will help you train your eye to remember what a reasonable portion looks like. Be sure you also have measuring cups and spoons, and follow all of your recipes to the letter.

Calculating Waist-to-Hip Ratio

To evaluate your risk of developing disease based on your fat distribution, determine your waist-to-hip ratio as follows:

1. Measure your waist at the navel, then your hips at the greatest circumference around the buttocks.

2. Divide the waist measurement by the hip size. This is your waist-to-hip ratio.

A waist-to-hip ratio greater than 1.0 for men and 0.8 for women indicates an increased cardiac risk. This means that, ideally, the circumference of a man's waist shouldn't exceed that of his hips; a woman's waist should measure no more than 80 percent of her hips.

For example, a woman who has a waist measurement of 28 inches and a hip measurement of 38 inches has a waist-to-hip ratio of 28 divided by 38, or 0.74. Since this is less than 0.8, it is considered a healthy waist-to-hip ratio.

energy for future use is one of the miracles of evolution. With fat in reserve, animals and, later, early humans could range through wide and inhospitable areas where food might be scarce.

The development of fat cells in the body is very precisely orchestrated, and their number (thirty to forty billion in the average adult) is carefully regulated. In the last trimester before birth, the fetus prepares for the uncertainties of life outside the womb by beginning to accumulate fat cells. For the first six months of infancy, the number of fat cells continues to increase. This rate slows through childhood, and the total number of accumulated cells depends on genetic and environmental factors, especially nutritional ones. (Although some data indicate that obesity in childhood predisposes a person to obesity for life, not all fat babies grow into fat adults.) At puberty, the body again significantly increases the number of its fat cells, with females taking on more than males, since the female body must be prepared for the possibility of pregnancy and the further demands of lactation.

By early adulthood the body has accumulated most of the fat cells it will ever have. Although people may subsequently gain a great deal of weight, their fat cells generally do not increase in number but only in size (in cases of extreme obesity, however, there is an increase in the number of fat cells). And while fat cells can shrink, they never disappear. In an experiment conducted at Rockefeller University in New York City, rats were put on a starvation diet. They lost some fat, but not their fat cells. As the diet continued, they lost muscle, organ, and connective tissue, but even at the point of death, their fat cells decreased in size but not in number and their brain cells remained intact. Clearly, fat cells are programmed to guard themselves zealously.

It is also speculated that the body has a "set point," or precise amount of fat it "decides" to maintain. Even if you cut down your caloric intake, this set point may be hard to change. This is one theory as to why it may be so difficult to diet and why people may be prone to put weight back on when dieting stops. There is also some evidence that people prone to obesity expend calories at a lower rate than others, even at the same level of activity.

The genetic factor

Why some people are fat and others are thin is a question that medical science is not yet able to answer. The old platitude that blames overweight on overeating is true, but doesn't tell the whole story about obesity. Food in the United States is plentiful, cheap, and available twenty-four hours a day, and many people not only overeat, but eat a lot of high-fat, high-calorie foods that contribute to weight gain. However, there are some people who eat anything they want and never gain weight, and studies show that obese people do not eat an inordinate amount of calories. In fact, they often eat less than nonobese people do. Perhaps more important than overeating, far too many Americans spend their leisure time inactively—shopping, driving around, or watching television, for instance. From an environmental standpoint alone, then, it is no wonder that obesity and overweight are as prevalent as they are in this country.

Yet there are other factors at work, including race, gender, economic status, and possibly genetics. African-American men between the ages of thirty-five and fifty-five are more likely to be overweight than white men in the same age group, and African-American women thirty-five to fifty-five are (text continued on page 36)

Does TV lead to weight gain?

Men who watch television for at least three hours a day are twice as likely to be obese as those who watch less than an hour. And an article in Pediatrics *stated that the prevalence of obesity in teenagers increased by about 2 percent for every additional hour of daily television viewing. Many researchers suggest that the relationship between excessive television watching and obesity is reciprocal—one reinforces the other. In addition, television viewers may be encouraged to eat more food, thanks in part to exposure to thousands of ads on television for high-calorie snacks. And viewers' attention is often so focused on what they're watching that they just keep eating automatically.*

Myths About Weight Control

Myth: Eating grapefruit burns away fat.

Fact: No food can cause fat to be burned away. Dozens of diets based on eating vast quantities of grapefruit claim that grapefruit, or grapefruit concentrate in the form of a pill, contains enzymes that digest fats and so burn them away. There are no known ingested enzymes that will increase the rate at which the body burns fat.

Adding fruit to your diet can be good for you. But there is nothing in grapefruit that will digest calories or cut appetite. In addition, a crash diet of grapefruit and eggs, or grapefruit and bacon and eggs, or some of the other high-fat, high-protein foods that are often recommended along with grapefruit, can raise your cholesterol level.

Myth: Taking diet pills is a good way to lose weight.

Fact: Weight lost with artificial reducing "aids" usually comes right back. Only reformed eating habits can take weight off and keep it off. The major ingredient of many reducing pills is a drug called phenylpropanolamine (PPA), which is a stimulant. When PPA is taken in large doses, its effects resemble those of amphetamines, or "speed." Even in low doses, the immediate effect of PPA is to constrict the blood vessels and speed up the heart, resulting in acute elevation of blood pressure. It can produce such side effects as anxiety, sleeplessness, headaches, irregular heart rhythm, and even lead to strokes or seizures.

Although many health authorities feel uneasy about recommending PPA, the Food and Drug Administration (FDA) has approved it as an over-the-counter reducing aid. It does tend to suppress appetite, and some studies have shown that over the short term, its use can result in slightly greater weight loss than if a placebo is taken. But results are minimal at best—and there's no evidence that it helps to promote long-term weight loss.

Myth: Your stomach shrinks when you eat less.

Fact: Your stomach cannot shrink, no matter how little you consume. If you eat enormous amounts of food, it can expand, but once empty it returns to normal size. If you diet for several days, your appetite level does indeed drop for reasons that medical science does not yet understand. However, this has nothing to do with the size of your stomach.

Myth: Fasting can lead to permanent weight loss.

Fact: As part of a fad diet, fasting is usually ineffectual. Total fasting as a medical treatment for severe obesity was first introduced about thirty years ago. A drastic method that is both risky and usually uncomfortable for the patient, fasting indeed results in a rapid initial weight loss, but most of the loss is fluid and minerals, rather than fat. As the fast continues, the person does lose body fat, but also considerable lean body mass (especially muscle) and more minerals. However, after a certain point in the fast, the body's energy production slows and the rate of loss of both fat and lean body mass decreases.

Depending on the duration of the fast, the amount of muscle and electrolyte (mineral) loss can become critical and usually represents a significant portion (30 percent or more) of the weight loss. Because of the dangers of a prolonged fast, this technique is rarely recommended any longer, even for the morbidly obese. Few people who actually lose weight by this means maintain their loss, and some may sustain permanent injury.

Myth: Toast is less fattening than bread.

Fact: Toast retains all of the calories of the bread it is made from. Many diet plans call for a slice of dry toast with a meal, as though toast were a special diet food. It may look more austere, but a slice of toast has the same 60 to 70 calories that a slice of bread has. Toasting removes only moisture.

Myth: Celery has "negative calories" because it takes so much work to chew it.

Fact: Celery is very low in calories, but not so low that chewing it burns more calories than it contains. An eight-inch stalk has only 6 calories, but chewing celery or anything else burns about the same amount of calories per minute as just sitting. Basically, celery, as well as iceberg lettuce and cucumbers, are nearly calorie-free—not because of the energy required to

---

The truth about food combining

While some beliefs about food combining—eating specific foods in the right combinations—are religious or cultural in origin, most are pure faddism. There is no scientific evidence that any one food should not be combined with another. Many fad diet plans will tell you, for example, that starches shouldn't be eaten in the same meal as proteins, and that improperly combined foods "putrefy" the body. But what the advocates of food combining don't tell you is that all foods, even when eaten individually, are combinations of fat, protein, and carbohydrates to begin with.

chew them, but because of their high water content.

Myth: Potatoes are very fattening.

Fact: A five-ounce potato baked in its skin has about 130 calories—no more calories than a serving of cottage cheese or tuna (water-packed) of the same weight, and 20 percent fewer calories than a serving of brown rice. Moreover, potatoes have no fat and no cholesterol, are low in sodium and high in fiber, vitamin C, niacin, and potassium. They are also a good source of complex carbohydrates. Potatoes become a problem food only when you fry them in oil or slather them with butter, gravy, sour cream, or melted cheese. Like other high-carbohydrate foods, such as pasta and bread, it's not the potato (or a sweet potato, for that matter) that's fattening, it's what you top it with.

Myth: Removing cellulite requires special treatment.

Fact: The whole idea of cellulite is nonsense. Cellulite is simply plain old fat asserting itself. Much of the body's fat is stored directly beneath the skin, where strands of connective fiber separate fat cells into compartments. When the cells increase in size, they bulge out of these compartments, giving the skin a crosshatched appearance in some individuals. Whether you develop this condition depends mainly on the amount of fat in your body, the strength of the connective fibers, and the thickness of the skin. In women, the fibers are taut, the skin is thin, and the fat between fibers tends to bulge. In men, the fibers are more flexible and the skin thicker, so the fat is more evenly contained.

Special creams, brushes, lotions, rub-downs, or rubber pants won't get rid of cellulite. It will, however, yield to the same regimen that gets rid of any fat—proper diet and regular aerobic exercise.

Myth: Electric muscle stimulators can make you trim.

Fact: The ads for electric muscle stimulators—claiming that you can lose weight and firm up without moving a muscle—sound too good to be true, and they are. Electric stimulators, devices that claim to provide "passive exercise" ("3,000 sit-ups without moving an inch," as one ad says) are only "the latest in vanity-type quackery," according to the Food and Drug Administration.

Electric muscle stimulators contract muscles by passing a current (from batteries or line current) through electrodes applied to the skin. Study after study has shown that regular use of electric stimulation produces no significant change in body weight or body fat. Researchers at Northeastern University in Boston found that this treatment burned only six calories in thirty-five minutes when applied to the buttocks, thighs, and abdomen.

Even if electric muscle stimulators burned a lot more calories, they wouldn't trim the treated areas, since spot reduction is a myth. The body draws energy from fat stores located throughout the body, not selectively from the parts that are being exercised or electrically stimulated at that time.

Myth: In order to lose weight, you need to give up all sweets.

Fact: Including a reasonable amount of sweets in a weight-loss plan may help to ensure that a diet will succeed.

The key to losing weight and keeping it off is to adopt healthy eating and exercise habits that you can stick to for a lifetime. It is unrealistic to expect that you will never again for the rest of your life eat a piece of chocolate or a slice of cake. In fact, there is some evidence that a craving for sweet foods is not a matter of flabby willpower, but has a chemical basis in some individuals. Nutritionists at the Massachusetts Institute of Technology have suggested that the hunger for sweets may be regulated in part by serotonin, one of several brain chemicals that appear to control many physiological functions. When we eat sweets, our brains normally respond by releasing increased amounts of serotonin. This causes us to feel satisfied.

Researchers speculate that some obese people crave carbohydrates because they "need" extra serotonin. Whether this theory is borne out by further research or not, you can include small amounts of dessert-type foods in your diet and still lose weight, provided that you don't do it too often and that you control your portion sizes.

almost twice as likely to be overweight as their white counterparts. For reasons not well understood, those who live below the poverty line, particularly women, are more likely to be fat than people at the top of the economic heap.

Although the tendency to be overweight appears to run in families, until recently no one was sure whether this is a matter of eating habits or heredity. But a study reported in the *New England Journal of Medicine* by Dr. Albert Stunkard and his colleagues concluded, "Genetic influences have an important role in determining human fatness in adults, whereas the family environment alone has no important effect." Dr. Stunkard studied 540 middle-aged adults who had been adopted as children. Their body mass index bore little relation to their adoptive parents' index; instead, the daughters tended strongly to follow the pattern of their biological parents, particularly of their mothers, although the sons showed no such relationship to either set of parents. This again emphasizes the complex relationship of genetics and environment to obesity.

Still, a genetic tendency toward being overweight does not doom a person to be fat—any more than a familial tendency in the other direction guarantees thinness. Studies have shown that rats bred for thinness can still get fat on a diet of snack foods; animals genetically prone to be fat will get fatter on the same diet. But both groups lose weight if returned to a normal maintenance diet. Furthermore, even fat-prone rats can be saved from obesity if their physical activity is increased.

If you know that overweight runs in your family, you can use the knowledge preventively. Because Americans, as a whole, live a relatively sedentary lifestyle and have plenty of food available to them, individuals looking to lose weight have to make an effort to keep active and eat a low-fat, high-carbohydrate diet that is moderate in calories.

Why crash diets don't work

Still, the advice "eat less and exercise more" is often too simplistic to be of much help. Furthermore, you already know that if through some feat of self-denial you manage to lose a few pounds, you'll almost certainly gain them back within six months. Or you may suffer through two weeks of deprivation only to find that you haven't lost a pound. What advice do the experts have for such problems?

No matter how much weight you want to lose, the reducing process has two phases: first, the time it takes to drop the desired number of pounds, which most people want to do as quickly as possible; and second, the development of a lifestyle that will keep the weight off. The second is the hard part because it has to continue for the rest of your life. That's why most diets emphasize the first phase only—the easy part. But the truth is that diets meant to lose weight fast won't keep you thin and may be harmful.

Three factors work against the dieter. One is that the body rather quickly adapts to a lower food intake by lowering its metabolic rate and thus resists burning off fat. When you restrict your diet and lose ten pounds, the body "becomes used to" that restricted diet. Then, if you increase your food intake, even though you still eat less than before your diet, the body treats the increase as an excess, and you gain weight. According to a recent National Institutes of Health panel, *about 90 percent of dieters regain all or most of their lost weight within five years.*

The second element working against the dieter is the fact that the weight lost in the early part of a strict diet program is not fat, for the most part, but water.

Weight and metabolism

Your metabolic rate is the total amount of energy your body uses in a given period of time—that is, the number of calories it burns, either at rest or while active. In general, if your resting metabolic rate (RMR) is high, you may find that you can eat a lot, exercise little, and not gain weight. Conversely, if your RMR is low, you may eat relatively little and be fairly active but still not lose weight.

RMR depends on a variety of factors, including body size and composition (more muscle and less fat means more energy use by your body—which is why men tend to have a higher metabolic rate than women). Age is a factor (RMR tends to slow as you age), and activity level and diet temporarily affect metabolic rate.

To a large extent, you can't change your RMR since you can't change your age, genes, or sex. However, by exercising to gain muscle mass and by watching your weight, you will boost your overall metabolic rate.

Very-Low-Calorie Diets: Do They Work?

The very-low-calorie diet—400 to 800 calories a day in the form of powdered egg or milk-derived protein supplements mixed with liquid—is, in effect, a modified fast designed for the very overweight. These new "liquid diets" are administered by hospitals and physicians who keep close tabs on their patients' health—a far cry from the over-the-counter liquid protein supplements of the 1970s, withdrawn when the Centers for Disease Control and Prevention in Atlanta reported sixty deaths attributable to their use. Unlike today's diets, the protein in these early supplements was collagen-based; its inadequate amino-acid composition (plus possibly a lack of carbohydrates) led to a dangerous loss of lean muscle mass, including heart muscle. Also, these early diets didn't provide for adequate potassium intake, which may have resulted in serious disturbances of heart rhythm.

A new formula

In addition to protein, today's supplements contain varying amounts of carbohydrates and the Recommended Daily Allowance for most nutrients. At least one also has added fiber. Mixed with liquid, these supplements are taken three to five times a day at meal and snack times. Other than eight glasses of water or more a day, that's all you get. (Some programs do allow you to munch on raw vegetables to satisfy the need to chew.) Very-low-calorie diet programs usually last three months. After one to three months on a maintenance diet of 1,250 to 1,500 calories, the patient may repeat the program. Reportedly, hunger pangs are rarely a problem, possibly because low intakes of calories lead to the manufacture of substances called ketones that are thought to suppress hunger. More importantly, the programs include regular electrocardiograms (ECGs), blood and urine tests, and visits to the doctor, as well as exercise regimens, nutrition education, and support groups.

Medical supervision is key

Medical supervision is extremely important when you're on such a diet program. One complication that can occur is an increased incidence of gallstones probably due to the sluggish flow of bile on a very low-fat, low-calorie diet. This problem and others can be watched for and prevented when you're under a doctor's care.

The very-low-calorie diet, extreme though it is, has earned medical recognition as sound therapy for people whose obesity puts them at risk for such problems as diabetes, hypertension, and heart disease. On the other hand, such drastic dieting is generally regarded as overkill for people who simply want to lose a few pounds from their hips or thighs; most programs won't admit you unless you are 20 to 30 percent above your ideal weight. And no one should undertake a program that provides fewer than 1,200 calories a day without a doctor's advice. Not all researchers or physicians, though, agree that even seriously obese patients benefit from such austere diets.

Studies made by researchers conducting these diet programs indicate high rates of short-term success. Two- to five-pound losses per week are common, and over three months most patients lose forty to sixty pounds. As yet, there are few long-term studies to indicate how many people manage to keep the weight off permanently—and it is weight-loss maintenance that ultimately validates any weight-reduction program. A study at San Diego State University found that while people who actually completed a very-low-calorie program (45 percent) lost an average of 84 percent of their excess weight, they regained 59 to 82 percent of their initial excess within thirty months. "This is disappointing, but may be exactly what should be expected," commented the researchers, since overweight individuals "have learned to overeat and underexercise."

Learning to eat less

The best very-low-calorie-diet programs include a maintenance phase of up to eighteen months devoted to reeducating patients in long-term weight-management techniques—in short, to improving their eating patterns and changing their lifestyles. For everyone, these patterns, which include cutting back on calories and engaging in regular physical activity, are the only ways to control weight in the long run; you can't safely shed pounds overnight again and again. And for the obese, since their condition can be life-threatening, a carefully monitored very-low-calorie diet may well prove of real help.

Third, if the dieter consumes less than 1,200 calories a day, he may lose muscle tissue as well as fat. So even though the dieter loses weight, he is actually fatter than he was before the diet because the percentage of body fat goes up. This is not the goal of a good diet, which is to lose weight without losing much muscle tissue.

A new look at crash dieting

For years, research suggested that people who try one crash diet after another, losing weight only to regain it, may be doing themselves more harm than good. Some research suggested that people who get caught up in the "yo-yo" cycle take progressively longer each time to shed pounds, and gain them back progressively faster. Studies of groups as diverse as obese patients, high-school wrestlers, and laboratory rats all suggested that repeated loss-and-gain cycles trigger metabolic changes that make it a little harder to lose weight each time you start over. Other studies, including the long-term Framingham Heart Study in Massachusetts, pointedly suggested that repeated bouts of dieting and then regaining weight may increase the risk of heart disease and other health problems. Consequently, many obesity experts have even suggested that remaining overweight may actually be preferable to riding the diet roller coaster.

Recently, however, experts on a National Institutes of Health task force reviewed forty-three human studies on yo-yo dieting and found that the evidence for the claimed adverse health effects is not convincing or consistent. Most studies do *not* show that yo-yo dieting by itself lowers metabolic rate, increases percentage of body fat, makes it harder to lose weight the next time, raises blood pressure, cholesterol, or blood sugar, or increases the risk of dying from heart disease. The scientists admitted, though, that repeatedly regaining hard-lost pounds may result in depression and a loss of self-esteem.

Even though the hazards of yo-yo dieting have not been proven, maintaining a stable, healthy weight is obviously preferable. But given the serious, proven risks of obesity, it is better to have repeatedly lost and regained weight than never to have lost at all.

Here is what the experts advise:

If you are obese or seriously overweight, don't let worries about yo-yo dieting deter you from trying to lose weight. *Losing even five to ten pounds can have significant health benefits. But your goal should be to commit yourself to lifelong changes*—notably increasing physical activity and cutting your caloric intake. As with any attempt at changing habits, you may have to go through several cycles of success and relapse to finally succeed.

If you are not seriously overweight, avoid "dieting," especially if you don't have a medical rationale (such as high blood pressure or a high risk for heart disease). Many people, especially women, who go on diets aren't even overweight. The government's chart of "healthy weights" on page 30 lists a fairly wide range of weights for a given height and allows for modest weight gain as you grow older. And even if you are somewhat overweight, this may not pose much of a health risk if your extra pounds have accumulated at the hips rather than around the waist.

Your goal should be to maintain a stable weight. If you find yourself steadily gaining weight, that should send up a yellow flag to re-evaluate what you're doing.

Diet pills: magic bullets?

Appetite suppressants, or anorectic drugs, may make it easier to stick to a diet, and some studies have shown that they can aid in weight loss during the initial phase of a weight-loss program. But by themselves, these drugs, which are similar to amphetamines but are nonaddictive, do not cause weight loss—they just make it easier to stick to a diet. It's also not known what effects these drugs might have when taken for many years or if they will remain effective as a weight-control measure.

As for people who are not seriously overweight, but who want to shed five or ten pounds, taking such drugs for a lifetime would not be worth it. A sensible diet and a regular exercise program may be more arduous than taking a pill, but it's the safest, most reliable method available over the long term.

Evaluating a weight-control plan

For most people, nutritionists and doctors usually recommend a diet of no fewer than 1,200 calories a day, composed of nutritious, low-calorie, low-fat foods such as fruits, vegetables, whole grains, lean meats, fish, and low-fat dairy products. Although people get discouraged with these sensible diets because they work slowly, sticking to a sensible plan ensures that the weight will stay off.

Some of the popular diet plans from best-sellers, magazines, and organizations can help those individuals who feel they need a regimen to get started. Here's how to distinguish a good plan from ineffective or harmful ones:

Pass up any diet plan that:

• Emphasizes a particular food (for instance, grapefruit, wheat germ, or yogurt) above all others.

• Guarantees that you'll lose a certain number of pounds, especially a large number of pounds—for example, "Lose up to ten pounds a week."

Tactics and Strategies for Weight Control

- Eat slowly.
- Clear your refrigerator and pantry of high-calorie foods and snacks; stock only what you intend to eat on your new diet.
- Eat less fat and more complex carbohydrates (grains, fruits, and vegetables).
- Limit your intake of butter, ice cream, cheese, salad dressings, and oils.
- Avoid packaged snacks, cookies, and high-fat baked goods.
- Use nonstick cooking utensils.
- Bake, broil, or poach meats and steam vegetables (instead of frying or sautéing them in fat).
- Switch to using skim milk and low-fat dairy products.
- Exercise regularly.
- Take up enjoyable activities that don't involve food (such as gardening, adult education, or sports).
- Get counseling or join a support group on a long-term basis.

• Is described as "first," "new," "innovative," "easy," or "fast"—there's nothing new or quick about losing weight.

• Uses fanciful theories to explain how a combination of certain foods (such as fruits and grains only) can improve your health and lead to weight loss. Food-combining theories have been around for a long time and have never been shown to promote weight loss—unless the menus they suggest happen to be low in calories.

• Omits one food group or major nutrient, such as carbohydrates. To stay healthy, you need to choose foods that supply all nutrients. The once-fashionable high-protein, low-carbohydrate diets are high in fat. Furthermore, although they may lead to rapid weight loss initially, it comes mostly from water loss, followed by loss of muscle tissue rather than fat.

• Recommends a total daily intake of fewer than 1,200 calories, unless you're under medical supervision. Besides being hard to follow, minimalist diets don't ensure you of proper nutrition. (For the truly obese, liquid diets—400 to 800 calories—may be useful for immediate weight loss; these require strict medical supervision and can be quite expensive. See page 37.)

• Tells you to take megadoses of vitamin and mineral supplements to make up for losses in foods. Be especially suspicious if "special formula" supplements are sold along with the diet plan.

Look for a diet program that:

• Relies on low-calorie foods that are high in nutrients, particularly fruits, vegetables, and whole grains, and are low in fat.

•Offers variety so you don't get bored with the diet.

•Fits the way you live. Allowance should be made—and advice given—for people on the go or those who are not expert cooks.

•Emphasizes slow weight loss and long-term change of eating habits. It shouldn't promise weight loss exceeding two pounds weekly.

•Offers instruction in the principles of nutrition, in addition to daily menus and charts. If the diet is successful, the day will come when you won't need the plan anymore.

•Includes exercise as part of the weight-loss regimen.

•Has been designed, or at least carefully reviewed, by someone with good credentials in nutrition—for instance, someone with a degree in nutrition, dietetics, or a related academic discipline from an accredited college or university.

•Offers strict medical care by a trained nutritionist or physician, if you opt for a rigorous formula or special diet. Make sure the person who developed the program is well qualified.

Still, bear in mind that an extensive study of factors leading to long-term maintainenance of weight loss showed that most formerly obese individuals who lost weight and kept it off (a small percentage of the obese population) achieved this on their own, without being on a weight-loss program.

The diet key: eating low-fat

Recent studies now support the theory that it's not just the number of calories you eat that cause weight gain or loss, but also which type of foods those calories come from. A study from Harvard Medical School looked at 141 women (age thirty-four to fifty-nine) and found that after adjusting for age, physical activity, alcohol, and

Studies suggest that increasing the amount of gratification and fun in daily life that is unrelated to eating can help ensure that a weight-loss plan will succeed. Researchers have found that most of the pleasurable activities in an overweight person's life are related to eating. Normal-weight people, in contrast, have a wider spectrum of enjoyable activities, such as hobbies or work.

Calorie-Saving Substitutions

Instead of:	Have:	Calories Saved
¼ cup sour cream (125 calories)	¼ cup plain low-fat yogurt (70 calories)	55
3 oz beef, prime rib, untrimmed (360)	3 oz beef, lean round, trimmed (160)	200
3 oz French fries (270)	3 oz baked potato (80)	190
1 cup whole milk (150)	1 cup skim milk (85)	65
¹⁄₁₂ frosted chocolate cake (205)	¹⁄₁₂ unfrosted angel food cake (125)	80
1 cup canned plums, in light syrup (160)	3 fresh plums (110)	50
3 oz chicken, dark meat, with skin, coated, fried (260)	3 oz chicken, light meat, skinless, baked (150)	110
½ cup premium ice cream (175)	½ cup fruit sorbet (110)	65
2 eggs scrambled in butter (190)	1 whole egg and 1 white scrambled in nonstick pan (95)	95
1 bagel, 1 oz cream cheese (300)	1 bagel, with 1 oz cottage cheese, 1% fat (220)	80
2 cups fettuccine Alfredo (800)	2 cups spaghetti, with tomato sauce (450)	350
2 oz potato chips (320)	4 cups popcorn, no oil or butter (100)	220

smoking, there was virtually no correlation between calorie intake and body weight. The degree of excess weight was linked to fat consumption (notably saturated fat), however, independent of calorie intake. Another study, from Stanford University School of Medicine, followed the eating habits of 155 sedentary, obese men (age thirty to fifty-nine) and came to similar conclusions: the proportion of daily calories that came from fat, not the number of calories per se, was directly related to the degree of obesity (total body weight and percentage of body fat).

Is fat more fattening?

A gram of fat yields more than twice as many calories as a gram of carbohydrates (about 9 to 4). Scientists have assumed that one calorie is pretty much like another, and that if you eat more calories than you expend, those calories will be stored as fat, whether they came from fat, protein, or carbohydrates. That fact is not likely to change. But it is now complicated by the question of "efficiency": are some types of calories, depending on their source and the metabolic state of the individual consuming them, used more efficiently in chemical reactions in the body and stored more easily as fat?

Common Fat Foods

Most people have no idea of what 70 grams of fat might be. A standard way to think of fat is in terms of vegetable oil or butter, which are virtually pure fat. Five tablespoons of any vegetable oil would give you 70 grams of fat, as would three-quarters of a stick of butter. But who eats that much oil or butter in a day? Here are some commonly eaten foods—some in "binge" quantities, others not—that by themselves nearly or totally fill your entire daily fat allowance:

Food	Fat (g)
Double-stuffed sandwich cookies (10) & 1 cup whole milk	42
Salad dressing, commercial (6 tablespoons)	54
Cheese (5 oz) and high-fat crackers (10)	55
Fried chicken, fast-food, 1 breast, 1 drumstick, and 1 wing	55
Cheesecake (2 average 4-oz slices)	56
Cheese enchiladas (2) & refried beans	60
Porterhouse steak, untrimmed (10 oz, cooked)	63
Large fast-food hamburger, large fries, shake	64
Pork sausages (three 2.5-oz links)	65
Peanuts, oil-roasted (1 cup)	71
Potato chips (8-oz bag)	80
Super-premium ice cream, butter pecan (1 pint)	96

Myth: Eating before bedtime produces greater weight gain.

Fact: *Assuming that you eat the same foods and maintain the same activity level, it doesn't make a difference what time you eat your food. There is no evidence that when food is consumed at night, significantly more calories are stored as fat than when those same foods are eaten during the day. The calories you consume at night will simply be burned when needed.*

Of course, if what you eat at night is in addition to your normal diet, or if you tend to eat higher-calorie snack foods late at night, you may well gain weight. But don't blame the late hour.

In recent years investigators have found evidence that the body may be able to convert dietary fat into body fat with greater ease than it can convert carbohydrates (starches and sugars) into body fat. Experiments at the University of Massachusetts Medical School, for example, suggest that if you consume 100 excess carbohydrate calories, 23 of those calories will be used simply to process those foods, and thus only 77 of them will end up being stored as reserve energy (body fat). But, the studies suggest, only 3 calories are burned in the processing and storing of 100 fat calories—20 less than it takes to process 100 carbohydrate calories. Still, this small difference can't completely explain the substantial loss of weight that occurs on a high-carbohydrate diet, compared to a high-fat diet, as some studies have reported. For example, if you consume 2,000 calories a day and cut your fat intake from 40 percent of calories to 20 percent (exchanging 400 fat calories for 400 carbohydrate calories), your metabolic savings would be only about 80 calories per day. That could account for a loss of only about two pounds in three months.

No one knows precisely why one person gains more weight than someone else who eats similarly and is as active. Certainly, what goes in (caloric intake) must be used (caloric expenditure) or be stored. But though we can measure caloric intake, it's trickier to measure how many calories the body burns. Energy output depends on many variables, including your basal metabolic rate (the bare-necessity energy required for vital functions at rest), energy expenditure from activities, and the energy required for processing food. Caloric efficiency is another factor complicating the picture, and further studies are being conducted to determine its exact effects on body weight.

Does this prove you'll lose weight, as some people claim, on a diet high in carbohydrates and low in fat? There's no guarantee. Inevitably, to shed pounds, you must burn more calories than you consume. But the most efficient way to lose weight is to cut down on high-fat, high-calorie foods (such as whole milk, butter, ice cream, oils, salad dressings, fatty meats, and most cookies and cakes) and eat a greater proportion of foods with high bulk and low caloric density (fruits, vegetables, grains, and even such starchy items as potatoes).

How exercise helps

Restricting calories and fat is only part of the weight-loss story. For most people, a regular exercise or sports program is essential for losing weight and maintaining the loss. Not only are you likely to enjoy exercise once you get into the habit, but it will also dispose of a certain number of calories.

The only exercise that burns fat, and thus helps you to lose weight, is aerobic exercise—activities such as running, cycling, walking, and cross-country skiing, which use large muscle groups and can be maintained for an extended period, thus burning more calories than anaerobic activities such as weight lifting and sprinting. Moreover, aerobic exercise requires oxygen to fuel the muscles. Without oxygen, your body cannot burn fat for energy.

As well as expending calories, exercise helps in weight loss and maintenance by building muscle tissue. Ultimately, if you're trying to lose weight, what counts

Are you burning fat during a workout?

How many calories are burned in exercise and where that energy comes from are very individual matters. How long and how hard you work are two key elements; your state of training is another.

Second, if you are working at more than about 70 percent of your maximum aerobic capacity (a five-minute sprint, for example), your body relies chiefly on carbohydrates, not fat. If you've jogged a mile in about ten minutes, the calories you've burned probably still come mainly from carbohydrates. If you exercise less intensively but longer (more than one hour of brisk walking, for example), you would start to burn fat along with carbohydrates. In a marathon or other long endurance activity, the primary fuel is fat. In addition, the fitter you are, the easier it is for your body to burn fat.

Your Personal Fat Calculator

If you're following a low-fat eating plan, there's nothing wrong with an occasional high-fat, high-calorie treat. Yet some people get carried away while mindlessly munching in front of the TV, at business or holiday meals, or simply by indulging in too many and too large "occasional treats." The chart at right will give you a general idea of what your daily calorie needs might be based on how active you are; it is derived from data in the National Research Council's most recent edition of Recommended Dietary Allowances. The chart also lists how much fat (in grams) you could eat so that it would contribute no more than 30 percent of your total caloric intake (that's the recommended maximum fat intake, according to federal health officials and other experts).

Remember, however, that these are rough estimates, since calorie needs vary from individual to individual, depending not only on activity level, but also on age, body weight, body composition, and other factors.

ESTIMATED DAILY CALORIE NEEDS (age 19 to 50) AND FAT ALLOWANCE

Activity Level	Men		Women	
	Calories	Fat	Calories	Fat
Very light	2,200	73 g	1,700	57 g
Light	2,600	87 g	2,000	67 g
Moderate	2,800	93 g	2,100	70 g
Heavy	3,500	117 g	2,500	83 g

Calorie Burning: An Activity Guide

The following chart gives you the approximate number of calories burned per minute for a variety of activities. Exactly how many calories are expended by an individual depends on many factors. For example, the more you weigh, the more calories you'll burn because of the additional effort during physical activity. Other factors that influence calorie burning are: your level of fitness, your proportion of body fat to muscle, air temperature and humidity, and how efficiently you perform a particular activity. Still, this chart gives you a rough estimate. The first column of numbers represents the calories burned per minute per one pound of body weight; multiply this number by your weight to get an estimate that is correct for you. Calculations are provided for 110, 150, and 190 pounds. To determine how many calories you burn during an extended period of activity, simply multiply the per-minute calculation for your weight by the number of minutes you perform the activity.

CALORIES BURNED PER MINUTE

Activity	Per Pound	Per Body Weight		
		110 lb	150 lb	190 lb
Ax chopping, fast	0.135	14.8	20.2	25.6
Skiing, cross-country, uphill	0.125	13.7	18.7	23.7
Running, 6-min mile	0.115	12.6	17.2	21.8
Squash	0.096	10.6	14.5	18.3
Running, 8-min mile	0.095	10.4	14.2	18.0
Jumping rope, 145 jumps per min	0.089	9.8	13.4	16.9
Running, 9-min mile	0.087	9.6	13.1	16.6
Racquetball	0.081	8.9	12.1	15.4
Jumping rope, 125 jumps per min	0.080	8.8	12.0	15.2
Snowshoeing, soft snow	0.075	8.3	11.3	14.3
Jumping rope, 70 jumps per min	0.074	8.1	11.0	14.0
Swimming, breaststroke, fast	0.074	8.1	11.0	14.0
Swimming, crawl, fast	0.071	7.8	10.6	13.5
Skiing, cross-country, walking	0.065	7.1	9.7	12.3
Climbing hills, with 22-lb load	0.064	7.0	9.5	12.1
Basketball	0.063	6.9	9.4	11.9
Aerobic dance, intense	0.061	6.7	9.1	11.6
Field hockey	0.061	6.7	9.1	11.6
Running, 11.5-min mile	0.061	6.7	9.1	11.6
Climbing hills, with 9-lb load	0.058	6.4	8.7	11.1
Swimming, crawl, slow	0.058	6.4	8.7	11.1
Climbing hills, with no load	0.055	6.0	8.2	10.4
Tennis	0.049	5.4	7.4	9.3
Aerobic dance, medium	0.046	5.1	7.0	8.8
Cycling, 9.5 mph	0.045	5.0	6.8	8.6
Badminton	0.044	4.8	6.5	8.3
Weight training, circuit training	0.042	4.6	6.3	7.9
Weight lifting, free weights	0.039	4.3	5.9	7.4
Golf	0.038	4.2	5.7	7.3
Walking, normal pace, fields and hills	0.037	4.1	5.6	7.1
Walking, normal pace, asphalt road	0.036	4.0	5.5	6.9
Table tennis	0.031	3.4	4.6	5.9
Cycling, 5.5 mph	0.029	3.2	4.4	5.5
Mopping floors	0.028	3.1	4.2	5.4
Raking	0.025	2.7	3.7	4.7
Dancing, ballroom	0.023	2.5	3.4	4.3
Volleyball	0.023	2.5	3.4	4.3
Conducting music	0.017	1.9	2.6	3.3
Typing, electric	0.012	1.3	1.8	2.2

isn't just how many pounds you take off but what kind of body tissue is lost. The goal should be to shed fat while sparing important "lean body mass," such as muscle, organ tissue, and bone. The problem of losing tissue other than fat is especially serious in very-low-calorie diets. In one study conducted at the University of Minnesota, caloric intake of participants was cut by 45 percent, and changes in the dieters' weight and body composition were observed for a period of twenty-four weeks. During the first twelve weeks, 54 percent of the weight lost was lean body mass; in the second twelve-week period, a third of what was lost was lean tissue.

But research has shown that a proper low-calorie diet combined with exercise can help dieters maintain lean body mass while increasing the burning of fat. To maintain that increased body tone, your body uses more calories—even at rest—eventually drawing on fat. As a result, your percentage of body fat decreases and you improve your fat-to-lean ratio. Deposits of fat gradually decline, revealing contours of muscle that were there all along.

Exercise and appetite

Many people fear that exercise will increase their appetite and that the calories they burn while exercising will be more than made up for by the extra food they'll eat. But evidence shows that most people who work out moderately eat about the same as they would if they didn't exercise—or slightly more. Although competitive athletes in strenuous training eat more than they would otherwise, the extra calories seldom overtake their increased energy expenditure.

How your appetite will respond to exercise depends on many variables, such as frequency, duration, and intensity of exercise; initial accumulation of body fat; metabolic rate; as well as the amount and type of food available after exercise. Among the recent studies, one looked at a group of college men, none of them overweight. It found that the harder they exercised, the less hungry they were during the first few hours after their workouts; however, their hunger increased slightly during the next several hours. Another study found that lean women who exercised moderately compensated by eating slightly more—but only enough to maintain their caloric intake/expenditure equilibrium. Yet when the same researchers conducted two studies of obese women, they found that the women did not compensate for exercise by eating more, despite free access to food.

Remember, however, that the results of such short-term experiments cannot explain the body's regulation and adaptation processes during a long-term exercise regimen. But it is probable that, over the long haul, the calories burned during regular exercise will more than make up for any slight increase in appetite.

Keeping weight off

Most people who lose weight regain it—and more. But some people succeed in keeping it off. What's the secret of their success? No one knows, but recently the experts have tended to downplay the "willpower" aspect. Overeating is similar to other forms of addiction. To understand it, you must ask why the addiction exists. Keep in mind that losing weight is not a moral issue. You may hear foods described as "sinfully rich" or "wickedly delicious," but food is not sinful. Nor are you morally deficient if you fall off the wagon. Most people do fall off occasionally, or get pushed off by circumstances. Remember that people trying to change other lifelong habits—smoking, for example—usually have two or three relapses

The pros and cons of grazing

Many diet plans suggest that grazing—eating six or more small meals over the course of the day rather than three normal-sized ones—can promote weight loss. While some studies have suggested that food may be more efficiently stored as fat when eaten in larger batches and infrequent eating may encourage excessive between-meal hunger and thus over-eating, there is no conclusive evidence for this. Other studies have found that it didn't matter whether people ate two large daily meals or ate the same amount of food at several small meals—the rate at which their bodies used the calories remained the same. And some obesity experts recommend that overweight people not graze, since that makes it harder to keep track of food intake and may promote mindless eating. The bottom line is: it's not how or when you eat your calories, but how many you consume and how many you burn in activity.

(returns to the old habits) before they succeed. Such relapses usually occur within the first three months. The same is true about eating lapses. But lapses and relapses simply mean that it's time to start over. In fact, according to many studies, analysis of what triggers your relapses can stiffen your resolve.

Researchers believe that emphasis should be placed on techniques to maintain change, rather than on the initial commitment to change. Sometimes, breaking a hard-to-keep vow can lead to feelings of inadequacy and guilt that in turn lead to further relapses. Slips may signal an emergency, but they aren't the end of the world. A slip should be viewed as an opportunity from which you can learn a lesson and then try to do better the next time.

It isn't enough just to say no: you have to plan ahead so you can see temptation coming. This is easier to do in light of an increased awareness of why some situations are particularly dangerous for you. As soon as you realize that you've gone overboard on your eating, take a hard look at what you've done and why. Ignore the feelings of guilt and inadequacy and concentrate on the reasons why you decided to control your eating in the first place.

Then review the conditions that led to your slip so you can recognize the warning signs next time and stiffen your resolve. Studies by psychologist G. Alan Marlatt of the University of Washington have identified three primary high-risk situations that account for 75 percent of all relapses:

Negative emotional states. Watch out if you are bored, tense, angry, or frustrated. That's when you are most likely to return to old habits.

Interpersonal conflicts. If you've had an argument at home or at work, you may return to old eating habits in compensation or in revenge.

Social pressures. It may not be easy to stick to your newly developed eating patterns at a business lunch or a party.

Plan strategies to cope with the type of situations that are the most dangerous. The details will differ from person to person, but there are three basic strategies for structuring your resistance:

1. Develop a positive addiction. Rather than rewarding yourself with ice cream or potato chips, become "addicted" to a healthful habit. Take up anything from gardening to jogging that leaves you feeling deprived if you don't get your daily fix.

2. Stay away from temptation. If you always have cake and coffee when you play bridge, don't play bridge for a while. Don't wander "aimlessly" through the baked goods section of the supermarket.

3. Learn to wait out the urge. Ride it like a surfer rides a wave: you know that all waves subside. And see through your own stratagems. Don't keep goodies around in case friends drop in when you know your own cravings will be hard to suppress.

Finally, be prepared to rehearse all or parts of these strategies several times: only practice will make perfect. And have confidence in your ability to change. Studies show that if you believe in your ability to reach a particular goal—a concept defined as self-efficacy—you are more likely to reach it. When beset with difficulties, people who entertain serious doubts about their capabilities slacken their efforts or give up altogether, whereas those who have a strong sense of self-efficacy exert great effort to master the challenges. Nonetheless, allow plenty of leeway for mistakes, and regard each of them as a fork in the road. One path leads to total relapse, the other to continued change for the better.

Boosting self-efficacy

Self-efficacy—your perception of your own ability to do a specific task—can be affected by past performance. If you've tried to break a bad habit and succeeded, breaking other bad habits will be all the easier. If you've tried and failed, however, you may find it more difficult. Here are some suggestions for boosting self-efficacy:

1. Think about a similar thing you have succeeded in doing. Maybe you haven't been able to give up potato chips or stick to an exercise program, but you did quit smoking.

2. Recruit your family and/or friends as a support group. Tell them what helps you and what does not.

3. Find a role model or join a support group.

4. Don't undertake too much at one time. Start with the easiest tasks first, or parts of tasks. Use a one-day-at-a-time philosophy. Instead of saying, "I'm going to lose weight," say, "I'm going to lose one pound this week," and outline a plan for doing it.

Cholesterol

How important is your blood cholesterol level? Very—but it does need to be put in perspective. Although some experts question whether high blood cholesterol levels cause heart disease in everybody, there is substantial evidence that, in most cases, the connection between high blood cholesterol levels and heart disease is as incontrovertible as the link between smoking and lung cancer. This connection is strongest in men under fifty. For young women and for everybody over fifty, the link is weaker, but still significant.

Still, your cholesterol level needs to be put in perspective within your total risk scenario for heart disease, based on such factors as age, sex, and health habits (see page 18). And the single number for total cholesterol tells only part of the story regarding your risk for coronary artery disease (CAD). This section covers updated recommendations for assessing and controlling cholesterol levels, along with background about cholesterol.

What is cholesterol?

Cholesterol is a white, waxy, fatlike substance. Although we usually think of it as found only in the bloodstream, it is actually present in all of the body's tissues. Cholesterol is essential to life: among other things, it is used in the outer membrane of cells; as a fatty insulation sheath around nerve fibers; and as a building block for certain hormones.

Despite its importance to life, cholesterol isn't an essential nutrient—you don't have to consume any to stay healthy. Most of the cholesterol in your bloodstream is manufactured in your body—primarily by the liver—from the fats, proteins, and carbohydrates you eat. The body produces varying amounts, usually about 1,000 milligrams a day. In addition, the average American consumes 400 to 500 milligrams of cholesterol in food every day. In foods, cholesterol is found only in animal products—meats, eggs, fish, poultry, and dairy products. (No plant-derived food contains cholesterol.) So, in a sense, there are two different "types" of cholesterol, though chemically they're the same—the type that comes from food (called dietary, or preformed, cholesterol), and that made by the body, both of which end up in the blood.

The "good" and the "bad"

Just how cholesterol is distributed throughout the body is not entirely clear, but researchers now hypothesize that the mechanism works like this: the liver puts together packages called lipoproteins, made of proteins, cholesterol, and triglycerides (fats either made by the body or derived directly from foods). The largest of these are called very-low-density lipoprotein, or VLDL. As it circulates through the bloodstream, VLDL drops off the triglycerides to the muscle and fat cells to be used for energy or stored for later use. When VLDL drops off its triglycerides, it breaks up into smaller low-density lipoprotein, or LDL. LDL carries cholesterol throughout the system, dropping it off where it can be used for cell metabolism.

Cholesterol carried by LDL that is not used, broken down by the liver, or excreted, is left to circulate in the bloodstream where it accumulates in the arterial walls. Nodules, called plaques, are eventually formed, decreasing the flow of blood over time—a condition known as atherosclerosis—and favoring the formation of blood clots. This may ultimately cut off the flow of blood: in the coronary arteries, this leads to a heart attack, and in the cerebral arteries, a stroke.

The liver makes another type of molecular package known as high-density lipoprotein, or HDL. Like the other lipoproteins, HDL is composed of proteins, fats, and cholesterol, but HDL carries less cholesterol than LDL. As it circulates through the bloodstream, HDL seems to have the beneficial capacity to pick up cholesterol and bring it back to the liver for reprocessing or excretion. In simple terms then, LDL brings cholesterol into the system, so it's often called "bad" cholesterol, and because HDL clears cholesterol out of the system, it has been dubbed "good" cholesterol. (If you have trouble remembering which is which, think "lousy" for LDL and "helpful" for HDL.) *HDL (as well as LDL) is formed only in the body. You can't eat "good" cholesterol; no type of cholesterol you eat is good for you.*

The cholesterol/heart disease link

Blood cholesterol levels are measured by withdrawing a small amount of blood—usually from your arm—to be analyzed in a lab. The result, a number that is usually between 150 and 300, is the number of milligrams of cholesterol per deciliter of blood (that's about a tenth of a quart, or a little less than half a cup). Recent surveys show that cholesterol levels dropped about 4 percent over a twelve-year period among Americans—to the current average of 205 milligrams per deciliter (mg/dl). That drop has meant a substantial number of prevented heart attacks. But about half of adult Americans have cholesterol levels that are far too high to be healthy—and this partly explains why Americans continue to have such a relatively high incidence of heart attacks and strokes.

A number of studies have provided more exact information about the relationship between cholesterol and heart disease. One large-scale study, called the Multi-

Different types of HDL?

Research into blood lipid chemistry—the fats that circulate in your bloodstream—has become increasingly complicated in recent years. Scientists now know, for instance, that different types, or "subfractions," of HDL and LDL interact in complex ways and appear to have different effects on coronary risk. For instance, HDL-2 seems to be more protective than HDL-3. Furthermore, HDL and LDL contain one or more kinds of proteins called apolipoproteins, which "carry" fatty particles in the blood and are involved in a host of metabolic processes.

Some of these proteins may play a role in the risk of heart attack. For instance, recent studies have found that low levels of apolipoprotein A-1 increase the risk of CAD, at least in men. But the role of these proteins is not well understood yet and they are not measured in routine screening tests.

Nine Factors That Influence Blood Cholesterol

Positive:

Soluble fiber. This lowers cholesterol. Oats, beans, fruits, vegetables are good sources.

Polyunsaturated fat. This lowers LDL, or "bad," cholesterol. Safflower, sesame, and soybean oil are good sources.

Monounsaturated fat. Studies have shown that this also lowers cholesterol. Olive oil is a good source.

Fatty fish. These contain special polyunsaturated fatty acids called omega-3s, which may lower cholesterol.

Aerobic exercise. Although overall cholesterol remains the same, regular exercise helps increase HDL ("good") cholesterol.

Negative:

Foods high in saturated fat. More than any other factor, a diet high in saturated fat raises blood cholesterol levels. Sources of saturated fat include beef, butter, whole-milk dairy products, dark meat poultry, poultry skin, and coconut, palm, and palm kernel oils.

Excess weight. In most overweight people, each pound of excess weight adds to total blood cholesterol.

Foods high in cholesterol. Only animal products contain cholesterol. Eggs and organ meats are the richest sources.

Smoking. Increases LDL ("bad") cholesterol and decreases HDL cholesterol.

ple Risk Factor Intervention Trial, or MRFIT, followed 361,000 healthy men who ranged in age from thirty-five to fifty-seven. The researchers found that, over a ten-year period, the likelihood of dying from CAD was almost five times higher in men with total cholesterol levels above 300 mg/dl compared with those whose levels were below 180 mg/dl. Numerous studies confirm that the risk of dying from CAD increases as total cholesterol levels rise.

In addition, several major studies have shown a reduction in CAD risk when total cholesterol levels are lowered. In a ten-year study conducted by the National Heart, Lung, and Blood Institute, almost 4,000 men between the ages of thirty-five and fifty-nine were divided into two groups. One group was given the cholesterol-lowering drug cholestyramine; the other group was given a placebo. By the end of the study, the drug-taking group lowered their blood cholesterol levels 8.5 percent below that of the control group—and those who reduced their cholesterol levels also reduced their incidence of heart attack by an astonishing factor: they had 19 percent fewer heart attacks than the control group. The study's conclusion: for every 1 percent drop in cholesterol levels, there is a 2 percent reduction in heart disease risk.

Experts now believe that to be at low risk for heart disease, adults should reduce their total blood cholesterol levels to less than 200 mg/dl (see box opposite). While there is no magic number—a point at which your blood cholesterol level automatically passes from safe to dangerous—the risk of heart disease rises continually with increasing levels of blood cholesterol, though it doesn't rise markedly until levels exceed 200 mg/dl. And the rate of coronary heart disease begins to accelerate rapidly above the 220 level. *Thus, many researchers believe that cholesterol levels should be as low as possible; well below 200 mg/dl is excellent.*

New guidelines: the importance of HDL

In 1993, the National Cholesterol Education Program (NCEP), the coalition of government and private health organizations in charge of persuading Americans to control their cholesterol levels, updated its guidelines to place new emphasis on HDL. Until recently, physicians have focused primarily on high total cholesterol and high LDL ("bad") cholesterol as cardiac risk factors. But accumulating research indicates that HDL is an independent risk factor of CAD—that is, a low level of HDL ("good") cholesterol increases the risk of a heart attack. For instance, the well-known Framingham Heart Study found that every 1 mg increase in HDL reduced the risk of CAD by 2 to 3 percent. Moreover, other studies have shown that people with a "safe" total cholesterol level—below 200 mg/dl—may still be at high risk for a heart attack if their HDL level is also low; and, conversely, some people with elevated total cholesterol (usually women) may not be at high risk if their HDL level is high. Thus HDL should be routinely measured along with total cholesterol. The same blood sample is used; you don't have to fast beforehand.

Low HDL, defined as 35 mg/dl or below, is now considered a risk factor for CAD. A high HDL level, defined as 60 mg/dl or more, is considered protective against CAD. Female sex hormones tend to raise HDL; this may help explain why women are usually protected against atherosclerosis during their childbearing years, when estrogen production is high. That's also why hormone replacement therapy helps lower cholesterol levels after menopause.

Who's at Risk?

In the past, experts focused on the ratio of total cholesterol to HDL (or LDL to HDL), but recent guidelines from the National Cholesterol Education Program (NCEP) have de-emphasized this, and consider HDL and LDL as separate risk factors for heart disease.

The parameters for total cholesterol and LDL cholesterol levels—shown below—remain unchanged for people free of coronary artery disease (CAD). (If you have CAD, your total cholesterol level should be below 160, and your LDL level should be kept below 100.) These values, as well as the levels for HDL shown in this box, must be interpreted in the context of other risk factors, as noted in the text below.

	Total Cholesterol (mg/dl)	LDL Cholesterol (mg/dl)		HDL Cholesterol (mg/dl)
Desirable	under 200	under 130	Risk factor	35 or less
Borderline-high	200 to 239	130 to 159	Protective	60 or more
High	240 or more	160 or more		

Testing guidelines

All adults over age twenty should be tested for HDL and total cholesterol at least once every five years. But some people should be retested more frequently, depending on their total and HDL cholesterol results and other risk factors:

•If your total cholesterol is in the desirable range (see chart above) and your HDL is above 35, you can wait up to five years to have them rechecked. If your total cholesterol is borderline-high and your HDL is above 35, you should be rechecked in a year or two.

•If your total cholesterol is borderline-high or high *and/or* your HDL is below 35, especially if you have two or more CAD risk factors, you should have a complete "lipid profile" (which requires fasting overnight) to determine LDL. Then, if your LDL is in the desirable range, you can wait up to five years to be retested. But if your LDL is borderline-high or high, and depending on your other risk factors, you'll need to be retested annually as well as to modify your diet and take other steps to reduce your risk of CAD.

Risk factors. The recommendations are more stringent if you have other risk factors for CAD besides high cholesterol and/or low HDL. These risk factors are age, family history of premature CAD (a heart attack in your father before age fifty-five, in your mother before age sixty-five), smoking, high blood pressure, and diabetes. The guidelines are even stricter for those who already have CAD: for instance, your LDL should be below 100, rather than 130.

Men and women. Women need to be monitored as carefully as men. But women tend to develop CAD about a decade later than men do, so while age is considered a "risk factor" for men starting at age forty-five, for women it's at age fifty-five. Women over that age who have high cholesterol should make as great an effort as men to reduce it. (Of course, younger women can also develop CAD, particularly if they have other risk factors for CAD.) In addition, since estrogen is known to raise HDL, the NCEP now recommends that such postmenopausal women consider taking hormone replacement therapy to lower their cholesterol rather than cholesterol-lowering drugs.

The elderly. People in their seventies or even older should be treated just like peo-

Triglycerides and risk

*The link between high levels of triglycerides—fats that circulate in the blood along with cholesterol and other lipids—and CAD remains unclear. Some leading scientists have proposed that elevated triglycerides may contribute to CAD, especially in women and diabetics. The problem is that triglyceride and HDL levels tend to be inversely related—that is, high triglyceride levels are usually accompanied by low HDL levels, and vice versa. Most researchers have found that elevated triglyceride levels are **not** predictive of heart disease independent of a low HDL level and other risk factors. In other words, if your HDL level is in the healthy range, it probably doesn't matter if your triglycerides are somewhat high.*

The recent NCEP guidelines state that a level below 200 mg/dl is desirable; between 200 and 400 is borderline-high, and over 400 is high. The same measures that help lower total cholesterol also help lower triglyceride levels.

ple in their fifties of sixties, according to the new guidelines. But in practice, it varies from person to person. If someone over seventy-five without heart disease is found to have a cholesterol level of 250, it probably doesn't make sense to take aggressive steps—such as a very strict diet or medication—to lower it. More moderate measures, such as daily walking, may make more sense. In any case, blood cholesterol levels naturally start to decline after age seventy-five.

Children. According to the NCEP, only children who have a family history of very high cholesterol levels and/or heart disease—particularly those with a parent who suffered a heart attack before age fifty—should have their cholesterol levels measured. That includes as many as one-quarter of the nation's children. Many authorities have concluded that screening *all* youngsters is unnecessary, since high blood cholesterol levels do not necessarily predict high levels in adulthood. But all children, whatever their family history, can benefit from a low-fat, heart-healthy diet after age two.

Cholesterol and diet

A diet rich in cholesterol and—even more significantly—in saturated fat can increase your blood cholesterol level. There are many other factors that affect your blood cholesterol level, and some people, no matter how little fat and cholesterol they eat, may continue to have high blood cholesterol levels because of genetic disorders, diabetes, or other metabolic diseases. For most people, though, diet remains the first defense against elevated blood cholesterol.

The connection between diet and cholesterol levels was shown as early as 1913, when the Russian pathologist Nikolai Anitschkow demonstrated that rabbits would develop atherosclerosis if they were fed a diet rich in cholesterol. And in the following years, other studies showed clear links between elevated blood cholesterol levels and atherosclerosis in humans.

Other evidence has indicated that high blood cholesterol levels are related to high intakes of saturated fat. The Finns, for instance, who have the highest levels of saturated fat in their diets of any national group, have the highest cholesterol levels, and the highest rate of heart disease, too. Americans, with a slightly less rich diet, have the second highest level of heart disease. And the Japanese, who eat a diet very low in saturated fat, have the lowest levels of blood cholesterol and cardiovascular disease of any developed nation.

In addition, studies have demonstrated that blood cholesterol can be lowered by diet. In one study, a group of physicians in Holland put thirty-nine subjects on a strict diet that contained only 100 milligrams of cholesterol a day. The diet also called for two parts polyunsaturated fat for every one part saturated fat. By the end of two years, the subjects had lowered their cholesterol levels by an average of 27 milligrams. Diet alone, it was demonstrated, could lower cholesterol levels and keep them low for at least two years.

In a more recent study conducted by Dr. Dean Ornish and other researchers at the University of California at San Francisco, subjects with severe heart disease who were put on very-low-fat vegetarian diets (10 percent calories from fat) and moderate exercise programs were able to lower their total cholesterol levels by about 30 percent and their LDL levels by 40 percent. Not only did the dietary and other lifestyle changes lower cholesterol, they actually decreased the extent of coronary-artery narrowing—on average by about 10 percent.

Fatty meat has about the same amount of cholesterol as lean cuts, since cholesterol is found primarily in the lean tissue, not the fat. Untrimmed fatty beef has about 82 milligrams of cholesterol in three ounces, while well-trimmed lean beef has about 79 milligrams. Untrimmed, high-fat cuts of beef, however, can still contribute to high cholesterol levels, since they are high in saturated fat.

Controlling cholesterol

If you are trying to control your blood cholesterol level, you must limit not only the amount of cholesterol you consume, but also the amount of saturated fat, which appears to stimulate the body's production of cholesterol. *Experts now recommend that you reduce dietary cholesterol to no more than 300 milligrams per day and keep your total fat intake at 30 percent or less of your total daily calories, with no more than 10 percent of those calories coming from saturated fat.*

Although they're often mentioned together, cholesterol and fat are not the same thing. Cholesterol is found only in animal products, while plant foods—vegetables, fruits, nuts, grains, and vegetable oils—contain no cholesterol at all. Both plant and animal products can contain fat, however. Saturated fat is found primarily in animal products—beef, pork, whole milk products, and poultry skin—and in three vegetable oils, coconut, palm, and palm kernel. Although foods high in saturated fat tend also to be rich in cholesterol, some foods are high in one but not the other. Organ meats (liver and kidney, for example) and eggs have lots of cholesterol but only moderate amounts of fat. Sour cream, butter, and lard, on the other hand, are rich sources of fat but not particularly high in cholesterol.

In addition to reducing the amount of saturated fat and cholesterol in your diet, there are other steps you can take to lower total and LDL cholesterol. HDL is harder to modify, but these measures tend to raise HDL levels, or may at least stabilize HDL while bringing down LDL:

Substitute unsaturated fats for saturated fats. Studies have shown that polyunsaturated fats (such as safflower and corn oil) and monounsaturated fats (such as olive oil) help to lower blood cholesterol levels. Monounsaturated fats may help maintain or increase the level of HDL cholesterol as well. But this doesn't mean you should add any of these fats to your diet—you should still keep your total fat intake at or below 30 percent of your daily calories. Less than one-third of these calories should come from saturated fat, and less than one-third should come from polyunsaturated fat; monounsaturated fat should make up the rest. To achieve this, for example, replace butter in cooking with olive or corn oil. Or substitute fish for some of the red meat and poultry in your diet. Some types of fish are high in a polyunsaturated fat known as omega-3 fatty acids, which have been shown to have cholesterol-lowering benefits.

Lose weight, if you're overweight. Not only does excess body fat raise your total blood cholesterol and LDL levels and reduce HDL, but it is also an independent risk factor for heart disease. On average, each two pounds of excess body fat contributes 1 mg/dl of total cholesterol. Where the fat accumulates is also important: excess weight around the waist (the so-called apple-shape body) seems to reduce HDL more than weight in the hips and thighs (pear shape).

Exercise more. Results of studies have been inconsistent concerning the effect of aerobic exercise or strength-training exercise on total cholesterol and LDL. But the evidence is stronger that an exercise program can help raise HDL, and its effect on lowering the risk of CAD is overwhelming. The exercise doesn't have to be strenuous—walking a mile or two or even gardening several times a week can help.

Increase your consumption of foods high in soluble fiber. Eat more legumes and other vegetables, such as black-eyed peas, kidney beans, carrots, split peas, corn, and prunes. Sweet potatoes, zucchini, and broccoli have some soluble fiber, as do bananas, apples, pears, and oranges, as well as many other fruits and vegetables. No

Progress on the cholesterol front

Between 1978 and 1990, the average cholesterol level in the U.S. declined from 213 to 205 mg/dl, a 4 percent decline, according to recent data from the National Center for Health Statistics. In addition, the proportion of adults with "high" total cholesterol dropped from 26 percent to 20 percent of the population, while those with "desirable" levels rose from 44 percent to 49 percent (those with "borderline-high" levels stayed about the same). This continues a thirty-year trend, which has coincided with a 54 percent decline in CAD mortality rates. It's impossible to say whether the drop in cholesterol levels is due primarily to lifestyle changes, such as diet and exercise, or to wider use of cholesterol-lowering drugs. Similarly, no one knows how much of the drop in CAD mortality is due to lower cholesterol levels and how much is due to declines in blood pressure and smoking rates and improved treatment of CAD.

one can say just how much soluble fiber you need to eat each day to lower your blood cholesterol, but if you regularly eat a high fiber, low-fat diet that includes a variety of the vegetables and fruits listed above and some oatmeal or oat bran daily, you may see results next time you have a cholesterol check—particularly if the level was previously elevated. Studies indicate that soluble fiber has a greater cholesterol-lowering effect on individuals with elevated cholesterol levels than on those with levels within the "safe" range.

Don't smoke. Smoking increases total cholesterol and reduces HDL, and is an independent risk factor for heart disease as well.

Consider alcohol. A drink or two a day may boost HDL. The health risks of heavier drinking, however, outweigh the potential benefit for the heart.

Cholesterol-lowering drugs

The new guidelines from the NCEP are even more cautious about medication than the old ones because of the potential side effects and the high cost (once you start drug therapy, you'll probably need to continue for the rest of your life). Whatever your age, if your cholesterol is high or your HDL low, you should first undertake the dietary and exercise measures outlined above. Drugs should be avoided or at least delayed in men under forty-five and women under fifty-five, unless they have additional risk factors.

Unfortunately, because of genetics, not everyone responds to a low-fat diet—but the vast majority do, and the higher the cholesterol level to begin with, usually the greater the response. But many others simply can't stick to a low-fat diet. If, after several months, all else has failed and your cholesterol level remains high, your doctor may prescribe a cholesterol-lowering drug, particularly if you have other risk factors and/or symptoms of CAD. Even when drugs are used, individuals still need to follow a diet low in fat and cholesterol for the drugs to be most effective.

There are several drugs that can produce significant results in some individuals; however, none of these drugs are without some side effects. Cholestyramine and colestipol, for example, have an unpleasant taste and can cause nausea, gas, and bloating. According to one study, megadoses of niacin—taken under a doctor's supervision—can produce a 10 percent drop in cholesterol and a 21 percent reduction in nonfatal heart attacks, but can cause flushing, stomach irritation, irregular heartbeat, impaired regulation of blood sugar levels, and liver dysfunction.

Lovastatin and several other cholesterol-lowering "-statin" drugs appear to be effective and also less likely to cause unpleasant or serious side effects. In a Scandinavian study published in 1994, subjects who took Simvastatin not only lowered their levels of LDL cholesterol, but also had a 42 percent lower coronary death rate and a 30 percent lower overall death rate than subjects who took a placebo.

Psyllium-containing over-the-counter laxatives—which are rich in soluble fiber—also appear to lower total cholesterol and improve the ratio of LDL to HDL. But these laxatives can cause bloating, gas, diarrhea, and abdominal cramping, and may result in a dependency on the laxative for normal bowel function. In addition, an excessive fiber intake may interfere with the absorption of certain minerals. (This is less likely to be a problem with high-fiber foods, since they tend to be rich in minerals and more than make up for any losses.) For these reasons, it is unwise to use this type of laxative to lower cholesterol without a doctor's recommendation and advice.

No one should elect to take any type of prescription or over-the-counter drug to lower cholesterol without first consulting his or her doctor. Individuals taking these drugs need to be monitored by a physician to check for side effects, regulate dosages, and judge the effects of the drugs on cholesterol levels.

What you need to know about cholesterol testing

Having your blood cholesterol measured is a relatively simple and inexpensive process. The problem is in getting accurate results and then a sound interpretation of the figures. This blood test is complicated to run in a laboratory. Different labs use a variety of methods that yield differing results. Analyses done in doctors' offices—especially by someone not trained in laboratory techniques and on machines that are poorly standardized—may be particularly unreliable. And not all clinical lab methods for determining blood cholesterol levels end up with values that are comparable to those used by the Lipid Research Clinics (LRC). This nationwide research group, working with experts at the National Institutes of Health (NIH), has developed a standardized method for determining blood cholesterol concentrations and has used it on a large group of patients. Based on these numbers, national estimates of the risks of elevated cholesterol have been made. Research has found that two commonly used clinical lab instruments indicated significantly higher cholesterol levels than those obtained when the same sample was analyzed by the LRC method.

Ask your doctor if the values his lab gives are comparable with those obtained by the LRC and if the lab participates in any recognized quality-control program to ensure the accuracy of their cholesterol determinations. Even under the best circumstances, different labs and different equipment can yield different results from the same blood sample.

Other factors that affect your test

In addition, various factors unrelated to the lab can affect blood cholesterol levels. If it's winter, your reading will probably be higher. The cause of this seasonal shift is unknown, but it may be because people tend to eat fattier foods and to exercise less in winter. Even your body position at the time of blood withdrawal can influence the measurable concentration of blood lipids. When you are prone, your blood becomes diluted. Still, there are measures you can take to ensure you are getting the best possible result from your cholesterol test:

•Don't exercise before your test. Exercise can cause a temporary rise in cholesterol levels—as much as 10 to 15 percent—for up to an hour after you've stopped.

•Cholesterol levels can be affected by illness, some medications, pregnancy, and recent heart attack or surgery. If any of these conditions apply to you, discuss them with your doctor.

•Sit down for at least five minutes before your blood is taken. Having blood taken while you are standing or lying down can skew the results.

•Don't eat anything for twelve hours prior to your blood test, if you are having your HDL/LDL levels measured.

•Have at least two tests performed and schedule them a month or two apart. Since cholesterol levels fluctuate, the average of two tests will give a more accurate picture, provided both results are within thirty points of each other.

Milligrams vs. millimoles

In Canada, as in many other countries, blood cholesterol is measured in millimoles per liter of blood (a millimole, one-thousandth of a mole, is a chemical measure based on the molecular weight of a substance), abbreviated as mmol/L. This is called the International System. In the United States, blood cholesterol is usually measured in milligrams per deciliter (one-tenth of a liter) of blood, or mg/dl—though the International System is also increasingly being used here.

To convert a result from the International System to the American system, multiply it by 38.67. Thus 6.5 mmol/L equals 251 mg/dl.

To convert an American number to the International System, multiply it by 0.0259.

Hypertension

The typical image of a person with hypertension (high blood pressure) is an overweight, overworked male executive with a very short fuse. The truth is, high blood pressure affects people of all ages, races, social classes, sizes, and shapes, women as well as men, and even children—a total of more than 60 million Americans. Moreover, at least 20 million of them are currently on antihypertensive drugs, spending more on such medications (approximately 2.5 billion dollars a year) than on drugs for any other diagnosis. Although great strides have been made in recent years to control this condition, often it still goes untreated or uncontrolled.

What is blood pressure?

Every cell in the body needs a constant supply of blood to bring in oxygen and nutrients and to remove waste products. The force that keeps blood moving comes from the heart, but a complex system of nerve signals, hormones, and other elements regulates the blood flow to each organ by widening or constricting small muscular blood vessels called arterioles, much like a faucet controls the flow of water. Blood pressure thus depends on a number of factors, including how much blood is flowing through the arteries, the rate of blood flow, and the resiliency of the arteries' walls.

Blood pressure fluctuates from moment to moment. Among the factors influencing it are the time of day (it is lowest in early morning) and your degree of physical exertion or anxiety. Although blood pressure tends to go up with age in industrial societies, population studies have found that in nonindustrialized countries, there is actually little increase in blood pressure with age.

Measuring blood pressure

Blood pressure is commonly measured with a sphygmomanometer, which consists of either a gauge or a column of mercury in a glass tube, an inflatable cuff, and a stethoscope. The cuff is wrapped around the upper arm, and air is pumped into the cuff until circulation is cut off. The column of mercury rises as the air is pumped in. When a stethoscope is placed over an artery below the cuff, there is silence. Then as the air is slowly let out of the cuff, blood begins to flow again through the constricted artery and can be heard through the stethoscope. The height of the mercury is recorded at that moment, which is the point of greatest pressure (called systolic). At its highest normal pressure, the heart would send a column of mercury to a height of about 120 millimeters. As more and more air is let out of the cuff, the pressure exerted by the cuff is so little that the sound of the blood pulsing against the artery walls subsides into silence. This is the point of lowest pressure (called diastolic), which normally raises the mercury to about 80 millimeters.

Normal blood pressure is thus usually said to be 120/80 (systolic/diastolic) or less, measured in millimeters of mercury (abbreviated as mm Hg).

Both systolic and diastolic readings are important, but diastolic pressure has traditionally been emphasized because it is less subject to fluctuations. However,

New Blood Pressure Classifications

Blood pressure is indicated by two numbers, each referring to how high in millimeters the pressure of the blood in your arteries can raise a column of mercury (Hg). The first number, the systolic pressure, represents the force of blood during a heartbeat. The second number, the diastolic, indicates the pressure between heartbeats.

In 1993, experts at the National High Blood Pressure Education Program (NHBPEP) reclassified blood pressure levels, replacing the terms "mild," "moderate," and "severe" with stages gradated from 1 to 4. The reason: The terms "mild" and "moderate" failed to convey the major impact of high blood pressure on risk of cardiovascular disease, according to the NHBPEP report.

In addition, blood pressure measurements for establishing hypertension now reflect equal emphasis on systolic and diastolic pressure, whereas previously only diastolic pressures had been emphasized.

When determining what category a person falls into, use the higher category indicated by systolic and diastolic readings. For example, someone with a reading of 140 mm Hg systolic and 100 mm Hg diastolic would fall into the Stage 2 (moderate) category.

Category	Systolic (mm Hg)	Diastolic (mm Hg)
Optimal	<120	<80
Normal	<130	<85
High Normal	130-139	85-89
Hypertension		
Stage 1 (Mild)	140-159	90-99
Stage 2 (Moderate)	160-179	100-109
Stage 3 (Severe)	180-209	110-119
Stage 4 (Very Severe)	≥210	≥120
Isolated Systolic Hypertension	≥140	≤90

recent studies, including the ongoing Framingham heart study, have revealed that systolic pressure may be as significant a heart attack predictor as diastolic pressure.

What causes hypertension?

In some people, the system that regulates blood pressure goes awry: arterioles throughout the body stay constricted, driving up the pressure in the larger blood vessels. Sustained high blood pressure—above 140/90 mm Hg, according to most experts—is called hypertension. About 90 percent of all people with high blood pressure have "essential" hypertension—meaning that it has no identifiable cause. In the remaining 10 percent of cases, the elevated blood pressure is due to kidney disease, diabetes, or another underlying disorder.

About 70 percent of people with high blood pressure have relatively "mild" hypertension—systolic pressure between 140 and 159, diastolic pressure between 90 and 99. This is usually only the first stage, since many cases worsen over time if untreated. And many researchers believe that even slightly elevated blood pressure (85 to 89 diastolic), called borderline hypertension, can be a health hazard if it persists for years.

Hypertension is known as the "silent killer" because it doesn't produce any

Myth: Low blood pressure can be just as bad as high blood pressure.

Fact: Low blood pressure, also known as hypotension, can, in rare cases, be a sign of underlying disease, but most of the time it is something to be grateful for.

However, one form of temporary low blood pressure can cause lightheadedness. Known as orthostatic hypotension, it occurs when you stand up suddenly. Your cardiovascular reflexes work quickly to prevent blood from pooling in your ankles and legs, but a too rapid change in position may tax these reflexes, especially in older people.

If you get dizzy frequently, ask your physician to help you discover the cause. If it's orthostatic hypotension, pace yourself when rising from a prone position, especially when getting out of bed. Sit for a moment before you stand, and stand a moment before walking. Walking in place briefly and pulling in your abdominal muscles several times before taking a step will aid in the return of blood from the legs.

symptoms—at least none that most people are aware of—until considerable damage has already been done. Untreated high blood pressure is the leading cause of strokes, which occur at a rate of half a million a year in the United States. As a result of hypertension, the heart, because it has to work harder, may become enlarged and less efficient. The added pressure also damages the artery walls, increasing the likelihood of fatty plaque being deposited, leading to scarring and hardening of these vessels (atherosclerosis). This in turn can reduce the flow of oxygen to the kidneys, heart, and eyes, or allow a blood clot to form in a narrowed artery. Life insurance studies show that untreated mild to moderate high blood pressure cuts life expectancy by three to six years on average; severe hypertension, by eight years or more. However, once detected, high blood pressure can usually be controlled.

There's no dispute that moderate or severe hypertension—Stage 2 or 3—needs immediate treatment. But doctors don't always agree on how to treat a person with a "mild" diastolic pressure between 90 and 99. Findings from several studies indicate that even such mild hypertension is associated with organ damage and a greater risk of atherosclerosis and heart attack. If left untreated, mild hypertension doesn't get better by itself. However, mild to moderate hypertension can often be effectively treated with simple lifestyle changes rather than drugs.

Risk factors you can't change
Certain unalterable conditions put you at greater risk for developing hypertension. If you fall into one of the following categories, you can avoid compounding your risk by making lifestyle changes.

Heredity. Those with a family history of hypertension are twice as likely to develop it as others. Many children of hypertensive parents have slightly elevated blood pressure even as infants.

Race. Hypertension is more common and generally more severe among African Americans than among whites. For reasons not completely understood, African Americans—especially males—tend to develop high blood pressure earlier in life, and much more often with fatal results.

Age. Blood pressure increases with age.

Pregnancy. Hypertension is not related to a person's sex. However, during pregnancy, some women—even those who have never had high blood pressure—develop it.

Six steps to reduce your risk
Although heredity, race, and age are unalterable, you can do something about other risk factors for high blood pressure. For some people, dietary and lifestyle changes may help prevent hypertension, or at least postpone it or reduce its severity. Such changes (under a doctor's supervision) are also the first step in treating people with mild hypertension, who may thus be able to avoid or postpone the need for antihypertensive drugs. If these steps fail to lower elevated blood pressure after three to six months, antihypertensive drugs will probably be necessary. And if you are put on such drugs, you should continue to modify your behavior, since this may help you get by on a lower dose and thus reduce any adverse side effects the drugs may cause.

There's no guarantee that the dietary and lifestyle changes described here will

Weight lifting and hypertension

Physicians usually warn people with high blood pressure against isometric exertion such as weight lifting because it can temporarily raise blood pressure to dangerous levels. But that may occur only if they lift the heaviest weights they can manage. Far safer is a more moderate type of weight lifting called circuit training. It calls for quickly lifting relatively light weights on a series of weight machines and actually provides a modest aerobic workout. In one study, for instance, subjects lifted 40 percent of the maximum load they could heft. Blood pressure readings taken immediately after circuit training were only slightly elevated—they were "within acceptable and safe clinical limits," according to the researchers.

Monitoring Your Own Blood Pressure

For some people, monitoring blood pressure at home can be a good idea. For example, if you're trying to lower your blood pressure by dieting or medication, you may be encouraged by frequent evidence that you're succeeding. Some medications require monitoring to minimize side effects. Equally important, a few people are "office" hypertensives—their pressure goes up just from being in a medical setting. The only way they get an accurate reading is by measuring at home.

Guidelines for measurement

You will need a health professional to teach you how to measure your blood pressure accurately. Remember, blood pressure varies from minute to minute. Body position and other factors, especially smoking, can cause pressure to rise. Prior to taking your blood pressure, you should avoid smoking for thirty minutes (or better still, do not smoke at all), and you should relax for about ten minutes beforehand in a quiet room. Take your pressure at the same time each day and under the same conditions so you can compare readings. One high reading should not alarm you, but consult your doctor if high readings persist. (Try to take your pressure occasionally when you are emotionally upset.)

Choosing the right equipment

Selecting accurate equipment may not be easy. You can buy a sphygmomanometer (a blood pressure measuring device) for as little as eighteen dollars, but many are wholly unreliable. Unfortunately, price is no guide to quality. Equipment comes in three types:

1. The old-fashioned mercury-filled glass column with cuff and bulb attached. This is very accurate but heavy and inconvenient for home use, and mercury will escape if the tube breaks. A stethoscope is required.

2. Mechanical-aneroid equipment with a cuff, bulb, and a clocklike gauge. This is also dependable and less awkward than the mercury column. You need a stethoscope for this one, too.

3. Electronic-digital equipment with cuff and bulb and with the gauge and stethoscope contained in one unit. This is easy to use and pleasingly high-tech in look; it is also the most costly and the least likely to give you an accurate reading.

Both the mechanical-aneroid and the electronic-digital equipment must be checked for accuracy against a mercury unit at least once a year, and possibly more often. Thus, it makes sense to buy from a medical supply house or other supplier who will perform this service for customers.

A reputable supplier should also be able to advise which kind of equipment will be accurate enough for your purposes. Make sure the cuff is the right size. If it's too tight or too loose, you won't get accurate readings. And you'll need a wider cuff if your arm is large.

High blood pressure, smoking, and elevated cholesterol increase the risk of heart attack more in middle-aged women than in men of the same age. While the average fifty-five-year-old woman who has none of these risk factors is slightly less likely to have a heart attack than a man of that description, her risk rises disproportionately as each risk factor is added.

prevent hypertension or lower elevated blood pressure. Still, even if they don't, they offer other potential health benefits, most importantly a reduction in risk factors for cardiovascular disease.

Exercise regularly. There is growing evidence that regular physical exercise can reduce mildly elevated blood pressure over the long term. One study looked at fifty-two men with mild hypertension. The subjects were divided into three groups: two groups took different hypertension medication and the third group took a placebo. The men, all of whom were previously sedentary, then started a ten-week exercise program, combining twenty minutes of aerobics (stationary cycling or walking/ jogging) and thirty minutes of weight training (in the form of circuit training) three times a week.

The nondrug group experienced a lowering of blood pressure as substantial as that of the two drug groups, dropping from 145/97 to 131/84 mm Hg on average in seven weeks. "There was no added benefit to the use of either drug in these patients," according to the researchers. However, the participants' exercise regimen was supervised by the researchers and the study lasted just ten weeks. The big "if" with exercise is commitment; treatment for high blood pressure is a lifelong endeavor. Under normal circumstances, the men may not have exercised as conscientiously. In addition, if the drug dose had been individualized rather than a standard amount, the drug therapy may well have had added results.

Nevertheless, other research has shown that even when exercise alone doesn't control hypertension, exercise may help some people get by on a lower dose of medication and thus reduce any adverse effects the drug may have.

Aside from its blood pressure-lowering potential, exercise is often accompanied by other healthful lifestyle changes, such as weight reduction and decreased sodium and alcohol consumption. Exercise strengthens the cardiovascular system and reduces the risk of heart disease. It can also help control diabetes, which is another heart disease risk factor. Most experts recommend aerobic exercise for twenty to thirty minutes at least three times a week. Hypertensives should avoid lifting heavy weights, since this can temporarily raise blood pressure to dangerous levels. (See marginal on page 56.)

Keep your weight at a desirable level. This is a factor in about 60 percent of all cases of hypertension. The obese (20 percent or more over ideal weight) are twice as likely to have high blood pressure as the nonobese. Even small weight losses can lower blood pressure significantly in overweight hypertensives.

If you drink alcohol, limit your intake to two drinks a day. One of the most common remediable causes of hypertension in the United States is alcohol consumption. Alcohol's effect on blood pressure appears to be completely reversible. (A drink equals one and a half ounces of eighty-proof spirits, five ounces of wine, or twelve ounces of beer) or less.

Don't smoke. Smoking briefly raises blood pressure (nicotine constricts small blood vessels), but the long-term effect of smoking on hypertension is not clear. Nevertheless, smoking is a risk factor for heart disease—as is hypertension. Therefore, smoking compounds the risk.

Moderate your daily sodium intake to the amount in a teaspoon of salt. Study after study has found that population groups consuming a lot of sodium (usually in the form of table salt) have a high incidence of hypertension. A high sodium intake does not promote high blood pressure in all people, nor does a low sodium intake always prevent it. Most people, in fact, are sodium resistant—that is, they can consume excess salt for a lifetime and remain healthy.

However, about 10 percent of the population are genetically "sodium sensitive"—that is, their blood pressure responds to the amount of sodium they consume. This group accounts for about half of the hypertensives in the United States. For them, restricting salt intake will usually lower their blood pressure.

Though you may think that you're sodium-resistant, there is no practical way to determine in advance who is sodium sensitive and who is not. Therefore, it makes sense to restrict your intake to about 2,400 milligrams of sodium daily—the amount in a teaspoon of salt. While there's no guarantee that this will protect you from hypertension, it's a sensible measure to take while you're still in good health. Genetic resistance to sodium may be weakened by high sodium intake over many years. And people who cut down on sodium are also likely to make other dietary changes that may lower blood pressure.

Eat a diet with adequate amounts of calcium, magnesium, and potassium. Some studies suggest that eating too little calcium may result in high blood pressure readings.

Do emotions raise blood pressure?

Yes, fear and anger, for example, raise it temporarily, but then it drops back to its prior level in most people. Contrary to popular belief, there's no evidence that any particular personality type is prone to high blood pressure.

However, psychology and social stress may contribute to chronic hypertension. According to Dr. Leonard Syme at the University of California at Berkeley, hypertension rates are high in people at the bottom of the social and economic ladder. Chronic anxiety may promote chronic high blood pressure.

Other researchers have noted that hypertension is more common in societies where change is the norm, where people are mobile and often insecure in their jobs, and where anxiety never seems to resolve itself.

This link is a weak one, however, and no long-term effect has been proven as yet. Maintaining your intake at the RDA for calcium is adequate (see page 137); there is no evidence that intakes higher than the RDA will have an influence on blood pressure.

Some studies suggest that a magnesium deficiency may be linked to hypertension. However, the evidence, again, is not sufficient to recommend a magnesium intake greater than the RDA.

An adequate potassium intake may help prevent or lower high blood pressure. By cutting down on high-sodium foods and substituting unprocessed foods, you'll probably consume more potassium.

Try to get these minerals from foods rather than supplements. For example, low-fat dairy products and some green leafy vegetables (such as broccoli and spinach) are not only the best sources of calcium, but are also high in potassium and magnesium. Avoid taking potassium supplements unless you are under a doctor's supervision.

Mild hypertension and medication

Doctors disagree about when to start drug therapy for people who have Stage 1, or "mild," hypertension—a diastolic pressure that consistently registers between 90 and 99. Some experts prefer to avoid drugs at first. In any case, you should be monitored by a physician, who will need to evaluate other factors, such as your age and family history. You will undoubtedly be told to adopt the lifestyle changes listed above. These changes may produce the desired result. If not, there is now a wide range of safe and effective drugs for controlling hypertension. Recent guidelines from the National High Blood Pressure Education Program panel recommend considering medication even for systolic pressures between 140 and 149 mm Hg, or diastolic pressures between 90 and 94 mm Hg.

If one drug doesn't work for you or produces unacceptable side effects, there are others you can try. If you do start taking antihypertensive medication, it's essential not to alter your dosage or quit on your own. Controlling hypertension with drugs and keeping side effects to a minimum require close cooperation between you and your doctor. And the goal should be to reduce the amount of drugs you take or even—on medical advice only—to discontinue them.

In addition to the preventive measures listed above and on the previous page, you may also want to try biofeedback, hypnosis, meditation, and other relaxation techniques, which may produce a modest reduction in blood pressure in some people. These reductions usually aren't predictable, and they are generally not useful as a first line treatment for hypertension. But they may be effective adjuncts to weight control, exercise, and medication. These and the other lifestyle changes can reduce the need for drugs.

Like smoking, caffeine causes a transitory rise in blood pressure, but the long-term effects on hypertension appear to be minimal. Habitual consumers may develop some tolerance to its effect on blood pressure. Hypertensives can try doing without caffeine to see if their blood pressure comes down.

Smoking

None of the habits that can damage the health of human beings has been as clearly documented—or as widely publicized—as smoking. There is simply no room for debate: smoking promotes heart disease and cancer, and is the major cause of premature, preventable deaths in the United States. Smoking can make you sick if you're healthy, and make it harder to recover if you do get sick.

By virtue of the massive evidence concerning the dangers of smoking, millions of Americans have given up the habit. Nearly half of all Americans who have ever smoked have quit. About 1.3 million Americans become former smokers each year, and more and more Americans now view smoking as socially unacceptable. At the same time, however, most heavy smokers continue to smoke. In fact, even after having a heart attack, many smokers refuse to give up the habit. And each year about one million young persons start—that is, about 3,000 each day. So there is a need to be reminded of smoking's risks, and to learn the most effective ways to break the life-threatening habit.

The harmful elements in smoke

There are three constituents in tobacco smoke that, in concert, cause most of the premature deaths in smokers. Smoke contains a number of gases, the most dangerous of which is carbon monoxide; when inhaled, it passes into the bloodstream, where it interferes with the ability of red blood cells to transport oxygen. Carbon monoxide may account for the breathlessness of some smokers, and also affects vision, hearing, and judgment.

Smokers also inhale tars—microscopic particles that form sticky, resinlike substances in the lungs. Not only do tars impair the function of the respiratory system, but some of the chemicals in them are carcinogenic—that is, they can produce cancer in tissues with which they come in contact.

The most insidious element in tobacco is nicotine, a powerful, central nervous system stimulant that is highly addictive. In the view of many experts, an addiction to nicotine is the leading reason (though not the only one) why smoking is so difficult to give up. In addition, nicotine directly affects blood pressure, heart rate, skin temperature, hormone production, muscle tension, and pain sensitivity.

The damage to your health

More than 350,000 premature deaths a year are attributable to smoking. Up to age sixty-five, people who smoke a pack a day (twenty cigarettes) or more die at almost twice the rate of nonsmokers in the same age group. Smokers suffer from nonfatal ill effects as well, particularly respiratory problems. If you smoke, you risk the adverse effects cited here. (Although smoking is clearly most harmful to smokers, evidence is mounting that the secondhand smoke generated by smokers can pose health risks for nonsmokers who are frequently exposed to it. The environmental considerations concerning "passive smoking" are explained on page 561.)

Cancer. The deadliest risks from smoking are cancer of the lungs, throat, and mouth. Pack-a-day smokers are fourteen times more likely to die from these cancers than nonsmokers. Lung cancer is largely a disease of smokers, and because it is difficult to detect until it reaches an advanced stage, over 90 percent of the cases are fatal. Most smokers tend to swallow small amounts of smoke, which puts them at higher-than-average risk for cancer of the esophagus. And carcinogenic chemicals that are absorbed into the blood increase a smoker's risk of bladder cancer.

Perhaps because the majority of smokers are men, lung cancer is often considered a man's disease. But while more men than women die of lung cancer, the incidence rate among men has leveled off, while that for women is rising. In 1994, an estimated 56,000 women died of lung cancer, compared with 46,000 from breast cancer. The reason more women are dying of lung cancer now is that so many of them began smoking after World War II. And while some adult women are quitting, among adolescents, tobacco use is not declining.

There is also mounting evidence that smoking may place young women at risk for cervical cancer, a disease that can strike them in their twenties or thirties. Nicotine and cancer-promoting agents in cigarette smoke have been detected in the cervical secretions of smokers. Studies indicate, however, that after two years, a former smoker's risk of cervical cancer is equal to a nonsmoker's.

Heart disease. Smoking is a major risk factor in heart attacks, to the extent that almost one fifth of the nearly one million deaths annually from cardiovascular disease are attributable to smoking—many more than the total number of smoking-related deaths from cancer and pulmonary disease. It's also estimated that 37,000 to 40,000 nonsmokers who have been exposed to environmental tobacco smoke die from cardiovascular disease each year.

Smoking contributes greatly to atherosclerosis in coronary arteries, which impedes blood flow to the heart. Smoking damages the lining of the arteries (which is thought to encourage the formation of arterial plaque); it raises total blood cholesterol and lowers HDL (the "good," protective cholesterol); and it increases the stickiness of blood platelets, making a clot in the narrowed arteries more likely. In addition, nicotine makes the heart beat faster, which requires more oxygen; yet the carbon monoxide in smoke cuts down on the amount of oxygen the

The long decline in smoking among Americans may be over temporarily. Between 1965 and 1990, cigarette smoking among adults decreased from 42.4 percent to 25.5 percent, or 46 million smokers. But the percentage then remained unchanged for two years in a row. This means that smokers who quit or die are being replaced by young people. We may also be getting down to the hard core of heavily addicted smokers.

Why Do You Smoke?

This test, based on one by the U.S. Department of Health and Human Services, will help you determine why you smoke. Jot down your answers as you go.

True or False: I smoke. . .
1. because I light up automatically and don't know I'm doing it.
2. because it's relaxing.
3. because I like handling cigarettes, matches, and lighters.
4. to help deal with anger.
5. to keep from slowing down.
6. because it's unbearable not to.
7. because I enjoy watching the smoke as I exhale it.

8. to take my mind off my troubles.
9. because I really enjoy it.
10. because I feel uncomfortable without a cigarette in my hand.
11. to give myself a lift.
12. without planning to—it's just part of my routine.

Results: "True" answers to 5 and 11 indicate that you smoke for stimulation; to 3 and 7, that pleasure of handling is important; to 2 and 9, that you seek relaxation; to 4 and 8, that you need a tension-reducing crutch; to 6 and 10, that you have a physiological addiction; to 1 and 12, that you smoke from habit. No doubt you smoke for a combination of these reasons.

blood can carry. Smoking also raises blood pressure temporarily, and it may constrict coronary arteries as well, which makes them less able to supply oxygen to the heart when increased physical effort demands it.

Together, these are perfect conditions for a heart attack, and people who smoke at least a pack a day are more than twice as likely to suffer a heart attack as non-smokers; even more sobering, they are as much as four times more likely to die from it within an hour.

Respiratory problems. The tars in tobacco smoke gradually impair the cilia, the tiny hairs in lungs and airways that sweep mucus and foreign particles toward the throat for clearing. At the very least, damaged cilia cause extra mucus to accumulate, producing a "smoker's cough." Heavy smoking will eventually destroy the cilia, making the smoker more susceptible to colds, chronic bronchitis, and other respiratory infections. Smoking is also the leading cause of emphysema, a condition that damages air sacs in the lungs and gradually destroys the lungs' elasticity, causing labored breathing and chronic shortness of breath.

The benefits of quitting

Smoking is an instance where your body—even after decades of smoking—will forgive you if you stop. The cardiac benefits start to accrue almost immediately such that, *in two years, much of your risk of heart disease will have disappeared.* Within five to ten years, your risk will be no greater than if you had never smoked. The risk of lung cancer and other malignancies begins to decrease steadily after you quit, and after ten years your risk is almost as low as that of nonsmokers—even if you had smoked for years. If you suffer from bronchitis or emphysema, you can expect an improvement in breathing almost at once. As an added benefit, non-smokers have stronger bones and less chance of getting osteoporosis.

Indeed, nothing you do for your health—not even dieting and exercise—pays as many dividends so quickly as giving up smoking.

No Safe Way to Smoke

In an effort to continue their habit, yet mitigate the risks, some smokers take up cigar and pipe smoking in the belief that these are less harmful. Studies are revealing, however, that cigars and pipes can be fully as risky as cigarettes, particularly for those who used to smoke cigarettes.

Smokers who have smoked only a cigar or pipe rarely inhale the smoke, which generally puts them at low risk of lung cancer (though they are at high risk for cancers of the mouth and lips). But former cigarette smokers who switch to cigars or pipes are at increased risk for lung cancer because they tend to inhale the smoke and to smoke a lot. Both habits are carryovers from cigarette smoking.

Studies of carbon monoxide levels in the blood indicate that virtually all former cigarette smokers inhale smoke from pipes and cigars—though many are unaware of it. By inhaling the smoke, they are able to maintain nearly the same level of nicotine in their blood as they had when they smoked cigarettes. And since pipe and cigar smoke is much higher in tar than cigarette smoke, these may actually pose a higher risk of lung cancer than cigarettes. In addition, studies indicate that the increased risk of heart attack associated with cigarette smoking may continue unabated in men who switch to cigar smoking.

Remember, too, that even if you don't inhale on your cigars or pipe and have never smoked cigarettes, the smoky environment that you are creating (known as "side-stream exposure") may increase your risk of both lung cancer and heart disease.

Why it's hard to quit

Although only about one in four Americans now smokes, each year an estimated 18 million smokers in the United States try to quit. Unfortunately, fewer than 10 percent of them have any long-term success. Psychology and physiology play complex roles in the smoking habit. Nicotine is a psychoactive, addictive drug that causes marked alterations in body chemistry. It acts through specialized cell formations in the brain and muscles, but unlike alcohol or other psychoactive drugs, it doesn't produce dramatic evidence of intoxication, and thus people underestimate its power.

Inhaled nicotine goes almost immediately to the brain, rapidly producing a sense of euphoria, particularly if you are smoking the first cigarette (or pipe or cigar) of the day. By taking more or fewer puffs, inhaling more or less deeply, and pacing your cigarettes, you unconsciously try to re-create this feeling again and again. What appears to be casual and random behavior is instead highly controlled. Nicotine not only affects blood pressure, heart rate, and other bodily functions, it also alters mood. You are not merely imagining that smoking a cigarette enhances your powers of concentration or soothes your anxiety. Yet the tense, uptight feeling that a cigarette supposedly relieves can itself be caused by nicotine. It's a vicious cycle.

Smoking is not just a matter of nicotine, however. Typically, an adolescent starts smoking to gain peer approval, to express his rebelliousness, or simply out of curiosity. What psychologists call "modeling" is a strong factor. If the people you admire smoke, you may emulate them.

As you begin to smoke, you learn that just handling cigarettes can be a pleasurable activity. You learn to associate them with such pleasures as mealtime, or the end of classes or work, or with the relief of tension. Smoking has cosmetic uses, too. A pipe makes a man look wise, a cigar is the mark of a connoisseur, a cigarette makes a woman look worldly—at least according to prevailing social stereotypes, which are largely created by advertising.

According to cigarette advertising, the brand you choose confirms your masculinity or your femininity, identifies you as avant-garde or as a risk-taker, and can lend you the appearance of being rugged or sophisticated. The charming, healthy, intelligent-looking young men and women in advertisements (who mostly aren't shown smoking) are swimming, playing tennis, sailing, or engaging in some other appealing activity.

All of this makes the smoking habit undeniably powerful: most people who smoke would like to break the habit, yet nine out of ten American smokers have tried to quit and failed on at least one occasion. On the other hand, an estimated 43 million people have succeeded—a sure sign that you can choose not to smoke.

Keys to quitting

Nearly every method—no matter how odd—has worked for somebody. If you know former smokers, interview them. Chances are you'll find some go-it-aloners, others who joined a group, and even one or two who swear by hypnosis or acupuncture. The important thing is to find a method that suits your needs. A previous failure is nothing to be ashamed of. If you've tried and failed, and are now trying again, that simply indicates the strength of your motivation. Giving up tobacco is a learning process and may take more than one try.

It's never too late to quit

Even for older, long-term smokers who already show signs of heart disease, the health risks from smoking are partly reversible by quitting. In the well-known Coronary Artery Surgery Study, researchers examined nearly 2,000 male and female smokers over age fifty-four, most of whom had coronary artery disease. They found that 807 people who quit smoking the year before the study and abstained for six years had substantially lower death rates than those who continued to smoke—largely as a result of fewer heart attacks. And the improved survival rate was seen even in the oldest abstainers.

Going it alone or joining a group. In the past, 95 percent of the millions of people who quit were thought to have quit on their own. Abstinence rates for formal programs were alleged to be quite low, and at least one study has claimed that self-quitters were two or three times more successful than people who sought professional help of some kind. But recent data shows that self-quitters and program-seekers are basically similar in their motivations; in their ability (or lack of it) to break the habit; and in their success rates at long-term abstinence. Go it alone if you wish, but don't ever forget that professional help and support groups do help some people—and you may be one of them.

If you want a group program, the local chapter of the American Cancer Society can supply information, and so can most public libraries. The yellow pages (look under "Smoker's Information and Treatment Centers") will also tell you what's available nearby. There are live-in programs and five-day plans. You will probably find a list of counselors, clinics, hypnotists, acupuncturists, and other self-proclaimed experts in behavior modification. Remember that there is no scientific evidence that hypnosis, acupuncture, or "total immersion" are effective. Whichever method you choose, ask in advance what the costs will be, what the dropout rate is, what percentage of people in the program succeed in quitting for an entire year, and whether there is any follow-up.

Drugs to cope with withdrawal. Clonidine, an antihypertensive drug, has been used to control alcohol and drug withdrawal symptoms, and although the Food and Drug Administration (FDA) has never approved it for such use, some doctors have prescribed it to cut down cigarette cravings. But a recent study failed to show that clonidine offered any benefits to people trying to quit. And a recent, exhaustive scientific review of the experimental use of various drugs to combat nicotine withdrawal concluded that the only effective treatment currently available is nicotine itself, in the form of nicotine chewing gum. Nicotine gum requires a prescription, and eventually you have to kick the gum habit. But nicotine gum combined with a stop-smoking program can be highly effective (close to a 50 percent success rate, according to some reports).

Assessing the patch. The nicotine patch is one of the hottest new pharmaceutical products, but how safe and effective is it? Sold only by prescription (at about four dollars per day), the patch is a two-inch adhesive pad that delivers a steady dose of nicotine through the skin for sixteen to twenty-four hours a day. The patches are used for eight to twelve weeks; the dose of nicotine is gradually reduced over time. Like nicotine chewing gum, the patch helps quitters minimize their withdrawal symptoms (such as intense cravings for cigarettes and irritability) by weaning them off nicotine. However, there are some caveats to consider:

The patch is not a cure for most smokers—but is certainly effective for some. Quitting rates for patch users have varied considerably in studies. While patches are being used, anywhere from 36 percent to 77 percent of people are able to abstain. Few studies, however, have looked at longer-term success rates off the patch. A major review of seventeen studies, published in the *Journal of the the American Medical Association* in 1994, found that the patch, when combined with counseling, can be about twice as effective as a placebo, allowing 22 percent of smokers to quit for six months. That's about as effective as many other methods.

The patch is only an adjunct in quitting. Patch users, like nicotine-gum chewers, are advised to receive counseling to help them overcome their psychological addiction to smoking (evident in habits such as lighting up after a meal or in stressful situations). The patch's directions point out the need for some sort of counseling program, but advertisements seldom mention this. It is unrealistic to expect most people to get adequate—or any—counseling. Several manufacturers supply booklets with their patches, which give tips on how to quit, or toll-free hotlines, but these are unlikely to be sufficient. The patch without continued psychological support may be only slightly more effective in the long run than a placebo.

The patch isn't for everybody. People who smoke more than a pack a day, are highly motivated to quit, and are willing to take part in counseling are the best candidates. People with heart disease and pregnant women shouldn't use the patch.

You must not smoke while using the patch or use more than one patch at a time. This can cause a nicotine overdose. Though the packaging warns against such misuse, the Food and Drug Administration (FDA) has received reports of at least thirty-three people having suffered heart attacks while using the patch; some of these patch wearers apparently continued to smoke. However, there's no direct proof that the attacks were related to use of the patch. The FDA is looking into the matter and may demand stronger warnings on the packaging.

Occasional adverse effects include mild skin irritation, insomnia, dry mouth, and nervousness.

Finding a substitute. The best way to quit smoking varies according to which kind of smoker you are, what you think you get out of smoking, and what it seems to do for you. See the box on page 61 to get a better understanding of what keeps you smoking; knowing why you smoke will help you find substitutes that enable you to quit. For example:

•If you smoke for stimulation or a lift, find a healthy substitute, such as a brisk walk or moderate exercise.

•If you smoke for pleasurable relaxation or to relieve tension (sometimes it's hard to tell which is which), physical exertion, social activity, a new hobby, deep breathing, or even eating and drinking can serve as a partial substitute.

•If the physiological addiction factor is high, you may need to go "cold turkey." Actually doing without nicotine may be the only way to teach yourself to do without it. To work up to quitting, set a final date, then smoke too much for a day or two, which should increase your distaste for cigarettes. Next, try cutting back by switching to a brand you dislike. This will decrease your nicotine intake and alleviate later withdrawal symptoms. Some people have quit by switching to low-tar, low-nicotine cigarettes for a week or two, then quitting completely. Others have found help in nicotine chewing gum, the only catch being that the gum is also addictive, so eventually you have to take the final step and quit the gum.

•If the habitual factor is strongest, work to alter your daily patterns. Cut down gradually—eliminate a certain number of cigarettes each day. Form the habit of asking yourself if you really want the cigarette you are about to light. You may be surprised at how often you say no.

•If handling the cigarettes is important, try doodling, or playing with some small object. Take up a craft such as embroidery that supplies tactile sensations.

A plan for quitting on your own

Choose a weekend (but not a holiday) or some time when you are under the least possible outside stress and have some time to devote to yourself. Throw out all

Some people, especially young ones, actually take up smoking as a way to stay slim. Researchers at Memphis State University found that among students who smoke, 39 percent of the women and 25 percent of the men do so as a dieting technique. As a means of staying svelte, this is a markedly poor bargain. The health risks from smoking just aren't worth it. Moreover, a recent Canadian study found that after quitting, most female ex-smokers (but fewer men) lose all or most of the extra pounds.

cigarettes, matches, lighters, and ashtrays. Visit the dentist and have the tobacco stains removed from your teeth. Steer clear of friends and family members who smoke. Plan lots of activity for the day you quit. Go places where smoking is not permitted—museums, department stores, theaters. Swim, jog, ride a bike, or play tennis. Try to avoid activities that you associate strongly with smoking.

It is realistic to expect unpleasant or even severe withdrawal symptoms, which may include headaches, constipation, productive coughing, drowsiness, a sore mouth, impaired concentration, irritability, mood swings, an increased desire to snack, and depression. However intense your symptoms may be, they are temporary and in no way threatening to your health and well-being. The worst symptoms should subside after a week or two. Intense cigarette cravings usually last only three to five minutes. When you feel the craving, take a break or a walk. Have something to eat or drink. Brush your teeth often, and use a tasty mouthwash. Breathe deeply or do stretching exercises.

Count the dividends. All the experts suggest plenty of self-congratulation in the first few days. As part of treating yourself well, add up the costs of smoking—just the short-term costs of tobacco and paraphernalia, throwing in a calculation for accidental damage to clothing and furniture. After a week or two, buy yourself a present with the money saved. Or calculate your savings for a month or a year (plus interest) and see what reward you will be able to give yourself or your family.

As your withdrawal pangs subside, the rewards will begin to accumulate. After only a week, your body will be free of nicotine. You will notice that your senses of smell and taste are a keen source of pleasure. Your food, breath, body, and clothing will smell better. Your cough will go away. Breathing will be easier. You will no longer have to go to the trouble of buying tobacco. Newly created nonsmokers are also pleased with the sense of mastery and accomplishment that accrues.

Smoking and weight gain

Researchers have known for some time that smokers generally weigh less than nonsmokers and that many people who quit smoking gain weight—an average of five to ten pounds. This weight increase may be caused by a difference in the number of calories smokers consume or by physiological differences between smokers and nonsmokers. The popular explanation for these weight swings is that smokers are jittery types who eat less than others and when they quit compensate by devouring candy bars and cookies. New evidence, however, suggests that people who stop smoking tend to gain weight not only because they turn to food as a substitute for the gratification once provided by cigarettes, but also because of metabolic changes that occur when they kick the habit.

Over the years studies have shown that nicotine slightly accelerates basal metabolic rate (the basic rate at which energy is expended to maintain essential body functions). That is, smokers burn more calories when they are at rest than nonsmokers. One study, at the University of Pittsburgh, found that nicotine causes your metabolic rate to increase to an even greater extent during light activity—by about 12 percent (compared to 5 percent during rest). Thus, when you quit smoking, your rate of energy expenditure—at rest and during everyday activities—slows back down, enough to promote weight gain.

The researchers themselves admitted, however, that this metabolic change would probably account only for a difference of 31 to 69 calories during an eight-

Is smoking a few cigarettes a day harmful?

Obviously it's worse to smoke a lot, but no amount of smoking is free of risk. The exact amount of damage depends on a host of variables: what type of cigarette you smoke, how long you've smoked, how deeply you inhale, as well as genetic factors. How much you smoke each day is also important, for there is a dose-response relationship between smoking and lung cancer, heart disease, and chronic respiratory disease. In other words, the more you smoke, the greater your risk. One study found that men who smoked from one to nine cigarettes daily had a nearly five times greater risk of dying from lung cancer than nonsmokers; for those smoking ten to nineteen cigarettes, it was nine times greater.

Bottom line: the smoke from even one or two daily cigarettes poses a greater cancer risk than anything else you're likely to be exposed to every day.

hour day—which would show up as only about an extra pound over the course of a month. That's within the normal weight range of most people and doesn't account for the five or ten pounds that the average smoker rapidly gains after quitting. So while these findings are interesting, they don't actually explain what happens in real life. We still don't know how much of the weight gain can be attributed to a change in eating habits, to activity levels, or to physiological changes.

If you smoke, don't put off quitting because you know it will probably cause you to gain weight. You can compensate for any shift to a lower metabolic rate that may occur when you quit by either consuming fewer calories or exercising more. In fact, by doing just that, a large portion of smokers maintain or eventually lose weight when they give up cigarettes.

•During the first week after quitting, which is likely to feature compulsive munching, eat raw vegetables and fruit instead of high-calorie snacks. In the next weeks, slightly reduce portion sizes and lower the proportion of fatty foods you eat.

•Aerobic exercise is a great calorie burner, and it helps keep your mind off cigarettes. At a slower pace, walking as little as an additional mile a day can completely make up for your slowed metabolism.

How to stay an ex-smoker

One of the myths about smoking is that quitting is mainly a matter of willpower. True grit is essential, but not sufficient in itself. Quitting is a "dynamic process, not a discrete event," according to a report in *American Psychologist*. That is, if smoking is central to your life (and for most smokers it is), you have to do more than just quit. After you've won the battle with acute withdrawal symptoms, you'll have to plan new activities and new ways to relax that don't depend on nicotine. Here are some tips for avoiding a relapse:

•The thought of never smoking again can sometimes feel overwhelming. When you have that thought, tell yourself that you are quitting just for today.

•The first three months are dangerous. Avoid smokers and smoking situations such as cocktail parties.

•When you feel the urge for a cigarette, try any of the relaxation techniques outlined on page 459.

•Be prepared for tough times. You'll find yourself making excuses to have "just one"—but having "just one" is never worth the risk. If you're tempted, remind yourself how hard it was to quit, and rehearse the benefits you've enjoyed as a nonsmoker: "I've saved money, I don't cough all the time, I'm proud of myself," and so on. Having a friend to confide in, especially a reformed smoker, can help.

•Don't be fooled into thinking you can become an "occasional" smoker, even after a year of not smoking. It's true that a few former smokers can smoke a cigarette on Saturday night and not get hooked again. But it's also true that some people, according to a study of 5,000 smokers and quitters, "cycle from smoking to nonsmoking and back again" most of their lives.

•Don't be alarmed or ashamed at falling off the wagon. If you do, quit again.

Myth: Snuff is a safe form of tobacco.

Fact: The tobacco industry implies in ads that snuff is safe as well as manly—and consumption of snuff and chewing tobacco has nearly tripled since 1972, with the biggest consumers being young men and teenagers. But no form of tobacco is safe. Snuff, which is powdered or ground tobacco, comes dry (for nasal use, most common in Britain) or moist (placed in the mouth). The chemicals in snuff are absorbed through the membranes lining the nose or mouth or through the intestinal tract. The final blood concentrations of nicotine are as high as if the tobacco had been smoked, and the addictive effect may be even greater because some moist snuff has a higher concentration of nicotine than the average cigarette.

Unlike smoking tobacco, snuff is not known to cause lung cancer, but it does lead to mouth, throat, and nasal cancers. In addition, some moist snuff is high in sugar, which causes tooth decay.

Alcohol

Alcohol, a natural product of fermentation, is probably the most widely used of all drugs. It has been a part of human culture since history began and part of American life since Europeans settled on this continent. "The good creature of God," colonial Americans called it. They and their descendants also called it "demon rum." At one time, beer or whisky may have been safer to drink than well water, but there have always been many other reasons for drinking: the sociability of drinking, the brief but vivid sense of relaxation a drink can bring, the wish to celebrate or participate in religious and family rituals where alcohol is served. In some cultures, abstention is the rule. In others, the occasional use of alcohol is regarded as pleasurable and necessary—but such use is carefully controlled and intoxication frowned upon. Tradition and attitude play a powerful role in the use of this drug.

Double messages about alcohol

Millions of people enjoy an occasional alcoholic beverage, and for most adults, moderate drinking—whether of beer, wine, or spirits—is not associated with any health risk. Some people, unfortunately, drink because of depression and/or addiction to alcohol. Apart from such needs, powerful social and economic forces encourage people to drink.

For starters, alcoholic beverages are everywhere—planes, trains, boats, bars, restaurants, county fairs, shopping centers, street corner stores, even school or church gatherings. Also, drink is cheap. The relative cost of alcohol has declined in the last decades. Since 1967 the cost of soft drinks and milk has quadrupled, the cost of all consumer goods has tripled, but the cost of alcohol has not even doubled. This is because the excise tax on alcohol is not indexed to inflation. Congress has raised the federal tax on beer and wine only once in forty years (in 1990). The tax on hard liquor has been increased only twice—small raises in 1985 and 1990. Opinion polls have shown that the public is in favor of raising federal excise taxes on alcohol, but the alcohol industry successfully fights increases. Furthermore, about 20 percent of all alcohol is sold for business entertainment and is thus partially tax deductible, making it that much less costly to whoever pays the bar bill.

Finally, the alcohol, advertising, and entertainment industries tirelessly promote the idea that it's normal, desirable, smart, sophisticated, and sexy to drink. In print, on television, and at the movies, we see beautiful, wealthy, healthy people drinking. Beer ads associate the product with sports events, fast cars, camaraderie, sex. Hollywood's most fabulous stars have always imbibed plentifully, on and off camera: "here's looking at you, kid," echoes down the ages.

Considering these pro-drinking forces, it's amazing that 35 percent of us over eighteen never drink, and another 35 percent drinks lightly and only occasionally. It's equally amazing that our drinking levels have been declining for the past ten years. But a tiny portion of the population consumes more than half of all the alcohol. Still, out-and-out alcoholism is only one factor in the grief caused by drinking, and alcohol problems are not a simple matter of the drunk versus the rest of us.

Alcohol's toll

When consumed in excess, alcohol acts as a toxic drug, with pronounced short-term and long-term consequences. After tobacco, alcohol abuse is the leading cause of premature death in the United States—and the drinker is by no means the only victim. Alcohol causes, or is associated with, the loss of more than 100,000 lives annually, often among the young. These include deaths not only from alcohol-related diseases (such as cirrhosis of the liver) but also from traffic accidents. In recent years, tougher laws and public campaigns against intoxicated drivers have reduced the incidence of alcohol-related traffic fatalities. Nonetheless, in 1992, about 18,000 people died and nearly one million were injured in traffic accidents involving alcohol. These include not only drivers, but also pedestrians, motorcyclists, and bicyclists who had been drinking. (Half the pedestrians killed by cars have elevated blood alcohol levels.)

Alcohol also contributes to serious hazards in the home, especially falls and house fires, and to drownings. People who drink habitually are more likely to smoke and hence to doze off and start fires with unextinguished cigarettes. Nor are the highways and the home the only places where trouble occurs. Reduced productivity and lost employment due to drinking cost an estimated 71 billion dollars annually. In addition to such statistics are the immeasurable emotional and psychological costs: the damage done to family life, for example, by a parent's drinking habits. Fetal alcohol syndrome, caused by drinking during pregnancy, is the leading known cause of mental retardation. After tobacco, in fact, alcohol is the leading cause of premature death in the United States.

Amid all the bad news about alcohol, there is definitely some good. For one thing, Americans have been drinking less alcohol—and lighter forms of it—since the mid-1970s, reversing the trend of heavier drinking in the post–World War II era. The number of intoxicated-driver fatalities has been decreasing steadily for almost two decades. And everywhere, even among people who regularly drink and serve alcohol, new attitudes prevail. Food writers in national newspapers and magazines urge party-givers to keep the cocktail hour short, not to serve alcohol before dinner, and even to deprive intoxicated guests of their car keys, if necessary, to keep them off the road.

Equally important, the abuse of alcohol is now being recognized as a complex biological and psychological disorder, and such recognition may help more heavy drinkers come to terms with their habit.

In a free society, banning alcohol is not acceptable. But government, schools, and other institutions could do much more than they do to protect the public health, to control the forces that promote alcohol use, to teach the young about the dangers of alcohol, and to treat alcoholics. As individuals and as citizens, we could all contribute to reducing the toll alcohol exacts in American life.

Alcohol in your bloodstream

Alcohol's effect on the mind and body depends on how much of it is consumed over what period of time. The amounts of different alcoholic beverages usually designated as one drink—five or six ounces of wine, twelve ounces of beer, and an ounce and a half of 80-proof spirits—all put the same amount of pure alcohol into the bloodstream, about two-thirds of an ounce.

How fast alcohol passes into the bloodstream depends on many variables.

In 1982, alcohol was involved in 57 percent of all fatal traffic crashes. In 1992, that figure was down to 45 percent, according to the National Highway Traffic Safety Administration. Reducing alcohol-related fatal crashes by just another 4 percent would save an additional 1,200 lives each year.

Effects of Alcohol in Your Blood

How drinking affects your physical and psychological state depends upon the concentration of alcohol in your blood—which, in turn, is related to the amount you drink in a given period of time and your body weight, as indicated below.

Percentage of Blood Alcohol Concentration*

Body Weight (lb)	Number of Drinks in Two Hours**				
	2	4	6	8	10
120	0.06	0.12	0.19	0.25	0.31
140	0.05	0.11	0.16	0.21	0.27
160	0.05	0.09	0.14	0.19	0.23
180	0.04	0.08	0.13	0.17	0.21
200	0.04	0.08	0.11	0.15	0.19

Resulting Condition

Blood Alcohol Concentration	Effect
0.05%	Relaxed state; judgement not as sharp
0.08%	Everyday stress lessened
0.10%***	Movements and speech become clumsy
0.20%	Very drunk; loud and difficult to understand; emotions unstable
0.40%	Difficult to wake up; incapable of voluntary action
0.50%	Coma and/or death

* These percentage values are approximate. ** 1 drink equals 1 ½ oz 80-proof alcohol, 12 oz beer, or 5 oz wine. .

*** Most states use 0.10 as the lowest indicator of driving while intoxicated. Some states use 0.08, while a few go as high as 0.12.

Unlike most other substances, alcohol can be absorbed through the stomach as well as the small intestine, allowing it to reach the bloodstream more quickly. Because the alcohol in beer and wine is less concentrated than in spirits, it is absorbed more slowly than the alcohol in, say, straight whiskey. But downing two beers in an hour raises blood alcohol content (BAC) more than one drink of whisky sipped for an hour. It's the alcohol that counts. A BAC of 0.10 is defined as legal intoxication in many states (some states have lowered this level to 0.08). It's hard to accurately predict BAC, since so many factors affect it. But a 150-pound man might reach a BAC of 0.10 if he had two to three beers in an hour. Any BAC impairs driving ability.

The carbon dioxide in champagne and in drinks mixed with soda seems to increase the absorption of alcohol (see the box at right for average blood alcohol levels per drink). Eating while or before drinking, particularly if you eat high-fat foods, slows down absorption. There is thus some rationale for eating rich hors d'oeuvres with drinks.

It takes the body about two hours to burn an ounce of pure alcohol (the amount in about one drink) in the bloodstream. Because alcohol is removed this slowly from the blood, even one drink per hour produces a steady increase in blood alcohol levels.

Once the alcohol is in the bloodstream, nothing can be done to hurry the process of metabolizing it. You cannot run or swim alcohol away or get rid of it by eating a meal, taking a cold shower, or drinking coffee.

Blood alcohol concentration can be estimated from intake and body size and accurately measured in body fluids and breath. The concentration is related not only to weight but also to the ratio of muscle to fat. Leaner individuals have more water in their bodies into which alcohol is distributed. Since males usually have proportionately less body fat than females, they will have lower blood alcohol concentration after consuming the same amount of alcohol for the same body weight over the same period of time. The general response to various concentration levels is shown in the box above. However, responses to a given concentration level vary from person to person and even in the same person under different circumstances.

Nine Ways to Drink Less (or Not at All)

1. Let your waistline be your incentive. For the same 215 calories in two seven-ounce gin and tonics, you can have three ounces of broiled, trimmed sirloin and get the meat's additional nutrients.

2. If you do drink, measure your consumption: five ounces of wine, twelve ounces of beer, or one-and-a-half ounces of spirits is the maximum that a 160-pound man should consume within an hour and a half to two hours. A lighter person should drink less. If the drink vanishes before the time is up, switch to a juice or soft drink.

3. At a restaurant, order food first, not a cocktail. That way you'll probably have time for only one drink before the meal is served.

4. Schedule your business meetings at breakfast time.

5. Avoid drinks made with carbonated mixers, especially if you're thirsty. You'll gulp them down.

6. If there is a convenient place to set a drink down, do that in preference to holding the glass constantly in your hand.

7. If you are drinking a glass of good wine, sip some water on the side. Make the wine last. Savor it.

8. Try a spicy Bloody Mary without the vodka.

9. Remember that the pressure to have a drink may be in your imagination. It is becoming more and more acceptable to say "no thanks" to alcohol.

Short-term effects of alcohol

Because all cells in the body can absorb alcohol, even its immediate effects (only partially described here) can be wide-ranging. Of all the changes it causes, none is more dramatic than the effect of alcohol on the central nervous system. Some experts have suggested that the effects of alcohol on human behavior are caused by "disorders" of cell molecules. At first the drinker gets a feeling of ease and exhilaration, usually short-lived. As BAC rises, judgment, memory, and sensory perception are all progressively impaired. Alcohol depresses the parts of the brain that integrate behavior. Thoughts begin to get jumbled; concentration and insight are dulled. The exhilaration of the first drink or two may turn into profound depression. Some people get angry or violent. Alcohol causes sleepiness, but at the same time disrupts normal patterns of sleeping and dreaming. It also adversely affects sexual performance.

Alcohol acts as a diuretic: it stimulates the kidneys to pass more water than is being consumed. The dehydration that results contributes to what is perhaps the most unpleasant short-term physical effect of too much alcohol—the hangover. No remedy has ever been found for this debilitating combination of dry mouth, sour stomach, headache, and exhaustion. The remedies for curing a hangover have ranged from eating cabbage—a palliative proposed by the ancient Greeks—to a stiff morning drink. In fact, passage of time is the only effective remedy; more alcohol will simply make matters worse.

The health effects of moderate drinking

Regularly consuming moderate amounts of alcohol—which is defined as averaging one or two drinks per day by the National Institute on Alcohol Abuse and Alcoholism—has not been linked to any significant health problems. In fact a number of studies support the idea that coronary heart disease is more likely to develop in nondrinkers than in those who have one or two drinks a day. In addition, X-ray studies show that moderate drinkers are less likely to have clogged coronary arteries than nondrinkers. Why this is so remains uncertain. Supposedly, this beneficial

Nonalcoholic beers; pros and cons

People who like the taste of beer but want to avoid the alcohol or cut down on the calories can now turn to any of dozens of brands of nonalcoholic beers. Bear in mind, though, that "nonalcoholic" on a label does not mean alcohol-free, but simply that a beverage contains less than 0.5 percent alcohol per volume. (Only a product labeled "alcohol-free" must contain none at all.) For most people, 0.5 percent is an undetectable trace. But for a recovering alcoholic, many researchers fear that these beverages may be the first step back to drinking. If strict abstinence is your goal, fruit juices, seltzer, and similar beverages may be the wisest choice. These beers are also not designed for children: some experts in addiction think that such beverages may serve as "training beers" for kids.

Nonalcoholic beers are truly "lite," with anywhere from 50 to 95 calories in twelve ounces—about one-third to one-half the calories of regular beer.

effect comes from alcohol's ability to raise HDL cholesterol, the "good" type that protects against atherosclerosis. Some researchers have suggested that only one kind of beverage—for example, red wine—is protective, but it's more likely to be alcohol itself.

Still, it's only moderate drinking that's helpful, and some people can't stick to moderation. Because of the other potential health risks associated with alcohol, few doctors suggest that nondrinkers begin drinking as a preventive for coronary heart disease. However, moderate drinkers who have recovered from a heart attack may be advised that they can continue to have one or two drinks a day. And healthy people who drink small amounts need not worry that they are increasing their risk of a heart attack. Choosing beverages with a lower alcohol concentration, and sipping them slowly with meals (as is the case with wines, for example), are among the better ways of achieving this.

Breast cancer risk. Some studies have indicated that drinking alcohol increases a woman's risk of developing breast cancer, while other studies have not demonstrated any relationship between this disease and drinking (see page 14). If you're a woman wondering whether an occasional drink will do you harm, the answer is still up in the air: no cause-and-effect relationship between alcohol and breast cancer has yet been demonstrated. Certainly, more medical research needs to be done. In the meantime, if you are a woman who drinks occasionally, you needn't be overly concerned that you are exposing yourself to risk unless you are planning to become pregnant or are a nursing mother.

Risks during pregnancy and breastfeeding. Pregnant women who drink heavily risk giving birth to children who suffer from fetal alcohol syndrome, characterized by mental retardation, poor coordination, hyperactivity, heart defects, and structural abnormalities of the face or limbs. Because no safe level of alcohol consumption during pregnancy has been determined, pregnant women (and those likely to become pregnant) are advised not to drink and to continue to abstain during breastfeeding. The amount of alcohol that passes into breast milk is smaller than the amount that crosses the placenta during pregnancy, but recent studies suggest that even a small amount can inhibit motor development in an infant. The idea that drinking beer promotes milk supply and benefits the baby is a myth.

Risks of heavy drinking

According to the National Institute on Alcohol Abuse and Alcoholism, a person who averages more than two drinks a day can be considered a heavy drinker. As consumption increases beyond two drinks, so do the risks to health; indeed, chronic, excessive use of alcohol can seriously damage nearly every function and organ of the body. These physical consequences of drinking cannot be reversed, but many of them can at least be halted once drinking is discontinued.

The brain. One of the organs most damaged by alcohol is the brain. CAT (computerized axial tomography) scans of the head show that heavy, prolonged alcohol consumption can actually cause the brain to shrink and the ventricles, or cavities, within the brain to enlarge.

The gastrointestinal tract. Alcohol is a stomach irritant, and it also adversely affects the way the small intestine transports and absorbs nutrients, especially vitamins and minerals. Added to the usually poor diet of heavy drinkers, this often results in severe malnutrition. And though alcohol is not a food, it does have calories and

Is there an addictive personality?

Some researchers claim that low self-esteem, antisocial behavior, an inability to control strong feelings, and an inability to turn to others for comfort may dispose a person to addiction. Yet many people display all of these characteristics without becoming addicts. A score of studies have been unable to link personality traits to a predisposition for alcoholism, for example. Alcoholics can be sociable or shy, impatient or easygoing. Partly, it's a matter of labeling: the executive who drinks heavily and uses cocaine at parties is less likely to be branded an "addict" than the panhandler at the corner. According to Peter Nathan of the Center for Alcohol Studies at Rutgers University, the personality disorders and antisocial behavior that accompany alcohol and drug abuse are the result of abuse, not the cause. There's no way to predict who will become an addict.

Hangover Facts

Short of not drinking alcohol, no preventive or sure-fire remedy for the hangover has ever been found. Perhaps that's fortunate; if there were a cure, some people might drink more, with disastrous results.

Some hangover symptoms are caused by the alcohol (or its breakdown products) remaining in the body. Other symptoms occur even after the blood alcohol level has returned to zero—these may be the after-effects of alcohol toxicity. Here are some hangover facts:

Taking aspirin before drinking won't fend off a hangover. In one study, men who took two aspirin an hour before drinking ended up with alcohol levels 30 percent higher than without aspirin. Aspirin may interfere with the enzyme that breaks down alcohol, scientists theorized.

Not everyone gets hangovers. Individual susceptibility varies. The morning-after scenario depends not only on what and how much a person drinks, but also on who that individual is and his drinking history. There are genetic factors—for instance, some people process alcohol somewhat better than others. Some people rarely, if ever, get headaches, even after drinking. Psychological factors are also involved—if a person expects to feel sick after drinking, he may be more likely to focus on symptoms.

Some alcoholic beverages are more likely to produce a bad hangover. To a large extent, booze is booze: 12 ounces of beer, 5 ounces of wine, and 1.5 ounces of 80-proof spirits all contain the same amount of alcohol (ethanol). But some beverages, notably red wine and brandy, also contain small amounts of methanol (which is broken down much more slowly by the body) and other substances that may worsen the severity of a hangover.

Coffee and other stimulants won't speed the elimination of alcohol from the body or alleviate hangover symptoms, though they may perk you up. Alcohol causes fitful sleep.

Eating (particularly fatty food) while or before drinking can slow the rate at which alcohol is absorbed into the bloodstream. But whatever you eat with your drinks, don't drive.

Drinking water helps counter dehydration caused by alcohol. Alcohol has a diuretic effect—that is, it stimulates urine production.

If you're looking for a preventive or remedy for a hangover, you're drinking too much.

can contribute to obesity. Heavy drinking also produces a whole spectrum of pancreatic disorders and can inflame the large and small intestines.

The liver. Alcohol is metabolized in the liver, and so excessive alcohol consumption directly interferes with the liver's cell function. Initially, alcohol causes fatty deposits to accumulate, resulting in an enlarged liver. Ultimately, damage to the liver can cause cirrhosis, which is estimated to affect one in five chronic heavy drinkers. In cirrhosis, healthy cells are destroyed and there is an overgrowth of scar tissue. The various functions of the liver, including the elimination of normal products of metabolism from the bloodstream and blood flow through the liver, gradually deteriorate. Though incurable and often fatal, the disease can be slowed if it is detected at an early stage and if the patient stops drinking.

The cardiovascular system. For many years doctors have observed that high blood pressure and alcohol abuse go together; moreover, according to a number of recent studies, heavy drinkers are indeed more likely to have high blood pressure than teetotalers. Heavy alcohol consumption also damages healthy heart muscle or adds extra strain if the heart muscle is already damaged, and increases the risk of heart attacks and heart disease.

Other effects. The direct effects of alcohol abuse are only part of the story. In the words of one study, "the alcoholic abusing only alcohol is very rare." Heavy drinkers also tend to be heavy smokers and are also more likely to take and misuse other drugs, such as tranquilizers. Alcohol itself is not a carcinogen, but excessive use of it, particularly in combination with tobacco, increases the chance of cancers of the mouth, larynx, and throat. Alcohol abuse appears to play a role in stomach and colorectal cancers and possibly in liver cancer as well. It can complicate and interfere with the treatment of cancer and other diseases.

Women drinkers and health risks. Though men have long outnumbered women as problem drinkers, studies have shown that drinking and drinking-related problems among women are on the rise. Today, 55 percent of women drink alcoholic beverages, the highest percentage ever. Perhaps as many as 25 percent of those women are heavy drinkers, and certainly they are susceptible to the consequences. In fact, women who drink the same amount as men—or even less—appear to be more vulnerable than men to medical problems, and to develop them more quickly than men. One study showed that women who had been drinking for a shorter period of time than men (fourteen versus twenty years) had nearly the same rates of alcohol-related diseases as the men. Women apparently develop liver disease at lower levels of alcohol intake and with shorter drinking histories than men, even correcting for their lighter body weight and smaller lean body mass.

Heavy drinking in women also puts them at greater risk of osteoporosis, the shrinking and weakening of bone tissue.

Alcohol and alcoholism

An estimated 15 million adults have more than two drinks a day. About 18 percent of that group have more than four drinks a day, and this group is at risk for becoming seriously addicted to alcohol. At which point someone becomes alcoholic is widely debated, as is what causes alcoholism or to what extent it is a disease. One official definition, recently devised by a twenty-three-member committee of experts, is "a primary chronic disease with genetic, psychosocial, and environmental factors influencing its manifestations. The disease is often progressive and fatal. It is characterized by impaired control over drinking, preoccupation with the drug alcohol, use of alcohol despite adverse consequences, and distortions in thinking, most notably denial."

Alcohol use, by itself, is not the cause of alcoholism. Paradoxically enough, most people can drink occasionally and sparingly throughout their lives and never succumb to alcohol abuse. Medical science cannot yet explain why one person has little or no interest in alcohol, while another habitually drinks to excess—or why some heavy drinkers are able to stop drinking, while others continue until they die of cirrhosis.

One area currently under intensive investigation is heredity. Studies have shown that a significant number of children of alcoholic parents, even when raised in a nonalcoholic household, become alcoholics. This suggests that the ability to handle alcohol may be in part genetically determined. Also, recent studies conducted in Japan have shown that 50 percent of all Asians do not produce the liver enzyme that metabolizes alcohol, so they cannot drink at all without becoming ill. Perhaps the chemistry of the body will prove to be the key to whether a person can drink moderately or not.

Still, this does not mean that everyone with the hereditary tendency must become an alcoholic. If there are alcoholism genes, they remain to be identified, and a test for potential alcoholism is a long way off. Researchers point to differences in blood enzymes among alcoholics and nonusers—but do not know whether the difference is responsible for the alcoholism or the result of it. Though most investigators believe that alcoholism has genetic, as well as environmental, causes,

Myth: You can always "sleep it off."

Fact: You can't. Everyone knows that a person's judgment and performance are impaired when under the influence of alcohol—but they can still be impaired the next day, too. According to a Swedish study, after an evening of heavy drinking, your driving ability may be diminished by as much as 20 percent the next morning, even though your blood alcohol level may have returned to zero. And it didn't matter whether the subjects felt fine or awful—driving performance tended to be equally impaired. In a more recent study, Navy pilots had impaired judgment up to fourteen hours after drinking heavily (about five to seven standard drinks or a bottle of wine in an hour or two). Anyone who has overindulged should avoid driving or operating heavy machinery the morning after.

Alcohol: Do You Have a Problem?

Alcohol problems occur at all educational and social levels, and in every age group. Although no objective definition exists for "problem drinking," there are general guidelines to indicate whether someone is having trouble controlling his or her alcohol intake. Ask yourself the following questions. If the answer to any of them is yes, you need to reexamine how alcohol is affecting your health, safety, and relationships with others.

1. When under pressure at your job, do you calm down with a drink at lunch?

2. Do you ever have hangovers?

3. Do family quarrels most often occur after you have had a drink or two?

4. Does your family think you drink too much?

5. Have you ever injured yourself or another person after drinking?

6. Are you often on—and off—the wagon?

7. If you drink regularly, do you know how much you spend at the liquor store or in restaurants, or do you avoid the calculation?

8. Do you avoid situations where you think it would be impossible for you to get a drink if you wanted one?

9. When pouring yourself a second or third glass of wine or beer, or mixing the additional highball, do you reassure yourself that you deserve it?

10. If you know that you have to drive home in an hour, do you go ahead and have a second drink anyway?

More than two-thirds of all American teenagers have used alcohol, and one-third drink enough to hurt their school performance or get in trouble with the law. The majority of these youthful drinkers start early, before they have even turned thirteen.

this does not mean that any individual is "doomed" to be an alcoholic. Alcoholic parents don't always produce alcoholic children. And many alcoholics come from families where no one ever drank.

Treating alcohol abuse

One problem in treating alcohol abuse is that, for health professionals as well as for the drinker, it is often hard to define when a person has crossed the line from moderate to heavy drinking. A person who is chronically drunk in public is obviously an alcoholic. But not all heavy drinkers advertise their problem by falling down in the street, losing their jobs, causing traffic accidents, or getting arrested. Many people drink secretly, or only on weekends, only in the evening, or even only once a month. Some may drink from depression, while others are sensation-seekers. They may successfully hold down a job or practice a profession. Yet at some point, whatever their drinking patterns may be, they have lost their ability to control alcohol intake.

There are several signals that a person is in danger from alcohol:
- drinking for relief of pain and stress;
- pattern drinking (drinking every day or every week at a certain time, particularly in the morning);
- making alcohol the center of life or of all pleasurable, relaxing activities.

Increasingly, alcohol abuse has become treatable. Therapists have devised many different approaches to alcoholism, and a number of organizations—particularly Alcoholics Anonymous and Al-Anon—can help you or a family member deal with a drinking problem. Whatever the approach, though, most experts agree that the crucial factor is for the *drinker to recognize that a problem exists* and wishes to seek the kind of treatment he or she needs.

NUTRITION

Part 2

Good nutrition is the cornerstone of good health. Not only is eating right crucial for the proper growth and functioning of your body, but there is strong evidence that it can offer protection from many chronic diseases as well. Scientists now estimate that 40 percent of all cancer incidence in men, and 60 percent in women, is related to diet. Diet has also been implicated in two of the three major risk factors linked to the development of heart disease—high blood cholesterol levels and hypertension. It is often a crucial aspect of being seriously overweight, and can aggravate the development of type II (non–insulin-dependent, or NIDDM) diabetes.

Fortunately, eating healthfully isn't as difficult as some people think. You don't necessarily have to make radical changes in the way you eat or give up your favorite foods. This part of the book outlines the steps you can take to achieve an optimal diet—one that supplies you with the nutrients you need and promotes longevity by emphasizing foods low in fat and high in complex carbohydrates. Guidelines and suggestions are provided for incorporating these steps into your daily meals.

The following chapters cover the various components of diet individually, sorting out the benefits and misconceptions and indicating which foods you should try to eat on a daily basis and which ones to limit. There is also a section that shows you how to decipher food labels and an extensive guide to help you select and prepare the healthiest versions of different foods.

The Healthy Diet

Americans are bombarded with a plethora of dietary advice. Every month, it seems, a new dietary recommendation is issued by one authoritative source or another, not to mention the "fad" diets that appear regularly on the best-seller list. As a result, many Americans are aware that making some changes in their diet would benefit their health, particularly with regard to lowering their risk of heart disease and cancer. Yet it isn't always clear to them which dietary guidelines are important or how to apply them on a day-to-day basis.

Actually, developing healthy eating habits isn't as confusing or as restrictive as many people imagine. The first principle of a healthy diet is to eat a wide variety of foods, rather than emphasize any one category. This is important because different foods make different nutritional contributions. Secondly, fruits, vegetables, grains, and legumes—foods high in complex carbohydrates, fiber, vitamins, and minerals; low in fat; and free of cholesterol—should make up the bulk of the calories you consume. The rest should come from low-fat dairy products, lean meats and poultry, and fish.

You should also try to maintain a balance between calorie intake and calorie expenditure—that is, don't eat more food than your body can utilize. Otherwise, you will gain weight. The more active you are, therefore, the more you can eat and still maintain this balance.

Following these three basic rules doesn't mean that you have to give up your favorite foods. As long as your overall diet is low in fat and high in complex carbohydrates, there is nothing wrong with an occasional cheeseburger or ice cream cone. Just limit how frequently you eat such foods, and eat small portions. You can also view healthy eating as an opportunity to expand your repertoire by trying foods—especially vegetables, grains, or fruits—that you don't normally eat. A healthy diet doesn't have to mean eating foods that are bland or unappealing.

Keys to a healthy diet

1. Keep your total fat intake at or below 30 percent of your total daily calories. Limit your intake of fat by choosing lean meats, poultry without the skin, fish, and low-fat dairy products. In addition, cut back on vegetable oils and butter—or foods made with these—as well as on mayonnaise, salad dressings, and fried foods.

2. Limit your intake of saturated fat to less than one third of the calories derived from fat. A diet high in saturated fat contributes to high blood cholesterol levels. The richest sources of saturated fat are animal products and tropical vegetable oils, such as coconut or palm oil.

3. Keep your cholesterol intake at 300 milligrams per day or less. Cholesterol is found only in animal products, such as meats, poultry, dairy products, and egg yolks.

4. Eat a diet high in complex carbohydrates. Carbohydrates should contribute *at least* 55 percent of your total daily calories. To help meet this requirement, eat five or more servings of a combination of vegetables and fruits, and six or more servings of whole grains or legumes daily. This will help you obtain the *twenty to thirty grams of dietary fiber* you need each day, as well as provide important vitamins and minerals. Make sure to include green, orange, and yellow fruits and vegetables, such as broccoli, carrots, and cantaloupe, and citrus fruits. These foods are thought to help protect against developing certain types of cancer.

5. Maintain a moderate protein intake. Protein should make up about 12 percent of your total daily calories. Choose low-fat sources of protein.

6. Eat a variety of foods. Don't try to fill your nutrient requirements by eating the same foods day in, day out. It is possible that not every essential nutrient has been identified, and so eating a wide assortment of foods ensures that you will get all nutrients. In addition, this will limit your exposure to any pesticides or toxic substances that may be present in one particular food.

7. Avoid too much sugar. Besides contributing to tooth decay, sugar is a source of "empty" calories, and many foods that are high in sugar are also high in fat.

8. Limit your sodium intake to no more than 2,400 milligrams per day. This is equivalent to the amount of sodium in a little more than a teaspoon of salt. Cut back on your use of salt in cooking and on the table; avoid salty foods; check food labels for the inclusion of ingredients containing sodium.

9. Maintain an adequate calcium intake. Calcium is essential for strong bones and teeth. Get your calcium from low-fat sources, such as skim milk and low-fat yogurt.

10. Try to get your vitamins and minerals from foods, not from supplements. Supplements cannot substitute for a healthy diet, which supplies nutrients and other compounds besides vitamins and minerals. Foods also provide the "synergy" that many nutrients require to be efficiently used in the body—for example, vitamin C helps you utilize iron.

11. Consider taking supplements of the antioxidant vitamins—E and C, as well as beta carotene—and, if you are a premenopausal woman, the B vitamin folacin. The role these substances play in disease prevention is well established, and even if you eat a healthy diet, it's unlikely you will get the amounts that many authorities think you need. For advice on how much supplementation is recommended, see page 126.

12. Maintain a desirable weight. Balance energy (calorie) intake with energy (calorie) output. Eating a low-fat diet will help you maintain—or lower—your weight, as will regular exercise.

13. If you drink alcohol, do so in moderation. Drink no more than the equivalent of one ounce of pure alcohol per day—the amount in two 12-ounce beers, two small glasses of wine, or 1½ fluid ounces of spirits. Excess alcohol consumption can lead to a variety of health problems. And alcoholic beverages can add many calories to your diet without supplying nutrients. (Pregnant women should avoid all alcoholic beverages because of the damage alcohol can cause to the developing fetus.)

Do you need to worry about meeting the RDAs?

The Recommended Dietary Allowances (the RDAs) were developed by the Food and Nutrition Board of the National Research Council, a committee funded in part by the federal government. This group, made up of scientists from a variety of specialties, evaluates the current research on nutrition to establish estimates of nutrient requirements for protein, calories, eleven vitamins, and six minerals. In addition, the committee has established a range of safe and and adequate intakes for two more vitamins and five more minerals for which *(text continued on page 82)*

(text continued on page 82)

The "high five"

The National Cancer Institute recommends that all Americans eat at least five servings of fruits and vegetables , in order to help protect against not only cancer, but also a wide range of other diseases.

A serving doesn't have to be huge. Allow about a cup of raw leafy vegetables, 1/2 cup of cooked fruits and vegetables, 1/4 cup of dried fruit, one raw carrot, one whole fruit, one slice of melon, or 6 ounces of juice for each serving.

All fruits, melons, and berries count as appropriate foods, and so do fruit and vegetable juices. Jams and sweet fruit preserves don't count, nor do fruit flavored yogurts, since they contain only a little fruit.

How the Body Uses Food

Food—or more accurately, the nutrients it contains—is essential to life. These nutrients are broken down into three types: *macronutrients*—carbohydrates, protein, and fats—present in foods in large amounts; *micronutrients*, the vitamins and minerals, present in much smaller amounts; and *water*, a basic component of all foods.

Each type of nutrient has primary functions, but they all interact to carry those functions out. The macronutrients provide energy and help maintain and repair the body. Vitamins regulate the chemical processes that take place in the body. Minerals assist with this, and play a role in body maintenance as well, notably in the formation of new tissue, including bones, teeth, and blood. Water—perhaps the most essential nutrient—is present in all cells. Among other things, it provides a fluid medium for all chemical reactions in the body, and for the circulation of blood and removal of waste; serves as a lubricant in joints; and plays a critical role in regulating body temperature.

ATP: the body's fuel

The ability of the body to perform all its various functions—from nerve transmission to digesting food to strenuous exercise—depends on the presence of a substance called adenosine triphosphate, or ATP. The body produces ATP from the nutrients supplied in foods. As nutrients are broken down, the chemical bonds holding them together are split apart, releasing energy. About 60 percent of that energy is disseminated as heat; the rest is stored in the form of ATP and is released gradually in reactions regulated by special enzymes. If the body were not able to store energy in the form of ATP, all of the energy provided by foods would be released at once and we would have to consume food constantly in order to survive. The body's supply of ATP, in turn, must be continually renewed either from foods or from stores of carbohydrates or body fat.

Getting energy from foods

Your body is always burning a mixture of the macronutrients for energy. At rest and low levels of activity, carbohydrates provide 40 to 50 percent of the body's energy needs. Carbo-hydrates are the most efficient fuel for the body because they can be broken down to produce energy almost instantly. The body breaks down the carbohydrates you eat into their simpler form, glucose, which must be present in order for the cells to produce ATP. Excess glucose is converted to a substance called glycogen and stored in the muscles and the liver; glycogen in the liver can readily be transformed back to glucose as needed by the body. When the muscles and liver contain as much glycogen as they can hold, any excess is converted to body fat.

Fat—either from foods or from body fat stores—also provides energy, but not as readily as carbohydrates. During digestion, fats are broken down into glycerol and fatty acids. Glycerol can quickly be converted to glucose, and the fatty acids, in the presence of sufficient amounts of oxygen, can be metabolized to produce ATP. During continual activities of moderate intensity—such as long-distance cycling or brisk walking—your body begins to rely more on fats and less on carbohydrates for energy. After twenty to thirty minutes of activity, fats begin to contribute more to the energy supply. The longer the activity, the more your body uses fat for fuel. Any dietary fat that is not burned is converted to body fat.

Protein is metabolized into amino acids, which are used to build and repair the body's tissues. Some protein can be, however, used for energy, especially during intense endurance or strength training regimens. Excess protein, like excess carbohydrate or dietary fat, is converted to body fat.

Measuring energy

The energy that food provides is usually measured in kilocalories, which are more commonly refer-red to as calories. Scientists determine the number of kilocalories in a food by burning it in a laboratory device called a calorimeter and measuring the amount of heat produced. A kilocalorie represents the amount of heat necessary to raise the temperature of one liter of water one degree Celsius. Carbohydrates and proteins contain four kilocalories per gram. Fat contains nine kilocalories per gram and alcohol contains seven per gram.

Nutritional Needs Through the Years

Calorie and nutrient requirements vary according to age and growth rate, as the chart below indicates. For women, they also change during pregnancy and lactation. To satisfy an increased need for calories at different stages of life, it is important to choose foods that are nutrient-dense—that is, foods that provide a good amount of vitamins and minerals for the number of calories they contain. RDAs and other recommendations for specific nutrients are provided in the chapters that follow.

Age Group	Special Concerns	Recommendations
Infants to age 2	High metabolism and rapid growth rate make it especially important to meet proper calorie and nutrient requirements of this age. Enough water is essential, since a greater percentage of an infant's body weight consists of water.	Breast milk is the best food for infants; it provides enough nutrients, calories, and immune and growth factors. Vitamin D, fluoride, or iron supplements may be prescribed by a pediatrician. If unable to breast feed, infant formula is satisfactory. Supplemental water is not necessary in hot weather for a breast-fed baby, but may be needed if vomiting, diarrhea, or high fever occur (continue breast feeding). Check with pediatrician on when to add solid foods. Don't restrict fat intake.
Children age 2 to adolescence	These children need to consume enough calories to sustain periods of rapid growth. Pay special attention to ensuring proper intake of calcium and iron.	Teach children healthy eating behavior. Start them on a low-fat, high-complex-carbohydrate diet. Switch to low-fat dairy products, lean-meats, and offer plenty of fruits, vegetables, and whole grains. Limit intake of sugary snacks. Patterns of growth affect appetite. Teach children to stop eating when full. Ensure proper nutritional intake by offering a few healthy food choices, not by encouraging a child to eat everything on plate.
Adolescents	There is variation in the rate of growth of adolescents and therefore in their caloric needs. Maintain the proper intake of calcium and iron. Dieting—common in this age group—can shortchange teens on nutrition.	Adults can help ensure that teens get adequate nutrition by stocking healthful foods—low in fat, cholesterol, and sodium, and high in nutrients. On average, about 25 percent of a teen's calories come from snacks, so keep healthy snack foods on hand, such as low-fat yogurt, rice cakes, bread sticks, sliced raw vegetables, low-fat cottage cheese, and part-skim mozzarella. Encourage increased physical activity over dieting to help control weight.
Adults	Growth stops, so energy needs decrease. Maintain adequate intakes of nutrients, especially calcium and iron and eat foods low in fat, cholesterol, and sodium, and high in carbohydrates and fiber.	Balance calorie intake with energy expenditure. Choose foods that are high in complex carbohydrates and low in fat. Get the bulk of your vitamins and minerals from foods, not from supplements. For vitamins C, E, beta carotene, and folacin, supplements may be beneficial (see page 125). Consume alcohol and caffeine only in moderation.
Older individuals	With age, caloric needs may decrease, depending on level of activity. Constipation may be a problem. Some prescription drugs can hamper the absorption or modify effects of certain nutrients, so check with your doctor or pharmacist.	As individuals grow older, nutrient needs remain virtually the same as for younger adults. However, some individuals over the age of sixty-five do not get enough vitamin D. Be sure to consume low-fat dairy products fortified with vitamin D or spend some time outside each day so that sunlight can stimulate the body's production of this vitamin. Inadequate zinc intake is also common; good sources of zinc include lean meats, whole grains, and legumes.
Pregnant women	More calories are needed to support the mother and fetus. Increased need for protein, vitamins B_6 and B_{12}, folacin, calcium, iron, zinc, and fluoride.	A weight gain of twenty-five to thirty pounds is recommended during pregnancy; two to four pounds per month during the first trimester and about a pound per week after that. (A large majority of this weight gain is from the baby, the placenta, and the increased volume of fluid in the woman's body.) Avoid alcohol and smoking completely. Drugs—prescription or over the counter—should be taken only on the advice of a physician.
Lactating women	About 500 extra calories per day are needed to maintain the production of milk. There is an increased need for calcium, protein, magnesium, zinc, and fluids.	Lactating women should eat nutrient-dense foods and consume approximately two quarts of liquid daily. Avoid alcohol and decrease caffeine. Drugs should be taken only after consulting a physician.

Daily Food Guide

Nutrient and calorie needs vary from person to person, depending on age, sex, body size, and level of physical activity. The chart here presents recommendations from the USDA for planning daily menus. Adults of all ages should consume at least the lower number of servings from each food group. However, most adults will need more calories than this, depending on body size and degree of physical activity. Most men, for example, can have the middle to upper number of servings that are shown.

The needs of children vary widely, but they, too, should eat at least the lower number of servings from each group. Teenagers need at least three servings of milk, cheese, or yogurt each day to meet their calcium needs. Adolescent boys can eat the higher number of servings from each food group, while girls usually can eat a middle range of servings, and more if they are quite active. Very young children, pregnant or lactating women, and other people with special needs may have higher nutritional requirements.

Food Group	Suggested Daily Servings	What Counts as a Serving?
Breads, Cereals, and Other Grain Products *(whole-grain; enriched)*	6 to 11 servings Include several servings of whole-grain products daily.	1 slice of bread; ½ hamburger bun or English muffin; a small roll, biscuit, or muffin; 3 to 4 small, or 2 large crackers; ½ cup cooked cereal, rice, or pasta; 1 ounce of ready-to-eat breakfast cereal
Fruits *(citrus; melons; berries; other fruits)*	2 to 4 servings	A whole fruit such as a medium apple, banana, or orange; a grapefruit half; a melon wedge; ¾ cup of juice; ½ cup of berries; ½ cup of cooked or canned fruit; ¼ cup of dried fruit
Vegetables *(dark green leafy; deep yellow; dry beans and peas; starchy vegetables; other vegetables)*	3 to 5 servings Include all types regularly; eat dark green leafy vegetables and dry beans and peas several times a week.	½ cup of cooked vegetables; ½ cup of chopped raw vegetables; 1 cup of leafy raw vegetables, such as lettuce or spinach
Meat, Poultry, Fish and Alternates *(eggs; dry beans and peas; nuts; seeds)*	2 to 3 servings	Amounts should total 5 to 7 oz of cooked lean meat, poultry, or fish a day. Count 1 egg, ½ cup cooked beans, or 2 tablespoons of peanut-butter as 1 oz of meat.
Milk, Cheese, and Yogurt *(low- or nonfat types)*	2 servings 3 servings for women who are pregnant or breast-feeding, and for teens; 4 servings for teens who are pregnant or breast-feeding	1 cup of milk; 8 oz of yogurt; 1½ oz of natural cheese; 2 oz of process cheese
Fats, Sweets, and Alcoholic Beverages	Avoid too many fats and sweets. If you drink alcoholic beverages, do so in moderation.	One ounce of pure alcohol equals: two 12-oz beers, two small glasses of wine, or 1½ fluid ounces of spirits.

insufficient scientific evidence exists to establish an RDA, but which are known to be toxic at levels only several times the upper limit of the committee's recommended range. The RDAs are designed to apply to healthy individuals and are adjusted for men, women, and children, and for different age groups, as well as for pregnant women. They are revised about every five years to include any new information about human nutrient needs.

It is important to note that the RDAs are *recommendations*, not *requirements*. Individual dietary needs vary greatly, and the RDAs are set at a level that is assumed to cover the nutrient needs of most people, plus a generous margin of safety. Therefore, the RDAs should not be viewed as the minimum amount of a nutrient required, but as an estimate of a safe and adequate intake; over a period of time, an intake below the RDA may leave some people deficient in a particular nutrient and in some cases, and for some nutrients, a regular intake far in excess of the RDA may have unpleasant side effects, or even be toxic.

The Recommended Dietary Allowances should serve as a rule of thumb; most people should aim at getting 100 percent of the RDA for each nutrient daily, but not worry too much if on any particular day they fall slightly below or above it. Without even trying, most Americans meet the RDAs from their regular diets. The only exceptions may be getting enough calcium and iron since these nutrients can be difficult to get and are not always absorbed readily by the body. Good sources of these two minerals are covered on pages 138 and 142.

In recent years, the principal basis for establishing RDAs—the prevention of diseases linked to deficiencies of nutrients and maintenance of good health—has been questioned. There is increasing evidence that higher doses of some nutrients may offer long-range protection against some chronic diseases (see pages 22-24). This evidence will probably result in changes in the RDAs. But any changes will *not* change this basic premise—namely, that the basis of a healthy diet is eating the right foods, rather than some combination of foods and vitamin and mineral supplements. Supplements are no substitute for a healthy diet, which not only supplies vital nutrients, but also contains potentially protective elements that scientists haven't yet discovered.

Breakfast

Most of us were brought up believing that breakfast is an important meal—perhaps the most important. Yet about one out of every four adults usually or always skips it. Is this a problem? What do nutritionists know about breakfast?

Some of the best and worst foods in the American diet are served at breakfast. Such foods as bacon, sausage, butter, and cream cheese add considerable amounts of saturated fat to traditional breakfasts, while doughnuts, Danish pastries, syrupy pancakes, and store-bought muffins add sugar, fat, and calories. Many breakfast cereals also supply hefty doses of sugar and sodium, especially for children. And eggs, a staple of the American breakfast, provide one-third of all the cholesterol consumed in the United States. If your breakfast supplies all the cholesterol or most of the sodium you should eat for the entire day, you may not be able to compensate for these excesses later on in the day, since it would be difficult to consume only foods that contain none of these substances.

On the other hand, it is probably easier to incorporate wholesome foods into your diet at breakfast than at other meal. Many low-fat, low-cholesterol foods are ideal morning fare, supplying nutrients that may be hard to get in later meals. Breakfast is also an important source of fiber.

Does breakfast affect performance?

Researchers have never proven that skipping breakfast is harmful to the health of adults. It may be possible that suddenly starting to skip breakfast has negative effects on those who normally eat in the morning, but that routinely omitting breakfast may have little or no effect on adults. Although there are no adequate studies on whether physical or mental performance is altered by skipping breakfast, there's considerable anecdotal material reporting that children who skip breakfast have a decreased attention span.

The argument for eating a good breakfast revolves around the idea that the body needs refueling after the twelve or so hours of overnight fasting. Foods do

A Better Breakfast

Eggs
Egg yolks are high in cholesterol, so most people should eat no more than four per week. For a cheese omelet, use one whole egg with one to three whites, low-fat cottage cheese, and chopped, cooked vegetables. Season with thyme, basil, dill, or a combination of herbs.

Butter
This spread is high in fat and cholesterol, so you should limit your intake. For cooking, use a nonstick pan or a pan lightly coated with vegetable oil. On bread, substitute apple butter or all-fruit spreads that have little or no added sugar.

Margarine
It has the same fat and calorie content as butter, but it is rich in polyunsaturates and free of cholesterol. However, those listing a hydrogenated oil first are usually higher in saturated fat. Diet margarine contains more water, so it has half the calories and fat.

Cream cheese
Not a good choice, since it is very high in fat and cholesterol, and low in calcium and protein for a cheese. Substitute low-fat cottage cheese, pot cheese, or farmer cheese; you can blend these with low-fat yogurt, dry mustard or dill, and pepper.

Whole milk
Substitute low-fat or skim milk; blend in strawberries, bananas, or low-fat yogurt if desired. You can also thicken skim milk, and boost its nutrients, by adding dry nonfat milk.

Bread
Almost all bread has 70 to 80 calories per slice (about an ounce). Bread made from 100 percent whole-wheat flour is the most nutritious. Commercial pumpernickel and rye usually contain mostly white flour; look for whole-grain varieties.

Bagels
These are made from high-protein flour and little fat.

Croissants
These rolls contain butter and sugar, which add saturated fat, cholesterol, and calories. They are also low in fiber.

Bran muffins
Rich in fiber, niacin, and iron. Store-bought muffins are usually high in fat and sugar (honey is just as high in calories). If you make muffins, use whole-grain flour, bran, one egg plus one white, dried fruit or fruit juice (instead of sugar), skim milk or low-fat yogurt. Add bananas, carrots, or cranberries, if desired.

Pancakes
Use whole-wheat flour instead of white. Or, try buckwheat pancakes. Use skim milk and low-fat yogurt instead of whole milk, and substitute an egg white for at least one egg.

Pancake syrup
Substitute fresh or puréed fruit, applesauce, or juice concentrate blended with tapioca.

French toast
Use whole-wheat bread and egg whites with skim milk and vanilla (or grated orange rind).

affect blood sugar (glucose) levels, but the links between blood sugar and performance, mood, and feelings of hunger and fatigue are not fully understood. In any case, the effect on glucose levels will depend on the specific food and the individual. So there's no reason to believe that you should eat anything for breakfast just to get something in your stomach in the morning. Eating a nutritious breakfast of food that maintains you through the morning does make sense, however, particularly for children and adolescents.

Weight control

Some people skip breakfast because they are trying to lose weight and this is an easy place to cut calories. Others skip it because they think eating breakfast increases their appetite later. But, in fact, studies suggest that eliminating breakfast does not help in weight control. Many people who skip meals "starve and stuff" themselves, and are more likely to eat snacks—usually high in calories and low in nutrients—and be obese than those who eat three balanced meals. In any case, a healthful, high-fiber breakfast will of course be much more conducive to weight control than one loaded with fat, sugar, and thus calories.

A fast-food cheese Danish can contain more calories and twice as much fat as a fast-food hamburger.

What to eat

The foods that provide a good breakfast—and suit most Americans' eating patterns—are some form of complex carbohydrates (such as breads or cereals containing fiber, protein, vitamins, and minerals), which will help provide a steady supply of blood sugar. Also recommended is fruit or fruit juice high in vitamin C, and low-fat or skim milk or other dairy product. A small amount of fat helps provide a sense of satiety. Most adults enjoy coffee or tea, which is harmless in reasonable quantities.

If you prefer chicken and vegetables, there's no harm in that. What people eat for breakfast is largely a cultural matter. In Japan, for instance, it often includes salad and soup, and in Norway, smoked fish and bread. But you should try to get fruit juice, whole grains, and milk products at lunch or dinner if you leave them out at breakfast. Try to avoid foods high in sugar, which tend to be low in nutrients. Also, limit traditional breakfast foods that are high in fat, cholesterol, and sodium because of the damage they do to your heart, arteries, and waistline.

Lunch

For most people, lunch is a meal eaten hurriedly in the middle of a busy workday. As a result, people tend to choose foods that are quickly prepared and convenient to eat: a sandwich and a bag of chips from the local deli or coffee shop, a slice of pizza, or a fast-food burger and fries. Many of these foods, however, are high in fat and sodium and low in fiber. Fortunately, you don't have to give up convenience for health; most traditional lunch fare can be modified to be more healthful.

Sandwiches

At home, in brown bags, and at restaurants, sandwiches are a standard lunch. But some of the old favorites—ham and Swiss, egg salad, pastrami—may be dealing out more calories, cholesterol, and fat than most of us want to consume at one sitting—particularly if the ham and Swiss are on a croissant and the roast beef comes with plenty of mayonnaise. Any one of the classic sandwiches in the first half of the chart (see below) could put you over the limit of no more than 30 percent of your total daily calories from fat. The sandwiches in the second half are healthier alternatives. To create sandwiches that are more nutritious and lower in fat, follow these suggestions:

•Whole-grain breads give you more minerals and fiber than white breads or buns. Most bagels and pita breads (check labels) are low in sodium as well as fat. Open-faced sandwiches are a good way to economize on calories.

Comparing Sandwiches

	Ingredients	Calories	Cholesterol (mg)	Fat (g)	Fat Calories
CLASSIC SANDWICHES					
Roast beef and Swiss	3 oz roast beef (rib), 2 oz Swiss cheese, 1 tbsp Russian dressing, 2 slices rye bread	580	128	33	51%
Tuna, oil-pack	3 oz oil-pack tuna, 1 slice tomato, lettuce, 1 tbsp mayo, 2 slices white bread	400	53	23	52%
Turkey and ham club	2 oz turkey roll, 3 oz ham, 1 tbsp mayo, 2 oz Swiss cheese, 3 slices white toast	745	140	46	56%
Egg salad	1 egg, 1 tbsp mayo, 1 slice tomato, lettuce, 2 slices white bread	315	281	19	54%
Bacon, lettuce, and tomato	3 slices bacon, lettuce, 1 slice tomato, 1 tbsp mayo, 2 slices white toast	325	24	22	61%
Reuben	3 oz corned beef, 1 oz Swiss cheese, $\frac{1}{4}$ cup sauerkraut, 1 tsp mustard, 2 slices white bread	455	107	25	49%
Ham and cheese on croissant	3 oz ham, 2 oz Swiss cheese, lettuce, 1 tbsp mayo, 1 croissant	730	122	51	63%
Peanut butter and jelly	3 tbsp peanut butter, 1 tbsp jelly, 2 slices white bread	465	0	26	50%
HEALTHY SANDWICHES					
Turkey	3 oz turkey breast, 1 slice tomato, lettuce, 1 tbsp dressing*, 2 slices whole-wheat bread	290	60	5	16%
Tuna, water-pack	3 oz water-pack tuna, 1 tbsp dressing*, $\frac{1}{4}$ apple, lettuce, 2 slices whole-wheat bread	305	49	3	9%
Chopped ham and vegetable pita	1 oz extra-lean ham, chopped bell pepper, $\frac{1}{4}$ cup sprouts, 1 tsp mustard, 1 pita pocket	220	13	3	12%
Hard-boiled egg-white salad	2 egg whites, 1 tbsp dressing*, 2 tbsp diced celery, 2 tbsp chopped watercress, 1 bagel	245	1	2	7%
Chicken salad	3 oz chicken breast, 1 tbsp dressing*, lettuce, 2 tbsp alfalfa sprouts, 2 slices whole-wheat bread	315	74	4	11%
Roast beef	3 oz roast beef (round rump), $\frac{1}{4}$ cup shredded fresh cabbage, 1 tsp mustard, 2 slices rye bread	310	76	10	29%

* Dressing made from plain low-fat yogurt with added spices (curry, mustard, garlic, dill, etc.) to taste.

• Processed sandwich meats like bologna, liverwurst, and salami are usually high in saturated fat and cholesterol, and all have large amounts of sodium. Roasting your own chicken or turkey breast (and removing the skin) for sandwiches is worth the effort: you'll cut down on calories, fat, and sodium. Discard all the visible fat on roast beef, ham, or pork, and limit the amount of meat you use on a sandwich.

• Instead of cheese or mayonnaise, add slices of vegetables or fruit to make a sandwich moister and tastier.

• A tasty, low-fat sandwich dressing can be made with plain, low-fat yogurt, or by blending equal parts of low-fat cottage cheese and buttermilk, flavored with herbs and spices, or with mustard powder, horseradish powder, lemon juice, minced garlic, or ground ginger. A tablespoon of such a mixture has only 9 calories and a trace of fat.

• Ketchup and prepared mustard are low-calorie, low-fat flavor boosters—10 to 24 calories per tablespoon. But they are high in sodium, with 150 to 180 milligrams per tablespoon. You can make sodium-free mustard by mixing mustard powder with water. Prepared horseradish has half the calories and one-tenth the sodium of mustard or ketchup.

Salad bars

Offering much more than just lettuce and tomatoes, the salad bars found in many delis and restaurants can make a quick and nutritious lunch. Still, you must choose wisely; a study conducted at Mississippi State University found that students who ate a salad-bar lunch generally consumed more fat and calories than those who ate a hot meal. This isn't surprising when you consider that in addition to fresh vegetables and fruit, and legumes, salad bars are stocked with such high-fat items as coleslaw, cheese, potato salad, and bacon bits. And most people top their choices off with a few ladles full of salad dressing, which is also high in fat.

Still, the salad bar offers many options for the health-conscious diner. Just keep the following guidelines in mind:

• Choose your selections carefully. Stick to vegetables, fruits, and legumes for the most part. Cottage cheese can also be a good choice, provided it is the low-fat variety—but that can be hard to determine.

• Sodium is another problem at salad bars. Ask if salt or MSG (monosodium glutamate), a source of sodium, is used in preparing the selections.

• Be aware that such widely varied foods as avocados, olives, sunflower seeds, bacon bits, cheese, and diced ham are high in fat and sometimes sodium. If you want to include items such as these, use them sparingly—think of them as condiments rather than the main focus of your salad.

• Avoid salad dressings or limit the amount you use. A typical small ladle at a salad bar holds about two tablespoons of dressing, so two ladles full of Italian, French, or blue cheese dressing contain about 300 calories, almost all of them from fat. Try using mustard, salsa, lemon juice, or vinegar mixed with a small amount of oil instead.

• Pre-dressed selections such as pasta or three-bean salad, marinated vegetables, and tuna fish are often doused with oil or mayonnaise. These items are also more likely to contain added sodium.

• Some salad bars offer hot foods as well. Many, such as macaroni and cheese,

A safe salad bar

A salad bar should offer more than just nutritious foods. Items that require refrigeration should be sitting in enough ice to keep them cool. The bar should have an overhanging cover that keeps dust and other contaminants from settling on the food. And an employee should be on hand to make sure that customers do not touch food with their hands or with serving utensils that have dropped on the floor; otherwise, foods, especially high-protein foods like eggs and meat, can become contaminated.

The New Vegetarianism

In recent years, the vegetarian way of eating—high in fiber and usually low in saturated fat and cholesterol—has lost its bohemian image and entered the health mainstream. Studies show that vegetarians are less at risk for heart disease, diabetes, and various cancers (notably of the colon) than the average American. They tend to have lower blood pressure and cholesterol levels, and are closer to optimal weights in insurance companies' acceptable-weight tables. They are also less often afflicted with digestive-system disorders such as constipation. And they have a reduced risk for type II (adult-onset) diabetes and gallstones.

It's true, of course, that some of the benefits attributed to what vegetarians eat may accrue from how they live: many abstain from tobacco, drugs, and alcohol, as they do from flesh and fowl. And they tend to exercise more. But whether vegetarian health gains arise from diet or lifestyle, they are reassuring enough to have spurred the American Dietetic Association to issue a position statement approving vegetarian diets as "healthful and nutritionally adequate when appropriately planned."

Vegetarian is a catchall term that includes the following:

Vegans (total vegetarians) abstain from all foods of animal origin.

Lactovegetarians, a far more common group, include dairy products as protein sources. Such a diet isn't necessarily low in fat and cholesterol unless skim or low-fat milk products are used.

Lacto-ovovegetarians eat eggs as well as dairy foods. Most American vegetarians fall into this category.

Semivegetarians occasionally supplement a diet of vegetables, cereals, fruit, and dairy products with a little fish or chicken; some may eat red meat occasionally and still consider themselves semivegetarians. Eating lean meat from time to time doesn't undo the beneficial effects of a vegetarian diet. Most low-fat, "heart-healthy" meal plans—which suggest eating meat as side dishes or condiments in small amounts, rather than as main courses, and increased consumption of grains and beans as protein sources—are essentially semivegetarian diets. So are many ethnic cuisines.

Planning a diet

If vegetarians plan their diets with some care, they are no more prone to deficiencies than meat eaters. While lacto-ovo- or semivegetarians choose from most or all of the basic food groups, strict vegans may be shortchanged on certain essential nutrients. The potential deficiencies in strict vegetarian diets are:

Vitamins. Vitamins B_{12} and D are found only in animal products. A lack of B_{12} can bring on anemia as well as degenerative changes in the central nervous system. But these conditions are rare, even in strict vegetarians. If you're not eating meat, dairy products, or eggs, you'll have to get your B_{12} from fortified products or a supplement.

Vitamin D is necessary for calcium absorption, and a deficiency can cause rickets in children. But you need very little of this vitamin and, given adequate exposure to the sun, the body is able to synthesize it.

Riboflavin, one of the B-complex vitamins, is found primarily in meat, eggs, and dairy products, though broccoli and almonds are good sources.

Minerals. Calcium is found mostly in animal products, and the iron and zinc found in plant foods are not as well absorbed as those in meat and dairy products. Women, in particular, need to make sure they are consuming enough iron and calcium, which can be a problem if they are vegans.

Peas, lentils, and wheat germ are good sources of zinc; broccoli, kale, collard and mustard greens, and fortified tofu contain calcium (though it may not be as well absorbed as the calcium in animal products); beans, potatoes, dried fruit, and fortified cereals and breads supply iron; and you can enhance your body's absorption of iron by eating foods rich in vitamin C (berries, citrus fruits, tomatoes, red bell peppers, and broccoli) with your nonmeat iron sources.

Protein. Many grains and legumes are surprisingly good sources of protein, but unlike the protein in meat, fish, or eggs, that in plant foods is incomplete— that is, it has insufficient amounts of one or more essential amino acids. The trick is to combine proteins that complement one another so that together they form a complete set of amino acids—for instance, legumes (peas, peanut butter, lentils, beans) with whole-grain bread, rice, or other cereals.

Contrary to common belief, you don't have to combine complementary foods at the same meal to get the effects of a complete protein. If you eat a wide variety of foods (especially if you eat even a small amount of meat or dairy products), you will absorb a full complement of all the amino acids you need as long as complementary proteins are eaten within a few hours of each other.

Variety is the key

It takes only a little planning to keep a vegetarian diet healthful and nutritionally adequate. If you decide to follow a strict vegetarian regimen, the word to remember is variety. Eat a wide range of foods: fruits, vegetables, whole-grain breads and cereals, legumes (such as soybeans, chick-peas, lima beans, lentils), nuts, seeds, and soy products. Dairy products made from low-fat or skim milk, and an egg now and then, make it easier to get the full range of nutrients.

Some studies have found that children who were brought up as vegetarians or were breast-fed by vegetarian mothers are smaller than other kids. And vitamin and mineral deficiencies can be particularly harmful for children. It's a good idea to have a qualified nutritionist evaluate the diet of any infant or child brought up on a strict vegetarian diet.

fried chicken, and meatballs are high in fat and sodium. However, roast chicken or turkey would make a healthful addition to your salad. Soup can be another low-fat option if it is vegetable based, though it is likely to be high in sodium. Cream soups and those made with beef are often high in fat as well.

Fast food

One-fourth of all Americans eat in a fast-food restaurant on a typical day, and many people rely on these establishments to provide them with a quick, hot lunch. But they may be shortchanging themselves nutritionally. Between 40 and 55 percent of the calories in many fast-food meals come from fat, mostly in the form of saturated fat, the kind that raises blood cholesterol levels. Sandwiches can be very high in sodium—between 700 and 900 milligrams. Specialty items such as cheeseburgers with bacon may pack 1,300 to 1,950 milligrams. Add in salty french fries and other fixings and you easily consume the entire maximum recommended daily allowance of sodium (2,400 milligrams) in one sitting. In addition, fast food is low in fiber and calcium and high in calories. While fast food provides protein, this isn't a reason to eat it since most Americans get more than enough protein already. American children tend to eat enough protein to meet the RDA twice over.

Still, because of consumer pressure for more healthful choices, fast-food menus now typically offer lower-fat choices, and most restaurants have switched from beef fat to vegetable shortening for frying (though this fat is often partially hydrogenated and so may be high in trans fatty acids, as explained on page 108). There are usually healthy choices to be made at a fast-food restaurant—all you need are the numbers. A few chains provide nutritional information upon request, so you can get the specifics about the foods you choose, but in general, here are some fast-food guidelines:

•Look for a restaurant with healthy options. Some chains offer salad bars, low-fat salad dressings, fruit juices, low-fat or skim milk, and whole-grain buns. Salad bars and whole-grain buns can help compensate for the lack of fiber, and salad bars add vitamins A and C, which are scarce in typical fast-food fare.

•Choose roast beef—it's almost always leaner than burgers.

•Choose single plain burgers. Skipping the "special sauce" or mayonnaise can save 100 to 150 calories (though some restaurants have switched to low-fat mayonnaise). Skipping the bacon and cheese can cut more than 200 calories plus a good amount of saturated fat and cholesterol.

•Unless you know that a fast-food restaurant's chicken and fish offerings are low in fat, avoid them; they are almost always breaded and fried in fat. Chicken nuggets and sandwiches often contain ground chicken skin (very high in fat). Six of these nuggets have as much fat as one and a half cups of standard ice cream.

•Watch out for "extra crispy" fried chicken—its texture comes from extra fat.

•If baked potatoes are available, order one instead of french fries; just skip the sour cream, melted cheese, and butter.

The healthiest lunch

Packing your own lunch is the easiest way to retain control over what you eat—it can be as simple as a healthful sandwich and sliced raw vegetables or yogurt and a few pieces of fruit. If you choose, you can invest in a thermos, an insulated lunch bag (both of which will allow you to keep hot foods hot and cold foods cold) and

School lunches have often fallen short nutritionally: typically, they have gotten 38 percent of their calories from fat and 15 percent from artery-damaging saturated fat. However, new regulations call for no more than 30 percent of calories derived from fat, a maximum of 10 percent from saturated fat, and an increase in servings of fruits and vegetables.

various sized plastic containers. This way, foods such as soups, salads, pasta, stews, and chili, along with leftovers, can regularly be on your lunchtime menu. If you have access to a refrigerator or microwave oven, you have even more choices. For example, you can prepare a number of individual meals and freeze them at the beginning of the week so you have a selection to bring to work.

Dinner

For many people, dinner is the most important meal of the day. It is usually the largest; according to food consumption surveys by the United States Department of Agriculture (USDA), Americans consume 42 to 45 percent of their total daily calories at dinner. The foods eaten at dinner contribute a significant amount of nutrients to the diet, but also a large proportion of the day's fat, cholesterol, and sodium.

It can be difficult to change eating habits at dinner; it is the meal most likely to be shared with other members of the household, and therefore must accommodate everyone's tastes. One easy way to start is to make dinner a lighter meal; most nutritionists recommend that individuals spread their caloric intake more evenly throughout the day. Beyond that, however, creating a more healthful dinner doesn't mean you have to make drastic changes in the foods that you normally would eat.

A steady diet of dinners centering around red meat can contribute more fat, cholesterol, and protein than is healthy. Fortunately, there are many alternatives to traditional "meat and potatoes" fare:

*Try skinless, light-meat poultry or fish instead.

*Use meat as an adjunct to a meal rather than as the centerpiece. Add a small amount of beef or pork to flavor an oriental-style vegetable dish; make a beef stew using lots of vegetables and a small amount of beef; for a light dinner, sliver steak or roast beef and add to a salad.

*Go completely meatless—for example, serve pasta, rice and beans, or a vegetable stir-fry with tofu as a main course.

Healthy accompaniments

Choosing more healthful appetizers and side dishes can improve the nutritional quality of your meals as well:

*Good starter choices include: vegetable crudités—raw carrots, celery, and peppers, and steamed cauliflower and broccoli—with a dip made from low-fat yogurt, a green salad with low-fat dressing, a vegetable- or chicken-based soup (heartier soups, such as lentil, can often serve as a main course).

*Serve brown rice instead of white with your meal to add potassium, phosphorus, and fiber.

*Other healthful side dishes include: steamed vegetables; grains such as wheat pilaf; baked potatoes topped with salsa or low-fat yogurt rather than sour cream or butter; and legumes flavored with herbs and spices.

Healthy cooking

One of the easiest ways to begin to make your dinner more healthful is to alter your preparation techniques. If, for example, you plan to have chicken for dinner, you

Some fast-food chains specialize in roasted (or rotisserie) chicken, rather than fried. However, roasted chicken is often only a little lower in fat than fried. The most important thing is to remove the skin, which is almost pure fat. And order white meat, not dark.

Ingredient Substitutes

Many recipes call for inordinate amounts of sugar, salt, and fat. But these are not always essential components of delicious food; many dishes taste fine without them, or with less of them. Try the suggestions below. (Remember that baking recipes are more exact than other types of recipes, so you may have to experiment more.)

In place of:	Substitute:
Whole egg	2 egg whites
Whole milk	Low-fat or skim milk
Sour cream	Low-fat yogurt; low-fat cottage cheese puréed in a blender with a little lemon juice
Sugar	Half the amount in most recipes; for baking, reduce to $\frac{1}{4}$ cup of sugar for every cup of flour
Cream	Evaporated skim milk or nonfat dry milk with a little water added
Salt	Omit and/or substitute mixed herbs and spices, or lemon or lime juice
Ground beef	In casseroles: kidney beans; in lasagna or sauces: ground turkey breast
Bacon	Canadian bacon or boiled ham
Cream cheese, on bagels or toast	Neufchâtel cheese, part-skim ricotta, or low-fat cottage cheese
Mayonnaise	Imitation mayonnaise or plain low-fat yogurt flavored with a little mustard
Butter or oil (for sautéing)	Use nonstick cookware and/or sauté in broth or wine
White flour	Substitute whole-wheat flour for half the flour in the recipe

can keep it relatively low in fat by choosing light meat over dark, removing the skin before cooking, and baking, broiling, or poaching it instead of frying. Four ounces of chicken prepared in this manner has just 175 calories and five grams of fat compared with the 195 calories and eleven grams of fat in the two and a half ounces of meat on a fried drumstick.

Other easy preparation techniques can improve the health benefits of foods. Use a nonstick skillet, for example, or cook with wine or stock instead of butter—this eliminates the need for added fat. Steam or microwave vegetables instead of boiling them in order to preserve nutrients, and use lemon juice or herbs and spices in place of butter or salt to flavor them—this saves on fat, calories, cholesterol, and sodium. (Other healthy food preparation techniques for specific foods are outlined in the Wellness Food Guide that begins on page 156.)

Modifying your recipes to incorporate substitute for ingredients high in fat, cholesterol, sugar, and sodium is another way to make your meals more healthful (see chart above).

Dining out

Dining in a restaurant can pose some difficulties for those interested in eating healthfully. While many people make nutritious choices when eating at home, they often ignore healthy eating habits when eating out. It's no wonder; many dishes offered in restaurants are high in fat and calories and commonly used preparation methods can further increase the fat and calorie count. Still, it is possible to make nutritionally sound choices in almost all types of restaurants by following a few simple guidelines. (The chart on page 92 provides specific suggestions for what to order and what to avoid).

• Choose items that are poached, steamed, broiled, or roasted. Avoid creamed, pan-fried, and sautéed dishes, as well as buttery, cheesy, and crispy ones.

• Ask how foods are prepared. Many restaurants are willing to accommodate special requests in preparing foods. For example, ask that the meal be prepared without salt or MSG; broiled or baked instead of fried; cooked in margarine or vegetable oil instead of butter; served with dressings or sauces on the side. You can also request that the fat be trimmed from meats and the skin removed from poultry before cooking.

• See if substitutions are possible. For example, can you get a baked potato instead of french fries? A green salad instead of coleslaw?

• Start your meal with a low-fat appetizer such as a green salad, a tomato- or broth-based soup, shrimp cocktail, a raw vegetable platter, or an artichoke (minus the butter sauce). Appetizers can help fill you up so that you don't feel the need to order a rich entrée. A slice of bread or a couple of breadsticks (minus the butter) are also good low-fat appetizers.

• If your table is provided with a bowl of chips, fried noodles, or nuts, ask the waiter to take them away.

• Consider ordering a few appetizers for dinner instead of a main course.

• Stick to entrées that center on foods such as chicken breast, fish, pasta, shellfish, or other low-fat foods. If you want to order a richer entrée, such as a T-bone steak, order an appetizer and share the entrée with a dining companion.

• Many ethnic restaurants—such as Chinese or Italian—offer cuisines that tend to be healthier than ours. Chinese and other Asian diets are semivegetarian diets with less animal fat and more fiber than ours, often with rice as the basis, meat included only occasionally, and such dairy products as cream and butter omitted altogether. However, Americans eating Asian cuisine seem to prefer high-fat versions in which meats often push rice and vegetables out of the picture, and foods are frequently stir-fried in a wok—a cooking technique that is no different from sautéing in a skillet and can end up adding a lot of oil on your plate. See the chart of page 93 for comments and tips on ordering healthy dishes in a Chinese or other Asian restaurant.

Healthy Dining Out

BREAKFAST

Choose

Whole-grain cereals—such as shredded wheat, oatmeal or bran cereals—with skim milk; bran muffins, whole-wheat toast, bagels, or English muffins with jam or low-fat cottage cheese; pancakes or waffles with fresh-fruit toppings and low-fat yogurt.

Avoid

Eggs, bacon, sausage, ham, butter, cream cheese, fast-food biscuits or muffins, doughnuts, croissants, Danish pastries, hash browns, cereals high in fat or sugar (including granola).

LUNCH AND DINNER

	Choose	**Avoid**
Salads	Salads containing fresh vegetables or fruit, protein-rich chick-peas or kidney beans; for dressing, oil and vinegar, lemon juice, or low-calorie bottled dressing; ask for dressing on the side and use sparingly.	Marinated vegetables, bacon bits, eggs, cheese, butter-fried croutons, avocado, meats, pre-dressed pasta salads; creamy salad dressings, mayonnaise, or sour cream; coleslaw and potato, macaroni, chicken, or tuna salads made with mayonnaise.
Soups	Minestrone, chicken noodle, and vegetable soups in a non-cream base; split pea, lentil, or other bean soups; potato-leek soup.	Soups made with cream such as New England clam chowder or cream of tomato; most soups have a high sodium content and so should be avoided if you are sensitive to sodium.
Appetizers	Raw vegetables, steamed or broiled seafood.	Cheese, pâtés, nuts, corn or potato chips, pretzels, cream dips.
Main courses	Pasta or rice with vegetables or legumes and no cream sauce or butter; seafood that is steamed or broiled; white meat poultry and lean red meat (ask that fat be removed from meat and skin from poultry before cooking); food that is baked, steamed, roasted, or dry-broiled in lemon juice or wine; lean cold cuts such as turkey or chicken breast; pita and whole-grain breads and muffins.	Liver, duck, goose, poultry with skin, and processed meats; food that is fried, sautéed, creamed, escalloped, marinated in oil, or basted; food in a cheese, butter, gravy, hollandaise, mayonnaise, or cream sauce; casseroles and quiches; fatty cold cuts such as bologna and salami; cheese, creamy dressings, or mayonnaise; "diet plates" consisting of a beef patty or high-fat (4 percent milk fat) cottage cheese; sodium-restricted dieters should avoid foods that are smoked, pickled, or in a broth.
Side dishes	Steamed, boiled, baked, or raw vegetables; low-fat yogurt topping for baked potatoes.	Vegetables or starches cooked or prepared with fats (oil, butter, mayonnaise, or sour cream) or cheese; coleslaw, potato and macaroni salad.
Desserts	Fresh fruit, sherbet, sorbet, skim or low-fat milk in coffee.	Cakes, pies, cookies, pastries, canned fruit in heavy syrup, ice cream, custards, and cheese made from whole milk.

The Best of Asian Cuisines

Rather than emphasize low-fat semivegetarian dishes, Chinese and other Asian cuisines prepared in America are often fried, then immersed in heavy sauces, with meats often favored over rice and vegetables, and with liberal doses of sodium and other flavoring agents added. Nevertheless, you can still get a healthy meal in an Asian restaurant if you choose wisely.

	Comments	Tips
Chinese	Rice should be the healthful center of any Chinese meal; brown rice is more nutritious than white and is now widely available in restaurants. Fried rice, however, can contain up to two tablespoons of oil per cup. "Crispy," deep-fried, and batter-coated items are almost always high in fat, as are fried egg rolls and spring rolls, even though they're filled with chopped vegetables. Spare ribs and sweet-and-sour dishes are high in fat and calories, too. Many restaurants offer low-sodium soy sauce, which has about half the 350 milligrams of sodium found in a teaspoon of regular soy sauce.	• If you want to avoid fat, don't eat the crispy deep-fried noodles that often arrive at your table along with the teapot. • If foods are cooked to order, ask to have them steamed instead of fried, inquire about the amount of oil used in cooking, and ask to have salty ingredients—such as soy sauce—reduced. • Pick main dishes with only small amounts of meat, and ask if the proportion of vegetables can be increased. Include a vegetarian dish or two, preferably steamed, in your order. • Choose a low-fat appetizer such as steamed dumplings or wonton soup. • Another good starter is cold noodles with sesame sauce. The sauce is high in fat, but it's mostly unsaturated fat.
Japanese	Like Chinese, Japanese cuisine generally relies on rice and vegetables (including seaweed, which contains small amounts of beta carotene and vitamin C). Foods cooked in broth, such as yosenabe (a seafood-and-vegetable soup/stew) or shabu-shabu (foods cooked in boiling broth at the table) are low in fat, although they may be high in sodium. In general, salt is more of a problem than fat. If you're on a low-sodium diet, Japanese cuisine may simply be too salty. Miso, a fermented soybean paste used in soups and other dishes, is very salty. Tempura and other deep-fried foods are greasy because the batter absorbs the cooking oil. Tofu (bean curd) is high in fat, though the fat is largely unsaturated.	• Start with soup made with fish or chicken broth, cucumber salad (substitute a squeeze of lemon for the dressing), or spinach with sesame seeds. • Yakitori (skewered, broiled chicken) and steamed dumplings are substantial but low-fat appetizers. • Skip sashimi (raw fish) and most sushi (seaweed wrapped around rice and usually raw fish), since raw fish may contain parasites or bacteria. • Stick to sushi made with vegetables such as cucumber or carrots or with surimi (processed fish, known as "crab leg"). • Ask the chef to reduce the amount of soy sauce. • Opt for steamed or broiled vegetables, fish, or chicken. Meats and fish broiled and served with teriyaki sauce should be low in fat. • Skip sukiyaki—beef and vegetables prepared at the table—since it is cooked in beef fat and served with raw egg as a dipping sauce.
Thai	Combines ingredients similar to those used in Chinese cooking with richer (high-fat) elements such as coconut milk and peanuts. Coconut milk, a frequent ingredient in curries, has more than four grams of fat per tablespoon, but a curry can still be low in fat if it contains vegetables, fish, or very lean meat.	• Choose clear broth with shrimp (tom yam kung) rather than coconut-milk-based chicken soup (tom ka gai). • Saté, skewers of grilled beef or chicken, are low-fat appetizers; go easy on the peanut dipping sauce. • Instead of deep-fried dishes, order steamed seafood in wine sauce; seafood stew; stir-fried chicken, beef, or vegetables; or grilled meats.
Indonesian	The most famous meal is the rijsttafel (the Dutch word for rice table)—mounds of rice served with a variety of small dishes and fiery chili sauces. Some other traditional dishes are gingery chicken or fish soup, broiled fish, broiled or stir-fried chicken, and saté (skewered grilled meats and fish).	• Deep-fried chicken and fish, spring rolls, and fried rice or noodles are all high in fat. • Ask to have dressing (such as peanut and coconut sauce) served on the side, and use it lightly as a dip.
Vietnamese	Notably lighter in flavor and often lower in fat than other Asian cuisines. Many foods are steamed, sauces are light, and many rolls are not fried. Fish and shellfish are staples, and in contrast to other Asian cuisines, salads and raw vegetables are widely used, along with flavorful herbs.	• Chicken, fish, or shrimp soups are low-fat starters. • Salads of chicken, beef, or shrimp with fresh vegetables and fruit can serve as main dishes, as can a large bowl of pho, soup made from beef broth with rice noodles, sprouts, herbs, and sliced beef added. • Other good choices include marinated fish and beef; meat and noodles wrapped in rice paper or lettuce; rice-noodle crêpes formed into "ravioli."

Carbohydrates

A decade or two ago, bread and potatoes had a bad name among weight-conscious people. Popular diet books were likely to warn you off these foods and guide you firmly toward broiled steak and salad. Today, however, carbohydrates, especially "complex" carbohydrates, are back in favor. Pasta is on the menu even in the most expensive restaurants; large helpings of meat on the dinner table are more likely to be blamed for their "fattening" properties than are baskets of bread.

Instead of just another dietary fad, the new attitudes may reflect a better understanding of what's good for us. For although carbohydrates (or any other single nutrient) are not a magic road to health, they are the body's largest source of energy. Moreover, carbohydrates are in bountiful supply on the American table, as in most parts of the world, and—unless purchased in highly processed forms such as breakfast cereals—are the most economical of foods.

What are carbohydrates?

The term covers an immense variety of edibles. Refined sugar, pears, strawberries, whole wheat bread, apple pie, popcorn, white flour biscuits, green peas, cole slaw, a hot dog bun, and sweet potatoes are all sources of carbohydrates. In fact, all sugars and starches that we eat and most types of fiber, too, are carbohydrates. However, fiber cannot be broken down by the body and used as energy. Varied though these foods may be in color, taste, texture, and nutritional content, the carbohydrates contained in almost all of them are transformed by the body into one essential substance—glucose, the main sugar in the blood and the body's basic fuel. For animals as well as humans, glucose serves as the primary source of energy.

Complex is best

There are two general types of carbohydrates:

Simple carbohydrates are the sugars, which include glucose and fructose from fruit and vegetables, lactose from milk, and sucrose from cane or beets, which is used for white table sugar (see page 97).

Complex carbohydrates, which are actually large chains of glucose molecules, consist primarily of starches as well as cellulose or other fiber that occurs in all plant foods. Starch takes other forms, too, including dextrin, which helps form the appetizing crust on bread when it is toasted or baked. Moreover, starches can be modified or refined, as in cornstarch, which is used for thickening sauces and other culinary purposes. Starch is the storage form of carbohydrates in plants; the storage form in humans and animals is glycogen.

In both humans and animals, unlike plants, the ability to store carbohydrates is limited, but small amounts of glycogen can be stored in the liver and in muscle. The body can quickly transform the glycogen in the liver into glucose for release into the bloodstream when needed for energy. Amounts of carbohydrates that are in excess of what can be stored as glycogen become fat.

Since the majority of carbohydrates are broken down into glucose, why does it matter which carbohydrates you consume? Complex carbohydrates are better for us than simple carbohydrates because foods high in sugars usually have a lot of added sugar, and are more likely to come in "empty packages." That is, they are what commercials are fond of calling "pure food energy," which means calories without added nutritional value.

By contrast, the calories in foods high in complex carbohydrates usually bring a lot of nutritional extras with them. Two slices of whole wheat bread, for example, may contain 130 calories—as compared with 150 in a soft drink. But in addition to carbohydrates, the bread also contains five grams of protein, one gram of fat, as well as small amounts of riboflavin, thiamine, niacin, calcium, iron, and, of course, dietary fiber. None of these nutritional benefits are available in the soft drink.

Fiber is a crucial item in the carbohydrate package, and comes from such plant foods as whole grains, fruits, and vegetables. Insoluble fiber provides bulk in the intestine and hence helps to regulate bowel movements. It may also protect against colon cancer. Soluble fiber also helps lower blood cholesterol levels and thus may reduce the likelihood of cardiovascular disease. Because of our high consumption of refined flours—which have less fiber than whole-grain flour—and our preference for high-protein and sugary foods over whole grains, fruit, and vegetables, fiber has tended to decrease in the average American diet. (For more information on fiber, see pages 102-106.)

Will carbohydrates make you fat?

If you are trying to control your weight or lose several pounds, you probably have heard contradictory things about carbohydrates. Dieters often shun starchy foods—beans, potatoes, pasta—in favor of high-protein foods such as lean meat, and stay away from soft drinks, candies, and rich desserts believing that sugar is fattening.

It may come as a surprise that—gram for gram—both simple and complex carbohydrates contain exactly the same number of calories as protein, 4 calories per gram. Fat, on the other hand, has 9 calories per gram.

Thus, if you have your choice of a five-ounce baked potato and three ounces of broiled lean hamburger, remember that the potato has fewer calories than the meat. This is because in addition to protein, the meat inevitably contains a fair amount of fat. And rich desserts aren't fattening because of sugar, but because they are loaded with fat. Foods high in complex carbohydrates tend to be low in fat and

A high-carbohydrate, low-fat diet can reduce the risk for five of the ten leading causes of death in the United States: coronary heart disease, stroke, atherosclerosis, diabetes, and certain forms of cancer. These chronic diseases are responsible for more than two-thirds of all deaths.

High-Carbohydrate Dishes

You should get 55 to 60 percent of the calories you eat each day from carbohydrates. No more than 15 percent of your total calories should come from simple carbohydrates; the rest should come from complex carbohydrates. The dishes below more than fulfill these requirements.

	Calories	Carbo-hydrates (g)	Carbo-hydrate Calories
Bean and rice salad, 6 oz	225	36	64%
Pasta with vegetables, 10 oz	310	49	63%
Pasta salad, 5 oz	160	25	63%
Potato-leek soup, 8 oz	100	17	68%
Cornmeal, pancakes, 6 oz	365	70	77%
Baked potato with ratatouille topping, 6 oz	95	16	67%
Apricot-banana-bran bread, 4 oz	290	47	65%

Foods High in Complex Carbohydrates

	Total Carbohydrates (g)	Sugars (g)	Complex Carbohydrates (g)
Bread, 1 slice	13	1	12
Corn flakes, 1 oz (low sugar)	24	2	22
Pasta or rice, ½ cup, cooked	20	0	20
Beans, 1 cup, cooked	40	0	40
Potatoes, corn, or peas, 1 cup	30	6	24
Carrots or beets, 1 cup	12	6	6
Broccoli, 1 cup, cut up	7	0	7

Potatoes are an excellent source of complex carbohydrates, but potato chips are not. Eating eight ounces of potato chips is like adding twelve to twenty teaspoons of vegetable oil (usually hydrogenated) to an eight-ounce potato.

are usually not fattening. They are likely to be high in nutritional quality as well; a diet that omits them will leave you seriously short of vitamins, minerals, and fiber.

. . .Or help you lose weight?

As for the claims that complex carbohydrates can actually help the dieter, the answer is a hopeful maybe. Because fruits and vegetables, which are usually rich in complex carbohydrates, have a high water content and relatively few calories, they are obviously useful in any weight-control program. For one thing, they allow you to vary your food intake in a satisfying way. They also satisfy your appetite. Foods high in fiber are particularly useful in this respect because fiber fills you up, but is not digestible and supplies no calories.

Furthermore, some studies suggest that carbohydrates are less effectively transformed into body fat than dietary fat is. Nevertheless, it is probably too much to claim that complex carbohydrates actually "help you lose weight."

Carbohydrates and the athlete

Since carbohydrates in the form of glycogen are stored in the liver and muscles and provide energy for muscle contraction, it is a commonly held belief among athletes that loading up on carbohydrates before a competition can postpone the time to exhaustion and improve their performance. The classic "carbo-loading" regimen took a week and called for depleting the body's stores of glycogen through exercise and a low-carbohydrate diet, followed by rest and a very high carbohydrate intake. Most sports nutritionists now advise against this dietary manipulation because it is hard to follow, may produce undesirable side effects (such as lethargy, weight gain, and cardiac rhythm abnormalities), and is unnecessary. Sports physiologists have devised a simpler version of carbohydrate loading; during the two to three days before an endurance event, simply increase your complex carbohydrate intake and slightly decrease your level of exercise.

However, studies have shown that, at best, any form of carbohydrate loading is of limited value, even in long-distance events, since muscles can store only so much glycogen. Anybody who eats a balanced, high-carbohydrate diet and is in reasonably good physical condition has enough glycogen stores in the muscles and liver to meet the demands of short-duration exercise of approximately one hour or so. Moreover, during long-duration, moderately intense exercise—such as cycling for two hours—the muscles are able to use more fat than carbohydrates as their main source of energy. The improvement in performance that comes from carbohydrate loading, if there is one, is usually small. So the best advice is to stick to the balanced, high-complex-carbohydrate diet that should be eaten on a daily basis.

Sugar

For many years sugar has had a bad reputation. At the very least, it has been considered a junk food and an indulgence. More seriously, it has also been said to cause heart disease, obesity, cavities, hyperactivity in children, and diabetes. While it's true that sugar per se is a source of "empty" calories—that is, it provides no nutritional value aside from energy—it certainly isn't the dietary villain it has been portrayed as. At the same time, many of us consume more sugar than we realize because of its prevalence in many of the foods we eat, particularly processed foods and soft drinks.

Types of sugar

To most people, sugar means white table sugar (sucrose) made from cane or beets. However, there are actually dozens of sugars: in their pure form they have such names as fructose, glucose (also called dextrose), maltose, lactose, and sugar alcohols like sorbitol and xylitol. In addition, sugars are often identified by their sources, such as maple syrup, honey, corn syrup, and molasses.

All sugars are essentially the same and none offers significant nutritional advantages over another (except blackstrap molasses, which is rich in iron). Therefore, there is no difference between honey or brown sugar and table sugar. And the sugar in fruit is no better than the sugar in a candy bar. Fruit actually contains a combination of fructose, sucrose, and glucose. In fact, sucrose is the main sugar in some fruit, such as oranges, melons, and peaches. The health bonus that comes from eating fruit lies in their vitamin, mineral, and fiber content, not in the type of sugar they contain.

Some differences do lie in the degree of sweetness, however. Fructose, for example, is much sweeter than other sugars, so far less of it is needed to make foods taste sweet. On the other hand, xylitol and sorbitol are much less sweet than other types, so more of them has to be used to produce a sweet taste.

Glucose: an essential element

The body needs sugar. Glucose, the main sugar in the blood and a basic fuel for the body, is essential to the functioning of all cells, particularly brain cells. But you don't need to eat any sugar to supply your body with glucose. All you need is complex carbohydrates, also known as starches, which are found in foods derived from plants—grains, vegetables, and fruits. In some circumstances glucose can be derived from the breakdown of protein or fat.

When you eat something sugary, it is broken down to the simplest sugars (unless the food's sugars are already in their simplest forms). For instance, during digestion sucrose is broken down into glucose and fructose, which enter the bloodstream through the walls of the small intestine and travel to the body's cells and the liver. With the aid of the hormone insulin, the cells absorb glucose and use it as energy. Some glucose is stored in the liver and muscle in the form of glycogen. Glycogen in the liver can be readily reconverted to glucose when energy is needed. Most of the fructose is also converted to glucose by the liver. The liver can also convert sugar into some of the building blocks of protein—amino acids. Any excess sugar, like any extra calories, is converted into fat and stored.

Myths about sugar

Obesity. Sugar alone is not to blame for obesity. Eating more calories than you burn up adds pounds to the body—and for most people the lion's share of excess calories comes from eating too much fat, not sugar. In fact, some studies have found, surprisingly, that lean people tend to eat more sugar (and less fat) than obese people. People often blame sugary foods for weight gain, forgetting that cakes, ice cream, chocolate, and cookies derive most of their calories from fat, not sugar, and that fat has more than twice the calories of sugar. Many a "sweet tooth" may actually be a "fat tooth." This doesn't mean you won't gain weight if you add sugary snacks to your diet. But it's calories, not sugar, that cause weight gain, and fat provides far more of the calories in the American diet than sugar does.

Heart disease. A few studies had indicated that sugar could raise blood cholesterol levels in most individuals, but a task force of scientists convened by the Food and Drug Administration (FDA) concluded in 1986 that there was no conclusive evidence that a high sugar intake is a risk factor for heart disease, whether by raising blood cholesterol, triglycerides (a fat in the blood), or blood pressure, "in the general population." However, some researchers suggest that a small number of "carbohydrate-sensitive" individuals with insulin or triglyceride levels that are high to start with may be particularly sensitive to sugar (especially fructose) and respond by increasing cholesterol and triglyceride levels.

Diabetes. Eating too much sugar is not the cause of diabetes. This misconception arises because diabetes is characterized by high levels of blood sugar (glucose). Excessive sugar consumption is indeed very dangerous for diabetics, who must curtail their sugar intake. But sugar doesn't cause this disorder. Obesity is probably the leading risk factor for non–insulin-dependent diabetes—and as stated above, sugar is not the major culprit behind most cases of obesity. Family history of the disease and advancing age are other important factors.

Hypoglycemia. Many people claim to suffer from low blood sugar, or hypoglycemia—and blame it for their fatigue, drowsiness, light-headedness, or anxiety, for instance—but true hypoglycemia is rare. Long-term severe hypoglycemia can be life threatening; it isn't a disease, but may be a warning sign of a serious disorder that can disrupt the body's ability to regulate sugar.

When low blood sugar occurs in response to food, it's called reactive hypoglycemia. Normally, however, the liver maintains a relatively constant level of blood sugar. After a meal, blood sugar rises and then returns to normal within two to three hours, as insulin allows the body's cells to utilize it. Some foods—sugary ones as well as

Pour eight ounces of water in a glass and add six teaspoons of sugar—that is the concentration of sugar in some soft drinks.

Other Names for Sugar

Sucrose—or table sugar—isn't the only form of sugar that can be added to a product. Even when a label claims "sugar free," it still can contain some type of caloric sweetener, and one form is no more nutritious than another.

Barley malt	Honey
Brown sugar	Invert sugar
Cane sugar	Lactose
Corn sweetener	Maltose
Corn syrup	Mannitol
Dextrose	Maple syrup
Fructose	Sorghum
Glucose	Sorbitol
Grape sugar	Sucrose
Grape sweetener	Sugar
High fructose corn syrup	

some starchy ones—tend to cause a greater rise in insulin, which may result in a rather precipitous drop in blood sugar.

Studies have found that few people with chronic fatigue or restlessness actually have a concurrent drop in blood sugar. Conversely, most people have no adverse symptoms when their blood sugar temporarily dips.

Quick energy. A drop in blood sugar can, however, cause problems when you are exercising. Sugar eaten right before exercise or an athletic event is likely to be counterproductive and may inhibit performance. Many people believe that eating a candy bar or some other sugary snack before an athletic event will give them quick energy. But you'd actually be better off offering a candy bar to your opponent rather than eating it yourself. Sugar indeed raises glucose levels and thus provides some energy for a short while. In response, however, the insulin released temporarily drops the glucose level even lower than it was to start. Thus, if you eat candy right before a long workout, it can cause you to become exhausted faster, since your body has to call on its energy reserves (glycogen) earlier than it normally would. In contrast, many complex carbohydrates, found in foods such as beans or whole wheat pasta, cause less of a glucose response in the body.

An exception: consuming a sugar snack or beverage during a workout lasting longer than two hours (such as a marathon) may help maintain your blood sugar level, stave off fatigue, and enhance your performance by supplying you with supplementary energy.

Behavior. It's a common belief that individuals can become addicted to sugar and that a high sugar intake can lead to all sorts of behavioral changes from hyperactivity in children to aggressiveness in adults. There is no evidence that sugar is addictive; people don't become physically dependent on sugar—that is, when they stop eating it they don't experience physical withdrawal symptoms associated with truly addictive substances. There is a popular belief that refined sugar, like drugs, causes a "high" or "rush"—in this case by boosting blood sugar. Other foods, however, such as bananas or dried fruit, may raise blood sugar just as much and no one claims they're addictive.

It is true that humans have an inborn preference for sweets. This may have evolved as a protective mechanism to ensure that our early ancestors ate enough high-calorie foods or tended to choose nontoxic foods such as fruit. And people do crave pleasurable foods, but this does not qualify as an addiction.

Despite the fact that many parents blame a high sugar intake for their children's uncontrollable behavior, nearly all well-designed studies have found that sugar intake does not cause or worsen hyperactivity, which affects as many as 5 percent of all children. For years many doctors prescribed strict diets for hyperactive children, but the cause of this condition—also called attention-deficit disorder—is unknown, even though it is one of the most studied of childhood disorders. Why do some children exhibit "hyper" symptoms—restlessness, a short attention span, and poor self-control—when they eat sugar? Scientists now believe that this is due, not to the sugar, but to parental expectations and the child's excitement over a sugary treat.

The jury is still out as to whether there's any consistent cause-and-effect relationship between sugar and behavior. Early investigators reported that eating excessive sweets may lead to aggressive and even criminal behavior in adults. However, some experiments during the last decade have found that a meal high in

Although the average American has cut consumption of table sugar (sucrose) to about 60 pounds a year, per capita intake of all types of caloric sweeteners, including corn syrup and all other forms of sugar, is up to about 150 pounds per year.

Sugar Substitutes

The ideal sugar substitute would have to be a chemical miracle: sweeter than sugar, with no bad aftertaste, calorie-free, colorless, odorless, water soluble, heat tolerant, nontoxic, noncarcinogenic, cheap, and safe for teeth. So far, no product meets all these demands.

The most widely used sugar substitutes are artificial sweeteners, the best known of which are saccharin and aspartame (brand names: NutraSweet and Equal). More recently, acesulfame-K (brand name: Sunette) has come on the market. It contains a small amount of potassium—thus the "K" (the chemical symbol for the element) in the name. A review of more than ninety studies by a Food and Drug Administration (FDA) study committee has given acesulfame-K a clean bill of health. Cyclamate, another artificial sweetener, is widely used in other countries, but has been banned in the United States. The effectiveness and long-term safety of all these products have been widely debated.

The two main groups of people who use sugar substitutes are diabetics and those trying to lose weight. And that would include almost everybody, since nearly everyone diets from time to time. Yet, according to the FDA, there is no evidence that drinking diet soft drinks or eating artificially sweetened foods will help a person lose weight. The consumption of diet sodas and other artificially sweetened products has dramatically increased and yet Americans are heavier than ever. Even for diabetics the need to avoid all sugar is open to question, since diabetic diets have been liberalized to allow a controlled amount of sugar.

Still, if you want to use sugar substitutes in cooking or at the table, or buy products that contain them, none of the three major substitutes (listed in the table below) are harmful when kept to a modest level. But one problem with artificially sweetened products is that you have no way to gauge the amount of artificial sweeteners they contain, since manufacturers are not required to list the amounts of sweetener used in foods on the label. For example, the FDA says it is safe for a healthy 150-pound adult to consume up to 3.5 grams of aspartame a day. A child weighing 50 pounds who downed a two-liter bottle of diet soda (containing 1.2 grams of aspartame) would have exceeded that. Since the aspartame content is not listed on the label, however, you would have no way of knowing.

Comparing Sugar Substitutes

	Safety	Who Should Not Use	Advantages	Disadvantages
Acesulfame-K	Nontoxic when used as intended. No allergic reactions noted to date. Does not carry a warning label.	Safe for all segments of the population, including pregnant women.	200 times sweeter than sucrose. No calories; no aftertaste. Suitable for use in cooking. Won't promote tooth decay.	
Aspartame	Allergic reactions, such as swelling of the larynx, have been reported. Can have a toxic effect on the fetal brain.	Pregnant and lactating women, children, and those with phenylketonuria (PKU).	180-200 times sweeter than sucrose. No aftertaste. Minimal calories. Doesn't promote tooth decay.	Loses sweetness when heated, so not good for hot drinks or cooking.
Saccharin	Found to cause bladder cancer in laboratory animals, but not proven to be a carcinogen for humans. Still, foods containing saccharin must carry warning labels.	Pregnant and lactating women, and children.	300 times sweeter than sucrose. No calories. Doesn't promote tooth decay. Can be used in cooking.	Tastes bitter.

carbohydrates (whether sugars or starches) and low in protein may lead to a relaxed feeling, sleepiness, and decreased alertness by boosting the level of a brain neurotransmitter called serotonin.

Sugar and tooth decay

The connection between sugar and cavities is the only well-substantiated argument against sugar. Still, just eating sugar isn't enough to cause cavities. Half of all children in the United States today have no cavities at all, though they're eating as much or more sugar than ever. Many factors play a role in tooth decay—including the strength of tooth enamel, which has been greatly improved by long-term fluoridation of most of America's water supply. In any case, while refined sugar remains the leading dietary cause of tooth decay, it is not the only food that promotes cavities. Sugars such as fructose in fruit and lactose in milk may promote decay, as may some foods high in fermentable carbohydrates, such as bread and rice. Other variables also affect tooth decay: the consistency of the food, how long the food remains on the teeth, and of course, how well and how often you clean your teeth.

Brown sugar is simply white sugar (sucrose) with small amounts of molasses or burnt sugar added for coloring; it offers no nutritional advantages.

Recommendations

There is no reason to severely restrict your consumption of sugar, unless you are a diabetic or carbohydrate sensitive (and even most diabetics are allowed occasional sweets). The best advice is the U.S. Department of Agriculture's vague admonition to "avoid too much sugar." This, however, may not be easy to do since sugar is a popular addition to many of the processed foods that are so commonplace in the American diet. While the amount of refined sugar (sucrose) we eat has dropped since 1975, the total amount of sugars in the typical American diet has remained the same. That's because there has been a large increase in the use of corn syrup, especially the very sweet and inexpensive high-fructose corn sweetener now used in most sodas and many processed foods.

Sugar is, in a sense, the number-one food additive; it turns up in some unlikely places such as soups, spaghetti sauces, fruit drinks, frozen dinners, cereals, and yogurts as well as in breads, condiments, canned goods, and of course, soft drinks and what we call sweets. Added to this are the sugars that are found naturally in fruits, vegetables, and dairy products. This amounts to each American consuming, on average, 133 pounds of sugar a year, which accounts for about 20 to 25 percent of all calories and 500 to 600 calories per day per person. Provided that an individual's overall diet provides the proper balance of nutrients, this isn't necessarily harmful. Ideally, however, sugar should contribute no more than 15 percent of your total daily calories.

Keep in mind, however, that most "sweets" are high in fat and calories and relatively low in other nutrients. If the cola you're drinking is taking the place of skim milk, it's a bad trade-off. But if you're eating a balanced diet that is low in fat and high in complex carbohydrates, there is no reason for you to go out of your way to avoid sugar. Indeed, by eating such a diet, you will automatically be restricting your sugar intake.

Fiber

A healthy diet is usually described negatively—eat less fat, cholesterol, and salt, for instance, or less red meat, eggs, and chips. Yet the same diet can be given a positive slant: eat more fiber in the form of whole grains, fruits, and vegetables. Though interest in high-fiber foods goes back to Hippocrates, our understanding of fiber's health benefits has been greatly enhanced by research done during the last twenty-five years. Formerly called roughage or bulk, fiber was once thought of primarily as filler—in other words, if you eat high-fiber foods, you'll have less room for high-fat, high-calorie items. That is still seen as one of fiber's potential benefits, as is the fact that it is generally found in foods rich in vitamins and minerals. But scientists now recognize that fiber itself may play a role in reducing the risk of the leading chronic diseases—heart disease, cancer, and diabetes.

To many people, fiber is synonymous with oat bran, thanks to all the ads for oat cereals in recent years. But if you depend on oat bran alone to create a high-fiber diet, you are short-changing yourself. Fiber is hard to peg down because it isn't a single substance, but rather a large group of widely different compounds with varied effects in the body. However, all types of fiber have two things in common: they are found only in plant foods and they are resistant to human digestive enzymes (that is, they pass through the digestive tract without being completely broken down). While other basic foods are nearly all digested and absorbed as they pass through the small intestine, fiber enters the large intestine more or less intact. Being indigestible, fiber also contributes no nutrients to the body, and for many years, no one thought removing it from food was bad (hence, the popularity of white bread over whole wheat). But nutritionists have discovered that fiber performs valuable functions precisely because it is not digested.

Insoluble vs. soluble

For simplicity, fiber compounds can be divided into two broad categories: those that are insoluble in water and those that are soluble. Most foods contain both types in varying amounts, but certain foods are particularly rich in one or the other.

Insoluble fiber — which includes cellulose, some hemicellulose, and lignin—is like a sponge: it absorbs many times its weight in water, swelling up within the intestine. Insoluble fiber is found mainly in whole grains and, in the form of cellulose and lignin, on the outside of seeds, fruits, legumes, and other foods. For example, wheat bran, which contains cellulose, is the outer protective layer of a grain of wheat. This outer material is often the chewiest part of foods, and for that reason it is often removed when food is processed by milling, peeling, boiling, or extracting. But it is best to eat unrefined foods, since insoluble fiber is crucial in promoting more efficient elimination by increasing stool bulk and may alleviate some digestive disorders. It is also thought to play a role in colon cancer prevention.

Soluble fiber — which includes pectin, gums, and some hemicellulose—is found in fruits, vegetables, seeds, brown rice, barley, oats, and oat bran. It can help pro-

Fiber Content of Foods

Better laboratory techniques now provide a measurement of fiber called "dietary fiber," which includes both soluble and insoluble fiber. (Previously, chemists could measure only insoluble fiber; the result was called "crude fiber.") And thanks to recent changes in labeling regulations, dietary fiber content has to be listed on more food labels. Still, there is as yet no single "correct" way to measure dietary fiber, so results from different laboratories can vary. But virtually all fruits, vegetables, and whole-grain products contain some of both types of fiber.

		Serving Size	Dietary Fiber (g)
Grains	Bread, white	1 slice	0.6
	Bread, whole wheat	1 slice	1.5
	Oat bran, dry	$1/3$ cup	4.0
	Oatmeal, dry	$1/3$ cup	2.7
	Rice, brown, cooked	$1/2$ cup	2.4
	Rice, white, cooked	$1/2$ cup	0.8
Fruits	Apple, with skin	1 small	2.8
	Apricots, with skin	4 fruit	3.5
	Banana	1 small	2.2
	Blueberries	$3/4$ cup	1.4
	Figs, dried	3 fruit	4.6
	Grapefruit	$1/2$ fruit	1.6
	Pear, with skin	1 large	5.8
	Prunes, dried	3 medium	1.7
Vegetables	Asparagus, cooked	$1/2$ cup	1.8
	Broccoli, cooked	$1/2$ cup	2.4
	Carrots, cooked, sliced	$1/2$ cup	2.0
	Peas, green, frozen, cooked	$1/2$ cup	4.3
	Potato, with skin, raw	$1/2$ cup	1.5
	Tomatoes, raw	1 medium	1.0
Legumes	Kidney beans, cooked	$1/2$ cup	6.9
	Lima beans, canned	$1/2$ cup	4.3
	Pinto beans, cooked	$1/2$ cup	5.9
	Beans, white, cooked	$1/2$ cup	5.0
	Lentils, cooked	$1/2$ cup	5.2
	Peas, blackeye, canned	$1/2$ cup	4.7

Sources: James D. Anderson, M.D., *Plant Fiber in Foods*; USDA, *Provisional Table on the Dietary Content of Selected Foods*

A food that is crunchy is not necessarily a good fiber source; cornflakes and lettuce, for example, contain only small amounts of fiber.

duce a softer stool, but does less to help the passage of food; rather, it works chemically to prevent or reduce the absorption of certain substances into the bloodstream. Soluble fiber appears to lower blood cholesterol levels and retard the entry of glucose into the bloodstream, an especially important factor for diabetics.

The benefits of fiber
In the late 1960s, the British epidemiologist Dr. Denis Burkitt began to link a high-fiber intake among rural Africans with a low incidence of diseases all too common in industrialized Western countries. It has been difficult, however, to prove the protective effects of fiber because fiber isn't consumed in isolation. High-fiber foods may be beneficial because they tend to be low in fat and calories and usually replace meats and other fatty foods that may increase the risk, for instance, of colon cancer or coronary artery disease. Foods rich in fiber also tend to be high in antioxidants (such as beta carotene and vitamin C) and other substances that may protect against a variety of cancers, and it is hard to separate the effect of

fiber from those of these other components. People who eat high-fiber diets may also make other healthy choices in their lives, such as exercising regularly and not smoking, that may lower their risk for some chronic diseases. In many studies, scientists use statistical techniques to adjust their data for some or most of these complicating factors, but even the best studies can't control for all known variables. Though extremely promising, the evidence concerning fiber's protective effects remains inconclusive, and research is continuing.

Here are some of fiber's proposed benefits:

Colon and rectal cancer. This is the second leading cause of cancer deaths in the United States, but is rarer in countries with a diet low in meat and rich in high-fiber foods. Dozens of studies have supported the hypothesis that a fiber-rich diet protects against colon cancer (a few studies have not). One of the strongest pieces of evidence came from New York Hospital in 1989 in a four-year study that found that a diet high in insoluble fiber significantly inhibited the development of pre-cancerous colon and rectal polyps (which tend to gradually enlarge and become malignant) in subjects with an inherited predisposition to them. More recently, the *Journal of the National Cancer Institute* published a large study also showing that a high-fiber, low-fat diet helps prevent the growth of precancerous polyps.

No one knows exactly how insoluble fiber may protect against colon cancer, but several theories have been proposed. By moving foods faster through the system, fiber may lessen the exposure of colon walls to potential carcinogens. Or fiber may dilute the carcinogens or inactivate them in some way. Studies have also confirmed that insoluble fiber reduces bile acids in the intestines as well as bacterial enzymes, both of which are possible cancer promoters.

Breast cancer. Research into the effects of fiber on the risk of breast cancer is still in its early stages. A recent study at the American Health Foundation in New York City found that wheat bran (rich in insoluble fiber) reduces blood estrogen levels, which, the researchers theorize, may affect the risk of breast cancer. However, there has been no conclusive evidence from epidemiological evidence to support this hypothesis. When people eat more fiber they tend to eat less fat, and it has often been proposed (though never proven) that a high-fat diet increases the risk of breast cancer.

Constipation. Insoluble fiber, consumed with adequate fluids, is the safest, most effective way to prevent or treat constipation—by increasing the frequency, bulk, and ease of bowel movements. This fiber is like a sponge: it absorbs many times its weight in water, swelling within the intestines and producing a larger, softer stool that the digestive system can pass quickly and easily. Also, when fiber enters the large intestine, some of it is broken down by bacteria, yielding compounds that in turn produce intestinal gas and initiate bowel movements.

Diverticulosis. About one American in ten over age forty and at least one in three over fifty suffers from diverticulosis, a condition in which tiny pouches form within the wall of the colon. When the pouches trap food, they may become painfully inflamed (diverticulitis). Insoluble fiber may help prevent or relieve this painful condition by reducing constipation and strained bowel movements, thus reducing pressure in the colon.

Heart disease. Numerous studies have indicated that soluble fiber (as in oat bran, barley, and fruit pectin) helps reduce total blood cholesterol, primarily by lowering LDL ("bad") cholesterol. The debate continues, however, about how much soluble

---

Psyllium—is it soluble or insoluble?

Psyllium is a seed grain used used in some bulk-forming laxatives, and it illustrates how complex a group of substances make up dietary fiber. About 80 percent of the fiber in psyllium is soluble, which is why some of the laxatives that contain psyllium help lower blood cholesterol. Yet psyllium is also quite effective against constipation.

It's true that insoluble fiber (found in wheat bran and high-bran breakfast cereal) has the greatest immediate effect on the frequency, bulk, and ease of bowel movements. But certain kinds of soluble fiber (notably that in psyllium) also enhance regularity in several ways—for instance, by forming emolient gels that facilitate the passage of intestinal contents.

Soluble fiber is relatively slow-acting: it usually takes twelve to twenty-four hours to enhance regularity, but may take up to three days in some people.

fiber you have to consume to get a significant reduction—and, again, the typical high-fiber diet is low in fat and that alone may reduce blood cholesterol. Most attention has focused on oatmeal or oat bran, thanks to research funding (and ad campaigns) from cereal companies, but there have also been studies about other sources of soluble fiber, such as grapefruit pectin and apples. Most have shown modest positive effects. But rather than looking at any single food as a magic bullet against cholesterol, you should get your fiber from a variety of sources. Reducing your intake of saturated fat (from fatty meats, whole milk, cheese) and maintaining a healthy weight are even better ways to control blood cholesterol.

Diabetes. Some studies have suggested that soluble fiber improves control of blood sugar and can thus reduce the need for insulin or medication in people with diabetes. Exactly why isn't clear, but soluble fiber (specifically gums and pectin) seems to delay the emptying of the stomach and slow the absorption of glucose in the intestine.

Obesity. Most high-fiber foods are also high in complex carbohydrates (starch) and low in fat—a good combination for weight control. Many take longer to chew, which slows you down at the table. Fiber also fills you up temporarily without adding calories.

Increasing your fiber intake—safely

Suddenly increasing the amount of fiber you eat can cause problems. One common consequence is intestinal gas due to fermentation of fiber and indigestible sugars in the colon. Usually this isn't serious and subsides once the bacteria in your system adjust to the fiber increase. You can reduce the chances of gas or diarrhea by adding fiber-rich foods to your diet *gradually*.

One of the potential adverse effects of a high-fiber diet is the tendency of fiber to bind some minerals—such as magnesium, calcium, and in particular trace minerals, such as zinc and iron—and to lessen their absorption. There is some evidence that because of this mechanism an extremely high intake of fiber could create mineral deficiencies in people whose diet is nutritionally poor. This should not be a problem for most Americans who consume a wide variety of foods. Moreover, high-fiber foods are usually rich in minerals which compensates for any losses. In contrast, fiber pills, which contain no nutrients, are more likely to create mineral deficiencies in people whose diet is nutritionally poor (see box on next page).

The daily intake of fiber for Americans averages about twelve grams. Most authorities agree that we should be consuming at least twice that amount. The National Cancer Institute recommends eating foods that provide twenty to thirty grams of fiber a day. While it helps to be aware of the amount of fiber in various foods, you can ensure an adequate fiber intake by gradually adopting these steps:

Eat a variety of foods—the less processed the better. Bran, for example, is a superb source of fiber. However, consuming it in the form of whole-grain cereal is more nutritionally sound than merely adding bran flakes as a supplement to your food because in addition to the fiber, you get the vitamins, minerals, and flavor. There is no evidence that bran or other fiber supplement can compensate for an otherwise unhealthy diet.

Eat more fruits and vegetables—at least five servings per day—and three to six servings of whole-grain breads, cereals, and legumes (beans). This may sound like a lot of food, but one serving is the equivalent of a slice of bread, one ounce of cold

Fig bars contain twice as much fiber and less than half the fat calories of many cookies. Still, they are high in sugar and calories, so save them for occasional treats.

Fiber Supplements

Can fiber in a bottle play the same role in weight reduction that a diet high in fiber can? Manufacturers of fiber supplements would like you to think so. And they may be right; there have been few studies so far, but there is some suggestion that fiber pills might be helpful in producing the same feeling of satiety produced by high-fiber foods. Still, much more research is needed to determine the safety of the use of fiber supplements over the long term. Moreover, getting fiber from supplements rather than from food is a little like getting vitamins from pills instead of from food. Here are four reasons not to use fiber supplements:

•Fiber pills alone won't make you slim. First of all, there's no conclusive evidence that fiber by itself decreases appetite. Second, the diets described in the fiber supplement packages—which you must follow if you expect to lose weight while taking the supplements—usually add up to about 1,200 calories a day, and on that allowance you would lose weight without fiber supplements. Even with them, you'll still need willpower.

•Fiber pills actually have little fiber in them. Five pills, at the recommended premeal dose, usually supply 2.5 grams of fiber—about as much as an apple or three rye wafers, but at a greater expense. So even if you swallowed the recommended fifteen pills daily, you're not getting that much fiber.

•Fiber is a large group of widely different substances, and no one knows precisely their optimal combinations. The fiber in the supplements may be unbalanced or incomplete. In contrast, if you eat a wide variety of foods, you're likely to get all kinds of fiber.

•Fiber binds some minerals in the foods you eat. Foods high in fiber contain minerals, so you more than make up for any losses; fiber supplements contain no minerals.

The fiber values of cooked vegetables and fruits are frequently higher than their raw counterparts. That's because water may be lost in cooking, causing fiber to make up a greater proportion of the total.

cereal, or one-half cup of pasta, rice, or beans. These foods are not only excellent low-calorie sources of fiber, but provide essential vitamins and minerals as well.

Drink plenty of liquids. Otherwise fiber can slow down or even block proper intestinal digestion.

The less processed the food, the better. Opt for whole-grain products, such as whole-wheat flour and brown rice. And eat the skin of fruits and vegetables, when possible—a potato with skin has twice as much fiber as one without. Fruits with edible seeds, such as raspberries and figs, tend to contain lots of fiber. However, chopping or cooking fruits or vegetables, such as broccoli, won't affect fiber content to a significant degree.

Get your fiber from food, rather than from pills or powders (see box above). Bulk laxatives (high in fiber) may be safe and effective against constipation, but lack the nutrients found in fiber-rich foods.

Spread out your fiber intake. Getting all of your fiber at one sitting may cut the benefits and increase the chance of unpleasant side effects. As a rule of thumb, try to eat foods high in insoluble and soluble fiber at every meal.

This approach will not only increase your fiber consumption, but should also help you reduce the sugars and fatty meats that most of us eat too freely. That is another way in which fiber, though not a nutritional panacea, is an excellent form of health insurance.

Fat

As most people see it, fat is the villain in the nutritional scenario, clogging the arteries and settling around the waist. They forget that we need to consume some fat to remain healthy. As with many other nutrients and foods, the question about fat is how much and which kinds should we eat?

Americans have one of the fattiest diets in the world; about 37 percent of all calories consumed today come from fats, up from 32 percent at the start of the century. Most of this fat intake occurs at the expense of carbohydrates. The chief sources of fat in the diet include meats, poultry, and dairy products, as well as vegetable oils and shortenings. Most nutritionists recommend that only 30 percent of our total daily calories come from fat, and that we should try to get more of these calories from plant sources or fish, rather than animal sources.

A source of energy, and high in calories

Technically called lipids, fats come in solid or liquid (oil) form. All are insoluble in water. Although carbohydrates are the body's main source of food energy, fats are the most concentrated source, supplying 9 calories per gram; carbohydrates and proteins have 4 calories per gram. High-fat foods are thus always high-calorie foods. The important functions of fats in the body include:

•Storing energy. Fats serve as the storage substance for the body's excess calories, filling the balloonlike adipose cells that insulate the body. Extra calories from carbohydrates and proteins as well as from fats are stored as body fat.

•Maintaining healthy skin and hair.

•Carrying fat-soluble vitamins (A, D, E, and K).

•Supplying "essential" fatty acids, so named because the body can't make them and must get them from foods. Linoleic acid is the most important of these, especially for the proper growth and development of infants. Essential fatty acids are the raw materials for several hormonelike compounds, including prostaglandins, which help control blood pressure and other vital bodily functions.

•Regulating levels of cholesterol in the blood.

•Promoting satiety, because they slow the emptying of food from the stomach.

Fatty acids: saturated vs. unsaturated

Most fats in foods are triglycerides, which consist of three fatty acids attached to a glycerol molecule. These fatty acids vary in length and in degree of saturation by hydrogen atoms—and it is these variations that determine the properties of different fats. All fats are combinations of saturated and unsaturated fatty acids. Fats containing mainly saturated fatty acids are described as "highly saturated," while fats that are primarily polyunsaturated or monounsaturated are described as "highly unsaturated."

Saturated fatty acids are loaded with all the hydrogen atoms they can carry. Fats that are largely saturated come chiefly from animal sources and include butter, milk fat, and the fat in meats; two vegetable oils—coconut and palm oils—are also highly saturated. Highly saturated fats are usually solid at room temperature and keep well.

Unsaturated fatty acids do not have all the hydrogen atoms they can carry. Depending on the number of missing hydrogen atoms, these fatty acids are called either *monounsaturated* (olive, peanut, canola, and avocado oils are largely monounsaturated) or *polyunsaturated* (corn, safflower, and sesame oils are primarily polyunsaturated). The important dietary unsaturated fats come from plants and fish. They generally are liquid at room temperature and may become rancid quickly since the absence of hydrogen makes the carbon atoms very reactive with oxygen.

A manufacturing process called *hydrogenation* adds hydrogen atoms to unsaturated fats, thus making them more saturated. The fats in margarines and shortenings are often hydrogenated because this makes them harder and more stable. Depending on the degree of hydrogenation, these artificially saturated vegetable fats are no better for you than comparably saturated animal fats.

The trans fatty acids issue

More important, hydrogenation transforms many of an oil's unsaturated fatty acids, making them more saturated and changing their structure in other subtle ways—they are thus called *trans* fatty acids. Scientists have been concerned that trans fats may increase the risk of heart disease and perhaps other health problems. While a diet high in regular unsaturated fat lowers total blood cholesterol, a diet high in trans fats lowers it much less—or may even raise it—by increasing LDL ("bad") cholesterol. In addition, trans fats lower HDL ("good") cholesterol, which carries cholesterol out of the arteries. This may help explain why a study from Harvard published in the *Lancet* found that women who ate the most foods high in trans fatty acids (especially margarine) had a 50 percent higher risk of heart disease than women who ate these fats rarely. Another recent study, reported in the *American Journal of Cardiology,* found that people with coronary artery disease have significantly higher levels of trans fatty acids in their blood than healthy people.

A few years back, the National Academy of Sciences concluded that there was little or no cause for concern about trans fats because they make up only a small amount of our fat intake. Critics claim, however, that in recent years Americans have been consuming two to

Red meat, poultry, and fish provide about one-third of the fat in the American diet. Dairy products and eggs contribute about 15 percent. The bulk of fat—almost half—comes from vegetable oils, shortening, butter, and margarine.

Hidden Fats

Potatoes, rice, bagels—low-fat foods, right? Not if you're talking about some supermarket varieties. When buying processed foods, look at ingredients lists for hidden saturated fats in the form of tropical oils (coconut, palm, and palm kernel), hydrogenated or partially hydrogenated vegetable oils (hydrogenation makes an oil more saturated), as well as cheese and butterfat. The following is a sampling of unlikely places where saturated fats often lurk:

Side dishes
Packaged potato mixes
Packaged rice dishes
Stuffing/breading mixes
Frozen vegetables in sauce
Gravies (canned or bottled)
Refried beans

Snacks
Crackers
Bagel/pita bits
Microwave popcorn

Breakfast foods
Granola cereals
Nondairy creamers
Flavored instant coffee mixes
Toaster pastries

three times as much trans fat as was previously estimated—especially since food makers, pressured to reduce the use of highly saturated tropical oils (such as palm and coconut), have generally replaced them with hydrogenated oils. The fact is, no one really knows how much trans fat we eat. For one thing, food manufacturers often change the types of oils they use and the degree of hydrogenation of the oils. In addition, nutrition labels don't specify how much trans fat is in the foods.

Fats and heart disease

Many factors affect blood cholesterol levels and thus the risk of developing cardiovascular disease. Surprisingly, there does not appear to be a simple direct relationship between *dietary* intake of cholesterol and *blood* cholesterol levels in all people. Researchers estimate that only about 20 percent of the population is genetically hypersensitive to dietary cholesterol—that is, their blood cholesterol levels jump when they eat high-cholesterol foods. There's no simple test for cholesterol hypersensitivity. (For more information on cholesterol, see pages 46-53.)

Nevertheless, dietary changes, especially involving fats, *can* have a significant effect on blood cholesterol levels. In fact, the type of fat you eat influences blood cholesterol levels more than dietary cholesterol does. *Saturated fats* usually elevate the levels of LDL cholesterol and raise overall cholesterol levels. That's why limiting your cholesterol intake but not your consumption of saturated fats can result in high blood cholesterol.

In contrast, *polyunsaturated fats* tend to lower the amount of LDL cholesterol, thus reducing the amount of artery-clogging cholesterol in the bloodstream. For this reason, highly polyunsaturated vegetable oils—such as safflower, sunflower, and soybean—used to be considered the most healthful oils. However, some animal studies using large quantities of polyunsaturated fat have suggested that in addition to lowering LDL cholesterol, polyunsaturated fats also lower the beneficial HDL cholesterol—and scientists now believe that a *low* HDL level is an independent risk factor for heart disease. In addition, studies on animals have found that large amounts of highly polyunsaturated vegetable oils increase the risk of several types of cancer—but that's not necessarily true for humans.

Some studies have shown that *monounsaturated fats,* such as olive oil and canola oil, may be able to reduce total cholesterol by decreasing the amount of damaging LDL cholesterol in the blood without producing a reduction, or as much of a reduction, in heart-healthy HDL cholesterol. Monounsaturated fats may also result in less oxidation of LDL (this chemical process appears to trigger a chain of events that causes plaque to build up in artery walls and that subsequently leads to a heart attack). Though the evidence is weaker, some studies have also suggested that olive oil can help lower blood pressure and control blood sugar levels. Highly monounsaturated oils are especially good for cooking: when overheated, they develop fewer "free radicals"—chemical agents that may be dangerous to human cells—than polyunsaturated oils do.

Still, no responsible scientists recommend that Americans simply add olive or canola oil to their food. Like other oils, they are 100 percent fat and contain 120 calories per tablespoon, and thus may cause you to gain weight. The important part of the equation is to use olive oil to *replace* animal fats and highly polyunsaturated oils.

Whether *nut oils,* such as peanut oil and macadamia nut, which are high in

Butter—or margarine?

Butter, lard, and coconut oil contain more saturated fat than margarine, so they probably raise blood cholesterol more than margarine. Butter and lard also contain cholesterol, while margarine doesn't. Still, if your diet is otherwise low in fat, you needn't worry about occasionally eating small amounts of butter, margarine, or any high-fat food. If, however, you eat lots of margarine and many processed foods that contain hydrogenated oils, try to cut back.

In general, the more solid the vegetable oil, the more hydrogenated it is, and therefore the more trans fatty acids it has—which is why tub and liquid "squeeze" margarines are preferable to stick margarine. "Diet" margarines are even better, since they are very soft and contain more water and only half the fat of other margarines.

Another option is to rely on vegetable oils for cooking and baking, as well as at the table (for example, dip bread in olive oil instead of spreading margarine on it).

Fish Oil Supplements

Fish oil has a protective effect on heart disease because it lowers trigylceride levels and reduces the tendency of the blood to clot. Researchers speculate that this is why Eskimos and the Japanese, whose diets include vast amounts of fatty fish, have such a low incidence of cardiovascular disease.

In light of this, a wide array of fish oil supplements have come on the market appealing to those who want the advertised benefits, but not the fish. But these supplements are not the great nutritional breakthrough they are advertised to be. Here are a few reasons why you should get your fish oil from fish, not from pills:

•Many questions remain about the effectiveness, safety, and optimal dose of fish oil in its various forms. Not much is known about potential long-term side effects either. In other words, we have no idea what is an optimal and safe dose of fish oil.

•Those same Eskimos who have a low incidence of heart disease have a high risk of hemorrhagic stroke, perhaps because of the decreased clotting ability of their blood. Fish oil's anti-clotting effect can be dangerous in an accident or during surgery.

•Fish oil in liquid (such as in cod liver oil) or in capsule form may contain pesticides or other contaminants, especially if it is made from fish livers, where these compounds tend to concentrate. Furthermore, cod liver oil is overly rich in vitamins A and D, which can be toxic in high doses (no more than a tablespoon or two a day should be taken).

•Prolonged consumption of fish oil may result in a vitamin E deficiency. Some manufacturers have therefore added this vitamin to their supplements.

•It is unclear whether fish oil by itself provides all the health benefits of fish. These fatty acids may work with other elements in the fish not found in the supplements. On the other hand, some supplements contain ingredients of questionable value, such as lecithin.

•Besides its oil, fish is rich in protein, iron, B vitamins, and other nutrients. Also, it can take the place of meats that are high in saturated fat. Pills cannot cancel out the effects of a high-fat, high-cholesterol diet. You don't have to eat huge amounts of fish to improve your cardiovascular health. Studies suggest that two to three servings a week are enough.

Calculating Fat Calories

To determine the percentage of calories from fat in a food, follow these steps:

Example:
325 calories, 11 grams of fat (per serving or unit):

1. Multiply the number of grams of fat in a serving by 9 (the number of calories in a gram of fat).
11 x 9 = 99

2. Divide the result by the number of calories in a serving.
99 ÷ 325 = 0.3046

3. Multiply your answer by 100, then round to the nearest whole number.
0.3046 x 100 = 30.46 or 30

This food would get 30 percent of its calories from fat.

---

monounsaturated fat, also help to reduce heart disease risk is not clear at this time. Several studies have suggested that nuts may offer beneficial effects. For instance, a study published in the *Journal of the American College of Nutrition* in 1992 found that people on a low-fat diet lowered their total and LDL cholesterol levels significantly when they started eating 3.5 ounces of almonds a day. Another study, using walnuts instead of almonds and published in the *New England Journal of Medicine,* found similar results. And a study of Seventh Day Adventists suggested that those who ate nuts most often had the lowest risk of heart attack. These results are promising, but it is still too early to recommend a daily handful of nuts—which are very high in calories—as a way to ward off heart attacks.

Eating large amounts of any kind of fat increases your chance of becoming overweight or obese, which is another risk factor in cardiovascular disease. Reducing overall fat intake and raising the *ratio* of unsaturated to saturated fats is no guarantee of protection against heart disease, but it does increase the odds in your favor because it has the potential to lower blood cholesterol levels. *Such a diet is recommended to everyone, especially if you have elevated blood cholesterol levels, or if you smoke, have high blood pressure, have a family history of heart disease, or are in another high-risk group for heart disease.*

The special role of fish oil

Fish oil contains a unique kind of polyunsaturated fatty acid called omega-3, which fish get by eating certain plants, particularly (text continued on page 116)

Fat and Cholesterol Content of Foods

Fat. The amount of fat in a serving of each food is listed in grams (there are about 28 grams in an ounce). Foods high in fat are printed in BLUE; this indicates that more than 30 percent of their calories come from fat. While you should limit your intake of the foods in blue, you don't have to avoid them entirely. The key to a healthy diet is to balance high- and low-fat foods so that no more than 30 percent of your daily calories come from fat.

Saturated fat. This is the type of fat that can raise blood cholesterol levels. Foods high in saturated fat (more than 10 percent of the total calories) have an "S" printed next to their fat

content. The major sources of saturated fat are meat (notably beef, pork, lamb, and cold cuts), poultry skin, whole-milk dairy products (such as cheese and butter), and three vegetable oils—coconut, palm, and palm kernel.

Cholesterol. The second most important dietary factor in controlling your blood cholesterol level is limiting your intake of cholesterol from foods. You should consume no more than 300 milligrams of cholesterol a day. Cholesterol is found only in animal products, such as meats, fish, poultry, eggs, milk, and cheese. Plant foods—such as grains, fruits, vegetables, and vegetable oils—contain no cholesterol.

This chart is designed to help you reduce the amount of fat and cholesterol you consume each day. Charts elsewhere in the book provide you with more nutritional information.

DAIRY AND EGGS

	Calories	Fat (g)	Saturated Fat (g)	Cholesterol (mg)
Cheese				
American, 1 oz	105	9 S	4	27
American spread, 1 oz	82	6 S	4	16
Blue, 1 oz	100	8 S	5	21
Cheddar, 1 oz	115	9 S	6	30
Cottage, creamed, ½ cup	108	5 S	3	15
Cottage, low-fat, ½ cup	104	2	1	10
Cream, 1 oz	100	10 S	6	31
Feta, 1 oz	75	6 S	4	25
Gouda, 1 oz	101	8 S	5	32
Mozzarella, part skim, 1 oz	72	5 S	3	16
Mozzarella, whole milk, 1 oz	80	7 S	4	22
Muenster, 1 oz	105	9 S	5	27
Parmesan, 2 tbsp	50	4 S	2	8
Provolone, 1 oz	100	8 S	5	20
Ricotta, part skim, ½ cup	170	10 S	6	38
Ricotta, whole milk, ½ cup	216	16 S	10	63
Swiss, 1 oz	105	8 S	5	26
Milk and Cream				
Buttermilk, 1 cup	100	2	1	9
Chocolate milk, whole, 1 cup	208	8 S	5	30

	Calories	Fat (g)	Saturated Fat (g)	Cholesterol (mg)
Eggnog, 1 cup	342	19 S	11	149
Heavy cream, whipped, ¼ cup	103	11 S	7	41
Evaporated milk, skim, 1 cup	200	1	0	9
Half and half, 1 tbsp	20	2 S	1	6
Milk, 2% fat, 1 cup	120	5 S	3	18
Milk, 1% fat, 1 cup	100	3 S	2	10
Milk, skim, 1 cup	85	0	0	4
Milk, whole, 1 cup	150	8 S	5	33
Sour cream, ¼ cup	123	12 S	8	26
Yogurt				
Low-fat, fruit, 1 cup	230	2	2	10
Low-fat, plain, 1 cup	145	4 S	2	14
Nonfat, plain, 1 cup	125	0	0	4
Whole milk, plain, 1 cup	140	7 S	5	29
Eggs				
Egg, whole	75	5 S	2	213
Egg, yolk	60	5 S	2	213
Egg, white	15	0	0	0

FATS AND OILS

	Calories	Fat (g)	Saturated Fat (g)	Cholesterol (mg)
Butter, 1 tbsp	100	11 S	7	31
Cocoa butter, 1 tbsp	120	14 S	8	0
Coconut oil, 1 tbsp	120	14 S	12	0
Lard, 1 tbsp	115	13 S	5	12
Palm oil, 1 tbsp	120	14 S	7	0
Palm kernel oil, 1 tbsp	120	14 S	11	0
Vegetable oil, other, 1 tbsp	120	14 S	2	0
Margarine, liquid, 1 tbsp	102	11 S	2	0
Margarine, soft tub, 1 tbsp	100	11 S	2	0
Margarine, stick, 1 tbsp	100	11 S	2	0
Mayonnaise, imitation, 2 tbsp	70	6 S	1	8
Mayonnaise, regular, 2 tbsp	198	22 S	3	16
Tartar sauce, 1 tbsp	75	8 S	1	4

	Calories	Fat (g)	Saturated Fat (g)	Cholesterol (mg)
Salad dressings				
Blue cheese, 2 tbsp	154	16 S	3	0
French, low calorie, 2 tbsp	44	2 0	0	0
French, regular, 2 tbsp	134	13 S	3	0
Italian, low calorie, 2 tbsp	32	3 0	0	0
Italian, regular, 2 tbsp	137	14 S	2	0
Russian, low calorie, 2 tbsp	46	1 0	0	0
Russian, regular, 2 tbsp	151	16 S	2	0
Thousand island, low calorie, 2 tbsp	50	4 0	0	4
Thousand island, regular, 2 tbsp	120	12 S	2	8

BREADS AND GRAINS

Breads and pastries	Calories	Fat (g)	Saturated Fat (g)	Cholesterol (mg)
Bagel, plain	200	2	0	0
Bread, French, 1 slice	100	1	0	0
Bread, Italian, 1 slice	85	0	0	0
Breadcrumbs, dry, grated, 1 cup	390	5	2	5
Bread, (oatmeal, white, wheat, whole-wheat, rye), 1 slice	65	1	0	0
Croissant, 1	235	12 S	4	13
Danish, fruit, 2½ oz	235	13 S	4	56
Doughnut, glazed, 2½ oz	235	13 S	5	21
English muffin, 1	140	1	0	0
Pancake, from mix, 1 (4")	60	2	1	16
Pita bread, 1	165	1	0	0
Tortillas, corn	65	1	0	0
Waffle, from mix, 3 oz	205	8 S	3	59
Cereals, hot, cooked				
Corn grits, 1 cup	145	0	0	0
Cream of Wheat, 1 cup	86	0	0	0
Oatmeal, 1 cup	145	2	0	0
Wheatena, 1 cup	168	1	0	0
Cereals, ready to eat				
All Bran, 1 cup	204	2	0	0
Cheerios, 1 cup	88	2	0	0

	Calories	Fat (g)	Saturated Fat (g)	Cholesterol (mg)
Corn flakes, 1 cup	88	0	0	0
Granola, ⅓ cup	125	5 S	3	0
Raisin Bran, 1 cup	180	1	0	0
Rice Krispies, 1 cup	110	0	0	0
Shredded Wheat, 1 cup	176	2	0	0
Wheaties, 1 cup	100	0	0	0
Crackers				
Graham crackers, plain, 2	60	1	0	0
Melba toast, plain, 4	80	0	0	0
Rye wafers, 4	110	2	1	0
Saltines, 4	50	1 S	1	4
Snack type, round, 4	60	4 S	1	0
Wheat, thin type, 4	35	1 S	1	0
Whole-wheat, 4	70	4 S	1	0
Grains and pasta				
Barley, cooked, 1 cup	200	2	0	0
Couscous, cooked, 1 cup	201	0	0	0
Egg noodles, cooked, 1 cup	200	2	1	50
Noodles, chow mein, canned, 1 cup	220	11	2	5
Pasta, cooked, 1 cup	190	1	0	0
Rice, brown, cooked, 1 cup	230	1	0	0
Rice, white, cooked, 1 cup	225	0	0	0
Rice, wild, cooked, 1 cup	166	1	0	0

LEGUMES

	Calories	Fat (g)	Saturated Fat (g)	Cholesterol (mg)
Black beans, cooked, 1 cup	225	1	0	0
Great northern beans, cooked, 1 cup	210	1	0	0
Kidney beans, canned, 1 cup	230	1	0	0
Lentils, cooked, 1 cup	215	1	0	0
Lima beans, cooked, 1 cup	260	1	0	0

	Calories	Fat (g)	Saturated Fat (g)	Cholesterol (mg)
Navy beans, cooked, 1 cup	225	1	0	0
Pinto beans, cooked, 1 cup	265	1	0	0
Soybeans, cooked, 1 cup	298	15	2	0
Split peas, cooked, 1 cup	231	1	0	0
Tempeh, ½ cup	165	6	1	0
Tofu (regular), 4 oz	80	5 S	1	0

FISH AND SHELLFISH

(4 oz except caviar)	Calories	Fat (g)	Saturated Fat (g)	Cholesterol (mg)
Carp, cooked	185	8	2	96
Caviar, 2 tbsp	80	6 S	1	188
Cod, cooked	120	1	0	63
Clams, breaded, fried	231	13 S	3	70
Clams, cooked	169	2	0	77
Crab, Alaskan king, cooked	111	2	0	61
Crayfish, cooked	130	1	0	203
Haddock, cooked	128	1	0	86
Halibut, cooked	160	3	0	47
Lobster, cooked	112	1	0	82
Mackerel, cooked	299	21 S	5	83
Mussels, cooked	197	5	1	64
Oysters, cooked	157	6	1	125
Perch, cooked	134	1	0	131
Pike, cooked	129	1	0	57
Salmon, pink, canned	159	7	2	45

(4 oz)	Calories	Fat (g)	Saturated Fat (g)	Cholesterol (mg)
Salmon, sockeye, fresh, cooked	247	13	2	99
Sardines, canned in oil, with bones	238	13 S	3	162
Scallops, breaded and fried	245	13 S	3	70
Scallops, cooked	128	1	0	61
Shrimp, breaded and fried	277	14	2	202
Shrimp, cooked	113	1	0	223
Snapper, cooked	146	2	0	54
Squid, fried	200	8	2	297
Swordfish, cooked	177	6	2	57
Trout, rainbow, cooked	173	5	1	83
Tuna, light, canned in oil	226	9	2	21
Tuna, light, canned in water	150	2	0	21
Tuna, blue fin, fresh, cooked	210	7	2	56

POULTRY

Chicken (4 oz)	Calories	Fat (g)	Saturated Fat (g)	Cholesterol (mg)
Dark meat, with skin, roasted	289	18 S	5	104
Dark meat, without skin, roasted	234	11 S	3	106
Light meat, with skin, roasted	254	12 S	3	96
Light meat, without skin, roasted	198	5	1	97
Light meat, with skin, batter dipped, fried	316	18 S	5	96
Capons, with skin, roasted	262	13 S	4	98
Goose				
With skin, roasted	349	25 S	8	104
Without skin, roasted	272	14 S	6	110

Turkey (4 oz)	Calories	Fat (g)	Saturated Fat (g)	Cholesterol (mg)
Breast meat, without skin, roasted	154	1	0	95
Dark meat, with skin, roasted	253	13 S	4	102
Dark meat, without skin, roasted	214	8 S	3	97
Light meat, with skin, roasted	225	9 S	3	87
Light meat, without skin, roasted	179	4	1	79
Turkey roll, light meat	168	8 S	2	0
Duck				
With skin, roasted	385	32 S	11	96
Without skin, roasted	230	13 S	5	101

BEEF

(4 oz)	Calories	Fat (g)	Saturated Fat (g)	Cholesterol (mg)
Beef frankfurter (cured)	360	32 S	14	70
Bottom round, trimmed, select cut, braised	245	10 S	4	110
Bottom round, untrimmed, prime cut, braised	285	14 S	5	110
Brisket, trimmed, braised	275	14 S	7	106
Brisket, untrimmed, braised	447	37 S	15	106
Chuck, blade roast, trimmed, select cut, braised	293	16 S	6	121
Chuck, blade roast, untrimmed, choice cut, braised	443	35 S	15	118
Corned beef, cooked	287	22 S	7	112
Eye of round, trimmed, roasted	209	8 S	3	79
Ground beef, lean, baked (medium)	306	20 S	8	89
Ground beef, extra lean, broiled	291	18 S	7	113
Ground beef, regular, broiled	333	21 S	9	115
Liver, pan fried	248	9 S	3	551
Pastrami	399	33 S	12	106
Prime rib, trimmed, broiled	320	22 S	9	94
Rib eye, trimmed, choice cut, broiled	257	14 S	6	91

(4 oz)	Calories	Fat (g)	Saturated Fat (g)	Cholesterol (mg)
Rib eye, untrimmed, choice cut, broiled	337	24 S	10	95
Round, trimmed, select cut, broiled	210	8 S	3	94
Salami	299	24 S	10	74
Sirloin, trimmed, broiled	238	10 S	4	102
Sirloin, untrimmed, (all grades), broiled	320	20 S	9	58
T-bone steak, choice cut, trimmed, broiled	245	12 S	5	91
T-bone steak, untrimmed, choice cut, broiled	370	28 S	12	96
Tenderloin, trimmed, roasted	240	13 S	4	98
Tenderloin, untrimmed, prime cut, broiled	363	26 S	11	98
Top loin, trimmed, select cut, broiled	217	9 S	3	87
Top loin, untrimmed, prime cut, broiled	279	16 S	6	86
Top round, trimmed, select cut, broiled	192	4	1	96
Top round, untrimmed, prime cut, braised	271	13 S	5	97

PORK

	Calories	Fat (g)	Saturated Fat (g)	Cholesterol (mg)
Bacon, 3 strips	109	9 S	3	16
Bologna, 1-oz slice	70	6 S	2	14
Canadian bacon, grilled, 4 oz	211	9 S	3	66
Ham, fresh, trimmed, roasted, 4 oz	251	13 S	4	107

	Calories	Fat (g)	Saturated Fat (g)	Cholesterol (mg)
Ham, fresh, untrimmed, roasted, 4 oz	336	22 S	9	106
Pork loin, trimmed, roasted, 4 oz	238	11 S	4	92
Sausage, Italian, cooked, 4 oz	369	31 S	10	89

VEGETABLES AND JUICES

	Calories	Fat (g)	Saturated Fat (g)	Cholesterol (mg)		Calories	Fat (g)	Saturated Fat (g)	Cholesterol (mg)
Artichoke, cooked, 1 cup	55	0	0	0	Peppers, sweet, raw, 1	20	0	0	0
Asparagus, cooked,					Potatoes, baked with skin,				
4 spears	15	0	0	0	1 large	220	0	0	0
Beans, snap, cooked, 1 cup	45	0	0	0	Potatoes, french fried,				
Bean sprouts, raw, 1 cup,	30	0	0	0	in vegetable oil, 2 oz	160	8 S	3	0
Beets, cooked, 1 cup	55	0	0	0	Potatoes, mashed, with milk,				
Broccoli, cooked, 1 cup	45	0	0	0	and margarine, 1 cup	225	9	2	4
Brussels sprouts, cooked,					Potato salad, with				
1 cup	60	1	0	0	mayonnaise, 1 cup	360	21	4	170
Cabbage, raw, 1 cup,	15	0	0	0	Pumpkin, canned, 1 cup	85	1	0	0
Carrot, raw, 1 medium,	30	0	0	0	Sauerkraut, 1 cup	45	2	0	0
Cauliflower, cooked, 1 cup	30	0	0	0	Spinach, raw, 1 cup	10	0	0	0
Celery, 1 stalk	5	0	0	0	Squash, summer, cooked,				
Corn, cooked, 1 cup,	135	0	0	0	1 cup	35	1	0	0
Cucumber, 6 large slices	5	0	0	0	Sweet potatoes, baked,				
Eggplant, cooked, 1 cup	25	0	0	0	1 medium	115	0	0	0
Jerusalem artichoke,					Tomatoes, canned, 1 cup	50	1	0	0
raw, 1 cup,	115	0	0	0	Tomatoes, raw 1 medium	25	0	0	0
Kale, cooked, 1 cup	40	1	0	0	Tomato juice, 1 cup	40	0	0	0
Lettuce, 1 cup	10	0	0	0	Tomato paste, 1/4 cup	55	1	0	0
Mushrooms, raw, 1 cup	20	0	0	0	Tomato sauce, 1 cup	75	0	0	0
Okra, 8 pods	25	0	0	0	Turnips, cooked, 1 cup	30	0	0	0
Onions, chopped, 1/4 cup	14	0	0	0	Vegetable juice cocktail,				
Parsnips, cooked, 1 cup	125	0	0	0	1 cup	45	0	0	0
Peas, cooked, 1 cup	125	0	0	0	Water chestnuts, 1 cup	70	0	0	0

FRUITS AND JUICES

	Calories	Fat (g)	Saturated Fat (g)	Cholesterol (mg)		Calories	Fat (g)	Saturated Fat (g)	Cholesterol (mg)
Apple, 1 medium	80	0	0	0	Grapes, 10	35	0	0	0
Apple juice, 1 cup	115	0	0	0	Grape juice, 1 cup	155	0	0	0
Applesauce, unsweetened,					Honeydew melon,				
1 cup	105	0	0	0	4-oz slice	45	0	0	0
Apricots, 3	50	0	0	0	Kiwi, 1	45	0	0	0
Apricots, canned in juice,					Nectarines, 1 medium	65	1	0	0
1 cup	120	0	0	0	Orange, 1 medium	60	0	0	0
Apricots, dried, 5 medium					Orange juice, 1 cup	110	0	0	0
halves	42	0	0	0	Peaches, 1 medium	35	0	0	0
Avocado, 1 medium	305	30 S	5	0	Peaches, canned in juice,				
Banana, 1 medium	105	1	0	0	1 cup	110	0	0	0
Blackberries, 1 cup	75	1	0	0	Pear, 1 medium	120	1	0	0
Blueberries, 1 cup	80	1	0	0	Pineapple, fresh, 1 cup	75	1	0	0
Cantaloupe, 1/2	95	1	0	0	Pineapple, canned in juice,				
Cherries, 10	50	1	0	0	2 slices	70	0	0	0
Cranberry juice cocktail,					Pineapple juice, 1 cup	140	0	0	0
1 cup	145	0	0	0	Plums, 1 medium	35	0	0	0
Cranberry sauce, canned,					Prunes, 5	115	0	0	0
1 cup	420	0	0	0	Prune juice, 1 cup	180	0	0	0
Dates, 5	115	0	0	0	Raisins, 1 oz	80	0	0	0
Figs, 5	238	1	0	0	Raspberries, 1 cup	60	1	0	0
Grapefruit, 1/2 medium	40	0	0	0	Strawberries, whole, 1 cup	45	1	0	0
Grapefruit juice,					Tangerines, 1 medium	35	0	0	0
unsweetened, 1 cup	95	0	0	0	Watermelon, diced, 1 cup	50	1	0	0

NUTS AND SEEDS

	Calories	Fat (g)	Saturated Fat (g)	Cholesterol (mg)		Calories	Fat (g)	Saturated Fat (g)	Cholesterol (mg)
Almonds, 1 oz	165	15	1	0	Peanuts, roasted in oil, 1 oz	165	14 S	2	0
Cashews, dry roasted, 1 oz	165	13 S	3	0	Peanut butter, 2 tbsp	190	16 S	3	0
Chestnuts, roasted, 1 oz	69	1	0	0	Pecans, 1 oz	190	19	2	0
Coconut, dried, shredded, sweetened, 1 oz	143	10 S	8	0	Pistachios, 1 oz	165	14 S	2	0
Hazelnuts, 1 oz	180	18	1	0	Sesame seeds, 1 tbsp	45	4 S	1	0
Macadamia, roasted in oil, 1 oz	205	22 S	3	0	Sunflower seeds, 1 oz	160	14 S	2	0
					Walnuts, 1 oz	180	18	2	0

SWEETS AND SNACKS

	Calories	Fat (g)	Saturated Fat (g)	Cholesterol (mg)		Calories	Fat (g)	Saturated Fat (g)	Cholesterol (mg)
Cakes (2-oz slice)					**Frozen desserts**				
Angel food	125	0	0	0	Ice cream, ½ cup	135	7 S	4	30
Coffee cake	180	5	1	28	Ice cream, premium, ½ cup	175	12 S	7	44
Devil's food, with chocolate frosting	191	6 S	3	28	Ice milk, ½ cup	92	3 S	2	9
Gingerbread	156	4	1	0	Sherbet, ½ cup	135	2	1	7
Carrot, with cream cheese frosting	225	12	2	43	Sorbet, ½ cup	100	0	0	0
Cheesecake	170	11 S	6	103	Fruit and juice bars	70	0	0	0
Candy (1 oz)					**Pies** (2-oz slice)				
Caramels	115	3 S	2	1	Apple	146	6 S	2	0
Chocolate, milk, with almonds	150	10 S	5	5	Blueberry	137	6	1	0
Fudge	115	3 S	2	1	Custard	119	6 S	2	61
Jelly beans	105	0	0	0	Lemon meringue	142	6 S	2	57
Marshmallows	90	0	0	0	Pecan	230	13	2	38
					Pumpkin	115	6 S	2	39
Condiments					**Puddings**				
Chocolate topping, fudge type, 2 tbsp	125	5 S	3	0	Chocolate, ½ cup	150	4 S	2	15
Jam or jelly, 1 tbsp	55	0	0	0	Custard, baked, 1 cup	305	15 S	7	278
Honey, 1 tbsp	65	0	0	0	Rice, ½ cup	155	4 S	2	15
Maple syrup, 2 tbsp	122	0	0	0	Tapioca, ½ cup	145	4 S	2	14
Cookies					**Snack foods**				
Chocolate chip, 4 small	185	11 S	4	18	Cheese puffs, 1 oz	160	10 S	4	0
Fig bars, 4	210	4	1	27	Popcorn, 1 cup, air popped	30	0	0	0
Oatmeal raisin, 4	245	10 S	3	2	Popcorn, popped in oil, with 1 tbsp butter, 1 cup	155	15 S	8	31
Peanut butter, 4	245	14 S	4	22	Potato chips, 1 oz	150	10 S	3	0
Shortbread, 4	155	8 S	3	27	Pretzels, 1 oz	110	1	0	0
Vanilla wafers, 4	74	3 S	1	10	Tortilla chips, 1 oz	150	8	1	0

FAST FOOD

	Calories	Fat (g)	Saturated Fat (g)	Cholesterol (mg)		Calories	Fat (g)	Saturated Fat (g)	Cholesterol (mg)
Cheeseburger, single, plain, on bun	320	15 S	6	50	French fries, fried in vegetable oil, regular order	235	12 S	4	0
Cheeseburger, 2 patties, with condiments, on double-decker bun	649	35 S	13	94	Hamburger, single, plain, on bun	275	12 S	4	36
Chicken, fried, dark meat, 2 pieces	430	27 S	7	165	Pancakes, with butter and syrup	519	14	6	57
English muffin, with egg, cheese, Canadian bacon	383	20 S	9	234	Pizza, cheese, one slice	109	3	1	7
Fish sandwich, with tartar sauce	431	23	5	55	Potato, baked, with cheese sauce and broccoli	402	21 S	9	20
					Roast beef sandwich, plain	346	14	4	52
					Salad, tossed, with chicken	105	4	1	72

those growing in cold water. Omega-3s significantly reduce blood clotting. They make platelets less likely to stick together and adhere to blood vessels, lessening the chance of a heart attack due to a coronary artery clot. Fish oil may also prevent hardening of the arteries, since it appears to be even more effective than polyunsaturated vegetable oils in lowering triglyceride levels in the blood, while slightly raising HDL cholesterol.

The best way to get omega-3s is to include at least two servings of fatty fish, such as salmon or mackerel, per week in your diet. Fish oil pills, a highly advertised alternative, can actually be dangerous (see box on page 110). Vegetable oils are also being touted as alternative sources of omega-3s, but they contain only linolenic acid and not the longer-chain eicosapentaenoic acid (EPA) and docosa-

Most packaged microwave popcorn contains as much fat (partially hydrogenated soybean, cottonseed, or coconut oil) per ounce as most cookies, along with more than twice as many calories as conventional popcorn. It's also high in sodium. Make your own at home using a hot-air or microwave popper, which requires no oil, and use the salt-shaker sparingly.

Lower-Fat Substitutes

Instead of eating:	Substitute:	To save:
1 croissant	1 plain bagel	35 calories, 10 grams fat
1 whole egg	1 egg white	65 calories, 6 grams fat
1 oz cheddar cheese	1 oz part-skim mozzarella	43 calories, 4 grams fat
1 oz cream cheese	1 oz cottage cheese (1% fat)	74 calories, 9 grams fat
1 tbsp whipping cream	1 tbsp evaporated skim milk,	32 calories, 5 grams fat whipped
4 oz skinless roast duck	4 oz skinless roast chicken	53 calories, 8 grams fat
4 oz beef tenderloin, choice, untrimmed, broiled	4 oz beef tenderloin, select, trimmed, broiled	86 calories, 11 grams fat
4 oz lamb chop, untrimmed, broiled	4 oz lean leg of lamb, trimmed, broiled	250 calories, 32 grams fat
4 oz pork spareribs, cooked	4 oz lean pork loin, trimmed, broiled	180 calories, 18 grams fat
1 oz regular bacon, cooked	1 oz Canadian bacon, cooked	111 calories, 12 grams fat
1 oz hard salami	1 oz extra-lean roasted ham	75 calories, 8 grams fat
1 beef frankfurter	1 chicken frankfurter	67 calories, 8 grams fat
4 oz oil-pack tuna, light	4 oz water-pack tuna, light	76 calories, 7 grams fat
1 regular-size serving fast-food french fries	1 medium-size baked potato	125 calories, 11 grams fat
1 oz oil-roasted peanuts	1 oz roasted chestnuts	96 calories, 13 grams fat
1 oz potato chips	1 oz thin pretzels	40 calories, 9 grams fat
1 oz corn chips	1 oz plain air-popped popcorn	125 calories, 9 grams fat
1 tbsp sour cream dip	1 tbsp bottled salsa	20 calories, 3 grams fat
1 glazed doughnut	2-oz slice angel food cake	110 calories, 13 grams fat
3 chocolate sandwich cookies	3 fig bar cookies*	4 grams fat
1 oz unsweetened chocolate	3 tbsp cocoa powder	73 calories, 13 grams fat
1 cup ice cream (premium)	1 cup sorbet	150 calories, 24 grams fat

Fig bar cookies have 15 more calories.

hexaenoic acid (DHA) found in fish oils. While fish are able to convert the linolenic acid in algae and other sea plants into EPA and DHA, the human body cannot do this to any significant degree. Nor has it been shown that the fatty acids in these oils can reduce blood clotting as much as marine omega-3s.

Fats and cancer

Many scientists have noted that, with a few exceptions, countries with a high national fat intake also have the highest cancer rates. Some studies have suggested that a diet high in fat—saturated or unsaturated—increases the risk of cancer of the colon and breast, and possibly of the ovary, uterus, and prostate. Most recently, a study presented to the American Cancer Society found that among nonsmoking women, the risk of an uncommon form of lung cancer increases dramatically along with saturated-fat intake.

By far the strongest evidence concerns the link between a high fat intake and colon cancer. For other kinds of cancer, fat's role remains controversial. Nonetheless, a low-fat diet makes sense if you're concerned about cancer, particularly since it helps guard against becoming overweight or obese, which in itself is a risk factor for certain cancers, as well as diabetes and heart disease.

The mechanism for the link between a high-fat diet and cancer has not been determined, but there are theories. A diet high in fat affects the secretion of some sex hormones, which might cause cancer in the reproductive organs. Moreover, high-fat diets increase the amount of bile acids in the colon, which may be converted by bacteria into carcinogenic by-products.

How much fat should you eat?

Virtually all health organizations and government agencies recommend that Americans reduce their fat intake and blood cholesterol levels. The American Heart Association and American Cancer Society say that no more than 30 percent of all calories consumed each day should come from fats. While most Americans consume about twice as much saturated as polyunsaturated fats, the American Heart Association recommends approximately equal amounts: less than 10 percent of all caloric intake should come from saturated fat, up to 10 percent from polyunsaturated fats, and the remainder from monounsaturated fats.

Some health professionals advocate that total fat consumption should drop to 20 percent, and a few recommend that only 10 percent of calories come from fats. But eliminating that much dietary fat is difficult, and unnecessary for most people.

Should children follow a low-fat diet?

Cardiologists generally agree that limiting a child's fat intake *from age two onward* will help reduce the odds against eventually developing coronary heart disease. Since the average American is estimated to have one chance in three of a significant cardiovascular event (such as a heart attack or stroke) before age sixty, prevention is important.

The major symptoms of clogged coronary arteries seldom become manifest until adulthood. However, the fatty streaks and fibrous plaques that are probable precursors of atherosclerosis can appear in early childhood. Autopsies of young soldiers killed in battle during World War II and the Korean and Vietnam conflicts

Fat substitutes

Walk down the aisles of your supermarket and you'll get a glimpse of the future: foods made with fat replacers. For instance, there are now dozens of ice-cream clones with the taste and texture of real ice cream, but with little or no fat. To approximate the creamy texture of ice cream (or salad dressing or mayonnaise), they use fat substitutes such as Simplesse (made from whey), as well as a variety of carbohydrate-based compounds, such as maltodextrin and polydextrose, which trap water and thus create a moist texture. Food manufacturers are constantly experimenting with these and other compounds to get a better imitation fat. One of the newest of these carbohydrate compounds — called Oatrim (also called TrimChoice)—even contains the soluble fiber in oats and barley, and may lower blood cholesterol levels and have other modest health benefits. One thing is certain: it is better for you than the fats it replaces.

often revealed a significant accumulation of coronary plaque. It is estimated that 5 percent of all five- to fourteen-year-olds in the United States have blood cholesterol levels above 200 mg/dl. *All high-risk children—those with a parent who develops any form of cardiovascular disease before age fifty-five or a parent who has high blood cholesterol that is not controllable by diet—should have a cholesterol test.* The American Health Foundation and some pediatricians recommend routine testing of all children between the ages of two and five to get a baseline cholesterol reading.

You should limit fat intake to 30 percent of the total calories in a child's diet (over age two), with less than 10 percent of daily calories coming from saturated fat. Cholesterol intake should be no more than 100 milligrams for each 1,000 calories consumed, not to exceed 300 milligrams a day.

The overall diet must, of course, be nutritionally balanced, and its total calorie count adjusted to your child's growth rate so as to maintain a desirable body weight. Restricting the fat will help overweight children lose unwanted pounds, but that is not the diet's primary purpose.

More important, the diet is likely to produce a small, but noticeable, decrease (10 percent on average) in your child's cholesterol level. Best of all, the diet can start your child on a long life of healthful eating habits.

How to cut down on fat

These tips will help you reduce your intake of fat—especially saturated fat:

•Read labels carefully to determine both the amount and type of fats in packaged foods you buy. To determine the number of calories that come from fat, multiply the grams of fat in a serving by nine. Then divide this number by the total calories in the serving to get the percentage of calories coming from fats.

•Substitute fish or chicken (preferably light meat, skinless) for some red meat.

•Eat more meatless meals. Use vegetables or grains as the main dish.

•Select lean meats and eat smaller portions (three to five ounces). Trim off all visible fat.

•Use skim or low-fat milk and milk products.

•Limit your intake of fats and oils, particularly those high in saturated fat, such as butter, cream, lard, heavily hydrogenated fats (some margarines), shortenings, and foods containing coconut or palm oil. Choose a margarine that has at least twice as much polyunsaturated fat as saturated.

•Broil, bake, or boil foods instead of frying them in fat.

•Moderate your use of fat-laden snack foods, such as potato chips and corn chips as well as cookies, cakes, and pastries.

Protein

Much has been said about protein in our diets—that we need it (as of course we do), that athletes should load up on it, that not all proteins are created equal, that we eat too much protein and should therefore cut down our consumption of meat and dairy products and fall back on fruits and vegetables to maintain ourselves. How much protein do we need to be healthy?

The basic component: amino acids

Aptly enough, the word "protein" is derived from a Greek root meaning "of first importance," and protein—which constitutes about one-fifth of an adult's body weight—is the basic material of life. Muscles, organs, bones, cartilage, skin, antibodies, some hormones, and all enzymes (the compounds that direct chemical reactions in cells) are made of protein.

Yet protein is not a single, simple substance, but a multitude of chemical combinations. The basic structure of protein is actually a chain of amino acids that can form many different configurations and can combine with other substances. Twenty-two amino acids have been identified in the proteins of the human body. The possible arrangements can be almost infinite, and tens of thousands of different proteins have been identified.

Proteins are constantly being broken down in our bodies. Most of the amino acids are reused, but we must continually replace some of those that are lost. This process is known as protein turnover. Our need to keep this process going begins at conception and lasts throughout life. Without dietary protein, growth and all bodily functions would not take place.

While plants and some bacteria can manufacture all the amino acids they need, the human body can manufacture only thirteen. The amino acids we can make are known, somewhat confusingly, as the "nonessential" amino acids. They are in fact essential, but not as part of our diet. The nine "essential" amino acids are those we have to eat. They are histidine, isoleucine, leucine, lysine, methionine, phenylalanine, threonine, tryptophan, and valine. We can either get them from plant protein directly or by eating animals that consume plants and animals.

When we eat foods containing protein, the digestive system breaks it down to the constituent amino acids, which enter the body "pool" of amino acids. Each cell then assembles the proteins it needs using the building blocks available. If, however, one or more of the needed amino acids is in short supply or not available at all, others that may be on hand cannot be utilized to form a protein. This is why it is important to eat a diet that contains all of the essential amino acids plus enough additional amino acids to allow for synthesis of the "nonessential" amino acids.

Getting complete protein

Nutritionists use the phrases "complete protein" and "incomplete protein" to describe the proteins provided by various foods. If a food supplies a sufficient amount of the nine essential amino acids, it is called a complete protein. Virtually all proteins from animal foods are complete. Foods that lack or are short on one or more of the nine essential amino acids—such as some fruits, grains, and vegetables—are called incomplete proteins. Such plant-derived foods can nonetheless be excellent sources of protein if eaten in complementary combinations that supply all of the essential amino acids. For example, the amino acids missing in a vegetable can be provided by eating a grain product, another vegetable, or an animal-derived protein on the same day.

A more specific example: bread, a staple of the human diet for thousands of years, is rich in the amino acid methionine, but low in lysine. Legumes are rich in lysine, but poor in methionine; when legumes and bread are eaten together, however, you get a complete protein. That lunch box favorite the peanut butter sandwich is an example of this complementarity. The peanuts provide the amino acids that the grain lacks, and vice versa.

Without understanding the chemical reasons for what they were doing, cooks the world over have come up with complementary combinations of proteins: beans or peas or lentils and rice; beans and brown bread or cornbread; corn and lima beans. Most of the diets in the world contribute adequate amino acids and protein; an exception is a diet based mostly on tubers (such as sweet potato or manioc), common in some parts of Africa.

Animal vs. vegetable

That meat and other animal products are the most readily available sources of complete protein is perhaps the reason why humans have been such ardent hunters and fishers, as well as domesticators of animals. The protein content, by weight, of cooked meat, fish, poultry, and milk solids is between 15 and 40 percent. The protein content of cooked cereals, beans, lentils, and peas ranges from 3 to 10 percent. Potatoes, fruits, and leafy green vegetables come in at 3 percent or lower. Soybeans and nuts have a protein content comparable to meat, but, depending upon how they are prepared, their proteins may not be as easily digested. However, recent research suggests that in a mixed or even totally vegetarian diet, the issue of

Do you have to eat complementary proteins at the same meal?

No. Contrary to common belief, you don't have to combine complementary foods at the same meal to get a complete protein—you can eat them a few hours apart or even much later in the day. For example, a study at Loma Linda University in California found that animals fed rice and beans at separate meals grew as quickly as animals fed these complementary proteins at the same meal.

If you eat a wide variety of foods (grains, vegetables, legumes, and seeds each day, you're likely to absorb a full complement of amino acids.

Protein Requirements

The body cannot store protein, so it needs a fresh supply every day. The Food and Nutrition Board of the National Academy of Sciences has established a daily Recommended Dietary Allowance (RDA) for protein based on a person's age and weight. According to the Academy, because most people in the United States eat meat and dairy products regularly, the average protein intake is higher than what most people need. So you should easily meet the following RDAs:

•The RDA for adults is 0.8 grams of protein for each kilogram (2.2 pounds) of body weight. This works out to 44 grams for a 120-pound person, 55 grams of protein for a weight of 150 pounds, and 66 grams for 180 pounds. These allowances assume that you eat a mixed diet of proteins—some high-quality (complete), some low-quality (incomplete).

•If, like most Americans, you consume mostly high-quality protein, your total requirement will therefore be *slightly* less. If you get almost all your protein from plant sources, it will be *slightly* greater. The variation due to the type of diet is no more than approximately 15 percent.

•Children under eighteen need some additional protein to allow for growth, and the younger they are, the more protein they need per pound of body weight.

•Pregnant women are allocated an additional 10 grams of protein per day by the RDA, lactating mothers an extra 12 to 15 grams during the first six months.

digestibility is not too important. For someone eating a whole grain and vegetable diet, no more than 15 percent of the protein consumed would be unavailable because of problems with digestibility.

The fact that we are omnivorous, that is, we can eat both meats and plants, has contributed to the survival of the human species. But as anthropologists have pointed out, human beings have overwhelmingly preferred meat to other foods, when they could get it. And a number of experts attribute the general good health, increased height, and longevity of people in developed countries today to their high-protein diets (this theory, however, ignores other important environmental factors that have led to improved health).

Other authorities regard American's meat eating as excessive, since it is a source of saturated fat, which may contribute to coronary heart disease, cancer, and stroke. Moreover, a diet high in animal protein—typical for adult Americans—increases the loss of calcium in the body (though no long-term studies have been done to indicate whether a habitual high-protein intake increases the risk of osteoporosis). Another potential problem with such a high-protein diet is the strain it puts on the kidneys in having to excrete extra waste products from the protein breakdown.

Fortunately, nutritionists have found that adding even small amounts of animal protein to plant foods can boost their protein quality—for example, using a light meat sauce on spaghetti, sprinkling cheese on macaroni, or adding half a cup of milk to breakfast cereal.

Can extra protein make you stronger?
The cells of muscles, tendons, and ligaments have to be maintained with protein. Hemoglobin, which carries oxygen through the bloodstream, is a protein. Given these physiological facts, many people try to eat more protein in their quest for a stronger body or to improve athletic performance. Others actually want to add poundage, preferably in the form of muscle. In the old days, in their quest for added protein, athletes were likely to wolf down T-bone steaks or drink raw eggs. Today they often turn to high-tech, high-protein powders, liquids, tablets, wafers, capsules, and bars.

Don't swallow such claims for enhancing strength or adding muscle bulk: they have not been supported by studies on athletes. A basic understanding of how protein works in the body helps explain why. Protein is indeed needed to build and maintain not only muscles but all cells in the body. But consuming more protein won't by itself stimulate muscle growth. Excess protein simply breaks down in the body and is burned for energy (though carbohydrates and fats are the main energy sources) or, if not used, is most likely converted to fat. Thus, though many people believe the more protein they eat the better, this is simply not true.

Besides protein, the supplements usually contain isolated amino acids, vitamins and minerals, and sometimes more exotic ingredients such as ginseng and bee pollen. These products' protein sources include whey, soy, egg white, gelatin, yeast, and nonfat dry milk. Most contain thirteen to twenty-three grams of protein per dose, as much as two or three ounces of chicken or other meat, though some tablets and wafers have only a few grams of protein. While some of the supplements claim that their isolated amino acids are better absorbed by the body than whole protein, healthy individuals have no problem digesting and absorbing the amino acids from whole protein. Furthermore, consuming large quantities of isolated amino acids is

Protein supplements and extra pounds

The one promise that protein supplements are likely to deliver on is weight gain: they are meant to be consumed in addition to your regular food, and many of the supplements are calorie-dense. Consumed as directed in two glasses of whole milk, some powders can add more than 1,000 calories a day to your diet.

The weight you gain will probably be mostly fat, however, unless you start to exercise more. Only strength-building exercise, not supplements, builds muscles. Excessive amounts of protein offer no benefits whatsoever, but can produce serious negative effects, chiefly dehydration, diarrhea, and calcium loss, and may aggravate liver or kidney disease as well.

Sources of Protein

The foods below are all good sources of protein. The listed protein amounts are averages. Many foods that are relatively high in protein are also high in fat, so the chart indicates the percentage of fat accompanying each food. Try to limit your intake of protein sources that derive more than 30 percent of their calories from fat.

	Protein (g)	Fat Calories
Dairy and eggs		
Cheddar cheese, 1 oz	7	70%
Cottage cheese (2% milk fat), ½ cup	16	17%
Egg, 1 medium	6	68%
Ice cream, hard, vanilla, ½ cup	2	48%
Milk, skim, 1 cup*	8	5%
Mozzarella, part skim, 1 oz*	8	56%
Ricotta, part skim, ½ cup*	10	53%
Yogurt, low-fat, plain 1 cup*	12	25%
Meat and fish (4 oz)		
Chicken, light meat, roasted, no skin	31	26%
Ground beef, extra lean, broiled	33	56%
Sirloin steak, choice cut, trimmed, broiled	35	37%
Tuna, canned, in water	33	12%
Turkey breast, roasted, no skin	24	6%
Grains		
Oatmeal, 1 cup cooked	6	12%
Rice, brown, 1 cup cooked	5	4%
Spaghetti, 1 cup cooked	6	5%
Whole-wheat bread, 2 slices	6	13%
Legumes and nuts		
Almonds, 1 oz	6	82%
Cashews, dry roasted, 1 oz	4	71%
Lentils, ½ cup cooked	8	4%
Lima beans, ½ cup cooked	8	3%
Peanut butter, 2 tbsp	10	76%
Red kidney beans, ½ cup canned	8	4%
Soybeans, ½ cup cooked	10	38%
Tofu, 4 oz	9	55%

Low-fat dairy products often contain added milk solids, which increase the protein content slightly.

not advised, since the body needs a balanced mixture of amino acids in order to synthesize protein. The excessive intake of a single amino acid may interfere with the absorption of other amino acids, and as a result inhibit protein synthesis.

Other claims

Numerous claims have been made for the curative powers of various amino acids, and some are sold over-the-counter in drugstores and health food stores. One amino acid, lysine, has been touted as a treatment for herpes. Another, argenine, has been featured as a "growth hormone releaser" that makes you lose weight as you sleep. For more than twenty years, probably the most widely used amino acid supplement was L-tryptophan, which has been taken by millions of Americans. Some researchers have suggested that this amino acid relieves insomnia, but scientific studies are still inconclusive in that regard (see page 478). In fact, there is absolutely no scientific evidence to back up any of the health claims that have been made for amino acid supplements.

Moreover, unlike most vitamin supplements, for instance, amino acid pills are not on the Food and Drug Administration's Generally Recognized as Safe (GRAS) list. In fact, in December, 1989 the FDA halted all sales of L-tryptophan—and products in which it's listed as a major ingredient—because of the development of a blood disease in some people taking as little as one gram a day. Called eosinophilia-myalgia (EMS), the disease causes muscle pain and an abnormally high count of one type of white blood cell. It can result in high fever, weakness, joint pain, swelling of the arms or legs, rashes, shortness of breath, and death. More than 1,500 cases were reported at the time, and the FDA now estimates that the actual number was 5,000. At least thirty-eight people died, and more than 60 percent of the victims have remained crippled with painful nerve damage, severe joint pain, fatigue, and scarring of skin and internal organs. Most cases of EMS were associated with one particular manufacturer of tryptophan supplements—and evidence suggests that the EMS was caused by a contaminant. However, tryptophan itself hasn't been completely absolved as a cause of EMS.

Even though the FDA removed isolated amino acids from its GRAS list (which still includes vitamin and mineral supplements), the FDA did not enforce its ban because of legal wrangling. Consequently, over-the-counter amino acid supplements have remained in a regulatory limbo. But the EMS outbreak in 1989 forced the FDA to act on tryptophan—and to take a closer look at certain other dietary supplements as well. In 1993, an FDA task force recommended that tryptophan and other isolated amino acids be banned as food supplements (which need to meet less stringent government regulations) and instead be regulated as drugs. That makes sense, since they fit the FDA's definition of a drug: a product sold not for nutritional purposes, but to treat or prevent disease, or to affect the structure and function of the body.

Even if isolated amino acid supplements continue to be marketed in catalogs and health-food stores, taking the supplements is, as a general rule, unnecessary and potentially unhealthy, unless there is a deficiency in the digestive system. Studies with animals have shown that abnormally large intakes of amino acids can create imbalances of those substances in the body. Certainly much more information is needed about the safety and efficacy of isolated amino acids before they can be recommended.

A normal diet: more than enough protein

You need adequate protein intake to build muscles, but if you eat a normal, balanced diet, it is hard *not* to get enough protein. Even strict vegetarians get enough of it if they eat grains and vegetables in proper quantities and combinations. Government surveys show that the typical American consumes about 100 grams of protein per day, nearly twice as much as the Recommended Dietary Allowance. For most people, five ounces of fish or meat supplies more than half the RDA, for instance, and two cups of milk would take care of the rest. In general, the RDA is easily met when 12 to 15 percent of your total caloric intake comes from protein.

Regardless of how much they exercise, even professional athletes do not need to go out of their way to consume extra protein. Recent studies suggest that some endurance athletes or heavy-duty weight lifters may need more protein than the RDA, but since they are usually consuming more calories, they get the extra protein with little trouble. Say, for instance, a body builder or wrestler consumes 4,000 calories a day; if 12 percent of these come from protein, he's consuming a whopping 120 grams of protein, much more than enough for any exercise regimen.

Since the only way to build muscle is to exercise, you should eat the same healthful diet recommended for everybody—one high in complex carbohydrates (bread, cereal, pasta, fruits, and vegetables) and low in fat (poultry, fish, lean meat, and low-fat dairy products). If you're trying to gain weight, just eat larger meals plus additional healthful snacks.

Four ounces of dry pasta provides about 20 percent of the RDA for protein, as much as two large eggs. And some high-protein pastas have twice that much.

Vitamins

Among the achievements this century will surely be remembered for is the discovery of vitamins—a scientific advance truly beneficial to humanity. For hundreds of years, of course, people had noticed that some foods seemed to prevent some diseases—most famously, the limes or lemons that British sailors ate to ward off scurvy—but the first vitamin was isolated in the lab only in 1911. That was thiamin, a B vitamin. Now thirteen vitamins are known. In the past, vitamins were discussed in terms of preventing deficiency diseases (beriberi, caused by a lack of thiamin, for instance, or scurvy, by a lack of vitamin C). The RDAs (Recommended Dietary Allowances), devised by scientists in the United States and revised and updated over the years, were designed partly to prevent such deficiency diseases and partly to meet the needs, as they have been understood, of healthy people.

But we still have much to learn about the functions of these powerful chemicals. Indeed, in the last decade alone, hundreds of scientific studies have found that vitamins play a much larger role in health than was dreamed of even twenty years ago.

What vitamins do

Vitamins are organic substances that your body requires to help regulate metabolic functions within cells. They are absolutely essential to life. Among the myriad tasks they perform are: promoting good vision, forming normal blood cells, creating strong bones and teeth, and ensuring the proper functioning of the heart and nervous system. More recently, researchers have uncovered the role vitamins play in preventing the damaging effects of oxygen on essential chemicals in the body. While vitamins themselves do not supply energy, some do aid in the efficient conversion of foods into energy.

The thirteen vitamins needed by humans are A, C, D, E, K, and eight vitamins often referred to as the B-complex—thiamine, riboflavin, niacin, B_6, pantothenic acid, biotin, folacin, and B_{12}. These can be categorized as either fat-soluble (A, D, E, K) or water-soluble (the B vitamins and vitamin C.) The distinction is important because the body stores fat-soluble vitamins, usually in the liver and fat tissue, for relatively long periods (many months); water-soluble vitamins, which are stored in various tissues, remain in the body only for a short time (up to a few weeks).

Each vitamin carries out specific functions, and if a certain vitamin is lacking or is improperly used by the body, a particular deficiency disease usually results. In such cases vitamins have worked miracles. Vitamin C has cured scurvy; vitamin A has cured night blindness; B vitamins have restored stamina and alleviated mental disturbances—but only when the lack of these vitamins in the diet was the cause.

In general, you have to consume vitamins: as a rule, your body cannot manufacture vitamins (though it does synthesize some vitamin K, D, and B_{12}, and convert beta carotene into vitamin A).

For a description of the specific functions and recommended intakes of each vitamin, consult the chart on page 126.

Vitamin supplements: a special prescription

The editorial board of the University of California at Berkeley *Wellness Letter,* headed by Dr. Sheldon Margen, has been reluctant to recommend supplementary vitamins on a broad scale for healthy people eating healthy diets. However, the accumulation of research in recent years has prompted a change in attitude, at least where four vitamins are concerned. These are the three so-called antioxidant vitamins, plus the B vitamin folacin. The role these substances play in disease prevention is no longer a matter of dispute.

The antioxidant vitamins are E and C, as well as beta carotene, a plant form of vitamin A. (Beta carotene, one of the carotenoids, is not strictly classified as a vitamin; once thought to be effective only after being converted to vitamin A in the body, it now appears to have important functions of its own.) Acting at the molecular level, these antioxidants inactivate a class of particles known as free radicals, which in humans are most commonly "activated" oxygen molecules. Free radicals can damage basic genetic material, cell walls, and other cell structures, and eventually this damage can become irreparable and lead to disease. The antioxidant vitamins help mop up free radicals before they do their dirty work.

A high intake of vitamins C and E and beta carotene seems to be protective against many kinds of cancer, including oral, esophageal, and reproductive. Vitamin E, in particular, may lower the risk of heart disease by reducing the build-up of plaque in coronary arteries. Vitamins C and E seem to play a protective role against cataracts. Antioxidants may even delay some effects of aging. Indeed, we are only beginning to understand their importance and how they work.

Though not an antioxidant, folacin (also called folic acid or folate) has been shown to prevent certain birth defects, and increased intakes of folacin are now recommended to all women in their childbearing years, unless they are absolutely certain of not becoming pregnant. Folacin may also protect against cancer, at least cervical cancer. More discoveries about folacin will undoubtedly be forthcoming.

Ideally your vitamins should come chiefly or entirely from your diet rather than from pills. Indeed, supplements cannot substitute for a healthy diet. There's a simple reason for this: foods supply much else besides vitamins—minerals, fiber, carbohydrates, proteins, and fats, as well as elements we have not yet even discovered. Furthermore, many nutrients require synergy: vitamin C helps you utilize iron, for instance, and vitamin E helps you use vitamin K. But even if you do eat a very healthy diet, and most Americans do not, it's unlikely you will get the high levels of folacin and of the antioxidant vitamins many authorities think you need. A recent government survey found that only 9 percent of Americans are eating the recommended minimum of five servings of fruits and vegetables a day.

Optimal doses of these vitamins are still far from agreed on. Dr. Gladys Block of the University of California at Berkeley and other scientists have called for serious national debate on the issues of fortifying more foods with vitamins and recommending supplementation for more groups. Folacin may soon be added to breads and cereals, which are already enriched with other B vitamins.

What you should do

The first step is to eat a very healthy diet—at least five servings of fruits and vegetables daily, six to eleven servings of grains, especially whole grains, two or three servings of low-fat or nonfat dairy products, and small servings of meats and fish.

Myth: Vitamin B_{12} shots give energy.

Fact: *Only if you have a B_{12} deficiency, which can indeed cause pernicious anemia. Just a small portion of people who frequently feel run-down have anemia, however, and a B_{12} deficiency may not even be the cause.*

Since one sign of pernicious anemia is extreme fatigue, the notion arose that B_{12} injections could make weary people feel more energetic, even if they don't have a B_{12} deficiency. There is no good scientific evidence for this. Some studies have suggested that B_{12} shots can boost the energy of such people, but most of these studies were poorly designed.

Vitamin B_{12} is found only in animal products, so strict vegetarians may become deficient, though this is relatively rare (they can get B_{12} from supplements). If you have symptoms of pernicious anemia—extreme weakness and neurologic problems such as disorientation and weakness in limbs—ask your doctor about tests to measure B_{12} in the body. Don't try to treat such problems without a diagnosis.

Vitamins: Benefits and Sources

Vitamin/Food Sources	What It Does/Potential Benefits	Adult RDA*/Supplementation
Vitamin A. Liver, eggs, fortified milk, fish, and fruits and vegetables that contain beta carotene.	Promotes good vision; helps form and maintain healthy skin and mucous membranes. May protect against some cancers and increase resistance to infection in children.	800 RE (4,000 IU), women; 1,000 RE (5,000 IU), men. No supplementation recommended, since toxic in high doses.
Beta carotene. Carrots, sweet potatoes, cantaloupe, leafy greens, tomatoes, apricots, winter squash, red bell peppers, broccoli, mangoes.	Converted into vitamin A in the intestinal wall. As an antioxidant, it combats adverse effects of free radicals in the body. May reduce the risk of certain cancers as well as coronary artery disease (CAD).	No RDA; experts recommend 5-6 mg (milligrams). For supplementation, 6-15 mg (equal to 10,000-25,000 IU of vitamin A) a day for anyone not consuming several carotene-rich fruits or vegetables daily. Nontoxic.
Vitamin C (ascorbic acid). Citrus fruits and juices, strawberries, peppers (especially red), broccoli, potatoes, kale, cauliflower, cantaloupe.	Promotes healthy gums and teeth; aids in iron absorption; maintains normal connective tissue; helps in healing of wounds. As an antioxidant, it combats adverse effects of free radicals. May reduce the risk of certain cancers, as well as CAD; may prevent or delay cataracts.	60 mg. For supplementation, 250-500 mg a day for anyone not consuming several fruits or vegetables rich in C daily, and for smokers. Larger doses may cause diarrhea.
Vitamin D. Milk, fish oil, fortified margarine; also produced by the body in response to sunlight.	Promotes strong bones and teeth by aiding absorption of calcium. Helps maintain blood levels of calcium and phosphorus. May reduce the risk of osteoporosis.	5 mcg (micrograms), or 200 IU; 10 mcg, or 400 IU, before age 25. For supplementation, 400 IU for people who don't drink milk or get sun exposure, especially strict vegetarians and the elderly. Toxic in high doses.
Vitamin E. Nuts, vegetable oils, margarine, wheat germ, leafy greens, seeds, almonds, olives, asparagus.	Helps in formation of red blood cells and utilization of vitamin K. As an antioxidant, it combats adverse effects of free radicals. May reduce the risk of certain cancers, as well as CAD; may prevent or delay cataracts; may improve immune function in the elderly.	8 mg, women; 10 mg, men (12-15 IU). For supplementation, 200-800 IU advised for everyone (you can't get that on a low-fat diet). No serious side effects at that level, though diarrhea and headaches have been reported.
Vitamin K. Body produces most of daily needs; the rest is supplied by cauliflower, broccoli, leafy greens, cabbage, milk, soybeans, eggs.	Essential for normal blood clotting.	60-65 mcg, women; 70-80 mcg, men. No supplementation necessary or recommended.
Vitamin B₁ (thiamine). Whole grains, dried beans, lean meats, liver, wheat germ, nuts, fish, brewer's yeast.	Helps the body's cells convert carbohydrates into energy; necessary for healthy brain, nerve cells, and heart function.	1-1.1 mg, women; 1.2-1.5 mg, men. No supplementation necessary or recommended.
Vitamin B₂ (riboflavin). Dairy products, liver, meat, chicken, fish, leafy greens, beans, nuts, eggs.	Helps cells convert carbohydrates into energy; essential for growth, production of red blood cells, and health of skin and eyes.	1.2-1.3 mg, women; 1.4-1.7 mg, men. No supplementation necessary or recommended.
Vitamin B₃ (niacin). Nuts, meat, fish, chicken, liver, dairy products.	Aids in release of energy from foods; helps maintain healthy skin, nerves, and digestive system. Large doses lower elevated blood cholesterol.	13-19 mg. Megadoses may be prescribed by doctor to lower cholesterol. May cause flushing, liver damage, and irregular heart beat.
Vitamin B₅ (pantothenic acid). Whole grains, dried beans, eggs, milk, liver.	Vital for metabolism of food and production of essential body chemicals.	No RDA; experts recommend 4-7 mg. No supplementation necessary or recommended.
Vitamin B₆ (pyridoxine). Whole grains, bananas meat, beans, nuts, wheat germ, chicken, fish, liver.	Important in chemical reactions of proteins and amino acids; helps maintain brain function and form red blood cells. May boost immunity in the elderly.	1.6 mg, women; 2 mg, men. Megadoses can cause numbness and other neurological disorders.
Vitamin B₁₂. Liver, beef, pork, poultry, eggs, dairy products, shellfish.	Necessary for development of red blood cells; maintains normal functioning of nervous system.	2 mcg. Strict vegetarians may need supplements. Despite claims, no benefits from megadoses.
Folacin (folate or folic acid). Leafy greens, wheat germ, liver, beans, whole grains, broccoli, citrus fruit.	Important in the synthesis of DNA, in normal growth, and in protein metabolism. Adequate intake reduces risk of certain birth defects. May reduce risk of cervical cancer.	180 mcg, women; 200 mcg, men. Premenopausal women can benefit from supplements—400 mcg— to help prevent birth defects.
Biotin. Eggs, milk, liver, brewer's yeast, mushrooms, bananas, grains.	Important in metabolism of protein, carbohydrates, and fats.	No RDA; experts recommend 30-100 mcg. No supplementation necessary or recommended.

These figures are not applicable to pregnant women, who need additional vitamins and should seek professional advice.

In addition, you should consider taking supplements of the antioxidant vitamins and, if you are a premenopausal woman, folacin (see chart).

Most people do *not* need a daily multivitamin and mineral supplement, although millions of Americans take one. It can't be said too often that a pill a day won't turn a poor diet into a healthy one. However, the following groups of people may benefit from a daily multivitamin or have special needs that can be met through taking supplements.

Pregnant women. According to the RDAs, pregnant women should get at least 15 to 50 percent more vitamins each day (and 100 percent more vitamin D), and they should continue to consume extra amounts of folacin. Some physicians recommend supplements during pregnancy, though a woman can generally meet her increased vitamin needs through a good diet. Because pregnant women have special needs, they should seek professional advice.

The elderly. Some elderly people may need supplements because they reduce their consumption of foods that are good sources of vitamins.

Frequent aspirin takers. Aspirin interferes with the metabolism of vitamin C and folacin, so people who take aspirin regularly—arthritis sufferers, for example—should ask their physicians about supplements.

Heavy drinkers. Heavy alcohol consumption often depletes B vitamins and vitamin C in the body.

Smokers. People who smoke appear to use up vitamin C at a faster rate than nonsmokers. Thus, the RDA for smokers is 100 milligrams (as compared to 60 milligrams for nonsmoking adults). A balanced diet—indeed, even an eight-ounce glass of orange juice—easily satisfies this higher RDA.

Taking huge doses of most vitamins is not wise. Some vitamins—A and D, specifically—are toxic in large doses. Others, like niacin, have serious side effects in large doses. Excess amounts of the water-soluble vitamins, in particular, will simply be eliminated by the body. In planning your diet and in taking supplements, stick with amounts recommended in the chart.

Minerals

Scientists have been paying great attention to minerals in recent years, looking for links between them and the major chronic diseases—high blood pressure, osteoporosis, cardiovascular disease, diabetes, and even cancer. This research has been very promising. Encouraged by this, and by advertising, Americans now take a variety of mineral pills. But who really needs mineral supplements?

The minerals that are nutrients are absolutely essential to a host of vital processes in the body, from basic bone formation and enzyme synthesis to the regulation of the heart muscle and the normal functioning of digestion. Many are necessary for the activity of enzymes, proteins that serve as catalysts in the body's chemical reactions. Unlike the organic compounds we call vitamins, minerals are inorganic substances—that is, they do not contain carbon—that are basic constituents of the earth's crust. Carried into the soil, groundwater, and sea by erosion, they are taken up by plants and consumed by animals and humans. The minerals in food are indestructible—even if you burn your food to a cinder, it will retain all its original minerals. However, when food is boiled, some of its minerals may dissolve into the water and be discarded. Minerals can also be processed out of foods, as when whole wheat is refined to make white flour.

The essential twenty-two

While there are more than sixty different minerals in the body, those currently identified as essential number some twenty-two. Of these, seven—calcium, chloride, magnesium, phosphorus, potassium, sodium, and sulfur—are generally designated as "macrominerals," or major minerals; those that are present in the healthy body in quantities exceeding 0.005 percent of body weight. The other fifteen are termed "microminerals," or trace minerals, and include chromium, copper, fluorine (fluoride), iodine, iron, manganese, molybdenum, selenium, and zinc—to name those best understood at present. The daily intakes of these are miniscule; some are measured in micrograms, or one-millionth of a gram. Very possibly the list of recognized microminerals will grow as researchers succeed in mapping in greater detail the complex chemistry of life.

As components of the body, minerals are present in small amounts. All together, they add up to perhaps 4 percent of the body weight. But this amount is in no way indicative of the relative importance of minerals to the functioning body. The 0.00004 percent of your body that is iodine is no less critical to survival than the approximately 1.5 to 2 percent that is calcium.

Recommended intakes

Precisely how much of any mineral the body needs to maintain good health is still debated by experts. Consequently, the National Academy of Sciences has issued Recommended Dietary Allowances (RDAs) for just seven minerals; for five others, the National Academy of Sciences makes what are more cautiously termed "estimated safe and adequate daily dietary intakes." Both types of intakes are covered in

Maximizing Minerals

Selected Minerals/Major Food Sources	What It Does	Adult RDA or Estimated Safe and Adequate Intake
Calcium. Milk and milk products, sardines and salmon eaten with bones, dark green leafy vegetables, shellfish, some tofu, some fortified cereals.	Builds bones and teeth, maintains bone density and strength; helps prevent or minimize osteoporosis; helps regulate heartbeat, blood clotting, muscle contraction, and nerve conduction. May help prevent hypertension. See also pages 136-137.	1,200 milligrams (mg), age 11-24 and during pregnancy; 800 mg, age 25 and over (1,500 mg for women over 50, according to NIH panel).
Chlorine (chloride) Table salt, fish.	Helps maintain fluid and acid-base balance; component of gastric juice. Important in metabolism of carbohydrates and fats. Deficiency may impair action of insulin and the regulation of glucose in the blood.	None.
Chromium. Meat, cheese, whole grains, brewer's yeast, fortified cereals.	Important in metabolism of carbohydrates and fats. Deficiency may impair action of insulin.	50-200 micrograms (mcg).*
Copper. Shellfish, nuts, beans, seeds, organ meats, whole grains, potatoes.	Formation of red blood cells; helps keep bones, nerves, and immune system healthy.	1.5-3 mg.*
Fluorine (fluoride). Fluoridated water and foods grown or cooked in it, marine fish (with bones), tea,.	Contributes to solid bone and tooth formation; may help prevent osteoporosis.	1.5-4 mg.*
Iodine. Primarily from iodized salt, but also seafood, seaweed food products, vegetables grown in iodine-rich areas. Widely dispersed in food supply.	Necessary for function of the thyroid gland and thus for normal cell metabolism; prevents goiter (enlargement of thyroid).	150 mcg; 175 during pregnancy.
Iron. Liver, kidneys, red meats, eggs, peas, beans, nuts, dried fruits, green leafy vegetables, enriched grain products, fortified cereals. Cooking in iron pots adds iron, especially to acidic food.	Essential to formation of hemoglobin (which carries oxygen in the blood) and myoglobin (in muscle); part of several enzymes and proteins in the body. Heme iron, found in animal products, is better absorbed by the body than nonheme iron, found in plants. See page 142.	15 mg, women age 11-50; 10 mg, women age over age 50; 10 mg, men; 30 mg during pregnancy.
Magnesium. Wheat bran, whole grains, raw leafy green vegetables, nuts (especially almonds and cashews), soybeans, bananas, apricots, spices.	Aids in bone growth; aids function of nerves and muscles, including regulation of normal heart rhythm. Low intake has been linked to high blood pressure, heart-rhythm abnormalities, and heart attack.	280 mg, women; 350 mg, men; 320 mg during pregnancy.
Manganese. Nuts, whole grains, vegetables, fruits, instant coffee, tea, cocoa powder, beans.	Needed for energy production and reproduction. May also be essential for building bones. Excess may interfere with iron absorption.	2-5 mg.*
Molybdenum. Peas, beans, cereal grains, organ meats, some dark green vegetables.	Aids in bone growth and strengthening of teeth; important in energy metabolism.	75-250 mcg.*
Phosphorus. Meats, poultry, fish, dairy products, eggs, dried peas and beans, soft drinks, nuts; present in almost all foods.	Helps build bones and teeth and form cell membranes and genetic material. Vital for energy production.	1,200 mg, ages 11-24 and during pregnancy; 800 mg, age 25 and over.
Potassium. Most foods, especially oranges and orange juice, bananas, potatoes (with skin), dried fruits, yogurt, meat, poultry, milk.	Vital for muscle contraction, nerve impulses, and function of heart and kidneys. Helps regulate water balance in cells and blood pressure.	1,600-2,000 mg minimum.*
Selenium. Fish, shellfish, red meat, grains, eggs, chicken, garlic, organ meats; amount in vegetables depends on soil.	Part of enzymes that act as antioxidants to fight cell damage (see page 23). Needed for proper immune response. Large doses can be toxic.	55 mcg, women; 70 mcg, men; 65 mcg during pregnancy.
Sodium. Table salt, salt added to prepared foods (like cheese, smoked meats, and fast foods), baking soda.	Helps regulate blood pressure and water balance in the body.	2,400 mg maximum.*
Zinc. Oysters, crabmeat, liver, eggs, poultry, brewer's yeast, wheat germ, milk, beans.	Important in activity of enzymes for cell division, growth, and repair (wound healing) as well as proper functioning of immune system. Maintains taste and smell acuity.	12 mg, women; 15 mg, men and during pregnancy.

*No RDA established. Instead, because less is known about these nutrients, the National Academy of Sciences has proposed ranges of Estimated Safe and Adequate Daily Dietary Intake.

Chelated Minerals

The term "chelation" (pronounced "key-lay-shon") comes from the Greek for "claw" because this process binds a metallic element to another substance. The chelated minerals found on more and more drugstore shelves—most often iron, zinc, magnesium, potassium, or calcium—are generally bonded to amino acids, the chemicals which are the building blocks of protein.

The manufacturers claim that by being linked to amino acids, chelated minerals are absorbed more quickly by the body. Non-chelated minerals, they say, must wait in the intestine until they are combined with amino acids, which slows their absorption. In fact, when the chelated supplement reaches the intestine, the mineral is quickly separated from the amino acids and absorbed like nonchelated minerals. There is no evidence that chelated minerals are absorbed any quicker or better than other minerals.

Take away the amino acids from chelated minerals and you have ordinary mineral supplements, which most people don't need anyway, since a varied and balanced diet provides all the minerals they need. Unless prescribed by a doctor, no one should take doses of mineral supplements greater than the RDAs or estimated safe intakes because of the complex interactions between minerals and the dangers of overdosing.

Don't confuse chelated minerals with oral chelation products. These combinations of vitamins, minerals, and amino acids have been banned by the Food and Drug Administration (FDA) as unapproved drugs.

the chart on page 129. Because of the complex interactions between minerals and the dangers of overdosing, no one should self-prescribe mineral supplements in amounts greater than the RDAs or estimated intakes. (Too much calcium in supplement form, for example, can interfere with the absorption of iron and other minerals.) If you believe you ought to increase your mineral intake, make changes in your diet according to the chart or get professional advice.

Significant mineral deficiencies—or excesses—are rare among Americans. If anything, the problem is that we consume too much of some minerals. Excess phosphorus, which impairs the absorption of iron, may be a problem for people who habitually consume soft drinks. Americans also tend to consume sodium excessively, contributing to high blood pressure, kidney disease, and heart disease.

Iodine deficiency, which causes goiter and other thyroid disturbances, was once a major health problem in certain inland parts of the United States where iodine was absent from the soil and thus from food crops. But the widespread use of iodized table salt and the nationwide marketing of food products from areas that do have high iodine content make iodine deficiency a rare condition in developed countries today.

Of all minerals, Americans are most likely to consume too little calcium, iron, and zinc. A lack of zinc can delay puberty, impair the healing of wounds, and decrease sensations of taste and smell. And low levels of zinc in pregnant women may lead to fetal abnormalities. Calcium and iron deficiencies are more commonly found in women than in men and are frequently related to the physiological demands of childbearing and menstruation. (These two minerals are covered in greater detail in the following chapter.)

Sodium, Calcium, and Iron

Sodium, calcium, and iron are three minerals of particular concern in the American diet. On average, we consume too much of one (sodium), and too little of the others. This chapter explains the functions of each of these minerals and provides you with suggestions on how to alter your intake of them.

Sodium: Too Much

Many people do not realize that there is some sodium in nearly everything we eat. Chemically, sodium is a metallic element, and it is usable in the human system only when it occurs in combination with another element. Its most common form is table salt (NaCl, or sodium chloride), which is actually only about 40 percent sodium. A number of unprocessed foods contain salt, but usually not in significant amounts; much of the salt that we consume we add deliberately, usually to enhance flavor. Salt is also an effective preservative, and for thousands of years salted fish and meats and brine-treated vegetables have been staples of the human diet.

How much is too much?

For a number of years many doctors and public health officials have been warning people about the dangers of consuming excessive amounts of sodium, and the public has reacted to a remarkable degree. In the last several years our intake of salty foods has fallen off by 30 percent, and the food industry—alert to this trend—is introducing an increasing number of processed foods that are lower in sodium.

Yet our per capita sodium intake is still very high—between two and three times the recommended maximum daily intake of 2,400 milligrams.

The convenience foods and fast foods and snacks that Americans love are often storehouses of salt. But fast foods are not necessarily the worst culprits. A meal in the most expensive restaurant—or dinner on the airplane—may be loaded with salt. Many recipe books tell us to add salt to anything we cook. (See chart on page 135 for the sodium content of commonly eaten foods.) In addition, there is sodium in baking powder, in the flavor-enhancer MSG (monosodium glutamate), and in such widely used preservatives as sodium benzoate and sodium propionate. The milligram count goes up more if you drink beverages containing sodium saccharin or take any of dozens of over-the-counter medicines such as antacids and cough syrups. When you add up the sodium in a day's ration of liberally salted home-cooked foods and then factor in the snack foods Americans eat so casually, the sum can be staggering. What will this do to people in the long run?

In light of the broad antisodium trend that has recently emerged, it may come as a surprise to hear that there is still a debate within the scientific community about what sodium intake to recommend. Sodium intake appears to be linked with hypertension, an ailment that leads to heart attacks, strokes, and kidney failure. Yet, of the 18 percent of the population with hypertension (and another 12 percent with borderline hypertension), only about half are sufficiently sensitive to sodium that they can be adversely affected by a high salt intake. A number of experts therefore believe that the majority of people do not need to reduce their sodium intake. So, they ask, why badger them about it?

On the other side of the question are arrayed equally respected experts who maintain that sodium is used to dangerous excess in our modern diet. They add that even though some people may never be made ill by a high salt intake, all of us must be cautious.

Need vs. craving

Sodium is not merely a flavor enhancer; it is a mineral essential to health. Sodium permeates the body. All cells in the body are bathed in a fluid that maintains cell function; this fluid contains particles that are mostly (90 to 95 percent) sodium salts. The ratio of particles to fluid determines the fluid balance of the entire body. If the body is retaining more sodium, it must also retain more water to maintain a proper particle/fluid ratio.

The body's daily requirement for sodium varies with each individual, but in any case the amount is quite small. The minimum sodium requirement is about 115 milligrams per day—roughly the amount of sodium in one-twentieth of a teaspoon of salt. The National Academy of Sciences recommends a minimum daily sodium intake of about 500 milligrams to maintain good health (though if you are sweating profusely, your intake may need to be higher).

In a healthy body many organs interact to regulate the amount of sodium in the system. The chief monitors are the kidneys, adrenal glands, heart, and brain. They do their job with amazing efficiency and accuracy. Although your sodium intake may vary from day to day, the amount of sodium in your body generally does not vary by more than 2 percent. Your regulatory system will conserve sodium if you need it and excrete it if you have an excess. However, the total amount of sodium in the body can be influenced significantly by substantial changes in diet, climate, or level of physical activity.

Does sea salt contain extra minerals?

No. Sea salt and table salt are essentially the same thing—sodium chloride. By law, anything sold as salt must be at least 97.5 percent sodium chloride, and some products (including sea salt) are even higher. Unrefined sea salt may contain small amounts of magnesium, sulphur, and potassium. By the time it is processed for the table, it's identical to regular salt. Actually ordinary table salt often does contain an essential mineral that sea salt does not offer—iodine. Sea salt is a favorite at health-food stores and in specialty foods, but it has no nutritional advantages, nor is it any less or more salty tasting.

All salt, by the way, comes originally from the sea. Even the salt that is mined out of the earth comes from ancient sea beds. Some commercial salt is still evaporated from sea water or from the Great Salt Lake in Utah.

Iodized Salt

Iodized table salt has been part of the American diet since the 1920s, when it was introduced to counteract a type of goiter (an enlargement of the thyroid) caused by the iodine deficiency then widespread in some parts of the country. With the advent of adding iodine to salt, goiter has nearly disappeared.

If you cut down on your salt intake, is there any reason to worry about getting enough iodine? Not really. We get our iodine from a variety of sources; in fact, only about 55 percent of the salt consumed in the United States is iodized. Iodine is widely dispersed in the food supply. It occurs in seafood and in crops grown near the seacoast, but its chief source is dairy products (cattle take it in from iodized salt licks and iodine-supplemented feed). Iodine is also used in some preparations to condition bread dough.

As a result, iodine deficiency is rare. The daily RDA is 150 micrograms, and the Food and Drug Administration's Total Diet Study shows that the average 2,900 calorie-a-day diet contains more than two-and-a-half times the RDA, excluding the use of iodized table salt. Only in the northernmost states are there truly low levels of iodine in the soil. In these areas, you may want to add a daily pinch of iodized table salt to your food—though remember that all you need is half a teaspoon of iodized salt *from all sources*, including processed foods, to meet your needs.

Flavor Without Salt

People who are placed on a low-sodium diet or those who choose to cut down on salt as a sensible health precaution often complain that foods aren't as tasty as they used to be, and that salt substitutes taste bitter. But retraining your taste buds is not so difficult. Your gustatory system has resources that you may have overlooked up to now.

Combining tastes

We can distinguish only four main taste sensations—sweet, sour, salty, and bitter—which may seem like a small repertoire until you consider the possible combinations. Not only can these four basic tastes be combined, but the other senses can be brought into play as well. For example, taste and smell are two entirely different sensory systems, but they greatly influence one another. Indeed, expert cooks have known for centuries that taste, aroma, texture, visual appeal, and temperature are all important parts of the sensation we call flavor. By selecting interesting foods, serving them attractively, and using alternate methods of adding tang to your foods, you can often compensate for the lack of salt.

Boosting flavor

A few drops of lemon juice, for example, not only perk up flavor but also seem to give even small amounts of salt more bounce. Just why a sour taste should work as an enhancer of or substitute for a salty taste when they are so different has never been explained. (Kosher cooks discovered the salt-sour crossover generations ago when they began using "sour salt," a preparation of powdered citric acid or tartaric acid, in place of sodium chloride in some dishes.) And don't forget herbs and spices, particularly the various forms of pepper. Many cuisines use vinegar and pepper in combination to stimulate taste buds.

Some packaged vegetable and herb mixtures contain salt, so be sure to check the ingredients listed on product labels.

Finding the sodium

When most people think about cutting back on sodium, they think about cutting back on the table salt from a salt shaker. But salt (NaCl, or sodium chloride) comes from other sources, and sodium comes in forms other than table salt. A few of the more commonly added sources of sodium are listed below.

Baking powder
Baking soda
Brine
Garlic salt
Kelp
Monosodium glutamate (MSG)
Onion salt
Sea salt
Sodium citrate
Sodium nitrate
Sodium phosphate
Sodium saccharin
Soy sauce

If the sodium level in the body falls acutely, it can trigger an appetite for salty foods—for example, after severe vomiting or diarrhea, or as a result of the profuse sweating that accompanies sustained and strenuous exercise on a very hot day. In such circumstances the body can release a hormone called angiotensin, which acts on the brain and can stimulate an intense appetite for salt (as demonstrated so far only in laboratory experiments with rats).

But the salt craving that people experience daily is not based on a physiological need for more sodium. It is instead a self-perpetuating cycle caused by salt itself. People who eat a lot of salty foods experience frequent cravings for sodium because their systems are used to it. The cycle can be broken with relative ease. People who are cutting down on salt generally report that it is not hard, certainly easier than giving up cigarettes, and that after several weeks they no longer crave foods that are highly salted.

Sodium and hypertension

Despite advances in our knowledge of how sodium functions in the body, the mechanism of hypertension and how sodium affects it is still not clearly understood. About 5 to 10 percent of the people who have high blood pressure develop it as a result of having diabetes or kidney disease. Such cases, called "secondary" hypertension, can be alleviated by treating the underlying disease. The remaining 90 to 95 percent of hypertension cases have what is known as "essential" hypertension and it is this condition that continues to puzzle researchers. The cause is unknown. But researchers have identified factors that, either alone or working in combination with one another, increase the risk of developing high blood pressure:

Are salt substitutes better than regular salt?

If you have high blood pressure and your doctor has told you that salt may endanger your health, then the answer is yes. Instead of sodium, the substitutes contain potassium, which may make your food taste bitter. People with kidney disease or certain endocrine diseases should avoid these substitutes.

"Lite" salts are combinations of sodium and potassium that contain about 40 percent of the sodium in common table salt, but taste almost as salty; however, they are not really sodium substitutes, since they still contain some.

Actually, if you do without salt or salt substitutes for a few weeks, you'll be surprised how quickly your taste buds adjust. See the box on page 133 for alternative ways to season foods.

cigarette smoking, habitual alcohol intake, obesity, psychological stress, certain dietary factors, and genetics. Age is also a factor: in industrialized societies, blood pressure tends to go up with age.

Studies have found that population groups that consume a lot of sodium tend to have a high incidence of hypertension, and groups that consume little sodium have a relatively low incidence. In northern Japan, for example, salt consumption is enormous—about twenty to twenty-five grams per day, which is three to four times higher than average consumption in the United States—and the prevalence of hypertension is also very high. Among the studies conducted to test the salt/hypertension link has been one in Kenya, among the Luo tribe. The preliminary findings indicate that the Luo who live in the countryside, where the diet is low in sodium, tend to have a low incidence of hypertension. But when members of this tribe migrate to urban areas, where the diet is higher in sodium, the incidence of hypertension goes up.

Many experts are reluctant to draw conclusions from studies such as these because other factors aside from salt intake may have influenced the levels of hypertension in these groups. For example, some rural diets include large amounts of fresh vegetables that are rich in potassium, a mineral that may protect against hypertension. And in the Kenya study, the rise in blood pressure was also associated with weight gain and psychological stress. More recently, though, a large international cooperative project called the Intersalt Study has offered convincing evidence of the relationship between sodium intake and blood pressure. Among ten thousand participants from thirty-two countries, researchers found that, with few exceptions, a low sodium intake was significantly correlated with a low incidence of high blood pressure.

While acknowledging that the results of the study are subject to various interpretations, the committee that directed Intersalt concluded that the evidence strongly supports the contention that sodium intake is an important factor in the occurrence of hypertension. Studies in twenty-four countries worldwide where salt intake could be accurately estimated also found a strong connection. In addition, numerous clinical trials have shown that reducing salt intake can lower blood pressure in people with normal blood pressure as well as hypertensives—and even lowering blood pressure by a few points can decrease the risk of heart attack and stroke. Health authorities in at least fourteen countries, including the United States, France, Japan, and Britain, advise reducing salt intake as one way of preventing high blood pressure.

Are you sodium sensitive?

Heredity also plays a key role in determining a person's susceptibility to hypertension. For reasons that are not at all clear, some people seem to be "sodium sensitive"; that is, their blood pressure responds to the level of sodium intake. Others are "sodium resistant" and do not show a significant rise in blood pressure even if they consume a lot of sodium. Current estimates indicate that up to 90 percent of the population is sodium resistant. Only 10 to 20 percent of the U.S. population is sodium sensitive. This group encompasses about half of the cases of hypertension in the United States.

Two recent studies have revealed that salt sensitivity increases with age. Researchers at the Indiana University School of Medicine measured the blood pressure response of groups of hypertensives and healthy people (aged seventeen to seventy-two) to injections of a saline solution. Among the hypertensives the reaction to the increased salt intake varied directly with age—the older the subject, the more pronounced the reaction. Among those who were not hypertensive the salt solution raised blood pressure only among those older than fifty. With aging, kidney function tends to slow down, and the body generates less of the substances that promote sodium excretion.

A complementary study at Wayne State University suggested that as people grow older they experience a decline in their ability to excrete sodium. Thus their sodium intake may have a greater effect on their blood pressure, since the body can no longer get rid of the mineral as efficiently.

The fact that so many of us seem to be genetically sodium resistant is the crux of the public health debate over the usefulness of discouraging excessive salt intake. If the majority of us are not sodium sensitive, why do we have to restrict our salt? There are good reasons to do so. In the

---

Sodium Content of Foods

LOW SODIUM	
	Sodium (mg)
Coffee, 1 cup	1
Fruit juice, 1 cup	2-10
Fruit, 1 fruit or 1 cup	1-5
Tea, 1 cup	5
Broccoli, ½ cup	8
Tomato, 1	14
Soft drinks, 1 cup	10-60
Eggs, 1	69
Beef, pork, lamb, poultry, fish (fresh), 3 oz	60-100

MEDIUM SODIUM	
Clams, steamed, 3 oz	95
Butter, salted, 1 tsp	115
Margarine, 1 tsp	115
Milk, 1 cup	120
Cake, 2 oz	150-400
Ketchup, 1 tsp	180
Bread, 2 slices	200-600

HIGH SODIUM	
Yellow mustard, 1 tsp	188
Potato chips, 1 oz	250
Cheese, cheddar, 1½ oz	300
Tuna, canned, 3 oz	250-500
Lobster, steamed, 3 oz	326
Olives, black, 2 oz	385
Ham, cured, 2 oz	400-800
Cheese, cottage, ½ cup	425
Pancakes, 3 prepared	400-800
Soy sauce, 1 tsp	420
Parmesan, 1 oz	528
Frankfurter, 1	450
Roll, crescent, 2 oz	500
Tomato juice, 6 oz canned	500
Pizza, 1 slice	500-1,000
Cheese, American, 1½ oz	600
Pickle, dill, 2 oz	700
Hamburger, 1 prepared (Big Mac, Whopper)	1,000
Spaghetti and meatballs, canned, 7½ oz	1,000
Soup, canned, 10 oz	1,000-1,500
TV dinner, 11 oz	1,000-2,000

Salt and sodium are not interchangeable terms. By weight, table salt is only 40 percent sodium, the rest chloride.

first place, before hypertension develops it is difficult to determine who is sodium sensitive and who isn't. In the second place, even though you may not be salt sensitive at thirty or forty, your sensitivity may increase with the years. There is also the possibility that the genetic resistance to sodium can be weakened by very high sodium intake over a lifetime and by other lifestyle factors such as stress.

Recommended intake

The real worry is that we are getting far more sodium than we need—5,000 to 7,000 milligrams is still the average daily intake. The Food and Drug Administration (FDA) and various professional groups have been carefully reviewing the evidence for and against sodium and have decided that *a sodium intake of 2,400 milligrams per day is the maximum amount for healthy individuals.* People under a doctor's care for hypertension may be advised to consume less. And there are other medical conditions, such as heart or kidney disease, that may require an adjustment in sodium intake.

Although the case against salt is not ironclad, it is only prudent to heed the evidence that does exist. Hypertension is a life-threatening ailment. Unless you are under a doctor's orders to do so, you need not take drastic measures. But avoid reaching for the saltshaker automatically, and avoid snacks and processed foods loaded with sodium. The health risks are too great to justify an overload of salt.

Calcium: Too Little

Bones are active tissues, constantly taking up and releasing calcium to maintain skeletal strength and density. All individuals, therefore, need to consume calcium regularly. An adult's bones still need two-thirds of the calcium required when he or she was growing and presumably drinking a quart of calcium-rich milk each day. Yet it appears that, starting in adolescence, many individuals consume too little calcium, mainly because they decrease their intake of dairy products. Over the long-term, a decreased calcium intake contributes to the development of osteoporosis, a condition of bone thinness and fragility that primarily afflicts postmenopausal women. The condition also appears—rarely—in elderly men. (For information on other risk factors for osteoporosis, see page 429.)

American women, in particular, consume only about half as much calcium as is recommended. The reasons that women are particularly vulnerable to calcium deficiencies are complex. During pregnancy the fetus makes increased calcium demands on a woman's system, and the high demands continue during lactation. During and after menopause the decline in estrogen may impair the bones' ability to retain calcium, or actually lead to rapid loss.

The role of calcium: bones and blood pressure

Calcium is the essential factor in building bones and teeth; indeed, about 99 percent of the calcium in the body is found in the bones and teeth. The remaining 1 percent or so is found in the cells and in the fluid that surrounds them. This minute amount plays an important role. Adequate calcium intake is needed for proper clotting of the blood, for proper muscle contraction (and therefore helping to regulate heartbeat), and for proper nerve transmission. In addition, calcium

Children age six to twelve who consume nearly twice the 800-milligram daily Recommended Dietary Allowance for calcium—the equivalent of about five glasses of milk a day instead of three—develop stronger bones, according to a study published in the New England Journal of Medicine. The greater bone mass, if maintained over the years, could protect against future fractures.

helps to maintain normal blood pressure, and according to some studies, may play a role in preventing and alleviating hypertension by decreasing contraction of muscles in the walls of blood vessels or by affecting certain hormones. In order to perform these functions, the cells must have calcium available on demand. Bones serve as a bank for calcium, storing the mineral and then supplying cells with it when they need it.

The body begins to build bone mass in infancy and continues to do so throughout childhood and young adulthood. In order to achieve maximum bone density, the body must have a calcium intake high enough to maintain the structural integrity of the bones and to compensate for calcium losses through excretion. The exact age at which the body stops forming new bone is unclear, but it appears that peak bone mass is not reached until the age of twenty-five, and may extend into the third decade of life. During these formative years, therefore, it is important to get the proper amount of calcium to ensure maximal bone formation and to continue to meet recommended allowances thereafter.

The body continually reprocesses bone in a cycle of formation and resorption. During the early years, the primary activity is formation; in the latter years, resorption predominates, and bone mass begins to slowly decline in most individuals after fifty. This decline is not debilitating in individuals whose bone stores are adequate. However, an inadequate calcium intake throughout the first two or three decades of life can contribute, later in life, to the development of osteoporosis, a more drastic loss of bone mass and density that makes bones increasingly fragile.

We also lose the ability to absorb calcium efficiently as we age. During childhood, a period of rapid bone growth, the body may absorb up to 75 percent of the calcium ingested. As growth slows, so does the absorption rate. Adolescents absorb 20 to 40 percent of ingested calcium and adults, on average, only 15 percent. This is another reason that it is important to consume adequate calcium during the early years of life when the body can make the most efficient use of it.

While calcium is the primary factor in building strong bones, it is not the only one. Other minerals such as manganese, magnesium, fluoride, copper, zinc, and boron also contribute to bone formation. Vitamin D, lactose, and protein (at the recommended level) help the body absorb calcium. In addition, regular weight-

Optimal Calcium Intakes

A National Institutes of Health consensus panel that studied calcium intake among Americans recommended the following calcium intake levels, some of them higher than the RDAs. The panel also recommended that daily calcium intake not exceed 2,000 milligrams.

Age	Calcium (mg)
less than 6 months	400 (same as RDA)
6 months to 1 year	600 (same as RDA)
1-10 years	800 (same as RDA)
adolescents	1,200-1,500 (RDA: 1,200)
Men:	
25-50 years	800 (same as RDA)
51-65 years	1,000 (RDA: 800)
over 65	1,500 (RDA: 800)
Women:	
25-50 years	1,000 (RDA: 800)
over 50 years	1,500, or 1,000 with estrogen (RDA: 800)
pregnant and nursing	Additional 400 (RDA: 1,200)

Myth: Cottage cheese is a good source of calcium.

Fact: Compared to milk, yogurt, and other cheeses, cottage cheese is a meager source of calcium. Low-fat varieties of cottage cheese are a good source of protein. But all types of cottage cheese retain only 25 to 50 percent of the calcium in the milk they were made from, since the special curdling procedure used to make cottage cheese encourages the loss of calcium into the whey, which is then drained.

As a result, a four-ounce serving of cottage cheese has only 70 to 80 milligrams of calcium (dry curd has only 23). Just one ounce of most hard cheeses has two to four times as much—for example, cheddar has 205 milligrams. Hard cheeses, though, are too high in fat to serve as a daily supplier of calcium. Low-fat or skim milk and low-fat yogurt make excellent calcium staples. Yogurt retains all the calcium in the milk it was made from—about 300 milligrams per cup.

Sources of Calcium

The most plentiful sources of calcium are dairy products, which, unfortunately, can also be high in fat. However, low-fat dairy products often contain slightly more calcium than their higher fat counterparts; low-fat, nondairy sources of calcium are also available. This chart compares the calcium content of selected foods with their percentage of calories from fat.

DAIRY PRODUCTS			
	Serving Size	Calcium (mg)	Fat Calories
Milk, skim	1 cup	316	5%
Milk, 1%	1 cup	313	26%
Milk, 2%	1 cup	313	36%
Milk, whole	1 cup	291	48%
Yogurt, plain, low-fat	1 cup	415	25%
Yogurt, plain, nonfat	1 cup	452	3%
Yogurt, fruit, low-fat	1 cup	314-383	18%
Blue cheese	1 oz	150	72%
Brie	1 oz	52	70%
Cheddar	1 oz	204	74%
Feta	1 oz	140	72%
Mozzarella, part skim	1 oz	207	56%
Provolone	1 oz	214	72%
Ricotta, part skim	1/4 cup	167	53%
Swiss	1 oz	272	72%
American	1 oz	174	74%

VEGETABLES			
Beet greens, cooked	1 cup	164	0%
Broccoli, cooked	1 cup	178	0%
Swiss chard, cooked	1 cup	102	0%
Collards, cooked	1 cup	148	0%
Dandelion greens, cooked	1 cup	147	26%
Kale, cooked	1 cup	94	22%
Mustard greens, cooked	1 cup	103	0%
Turnip greens, cooked	1 cup	249	0%
Spinach, cooked	1 cup	244	0%

CANNED FISH			
Salmon, sockeye, canned, with bones	3 1/2 oz	237	38%
Sardines, canned, in water, with bones	3 1/2 oz	240	72%

MISCELLANEOUS			
Almonds	1 oz	75	79%
Figs	3	81	0%
Rhubarb, cooked, with sugar	1/2 cup	174	0%
Soybeans, cooked	1/2 cup	66	38%
Tofu	3 1/2 oz	90	56%

bearing exercise, such as walking, and not smoking help the body build and maintain bone density.

A National Institutes of Health panel has found that most Americans need to consume more calcium. Its recommendations are shown in the chart on page 137, alongside the Recommended Dietary Allowances (RDAs), which in some instances are well below the intakes recommended by the NIH panel. For Americans, satisfying these new recommendations may mean doubling the amount of calcium that many of them currently consume. It's estimated that about half of Americans consume less than 600 milligrams of calcium daily.

Getting enough calcium

The best calcium sources are dairy products, particularly milk, yogurt, and cheeses. Whole milk dairy products, however, are also concentrated sources of fat, and should be consumed in moderation. The solution is to consume adequate amounts of low-fat dairy products such as 1 percent or nonfat milk, low-fat or nonfat yogurt, and lower-fat cheeses such as part-skim mozzarella and ricotta—all are just as high, if not higher, in calcium than high-fat versions. For example, one cup of whole milk has 291 milligrams of calcium; nonfat milk has 316. The vitamin D added to milk and dairy products is thought to aid in the absorption of calcium.

If you do not like milk, try yogurt or kefir. If you have trouble digesting dairy products (a condition known as lactose intolerance), try yogurt, which is easier to digest, or milk treated with the enzyme lactase. There are also good nondairy sources of calcium: leafy green vegetables, such as turnip greens and broccoli, and canned salmon or sardines eaten with the bones. Other foods, while not considered good sources, do contribute some calcium in the diet. For example, one cup of cooked carrots contains 48 milligrams of calcium, and one orange has 52 milligrams.

When to consider calcium supplements

The Surgeon General, the National Research Council, and many nutritionists recommend that, first and foremost, calcium should come from food sources. Getting calcium through food ensures that you are also getting the other nutrients that work together to develop bone mass and help the body absorb calcium. In addition, calcium-containing foods are excellent sources of other vitamins and minerals.

But many women, especially older women who tend not to eat dairy products, simply don't get enough calcium. If you cannot get enough calcium through your diet, taking a supplement is better than ignoring calcium altogether. Until recently, there have been serious questions about whether calcium supplements do any good. But research has made it clear that supplements can help—even in women well past menopause who are not on hormone replacement therapy (HRT), which slows bone loss. Two well-designed studies published in the *New England Journal of Medicine*—one from Australia, the other from New Zealand—provided strong evidence that supplements slow bone loss and can even reverse osteoporosis in postmenopausal women.

If you decide to take calcium supplements or if your doctor recommends them, treat them as something you add to an already balanced diet, not something you consume instead of a mineral rich food. The best plan seems to be to get *at least* 750 milligrams of calcium from your diet. A pint of skim milk with a cup of broccoli or another leafy green vegetable would supply this much calcium. Then bring your total intake to 1,750 milligrams by taking a 1,000-milligram supplement.

Generally, the least expensive form of supplement is calcium carbonate; there is really no evidence that other, usually more expensive, supplements are better absorbed. Take it with meals to enhance absorbability.

Keep in mind that you should not take supplements in excess of the RDA or, if you are a postmenopausal woman, the National Institutes of Health recommendations. An excess of calcium may lead to the formation of kidney stones in susceptible individuals. Furthermore, while large amounts of calcium may not be toxic for healthy individuals, no one really knows what constitutes an overdose. Little research has been done on long-term intakes over 2,500 milligrams a day, since getting that much calcium from food has been nearly impossible. We do know, however, that large doses of calcium can interfere with the absorption of other nutrients, such as iron and zinc.

Iron: Too Little

Iron deficiency is one of the most common nutritional shortfalls in the United States today. Up to 15 percent of women of childbearing age have some form of iron deficiency. This deficiency is most common in women because of losses during menstruation and the physiological demands of childbearing. In some developing countries, where people eat less meat and where fewer foods are iron-enriched, half the population may be iron deficient.

Calcium and kidney stones

Doctors often recommend that people who have had kidney stones avoid calcium-rich foods. (The most common stones are made from calcium). Yet a Harvard study found, surprisingly, that men who consumed a calcium-rich diet had a nearly 50 percent lower risk of developing kidney stones over four years than men who consumed little calcium.

Should people who have had a stone already or who have a family history of kidney stones increase their calcium intake? Not on the basis of this single study. It is well known that some stone formers reduce their chance of a recurrence when they cut down on calcium. Also, kidney stones are a complex problem: different kinds of stones are caused by and affected by different factors. In addition, this study looked only at men who initially never had stones—the findings may or may not apply to men with a previous history of kidney stones, or to women. If you have a history of stones, talk to your doctor about what dietary measures you should take.

All cells in the body contain iron, which plays a vital role in many biochemical reactions. Most iron is incorporated in hemoglobin, the oxygen-carrying protein that gives blood its red color, and in myoglobin in muscle. Iron is stored in the liver, spleen, bone marrow, and other tissues. Low iron intake over a long period can gradually lead to a depletion of these stores, especially if the body is losing blood, as in menstruation.

Iron deficiency

The initial stage of iron deficiency usually has no symptoms. It occurs when the body's iron stores are depleted or exhausted, a condition reflected by a drop in the blood's iron levels and an increase in transferrin—a protein that transports iron through the bloodstream. As the iron supply to the bone marrow dwindles, so does the marrow's ability to produce healthy red blood cells, which require iron. If the iron balance worsens, full-blown iron-deficiency anemia—characterized by low hemoglobin levels—can gradually develop. Since iron is an essential component of hemoglobin, a shortage of iron can impair the transport of oxygen from the lungs to the body's cells; as a result, work performance will be impaired.

It can take months or even years for symptoms of iron deficiency—such as weakness, shortness of breath, paleness, poor appetite, and increased susceptibility to infection—to become evident. These usually disappear when iron stores are rebuilt.

Groups with higher iron needs

An iron deficit isn't necessarily due to poor eating habits. *An otherwise balanced diet may not supply adequate iron if you are in one of the following groups:*

Menstruating women. Because monthly blood losses increase iron needs, women aged nineteen to fifty have a higher RDA (see box on page 141). Women who bleed heavily should pay special attention to their iron intake.

Dieters, especially women. The average balanced American diet offers about six milligrams of iron per 1,000 calories. Thus, the less you eat, the less likely you are to get enough iron. In particular, women consuming less than 1,500 calories a day will find it hard to get their RDA.

Pregnant women. Iron needs increase due to higher blood volume and the demands of the fetus and placenta.

Endurance athletes. Long-distance runners tend to have a higher incidence of iron depletion, which may impair top performance. This iron shortfall has been attributed to a variety of factors, including the increased elimination of iron during prolonged exercise.

Strict vegetarians. People who eat no animal products, which are the richest sources of iron, have to make a special effort to eat other foods that contain fair amounts of iron, such as beans, dried fruits, leafy greens, and enriched cereals and grains. The iron in vegetables, grains, and beans is not nearly as well absorbed by the body. Dairy products have negligible amounts.

Infants and children. Youngsters need a high iron intake because of their rapid growth. Some studies have found that iron deficiencies even without anemia can adversely affect the learning and problem-solving capacity of children. Menstruating adolescents who are still growing are at high risk, especially if they eat poorly or go on crash diets.

Factors that affect iron absorption

Only a small amount of the iron you eat is absorbed by your body, so you must consume substantially more iron than your body actually needs. The absorption process is affected by dietary as well as physiological variables:

•The amount of iron you consume.

•The form of iron in your foods. Not all iron is the same: heme iron, which makes up about 40 percent of the iron in animal tissues, is much better absorbed than nonheme iron, which makes up the rest of the iron in animal tissues, and all of the iron in dairy products and eggs; in vegetables, fruits, and grains; and in the supplements used to enrich flour and cereals.

•Composition of your meals. Dietary factors such as vitamin C enhance the availability of iron in a meal. Others, such as oxalic acid in spinach, inhibit absorption of this mineral.

•Your body's needs. If your iron stores are low or you have a greater need because of rapid growth or pregnancy, you absorb more iron through the intestinal tract. When your stores are plentiful, the body reduces its iron absorption rate.

The RDA for iron is based on the rough estimate that 10 percent of all iron is absorbed. Thus the RDA for men is set at 10 milligrams to provide the estimated 1 milligram of absorbed iron they need each day. The recommendation for women varies by age (see below). Until recently, it was set at 18 milligrams for menstruating women—the recommendation specifies ages eleven to fifty—to provide the 1.5 to 2 milligrams they need. But in 1989, a committee of the National Academy of Sciences recommended that iron intake be reduced to 15 milligrams since it has been difficult for women to get 18 milligrams and the lower amount was found to be sufficient.

Increasing your iron intake

As iron absorption is a complex process—it varies according to the foods you eat, how you combine them, and your body's need—here are some steps that will help you get the most iron from your diet:

Eat red meats (lean, of course), since these are rich in heme iron, the most readily absorbed form. Liver is one of the best sources, but should be eaten no more than once a week because of its high cholesterol content. Chicken and fish usually contain one-third to one-half the iron in red meat.

Peas, beans and corn are relatively good plant sources of iron. You can also choose breads, cereals, and pasta labeled "enriched" or "fortified." Unrefined whole grains, such as whole wheat bread, supply a fair amount of iron, but this is removed during the refining process. Enrichment makes such foods comparable to their unrefined counterparts in nutrient value. Fortification adds more iron than was originally in the grain.

Try to eat foods high in vitamin C at most meals, since it helps the body absorb

Sodium, Calcium, and Iron

The iron content of a half cup of spaghetti sauce increases from 3 to 50 milligrams or more when simmered in a cast-iron pot for a few hours.

Daily RDAs for Iron

Age	Iron (mg)
less than 6 months	10
6 months-3 years	15
4-10 years	10
11-18 years	15
19-50 years (men)	10
(women)	15*
over 51	10

During pregnancy, the National Academy of Sciences recommends 30 to 60 milligrams of supplemental iron, as prescribed by a physician, continuing after childbirth for two to three months.

Sources of Iron

Any table listing the iron content of foods presents only part of the picture, since this mineral is absorbed better from some sources than others. About 15 to 30 percent of the iron in meat, fish, and poultry is absorbed, compared to an average of 5 percent from vegetables, fruit, grains, and eggs. In addition, some foods contain substances that hinder absorption.

The figures below are for the total iron content and don't take into consideration how well it is absorbed.

Sources of Heme Iron	Amount	Iron (mg)	Sources of Nonheme Iron	Amount	Iron (mg)
Beef liver, sautéed	3 oz	7.5	**Dried apricots**	3 oz	4.0
Clams	3 oz	5.2	**Molasses,** blackstrap	1 tbsp	3.2
Oysters, raw	3 oz	4.8	**Baked beans**	½ cup	3.0
Pork chop, broiled	3 oz	3.3	**Potato,** baked, with skin	1 medium	2.8
Steak, lean, broiled	3 oz	3.0	**Almonds**	2 oz	2.7
Sardines, canned	3 oz	2.5	**Lima beans,** dried, cooked	½ cup	2.1
Chicken, dark meat, cooked	3 oz	2.0	**Raisins**	3 oz	1.9
Lamb, broiled	3 oz	1.7	**Spaghetti,** enriched, cooked	1 cup	1.4
Tuna, canned	3 oz	1.6	**Brewer's yeast**	1 tbsp	1.4
Ham	3 oz	1.2	**Peas,** cooked	½ cup	1.2
Chicken, white meat, cooked	3 oz	1.0	**Breakfast cereal,** enriched or fortified	1 oz	1-10
Salmon or white fish, broiled	3 oz	1.0	**Egg**	1	1.0
			Broccoli, cooked, chopped	½ cup	0.9
			Peanut butter	3 tbsp	0.9
			Bread, enriched or whole-grain	1 slice	0.7

Spinach isn't a particularly good source of iron because oxalic acid in this vegetable hinders the body's absorption of iron.

iron, especially from a meatless meal. For instance, if you drink a glass of orange juice with iron-enriched breakfast cereal, you may double or triple your iron absorption. Besides citrus fruits and juices, other good sources of vitamin C include tomatoes, sweet peppers, broccoli, cauliflower, leafy greens, strawberries, and even potatoes (with skin). Try to distribute your vitamin C intake so that you consume some at each meal. Consider the effect of vitamin C, for instance, on a vegetarian meal of navy beans, rice, cornbread, and an apple. By adding seventy-five milligrams of vitamin C—as in a cup of steamed broccoli or five ounces of fresh orange juice—you could get three to seven times more *absorbable* iron from this meal.

To improve the absorption of the nonheme iron in vegetables, fruits, and grains, eat them with small amounts of meat and fish, which are rich in heme iron. Try chili beans with lean ground beef, for instance, or peppers and chicken. The body's absorption of nonheme iron can vary by up to tenfold, depending on the presence of heme iron and other inhibiting and enhancing substances in the meal.

Cook in cast-iron pots to increase the iron content of foods. The more acidic the food (such as spaghetti sauce) and the longer it cooks, the higher the increase in iron content.

Iron supplements

If you eat meat and combine foods wisely, you probably don't need an iron supplement, especially if you are a man or a postmenopausal woman. Even if you fall into one of the groups listed on page 140, however, consult a doctor before taking supplements. (The RDA now includes a recommendation for pregnant women.) Despite the claims made in some advertisements, don't expect iron pills or elixirs to "perk" you up or improve your athletic performance unless your body is chronically lacking in iron.

In any case, self-treatment with iron supplements is not recommended, even if you think you have an iron deficiency or anemia. If something is amiss with your blood, you should consult a doctor to find out why. Self-diagnosis is foolhardy for several reasons. First of all, weakness and fatigue can be symptoms of many other conditions besides anemia. Secondly, not all anemias are due to inadequate iron intake. Some result from other nutritional shortages (such as a lack of folacin) and won't respond to iron supplementation. Many cases of anemia are not due to diet at all. For instance, one of the most common causes of iron-deficiency anemia in older people is internal bleeding, which requires prompt medical care, particularly if it is due to a cancer of the gastrointestinal tract.

Over a lifetime, the average woman will need almost twice as much iron as a man.

Finally, if you really are suffering from iron-deficiency anemia, this should be corrected under a doctor's supervision. If your doctor prescribes iron supplements, take them on an empty stomach—one hour before or two hours after meals—for best absorption. However, if you are extremely sensitive to iron, you may need to take supplements with meals to prevent stomach upset.

Children are especially susceptible to suffering ill effects from excessive doses of iron. In fact, iron pills are the leading cause of childhood poisoning death. As few as five high-potency over-the-counter iron pills could be fatal for a child.

Self-prescribed supplements are also hazardous to a small number of individuals who are susceptible to iron toxicity because their bodies don't properly regulate iron absorption. While it's nearly impossible to get too much iron from diet alone, these people—about 0.35 percent of the population—may get an overdose from potent pills and elixirs, possibly damaging the liver, pancreas, heart, or immune system. Excessive iron intake can also impair the absorption of other trace minerals, particularly zinc and copper. As is true of other nutrients, you are always better off getting your iron from foods in a well-balanced diet than from pills.

Caffeine

Caffeine is a mind-altering drug, one of the most ancient, as well as one of the most popular. Whether they get their caffeine in coffee, tea, cocoa, headache remedies, or soft drinks, nearly everyone ingests at least some caffeine daily. Most adult Americans begin their day with coffee or tea; others, including many children, get their morning start with a cola. The average American coffee drinker consumes three cups a day.

Yet many people worry about caffeine's side effects. In sufficient amounts it can bring on the jitters, and at one time or another caffeine has also been accused of causing pancreatic cancer, heart disease, breast disease, high blood pressure, high blood cholesterol levels, and birth defects. But does it indeed play a part in all of these health problems?

Caffeine's positive effects

Caffeine occurs naturally in more than sixty plants and trees that have been cultivated by humans since the beginning of recorded history. It is one of a group of compounds called methylxanthines, which act directly to stimulate certain neurotransmitters in the central nervous system, with effects throughout the body.

People like caffeine because it wards off drowsiness and increases alertness. One of the documented effects of caffeine is that it shortens reaction time. It also helps people wake up and feel better in the morning, helps them stay awake on the road, and gives them something to drink socially that isn't alcohol. It may even increase aspirin's effectiveness as a painkiller, which is why it is added to some pain relievers. Some studies have found that caffeine improves reading speed, enhances performance on math and verbal tests, and produces an increased capacity for sustained intellectual effort in general. Other studies, however, have shown that caffeine does not significantly affect verbal fluency, numerical reasoning, or short-term memory.

Physical benefits

Over the years, coaches and athletes have reported beneficial effects of caffeine for endurance exercise such as cycling or cross-country skiing. Caffeine boosts athletic performance supposedly by helping the body break down fats for use as energy, thereby sparing glycogen for later use and delaying exhaustion. So far, however, research has produced inconsistent results. Several small studies have shown that the caffeine in two or three cups of brewed coffee (220 to 330 milligrams), taken within a few hours of endurance exercise, postponed exhaustion in well-conditioned athletes. But other studies have found little or no benefit from caffeine. Like so many effects of caffeine, the effect on exercise varies from person to person. If you're a regular coffee drinker, don't expect coffee to have dramatic effects on your athletic performance; to get a boost, you would have to abstain from caffeine for three or four days and then consume some before the event. If you're not accustomed to caffeine on a daily basis, be careful, since you may have an adverse reaction while exercising.

Adverse effects: how much is too much?

Aside from shortening simple reaction time, caffeine does not appear to help in the performance of more complex motor tasks, and it may even be slightly disruptive. Depending on how much you consume, caffeine can temporarily step up your heart rate and increase stomach-acid secretion and urine production. Such effects are minimal among healthy adults who consume moderate amounts of caffeine—about two or three cups of coffee a day. The most common of caffeine's ill effects is "coffee nerves"—trembling, nervousness, insomnia, muscle tension, irritability, headaches, and disorientation. This usually occurs only in people who don't normally consume caffeine. Your reaction depends not only on your habituation and sensitivity to caffeine, but also on the amount you consume, your body weight and physical condition, and your anxiety level in general.

Children run a special risk of coffee nerves, since one cola for a small child may have the same effect as two to four cups of coffee for an adult. But children who regularly consume caffeine are less affected than children who do not.

Many people who drink caffeinated coffee regularly have no trouble sleeping after a late-night cup. But those unaccustomed to it may have trouble falling asleep, followed by disturbed sleep patterns. Caffeine levels peak in your body within an hour of consumption; more than half the caffeine is metabolized (that is, broken down and rendered inactive) in three to seven hours. Thus an afternoon cup of coffee or tea is unlikely to keep anyone awake eight hours later. Of course, psychology plays a role, too: if you expect that something will keep you awake, you may not sleep well.

Caffeine and health: myths and facts

Caffeine's effects are hard to study because the response to caffeine varies considerably from person to person. In addition, many of the discrepancies can be explained by the fact that researchers have not consistently distinguished between habitual coffee consumers and non–coffee-drinking volunteers who ingest large doses of caffeine over the course of an experiment. A dose of 250 milligrams given to a regular coffee drinker usually has no significant effect on blood pressure, heart rate, respiration, metabolic rate, blood cholesterol, or anxiety level. But caffeine given to subjects who haven't been consuming caffeine for a week or so can temporarily raise all these. Another complication in evaluating caffeine's impact on health is that people who drink a lot of coffee also tend to smoke, exercise little, eat lots of fat, and have other habits that put them at risk for a variety of ailments. Keep up good health habits, and coffee drinking is seldom a problem.

Heart disease. Scores of studies on caffeine have failed to establish any conclusive link to coronary artery disease (CAD). Many studies that claimed to find such a link were flawed, often because confounding factors were ignored. Recently, a review of studies on the subject in *Heart & Lung* found no increased risk of heart attack in people who consume caffeine, even if they had heart disease. In fact, the researchers suggested that cardiac patients not have their caffeine restricted while in the hospital (up to five cups of caffeinated beverages a day). In addition, a recent report in the *Archives of Internal Medicine* found no association between coffee drinking—even more than six cups a day—and CAD.

Caffeine may boost blood pressure in those not accustomed to it, but only temporarily. Still, people with hypertension (diastolic blood pressure above 105)

Myth: Coffee stimulates your appetite.

Fact: Coffee doesn't make you hungry per se. If you're used to having breakfast or a snack with coffee, the association might lead you to eat. Coffee, both regular and decaffeinated, can stimulate the flow of stomach acids and may cause heartburn. This feeling of discomfort might also make you want to eat something. However, black coffee is calorie-free and so can be part of a restricted-calorie diet.

should ask their doctors about avoiding caffeine. There's little or no evidence that caffeine increases irregular heartbeats, or arrhythmias. But people subject to them, particularly if recovering from a heart attack, should also get medical advice.

Blood cholesterol. The effect of caffeine on blood cholesterol is murky. For every study that finds that caffeine boosts cholesterol, another finds the evidence inconclusive and several discover no effect at all. A study at the Johns Hopkins Medical Institutions in 1992, which found that healthy men who drank four cups of filtered coffee daily experienced a slight rise in total blood cholesterol, received lots of press. But HDL ("good") cholesterol rose proportionately with LDL ("bad") cholesterol, which means that the men's risk of heart attack was not increased. Two Dutch studies did show that four to six daily cups of unfiltered European-style coffee raised blood cholesterol levels, while filtered coffee did not. Why this should be is a mystery, but the researchers theorized that a standard paper filter (which most Americans use) may trap some unidentified cholesterol-raising substance.

Benign breast disease. The fibrocystic tissue that forms in the breasts of some women can be lumpy and painful. Some doctors advise women with fibrocystic breasts to limit their intake of caffeine. But several studies—including a report on more than 3,300 women issued by the National Institutes of Health— have found no relationship between caffeine consumption and fibrocystic disease. Nor is there any evidence that giving up caffeine by itself eases the discomfort some women experience.

Cancer. Despite reports of links between coffee drinking and cancer of the bladder and pancreas, studies have failed to confirm them. The authors of a 1981 study suggesting a link between pancreatic cancer and coffee reversed their findings in a second study carried out five years later. And an evaluation of more than 16,000 men and women who were observed between 1967 and 1979 found no correlation between coffee drinking and cancer at any body site, including the breast, bladder, and pancreas. More recently, in 1993, the Iowa Women's Health Study found no link between caffeine and breast cancer.

Stomach problems. Don't blame caffeine for an upset stomach. Coffee does stimulate the flow of stomach acid and thus potentially irritates the stomach lining and ulcers. It may also relax the sphincter at the end of the esophagus (as do alcohol and smoking), allowing

Does caffeine interfere with nutrient absorption?

Not caffeine, but other substances (such as polyphenols) in coffee and especially tea may interfere with the body's absorption of certain minerals, notably calcium and iron—especially nonheme iron, the kind found in plant foods. This is only rarely a problem. If you drink tea with every meal or drink many cups per day while eating a strict vegetarian diet, it's possible that the tea could promote iron deficiency, but only if you're eating minimal amounts of iron-containing foods. Tea and coffee in moderation can be part of a healthy diet, and there's no evidence that they lead to iron-deficiency anemia or calcium loss.

Caffeine Content

This chart will help you calculate your daily caffeine intake. But remember, caffeine content varies widely, depending on the product you use and how it's prepared.

BEVERAGES	Serving Size	Caffeine (mg)
Coffee, drip/brewed	6 oz	80-175
Coffee, instant	6 oz	60-100
Coffee, decaffeinated	6 oz	2-5
Tea, 5-minute steep	6 oz	40-100
Tea, 3-minute steep	6 oz	20-50
Hot cocoa	6 oz	2-20
Cola	12 oz	30-45

FOODS	Serving Size	Caffeine (mg)
Milk chocolate	1 oz	1-10
Bittersweet chocolate	1 oz	5-35
Chocolate cake	1 slice	20-30

OVER-THE-COUNTER DRUGS	Dose	Caffeine (mg)
Anacin, Empirin, Midol	2	64
Excedrin	2	130
NoDoz	2	200
Aqua-Ban (diuretic)	2	200
Dexatrim (weight-control aid)	1	200

Caffeine and Pregnancy

During 1993, a series of conflicting studies about the risks of consuming caffeine during pregnancy were published. On the basis of this evidence, most researchers decided that it wasn't necessary to prohibit caffeine during pregnancy, but to discourage excessive consumption (more than two or three cups of coffee a day). But in December of that year, a major study in the *Journal of the American Medical Association* found that pregnant women who drank from 1.5 to 3 cups of coffee a day doubled their chance of miscarriage. Women who drank more than 3 cups a day during pregnancy tripled their risk; even those who drank that much the month before conception had a doubled risk of miscarriage.

In an editorial accompanying the study, Dr. Brenda Eskenazi of the University of California at Berkeley presented possible explanations for the discrepant results of the earlier studies, including the variability of caffeine content of coffee and the huge range of cup sizes. Also, other sources of caffeine, such as tea and soft drinks, may not be as hazardous. The problem with coffee may be not only caffeine, but also other chemicals released during roasting.

Dr. Eskenazi recommended that we "must navigate between protecting the fetus and besieging women with excessive warnings." While it's clear that high levels of caffeine intake (more than 300 milligrams per day) during pregnancy are potentially harmful, "we cannot conclude that lower levels are safe." The potential risk to the fetus posed by caffeine is small—not of the same magnitude as the risks from alcohol, tobacco, or lack of prenatal care. But the risk is real, nonetheless.

Thus "pregnant women should limit their intake of caffeine to a minimum"—or, to be safe, should avoid it altogether, according to Dr. Eskenazi. Even women who may become pregnant should not exceed a moderate intake, since most women don't realize they are pregnant during the first few weeks, and excessive caffeine consumed even during the month before conception may put the fetus at risk. Prospective fathers should also consider limiting their caffeine intake, said Dr. Eskenazi.

A cup of coffee ice cream contains an average of 19 milligrams of caffeine. That's more than twice the amount found in chocolate ice cream, but far less than the caffeine levels in brewed coffee.

for the backup of stomach contents and thus increasing the chance of heartburn in some people. However, decaffeinated coffee seems to be almost as much of a problem as regular coffee. The principal culprits are either the beans' natural oils or substances apparently introduced during the roasting process. So people with ulcers or chronic heartburn should avoid both types of coffee. Even caffeine-free herbal teas and grain-based beverages can stimulate stomach acid.

Coffee or tea?

A cup of brewed tea has about 40 milligrams of caffeine on average, less than half of what you get in a cup of coffee. The exact amount depends on the type of tea and how long it is brewed. Green teas generally have less caffeine than black. And loose teas contain less caffeine than the same brands when brewed from tea bags.

Many people believe that tea contains tannins, which are known to interfere with the body's absorption of iron, protein, and other nutrients. It is true that tea contains a variety of substances called polyphenols, which give tea its astringent taste. Some of these polyphenols are chemically similar to tannins, but they don't have the nutrient-binding effect of true tannins. For many years tea polyphenols were marketed as bioflavonoids or vitamin P, with numerous medicinal claims made for them. The Food and Drug Administration (FDA) considers them ineffective, so they are no longer available for purchase in the United States.

Should you give it up?

If you're a healthy adult who enjoys coffee or tea, there's no evidence that caffeine will do you any harm. If it gives you a lift or a reason to relax, there's no reason to deprive yourself of caffeine's benefits. If you think caffeine may be robbing you of a sound night's sleep, by all means try cutting out caffeine in the evening. If you get jittery and nervous from it at any time of day, it makes sense to cut back.

Many people who occasionally suffer from nothing worse than coffee nerves may want to cut down on coffee drinking or stop entirely. Since caffeine is mildly habit-forming, some heavy coffee and tea drinkers may experience withdrawal symptoms twelve to sixteen hours after their final dose: drowsiness, headache, lethargy, irritability, the blues, nausea. Even passing up the regular after-dinner cup can cause morning-after headache. Such symptoms can be avoided simply by cutting back gradually. You can switch to drinking decaffeinated coffee or other caffeine-free beverages, which, however, may also have unwanted side effects.

Decaffeinated coffee

Many people, unwilling to give up the pleasures of coffee, choose decaffeinated coffee: it has much of the taste and aroma of "real" coffee, but almost no caffeine.

One worry, which turned out to be of little significance, was the use of the solvent methylene chloride to extract the caffeine in some brands. This chemical was shown to cause cancer when inhaled by laboratory animals, which is why its use was banned in hair sprays. But scientists found no carcinogenic effect when the animals drank the chemical. In any case, the residue in decaf is virtually nil, and the FDA has approved it for use in decaffeination. There are also plenty of water-processed decaffeinated coffees now available, though they usually cost more and offer no particular health advantages.

Another inflated concern about decaf grew out of a study conducted at Stanford University that suggested that decaf raises levels of LDL, the "bad" cholesterol in blood. At the end of the two-month study, decaf drinkers purportedly showed an average increase of 5 milligrams per deciliter in LDL, while regular-coffee drinkers and abstainers showed no significant change. Researchers had no idea why any of this had happened, but they doubted that it was the absence or presence of caffeine that caused the difference. One possibility they hazarded was that the type of coffee bean may have caused the rise since the regular coffee used in the experiment was made from a different type of bean than the decaf. In a well-designed study, though, both groups would have drunk coffee made from the same kind of beans. Moreover, this study was small (only 181 men), it was also brief, and the reported difference of 5 milligrams in blood cholesterol between the two groups is of no significance.

Percolated or drip coffee typically contains twice as much caffeine as instant.

Food Labels and Additives

In 1993, after years of debate, the Food and Drug Administration (FDA) announced its new labeling regulations for packaged foods. The old labels offered plenty to complain about: nutrient values presented in a vacuum; serving sizes that differed on nearly identical products; terms like "healthy" and "light" that were nebulous at best; and the absence of some important food substances, such as fiber, from many labels. The new label format was required as of May 1994. The United States Department of Agriculture (USDA) agreed to use the same label format on processed meat and poultry products such as cold cuts and canned chili beginning in July 1994.

Nutrients in context. To give a clearer picture of what's in a food, major nutrients will be listed not just in grams and milligrams, but also as a percentage of the total recommended intake (called the "Daily Value") for someone consuming 2,000 calories a day. This will take much of the work out of label reading. For example, the label will show that a food with thirteen grams of fat provides 20 percent of the suggested daily maximum (based on the FDA's recommendation that fat supply no more than 30 percent of your total calories). A small chart shows the suggested daily intake for the macronutrients —carbohydrate, protein, and fat—for a 2,000-calorie and 2,500-calorie diet.

To help complete the picture, the new label tells you that each gram of protein and carbohydrate supplies 4 calories, while a gram of fat has 9 calories. The label does *not* indicate the percentage of calories derived from fat—but you can easily obtain that figure with the formula shown on page 110.

Standardized serving sizes. Servings for various products will be set by the FDA, making it easier to compare different brands. No longer will one brand of ice cream claim that a pint yields five three-ounce servings while another states that one-half cup is a serving.

More on fat. In addition to total fat, the label must also give values for saturated fat (most responsible for raising blood cholesterol) and the number of calories supplied by the fat. The manufacturer has the option of listing poly- and monoun-

---

A Sample Label: Macaroni & Cheese

Nutrition Facts

Serving Size: 1/2 cup
Servings Per Container: 4

Amount Per Serving

Calories 260	Calories from Fat 120

	% Daily Value*
Total Fat 13g	20%
Saturated Fat 5g	25%
Cholesterol 30mg	10%
Sodium 660mg	28%
Total Carbohydrate 31g	11%
Dietary Fiber 0g	0%
Sugars 5g	
Protein 5g	

Vitamin A 4% • Vitamin C 2% • Calcium 15% • Iron 4%

* Percents (%) of a Daily Value are based on a 2,000 calorie diet. Your Daily Values may vary higher or lower depending on your calorie needs:

Nutrient		2,000 Calories	2,500 Calories
Total Fat	Less than	65g	80g
Sat. Fat	Less than	20g	25g
Cholesterol	Less than	300mg	300mg
Sodium	Less than	2,400mg	2,400mg
Total Carbohydrate		300g	375g
Fiber		25g	30g

1g Fat = 9 calories
1g Carbohydrate = 4 calories
1g Protein = 4 calories

saturated fats as well. (For definitions of these various fats, see pages 107-108.)

More on carbohydrates. Total carbohydrate content as well as dietary fiber and sugars is given.

Fiber content. The label may also break down fiber into soluble and insoluble, at the packagers' discretion. These values are good indicators of just how healthful a bread or cereal, for instance, might be.

New definitions. In what is truly a revolutionary change, a number of slippery terms—including "light," "free," "high," "low," "reduced," and "extra-lean"—have been assigned specific meanings (see below).

A Labeling Glossary

Until now, many nutritional claims on food labels—from "low in fat" to "high in fiber"—have more often than not been advertising hype. But the new food labeling regulations spell out which nutrient content claims are allowed and under what circumstances they can be used. Here are the core terms and their new definitions on food labels:

Free, as in "fat-free," means that a product is either absolutely free of that nutrient or contains an insignificant amount: less than 0.5 grams per serving of fat, saturated fat, or sugar; less than 2 milligrams (mg) of cholesterol; or less than 5 mg of sodium.

Fresh means that a food is raw, has never been frozen or heated, and contains no preservatives.

Fortified, enriched, added, or "more" are all claims that mean a food must have at least 10 percent more of the Daily Value for a particular nutrient (dietary fiber, potassium, protein, or an essential vitamin or mineral) that was not originally in the food, or was present in smaller amounts.

Healthy can be used on a label if a food is low in fat and saturated fat and a serving does not contain more than 480 mg of sodium or more than 60 mg of cholesterol.

High and good source focuses on nutrients for which higher levels are desirable—for example, fiber or calcium. "High" must equal 20 percent or more of the Daily Value for that nutrient in a serving. (The FDA has also approved "rich in" or "excellent source" as synonyms.) "Good source" means a serving contains 10 to 19 percent of a nutrient's Daily Value.

Lean and extra lean can be used to describe the fat content of meat, poultry, seafood, and game. "Lean" foods have less than ten grams of fat, four grams of saturated fat, and 95 mg of cholesterol per serving. "Extra lean" means less than five grams of fat and two grams of saturated fat.

Light or "lite," when applied to a nutritionally altered food product, means that it contains one-third fewer calories or half the fat of the food from which it was derived. In addition, the term "light in sodium" can indicate that the sodium content of a low-calorie, low-fat food has been reduced by 50 percent. Light can also refer to taste, color, and texture, provided any qualifying information is included.

Low can refer to total fat, saturated fat, cholesterol, sodium, and calories. It means that a relatively large amount of a food can be eaten without exceeding the Daily Value for the "low" nutrient. "Low-fat," for example, means three grams or less per serving (or per fifty grams of the food)."Low-sodium" equals 140 mg per serving (or per fifty grams of the food). Synonyms for "low" are "little," "few," "low source of," and "contains a small amount of." A claim of "very low" can only be made about sodium (35 mg or less per serving).

Reduced (or less) is a comparison claim applied to total fat, saturated fat, cholesterol, sugar, sodium, and total calories. To be labeled "reduced," a food must have 25 percent less of a nutrient (or of calories) than the regular product. The comparison must also be shown on the label.

Only a limited number of health claims—and these are scientifically established claims—are permitted. The food must contain a defined amount of the nutrient in question, and the claims must use the terms "may" or "might" to describe the risk-reducing or health-enhancing qualities of certain nutrients within the context of overall daily diet. Loose and unsubstantiated terms such as "heart-smart" and "health-wise" are no longer permitted. The seven approved claims concerning nutrient/disease relationships are:

- calcium and osteoporosis
- fat and cancer
- saturated fat and cholesterol in relation to coronary artery disease
- fiber and cancer
- fiber and coronary artery disease
- sodium and high blood pressure
- fruits and vegetables and a reduced cancer risk

Abridged versions. The full version of the new label must appear on all packages with forty square inches of surface area. Smaller packages (between twelve and forty square inches) are required to carry less information, and the very smallest—a pack of gum or a roll of hard candies, for instance—need not have nutrition labeling, but must provide a telephone number or address where the consumer can get nutrition information. Foods such as soft drinks, which contain limited nutrients, may use a simplified format that gives only calories, total fat, sodium, total carbohydrates, sugars, and protein.

Will the new labels help?

In a study published in 1993 in the *American Journal of Public Health*, researchers analyzed the potential health benefits to Americans of the new food labels—assuming that some consumers will make changes in their diets based on the label information. The researchers concluded that even if not every food is labeled (as the law stands now, labeling is voluntary—not required—for meat, fish, and poultry), and even if some consumers

New Safety Labels for Meat

The great majority of food poisoning cases could be avoided through proper food handling and cooking, according to federal officials. In an effort to increase consumer awareness of meat and poultry safety, the USDA mandated new labels for raw and partially cooked meat and poultry products. The instructions serve as a reminder to consumers about careful storage, thawing practices, preparation, and cooking. Some retailers are also offering brochures and other handouts to help shoppers handle meat and poultry more safely.

Ground meat (beef, pork, veal, and lamb) and ground poultry products were required to carry the new labels as of May 1994; the labels were required on all meat and poultry products as of July 1994. The new label is reproduced below.

Safe Handling Instructions

This product was prepared from inspected and passed meat and/or poultry. Some food products may contain bacteria that could cause illness if the product is mishandled or cooked improperly. For your protection, follow these safe handling instructions.

Keep refrigerated or frozen.
Thaw in refrigerator or microwave.

Keep raw meat and poultry separate from other foods.
Wash working surfaces (including cutting boards.)
utensils, and hands after touching raw meat or poultry.

Cook thoroughly.

Keep hot foods hot. Refrigerate leftovers
immediately or discard.

What is "natural"?

When applied to meat or poultry, the term "natural" means the food is minimally processed and free of artificial ingredients. But for other foods "natural" has no legal meaning. Many foods labeled as such are highly processed, and loaded with fat, sugar, and preservatives. A "natural" flavor must come from a juice, oil, leaf, herb, or spice, but something containing "all natural flavor" may still have artificial colors and preservatives. Perhaps "natural," like the term "health food," should be a warning rather than a reassurance.

don't understand the labels—or don't change their diets in response to label information—there should still be substantial improvements in the American diet.

In other words, even relatively small changes in nutrient intake can add up to large public health benefits: the researchers estimated that thanks to the label changes, in the first twenty years, Americans will gain at least 40,000 "life-years" under the worst-case scenario, and as much as 1.2 million "life-years" under the best-case scenario. For instance, the information provided about fat on the new labels might help some Americans cut overall fat intake or reduce consumption of saturated fat; the fiber information might alert some to the importance of a diet high in fiber. The new labels heighten awareness of the nutrient content of foods for consumers who are now oblivious to the links between diet and health; and people who are already trying to eat healthfully will now have more and better information on which to base their food purchases.

Labeling for fresh foods, too

Although fresh produce and seafood are not required to carry the new nutrition labeling, they are covered under voluntary labeling regulations. Voluntary labeling for the twenty most consumed fresh fruits, vegetables, and raw fish has gone into effect under the Nutrition Labeling and Education Act of 1990. If at least 60 percent of retailers participate in the program, it will remain voluntary; however, if participation drops, labeling will become mandatory.

Stores can display nutrient information on charts or labels or in brochures. Per-serving values for calories, protein, fat, carbohydrates, sodium, vitamins A and C, calcium, and iron are required. Information on other vitamins, complex carbohydrates, sugars, dietary fiber, saturated fat, and cholesterol is optional.

Voluntary labeling of raw meat and poultry went into effect in July 1994. The labels will list calories, fat, saturated fat, cholesterol, sodium, protein, calcium, and iron, plus total per-serving calories from fat and saturated fat. As with fresh produce labeling, this program will remain voluntary as long as more than 60 percent of retailers comply; mandatory labeling is under consideration.

There are also new FDA regulations covering labeling of waxed fruits and vegetables. As of May 1994, produce (such as apples, cucumbers, and tomatoes) sold with a protective coating of wax or resin must be identified on the shipping container and on the retail package if the product is sold packaged. For produce sold in bulk, the retailer must post a sign stating which products are waxed.

What's not covered

The new FDA labeling rules don't apply to food sold for immediate consumption at restaurants, bakeries, delis, or vending carts, so you're on your own when eating out. Foods produced by small businesses, such as locally baked cookies or muffins, may also be exempt from this labeling.

Food Additives

Food additives are hardly new: they have been with us for thousands of years, probably starting with the discovery that salted meat lasted longer. And they are not likely to go away, since Americans depend on an ever-wider variety of convenience foods that require additives. Some of these substances offer indisputable health benefits, but most additives are used solely to make foods more attractive and palatable to consumers. Surveys show that few things worry consumers more than additives, particularly "chemicals" or "artificial ingredients" in foods. Are these fears well founded?

Our food supply is more closely scrutinized and additives more strictly regulated than ever before. In the "good old days" a century ago, eating was really risky, since foods weren't well preserved or carefully handled. Adulteration of foods was common—for instance, toxic metals were used in food coloring, and copper sulfate in bread. No one claims that such acutely toxic compounds are being added to our foods today. Instead, consumers worry about long-term safety. Their fears have been heightened in recent years by the banning of the artificial sweetener cyclamate and other substances approved by the Food and Drug Administration (FDA) that were subsequently shown to cause cancer in animals. In addition, food scientists as well as consumers are concerned about the health implications of "indirect" additives—substances that find their way into foods during packaging and storage.

The most commonly used additives are sugar, salt, and corn syrup, which together with baking soda, pepper, and a dozen other substances, make up about 98 percent (by weight) of all additives in the United States. Notice that these are all "natural." Yet natural substances can be health hazards—just look at sassafras bark extract (known as safrole and formerly used to flavor root beer) or aflatoxin (found in a mold that grows on peanuts), both known carcinogens. On the other

Controversial Additives

Artificial colors

The most controversial food colors are the so-called coal-tar dyes, which were originally derived from coal tar but now come from other sources. Many have been banned by the FDA, including red no. 2 in 1976, then the most widely used food coloring in the United States. To ensure that it contains no harmful contaminants, each batch of food coloring has to be certified by the FDA. (Other dyes don't have to be certified; they are derived from natural products, such as caramel and annatto, or are pure chemicals.)

Only a handful of certified artificial dyes remain on the FDA's approved list, yet they account for most food coloring used today. All are under fire as suspected carcinogens, especially red no. 3, found in maraschino cherries, pistachio nuts, gelatin desserts, and other foods. In addition, yellow no. 5 can cause allergic reactions in a small segment of the population. Hence, it is the only dye that must be listed by name on food labels; others can be listed as "artificial coloring." Manufacturers seem to be aware of consumer concern, and a few have ceased adding artificial dyes to some of their products.

BHT and BHA

Like many forbidding-sounding chemicals, butylated hydroxytoluene and butylated hydroxyanisole are allowed to go by their initials: BHT and BHA. These preservatives are used to retard rancidity in vegetable oils, potato chips, candy, cereals, and many convenience foods. Though on the GRAS ("generally recognized as safe") list, they have been plagued by controversy for years. Some studies have shown that BHT causes cancer in rats, while a few have actually found that it may prevent cancer in certain circumstances. The FDA is still reviewing BHT and BHA. Meanwhile, some companies have stopped using these chemicals, substituting natural preservatives such as ascorbic acid, citric acid, or vitamin E. Going against this trend, the United States Department of Agriculture allows meat processors to add BHT and BHA to raw and cooked meat-based toppings for pizza and to meatballs.

A Food Additive Primer

Additives do many jobs—the Food and Drug Administration lists thirty reasons why they may be added. Most of the estimated 3,000 compounds deliberately added to foods fall into the following categories. The great majority of them are safe; safety questions are discussed under "comments."

Type	Functions	Common Uses	Comments
Preservatives Nitrates, nitrites, BHT, BHA, benzoic acid, ascorbic acid, sulfites, calcium propionate	Retard spoilage from bacteria, molds, and fungi; keep fats/oils from turning rancid; delay browning, as in cut fruit.	Most processed or prepared foods.	Nitrates and nitrites promote cancer in lab animals, so limit your intake of cured meats. Sulfites may cause allergic reactions, especially in asthmatics. BHT and BHA are under continuing review.
Nutrients Vitamins and minerals	Replace nutrients lost in processing, or add those lacking in the diet.	Processed flour, rice, cereals, salt, margarine, milk.	Most vitamins are either artificially synthesized or are derived from fermentation processes, but all are chemically identical to the natural substances.
Flavor enhancers MSG, hydrolyzed vegetable protein, maltol	Modify taste or aroma of food.	Gravies, oriental foods, canned vegetables, soup mixes.	Some people are allergic to MSG. Hydrolyzed vegetable protein can produce MSG when heated and combined with salt.
Flavors Vanilla, spices, seasonings, artificial flavorings	Improve flavor; restore flavor lost in processing.	Baked goods, soft drinks, and many other products.	Largest category of additives. Can be listed on labels in general terms, such as "artificial flavors."
Colors Annatto, carotene, caramel, fruit juice, synthetic colors	Make food appealing by giving an appetizing, characteristic color.	Used in virtually all kinds of processed foods.	Synthetic dyes are most widely used; their safety is under continuing review. Only yellow no. 5 must be listed by name on labels, because of allergic reactions.
Sweeteners Natural sugars (e.g. fructose, corn syrup); artificial sweeteners (saccharin, aspartame, acesulfame-k)	Give food a more agreeable flavor.	Candies, baked goods, soft drinks, and many processed foods.	Many consumers are concerned about artificial sweeteners because of questions about saccharin and the banning of cyclamates in 1970.
Emulsifiers (mixers) Lecithin, mono/diglycerides, polysorbate	Keep liquid particles evenly mixed and homogenous.	Baked goods, frozen desserts, puddings, gelatins, dressings.	Help disperse oils and flavors. Most come from natural sources.
Stabilizers, thickeners, texturizers Gums, carrageenan, gelatin, flour, pectin, cellulose, starch	Improve consistency and provide desired texture.	Most prepared desserts, sauces, baked goods, fruit products, soups.	Many are natural carbohydrates that absorb water. Affect "mouth feel" of foods—i.e., prevent ice crystals from forming in ice cream.
pH control agents Citric acid, acetic acid, other acids, alkalis, buffers	Control acidity or alkalinity, thus affecting texture and taste.	Soft drinks, confections, baked goods, fruit products.	Also used to prevent botulism in low-acid canned goods such as beets. Some acids help in the rising of dough.

hand, there's no reason to worry about the great majority of artificial ingredients. Laboratory-made vitamins and some flavors, for instance, are exact replicas of natural substances, and since they have identical chemical structures, the body can't tell them apart. Other chemicals have no natural counterparts, and while this isn't necessarily bad, they arouse the most fear in consumers.

Who is protecting you?

Food additives are extensively studied and regulated, primarily by the FDA. Legislation in 1958 and 1960 required manufacturers to prove the safety of any new additive; before that, the burden was on the government to prove the health danger of a substance.

Margin of safety. If manufacturer-sponsored tests prove an additive is safe, the FDA sets guidelines for its use. Generally, food manufacturers can use only one-hundredth of the least amount of an additive shown to be toxic in lab animals.

The Delaney clause. This is the most restrictive provision of the 1958 law, stating that a substance shown to cause cancer in animals or man may not be added to food in any amount. Food manufacturers argue against this rule on the grounds that in some cases the cancer risk is minuscule, or that any risk is outweighed by the benefits the additive may provide—as with nitrites and saccharin, weak carcinogens that are still on the market.

Testing for safety. Even under the best circumstances, absolute safety of an additive can never be proven. Any substance may be harmful when consumed in excess. Animal studies, which are our primary mode of testing, have limitations. They may not be effective in assessing the degree of cancer risk from long-term use because of the animals' short life spans. Moreover, it is hard to make precise comparisons between animals and humans. Other questions concern possible interactions of the hundreds of additives we consume.

GRAS. The 1958 law exempted about 700 "generally recognized as safe" (GRAS) substances from testing because of their long history of use without any harmful effect. This grandfather clause has turned out to be somewhat problematic. Many of the most widely used—and controversial—additives are on the GRAS list. The FDA has been re-evaluating all GRAS substances and has banned some or restricted their use.

Smart choices

•Eat fresh or minimally processed foods as much as possible, since they usually have few additives. Avoid junk foods (such as cookies, candy, and soda), which are not only chock-full of artificial colors and other additives, but are also of little nutritional value—high in calories, sugar, fats, and/or sodium. This is especially good advice for children, who are the main consumers of junk foods and are at increased risk if there are any health problems with additives.

•Read food labels. But remember, additives aren't always listed: more than 300 standardized foods don't have to list their ingredients. Ice cream, for example, can contain some twenty-five specified additives without having to list any of them.

•Limit your intake of foods listing "artificial colors." Substitute products colored by real fruit juice. Still, an occasional maraschino cherry won't harm you.

•Eat a variety of foods. This will limit your exposure to any one additive, should it turn out to have long-term risks.

Natural "non-nutrients" in food

Consumers tend to focus their concerns on the health impact of artificial additives. But edible plant foods contain many natural non-nutrient substances that can be considered "toxic"—in the sense that they kill off diseases and pests that can harm the plant. Others are there for purposes we can't understand. Some of these substances may be hazardous to humans—for example, hydrazines in mushrooms—while most probably aren't. Such substances are in the process of being studied, and hopefully we will soon know enough about some of them to convey the information on a food label.

The Wellness Food Guide

Which fruits and vegetables are the best sources of beta carotene? Is margarine better for you than butter? What's the difference between beef graded choice and beef graded select? Is goat's milk more nutritious than cow's milk? Answering these questions and many others, this chapter serves as a complete guide that covers a wide variety of foods in the following categories: Produce, Dairy and Eggs, Grains and Legumes, Meat and Poultry, Seafood, Fats and Oils, Snacks and Desserts, and Convenience Foods. Each entry provides you with nutritional information, shopping tips, and guidelines for preparing and storing foods.

PRODUCE

Fruit

Apples

Although there are 7,000 varieties of apples, only twenty are widely available in this country, and a mere eight varieties account for 75 percent of sales—Delicious, McIntosh, Rome Beauty, Jonathan, Granny Smith, and Stayman. They vary in taste and texture, but nutritionally are pretty much the same. A medium-sized apple has roughly 65 to 85 calories, depending on how sweet it is—the sweeter the apple, the more fructose (fruit sugar) it contains. While apples may not be as nutrient-packed as other fruits, the edible portion of a five-ounce apple provides about four grams of dietary fiber (most of it in the form of pectin, a soluble fiber that has been shown to help lower cholesterol levels), about 10 percent of your daily requirement for vitamin C (storage decreases the vitamin C content), and some potassium. These features, plus low-calorie content and varied sweet-tart tastes, make apples a very good snack and dessert choice.

Choose apples that are firm and free of wrinkles, soft spots, and bruised areas. Store apples in the refrigerator; apples stored at room temperature will deteriorate quickly and become mealy. Kept in the refrigerator, apples will stay fresh for two weeks or more depending on the variety.

Apricots

Apricots are rich in the antioxidant nutrient beta carotene. Three medium-sized apricots provide 2 milligrams of beta carotene—a third of the minimum recommended daily intake—and only 50 calories. Apricots are also rich in potassium and vitamin C, and they are a good source of fiber.

Choose fruits that are golden, plump, and juicy-looking. Ripe fruit gives slightly when pressed. Avoid apricots that are very soft (overripe), hard (underripe), or greenish-yellow in color. Ripe apricots should be stored in the coldest part of the refrigerator and eaten promptly.

Bananas

Bananas are the most popular fruit in the United States; Americans consume, on average, about 25 pounds per person, per year. It's no wonder: bananas are inexpensive and available year round. What's more, they are easy to chew and digest, making them ideal foods for babies and the elderly. Bananas are always picked green and allowed to ripen en route to the market, so it is not unusual to find very green fruit in the supermarket. In fact, allowing bananas to ripen on the tree would result in mushy, overripe, and damaged fruit by the time they arrived at the store.

Bananas are an excellent source of potassium; in fact, bananas have more potassium by weight than any other fruit, except avocados (which have a great deal more fat). They are also a good source of vitamin B$_6$, and provide some folacin and magnesium as well. A medium-sized banana has about 100 calories.

Choose bananas that are yellow, but green at the tips and free of dark spots, bruises, or gashes. These bananas will not be quite ripe, so store them at room temperature for a few days. Bananas are at their sweetest when they are solid yellow and flecked with brown spots. When they reach that stage, they can be put in the refrigerator to prevent further ripening; this will darken the skin, but this does not affect the fruit inside. Refrigerated, ripe bananas will keep for about two weeks. Overripe bananas can be mashed and used in breads, cakes, and muffins.

Blueberries

Blueberries are a perfect summer food. Light and flavorful, they can be eaten by the handful, in cereal, added to fruit salads, stirred into muffin mix, or used to top pancakes or yogurt. A cup of fresh blueberries has just 87 calories and supplies about one-third of your daily vitamin C requirement and provides small amounts of potassium, iron, and beta carotene. Blueberries are also an excellent source of fiber.

Choose berries that are dark blue, dry, plump, and uniform in size. The powdery finish on blueberries, called bloom, is a protective coating and a sign of freshness. Avoid those that are shriveled or moldy and those in boxes stained with juice. Before storing, pick over the fruit and discard stems, leaves, and any berries that are shriveled, squashed, moldy, or green. Do not wash the berries until just before eating. Blueberries will keep for about a week in the refrigerator, but are best used within a few days of purchase.

Cranberries

Cranberries are high in fiber and potassium. A half cup of chopped fruit contains just 27 calories and supplies 13 percent of the daily requirement for vitamin C. You enjoy all these benefits if you eat dishes prepared with raw berries and not much sugar, such as homemade cranberry-orange relish. But if you like cooked cranberry sauce, finding a low-calorie commercial product is virtually impossible (unless it contains artificial sweetener). The added sugar in store-bought cranberry sauce increases the calories to 209 per half cup and cooking significantly reduces the vitamin C content. Fresh cranberries are a wonderful addition to muffins, cookies, and pies, and are delicious in stuffing for baked apples, squash, and chicken.

Choose plump, well-formed berries with a deep red luster. Cranberries are almost always sold in clear plastic bags, which makes it easy to check the quality. It's rare to find bad cranberries, though, since inferior ones are sorted out during the packing process. Cranberries will keep for about a week in the refrigerator; about a year in the freezer. Do not wash them until ready to use. Frozen cranberries do not need to be thawed before using them in dishes or recipes.

Dried fruit

Drying is a time-honored method for preserving food; fruit is dried either in the sun or by forced hot air. This process reduces the fruit's water content, usually from about 80 percent to between 15 and 35 percent. As a result, the nutrients are concentrated, leaving the fruit high in minerals—especially iron, copper, and potassium—and sometimes beta carotene. Dried fruit is also a compact source of fiber.

The catch is that drying also concentrates the fruit's sugar—and calories. Dried fruit may contain as much as 70 percent sugar by weight, a higher per-centage than that of many cookies and approaching that of some candies. In return for the high mineral content, you are getting a relatively calorie-dense snack food, and, since dried fruit tends to stick to your teeth, an increased risk of tooth decay. (Try to brush and floss your teeth, or at least rinse your mouth with water, after eating dried fruit.) Fruit also loses most of its vitamin C when dried.

Choose dried fruit that has not been "glazed" or had sugar added. Sulfite preservatives are often added to light-colored fruit such as apples, peaches, pears, apricots, and golden raisins to keep them from turning brown. These preservatives can produce allergic reactions in some people—especially asthmatics—and many experience severe, sometimes even fatal reactions to them. Manufacturers are required to list these preservatives—usually sulfur dioxide—clearly on packages, shipping containers, and bulk bins.

Sulfite-sensitive people should be sure to check labels and ask whether or not the fruit has been treated when buying from an unlabeled bin. Fortunately, there are some sulfite-free, light-colored fruits; these are usually labeled as such.

Fruit and vegetable juice

Most people drink juice to get vitamin C. In fact, orange juice is the major source of this vitamin in the American diet. But orange juice isn't the only juice high in vitamin C, and vitamin C isn't the only reason to drink juice. The range of juices is wider than ever—from tart to sweet, prosaic to exotic, in old-fashioned bottles to unrefrigerated mini-boxes. How can you tell the good juices from the bad?

The next best thing to whole fruits and vegetables is their juice. Most of their nutrients are retained, but nearly

NUTRITIONAL CONTENT OF
Dried Fruit

Fruit (3½ oz)	Calories	Dietary Fiber (g)	Iron (mg)	Beta Carotene (mg)
Apples, 10 rings	240	10.6	1.4	0
Apricots, 12 halves	240	8.1	4.7	4
Dates, 12	275	8.7	1.2	0.03
Figs, 6	255	18.5	2.2	0.08
Peaches, 8 halves	240	N/A	4.0	1.3
Pears, 6 halves	260	11.0	2.1	0
Prunes, 12	240	16.1	2.5	1
Raisins, ⅔ cup	300	6.8	2.1	0

all fiber is lost. Here are some of the nutritional bright spots:

• All citrus juices are high in vitamin C, containing up to twice the daily Recommended Dietary Allowance (RDA) in an eight-ounce glass.

• Most red or orange-colored juices are rich in beta carotene. Thus red or pink grapefruit juice has more beta carotene than white. The champion is carrot juice: an eight-ounce glass supplies six times the amount recommended by most experts.

• Grapefruit, orange, and pineapple juices are good sources of folacin. Women of child-bearing age need 0.4 milligrams (400 micrograms) of this B vitamin—twice as much as other adults—in order to ward off certain birth defects.

• Potassium is abundant in nearly all fruit and vegetable juices, with carrot, prune, tomato, and orange juice at the top of the list.

• One juice is high in iron: a cup of prune juice provides 30 percent of the RDA for men, 20 percent for women.

• Calcium-fortified orange juice has nearly as much calcium as milk and may be worthwhile for people who don't consume enough dairy products.

Fresh vs. frozen vs. reconstituted. Do you sometimes wonder if the vitamin C is really there when you pick up a carton of orange juice? The amount of vitamin C in eight ounces of juice can range from about 80 to 140 milligrams. It depends on many factors over which you have no control: the variety of oranges (most brands are made from several varieties), their ripeness, the climate in which they grew, and how the juice was handled, processed, packaged, and stored (heat, including pasteurization, reduces vitamin content). Vitamin C deteriorates when in contact with oxygen, so the longer juices sit around exposed to air,

the less vitamin C they contain. Loss of flavor parallels loss of nutrients. Many studies have compared various types of packaging and brands for nutritional content. It has been found, for example, that since vitamin C deteriorates when in contact with oxygen, there's

Beta Carotene and Vitamin C in Juices

Juice (8 oz)	Calories	Beta Carotene (mg)	Vitamin C (mg)
Apple, canned/bottled	115	0	2*
Apricot nectar, canned	140	2	1*
Carrot, canned	95	38	22
Cranberry cocktail, bottled	144	0	90
Grape, canned/bottled	155	0	0.2*
Grapefruit, pink, fresh	96	0.7	94
Grapefruit, white, fresh	96	0	94
Lemon, fresh	60	0	112
Orange, canned	104	0.3	86
Orange, carton	110	0.2	82
Orange, fresh	110	0.3	124
Orange, frozen	112	0.2	97
Papaya nectar, canned	140	0.2	8
Peach nectar, canned	135	0.4	13*
Pineapple, canned	140	0	27
Prune, canned	180	0	11
Tomato, canned	40	0.8	45
V-8 vegetable, canned	47	1.8	36

Vitamin C may be added. If so, it will be listed on the label.

increased risk of vitamin C loss in plastic jugs and some wax-coated cardboard cartons, which are permeable to air (unless the cartons are foil-lined). Fortunately, because citrus fruit is so rich in vitamin C, you can generally assume that, as long as it tastes good, six ounces of any type of orange juice will supply at least 100 percent of the RDA.

Freshly squeezed juice usually has the highest vitamin C content, followed by juice made from frozen concentrate. Unopened canned and bottled juices are next best: stored at room temperature, they retain more than 75 percent of their vitamin C for a year or longer. Chilled cartons, especially if they have been reconstituted, and unrefrigerated mini-boxes usually contain less vitamin C and have a shorter shelf life. One study found that an unopened carton of orange juice lost 1 to 2 percent of its vitamin C a day when kept at 40° F. That's not much, but it can be a problem if juice is kept for long periods. So when buying a chilled carton of juice, check the date on it, which should indicate the last day it can be sold (an average of twenty-seven days after packaging). If the date is close or has passed, there may be significant loss of vitamin C — and of taste.

Once you get the juice home, store it properly. Refrigerated juice in a carton can last two to four weeks (depending on its "sell by" date) before there's a serious loss of vitamin C and taste. The same is true of frozen juice once it is reconstituted, and of canned juice once it is opened. To protect the vitamin C from air, store the juice in a tightly

Exotic Fruits

It used to be that fruit was just apples, pears, oranges, a few other delicious but pedestrian varieties, and maybe an occasional pineapple. But thanks to improved horticultural methods and shipping, dozens of tropical or otherwise exotic fruits are now sold in specialty shops and well-stocked supermarkets around the country, sometimes year-round. Some types are now grown commercially in California,

Hawaii, or Florida. All are expensive, however, so don't expect to replace your daily apple with a guava or persimmon.

Exotic fruits can be added to fruit salads, green salads, or cereal, made into jellies or preserves, or used in toppings or sauces for ice cream or for other fruits. Still, the best way to eat these fruits is by themselves—as low-calorie snacks and healthful desserts.

Fruit (3½ oz edible portion)	Calories	Beta Carotene (mg)	Vitamin C (mg)	Comments
Guava	51	0.4	184	Sweet and aromatic. Use in pies or tarts, or for preserves.
Kiwifruit	61	0.1	98	Sweet-tart flavor. Good in fruit salads and tarts. High in potassium.
Kumquat	63	0.1	37	Small orangelike fruit. Good in fruit salads and pies.
Lychee	66	0	72	Grapelike flesh. Use in salads.
Mango	65	2	28	Peachlike flavor and spicy aroma. Must be fully ripe before eating. Good source of niacin.
Papaya	39	1	62	Mellow flavor. Use over ice cream or in fruit salads.
Passion fruit	97	0.4	30	Intense sweet flavor. Good when scooped out as a topping for fruit or ice cream. High in iron and potassium.
Persimmon, Japanese	70	1.3	8	Sweet and spicy. Must be ripe. Good in puddings and cakes. American variety is higher in vitamin C.
Quince	57	0	15	Aromatic. Tart when raw, sweet when cooked. Use in preserves, pies, stews, or as a cooked dessert.

closed glass container and keep it at 40° F. or below.

Since nutrition isn't a major issue when choosing among orange juices, that leaves taste and price. Taste tests have found that nothing compares to fresh-squeezed; it is also most expensive. Frozen orange juice rates second in taste, and is usually least expensive. If you want orange juice in a carton that is closer in taste to fresh-squeezed, look for "premium" brands: they aren't made from concentrate and are less processed than reconstituted orange juice in cartons.

Read the labels. When buying fruit juice, watch the wording on labels. If something is simply called "juice," it must be 100 percent juice. But what kind of juice? Something labeled cherry or apricot juice, for instance, is usually more grape and apple juice (which are cheaper) than cherry or apricot. And anything called "drinks," "beverages," "punches," "juice blends," "-ades," "punch," and "juice cocktails" usually contain little fruit juice—the rest being water and sugar, such as corn syrup. So you would be hard put to know some brands of fruit punch are only 10 percent juice, for instance, or some types of cranberry juice cocktail are just 27 percent juice. (Pure undiluted cranberry juice is available in health foods stores, but it is extremely tart.) The Food and Drug Administration (FDA) acting on complaints by consumer groups recently directed manufacturers to disclose the type and percentage of juice in a fruit beverage on its label. As long as you know what you're getting, there's nothing wrong with some of these beverages. But in some cases these products cost more than real juices, so you're paying a lot for water. If you want diluted fruit juice, you're better off mixing real juice with water or seltzer yourself. You'll cut calories, and you'll know what you're drinking.

Grapefruit

Grapefruit comes in white, pink, and red varieties. All are good sources of vitamin C, and pink and red grapefruits supply 5 and 12 percent, respectively, of the minimum recommended daily amount of beta carotene. Grapefruit is low in calories—40 per half—and virtually fat free, but those are the only characteristics that qualify it as a diet food. It has no special properties that can help burn fat or otherwise cause you to lose weight. Grapefruit is, however, a good source of potassium and soluble fiber, the kind that helps lower blood cholesterol levels.

Choose grapefruit that feels heavy for its size and with a thin skin; this indicates that it is juicy. Minor blemishes on the skin do not affect the fruit inside, but avoid grapefruit with any soft spots. Grapefruit can be stored at room temperature if you plan to eat it within a few days, though you may find it tastier when it's been chilled. Stored in the refrigerator it will keep for several weeks.

Lemons and limes

These citrus fruits don't offer much nutritionally simply because unlike oranges or grapefruits, they are rarely eaten out of hand. Still, they are fairly high in vitamin C and they can make a significant nutritional contribution when used to replace salt or butter as a seasoning or used as a low-fat salad dressing. The juice of a lemon or lime will also serve nicely as a low-fat marinade. And, of course, you can use fresh lemons and limes to make your own lemon- or limeade; that way you'll be able to control the amount of sugar added. Lemons can also be squeezed over cut fruits to prevent browning.

Is it dangerous to eat moldy fruit?

Discard small fruits—such as grapes or berries—if they become moldy. Some molds produce toxins, but it's hard to tell which do and which don't. (If a few berries on top of the box are moldy, it's okay to eat the unaffected ones, but inspect them carefully.) Cutting mold out of an apple, pear, tomato, or cucumber and then eating it may be okay. But the visible mold may not be all the mold there is—the threadlike hyphae (the equivalent of roots) may have penetrated the fruit, so if you cut out any mold, cut widely.

Keep a few lemons and limes on hand; fresh-squeezed juice is more flavorful than bottled. To get the most juice from a lemon or lime, roll the fruit with light pressure between your hands—preferably under warm water—before squeezing.

Choose lemons and limes that are heavy for their size and feel firm to the touch. The skin should be glossy and rich-colored. Avoid spongy fruit or those with thick skins. Stored in the fruit bin of the refrigerator, they will keep for about two weeks.

Melons

Two of the most widely available melons are cantaloupe and honeydew. Orange-fleshed cantaloupe is one of the best nutritional buys in the fruit world. Just half a melon provides you with more beta carotene and vitamin C than you need daily. It is also a good source of potassium and contains only 95 calories. Honeydew melon is large and creamy- or yellowish-white on the outside and light green on the inside. One four-ounce slice of honeydew contains just 45 calories and 29 milligrams of vitamin C—nearly half the RDA.

Choose cantaloupes with rinds covered with thick, close netting; avoid those with any smooth areas. The ends should slightly yield to pressure, be free of any stem, and have a full, fruity fragrance. Honeydews should have a smooth velvety surface and give a little when pressed at the blossom end (opposite the stem end). Ripen melons at room temperature; once ripe, store in the refrigerator.

Nectarines

Nectarines are a member of the peach family but are not, as some people believe, a cross between a peach and a plum, or simply a fuzzless peach. One large nectarine has only 65 calories and

contributes one-fifth of your minimum daily requirement for beta carotene as well as some potassium.

Choose well-colored fruits—deep yellow with a red blush. In order to ripen properly, nectarines must come to maturity on the tree—once picked, they will get softer, but not sweeter—so avoid those that are hard and green or dull colored. Mature fruit will soften at room temperature. Nectarines are ready to eat when there is a slight softening along the seam. Store ripe fruit in the refrigerator, but for maximum flavor, serve at room temperature.

Oranges

Oranges are of two types: eating and juice. Popular eating oranges include: the navel, a large seedless orange that is meaty and flavorful; the temple, a juicy, sweet-tart cross between an orange and a tangerine; and the Valencia, a medium-sized, thin-skinned orange. Temples and Valencias also make good juice oranges. Relatives of the orange—tangerines, clementines, tangelos, and mandarins—are also good for eating. Varieties of oranges that are used primarily for juice include Hamlin, Pineapple, and Parson Brown.

Oranges, as most people know, are an excellent source of vitamin C—one orange more than fulfills your daily requirement. They are also a fair source of beta carotene. Tangerines have less vitamin C than oranges, but are a better source of beta carotene. Both are good sources of potassium. Oranges provide a small amount of calcium as well. A medium-sized orange has about 60 calories, a medium-sized tangerine, about 35 calories.

Choose oranges that are firm and feel heavy for their size. Lightweight oranges will be dry. A very rough surface often indicates a thick skin, and

Ripe oranges sometimes undergo a process known as regreening. This occurs when a ripe orange pulls some green chlorophyll from its stems and leaves back into its peel. Such greenish oranges are extra ripe and thus often sweeter than other oranges.

therefore little fruit inside. Color is not an indication of quality: many perfectly ripe oranges have green streaks through their skin. Tangerines and tangelos also should feel heavy for their size. Their skin is naturally loose, so the fruit will not feel firm. As with oranges, a slight greening does not mean the fruit is not ripe. Carefully check oranges and tangerines sold in plastic bags for mold before buying. Mold spreads quickly, especially in tangerines, and can spoil the whole bag. Store oranges in a cool place or in the refrigerator. Store tangerines in the refrigerator fruit bin.

Peaches

Peaches are a fair source of potassium, beta carotene, vitamin C, and fiber. A medium-sized peach has 35 calories.

Choose peaches that are just beginning to soften. A ripe peach will have a creamy yellow and red color and a peachy smell. Do not buy fruit that is rock hard or has a greenish tinge—it will not ripen. Ripe peaches are very susceptible to bruises and should be handled with care. Ripen peaches at room temperature and store ripe fruit in the refrigerator.

Pears

There are many varieties of pears sold. Bartlett and Comice pears are soft, juicy, and sweet. They are also very fragile. Bosc and D'Anjou are firmer, but still very sweet and juicy. Depending on size and variety, pears contain between 85 and 120 calories. They are excellent sources of fiber.

Asian pears—also called Chinese or Oriental pear, Nashi, or apple pear—look very much like a cross between an apple and a pear, but are true pears. They have the round shape of apples (though sometimes they are lopsided), and the texture—crisp, firm, juicy, and sweet—is like that of an apple. But the color is yellow-green or russet, and they have a more mellow flavor than either apples or any pear variety. A four-ounce Asian pear has 55 calories and a small amount of potassium and fiber.

Choose pears that are firm, but not rock hard, and ripen them at home. (Pears are never left to ripen on the tree.) To ripen, place the fruit in a perforated paper bag and leave at room temperature for a few days. Pears are at their best when perfectly ripe; they are ready to eat when the flesh around the stem gives to gentle pressure. Avoid those pears with gashes or bruises and those that have gone soft at the blossom end. Ripe pears should be stored in the refrigerator.

Asian pears do not yield to gentle pressure; the best indicator of ripeness is a sweet aroma. Most Asian pears are sold ready to eat, and they store very well even when ripe, keeping for a week at room temperature or up to three months refrigerated.

Pineapples

Pineapples are a good source of vitamin C—$3\frac{1}{2}$ ounces of the fresh fruit provide 25 percent of the RDA. Canned pineapple is lower in vitamin C—containing 16 percent of the RDA—and higher in calories. Fresh pineapple has 50 calories per $3\frac{1}{2}$ ounces. The same amount of pineapple canned in its own juice has 60 calories. For pineapple canned in heavy syrup the calorie count jumps to 79 per $3\frac{1}{2}$ ounces.

Choose fresh pineapples that are golden-yellow in color and heavy for their size. Pineapples do not ripen after they are picked, so they do not need any time to ripen at home. Contrary to popular folklore, you cannot tell if a pineapple is ripe by the ease with which a leaf is removed. A good indication of ripeness is a strong, pleasant

Some fresh fruits, such as pineapple and papaya, contain protein-digesting enzymes that may cause lip and mouth irritation. Cooking (which takes place prior to canning) inactivates the enzymes.

pineapple fragrance. Avoid any pineapple that has soft spots. Pineapples should be eaten as soon as possible, but will keep for three to five days if stored in the refrigerator. Cut up fresh pineapple stored in an airtight container in the refrigerator will keep for a week.

Plums
There are many types of plums that offer a variety of colors, tastes, and textures. Some popular varieties include: Santa Rosa, a deep red plum with yellow flesh; El Dorado, a large plum with reddish-blue skin and pink-tinged flesh; the mirabelle, a small aromatic, golden-yellow plum; and Italian prune, a small purple plum (this variety is dried to make prunes).

The nutritional content of plums depends on the variety, but generally they are good sources of potassium and fiber and contain some vitamin A and iron. One medium-sized plum contains about 35 calories.

Choose plums with good color for the variety you are choosing. Plums should be slightly soft. Avoid any plums that are very hard, bruised, those that are shriveled, or those that have gone too soft. Store plums in the refrigerator.

Raspberries
Raspberries, and their cousins, blackberries, are good sources of fiber, potassium, and vitamin C. They also contain small amounts of beta carotene and iron, and blackberries supply a small amount of calcium as well. A cup of raspberries has just 60 calories; a cup of blackberries has 75 calories.

Choose berries that are plump with good color. Avoid containers that are stained, or contain berries that are moldy or mushy. Raspberries and blackberries are best eaten on the day purchased. Do not wash the berries until you are ready to eat them.

Raspberries and strawberries, along with cranberries and loganberries, contain ellagic acid, a natural substance that preliminary research suggest may help to prevent certain types of cancer.

Strawberries
Strawberries are delicious, beautiful, and nutritious. Strawberries have just 96 calories per pint or 45 calories per cup, which also provides 141 percent of the RDA of vitamin C and more fiber than two slices of whole wheat bread. They are also a good source of potassium and folacin.

Strawberries retain most of their vitamin C only if the green stem caps are still attached. Don't remove the caps until just before you are going to eat the strawberries.

Choose strawberries that have a lustrous red color and are firm to the touch. Avoid boxes of berries that show signs of leakage, or contain moldy-looking berries (check the bottom of the box); mold will rapidly spread to the rest of the berries. Opt for small or medium-sized berries rather than large ones; though they may look pretty, large berries are often not as sweet and flavorful as smaller ones. Stored in the refrigerator, strawberries will keep for a day or two. Do not wash them until you are ready to eat them.

Watermelon
Watermelon has a very high water content, making it a good, flavorful, low-calorie thirst quencher. One cup of cubed watermelon has 50 calories, is a good source of beta carotene and potassium, and contains some vitamin C as well.

Choose whole melons with a smooth, dull, exterior and a creamy yellow underside. You can more accurately judge the quality of a watermelon if you choose precut sections. The flesh should be deep red, moist, and fresh-looking. Avoid pale-fleshed watermelons or those that look dehydrated. Store whole melons in a cool room; wrap cut watermelon in plastic and store it in the refrigerator. Use watermelon within a few days.

Vegetables

Artichokes

Globe artichokes are usually served as an appetizer rather than as a side dish since they take a lot of concentration to eat. To remove the edible flesh, each leaf must be pulled off and scraped along the front teeth. But the effort is well worth it, both for flavor and nutrition. One medium-sized artichoke contains, on average, 55 calories and is high in folacin and fiber. It also contains some vitamin C, calcium, iron, and potassium. To make the most of the low-calorie count, stay away from traditional high-fat dipping sauces and serve artichokes with fresh lemon juice or a light vinaigrette. Tomato sauce and puréed roasted red peppers also make good, low-fat dips for artichokes.

Choose artichokes with tightly closed, fresh-looking leaves. A few dark spots on the leaves do not indicate spoilage as long as the vegetable looks healthy overall, but avoid any with extensive spotting or discoloration. Artichokes are best used as soon as possible. They will, however, keep in the refrigerator for four or five days.

Asparagus

Asparagus is very low in calories: eight spears have just 30. Asparagus is an excellent source of folacin and also provides potassium, vitamin C, beta carotene, and iron.

Choose bright green asparagus with compact, pointed tips. The stalks should be round: flat stalks can be tough and stringy. Thick stalks are more tender than thin ones. After harvesting, asparagus deteriorates quickly if not kept cold, losing flavor and nutrients. In the market, asparagus should be refrigerated or standing in several inches of cold water. At home, trim the stem ends of the asparagus and wrap the bases in a damp paper towel. Store asparagus in the refrigerator crisper. Asparagus loses its flavor if kept too long, so use it within a few days of purchase.

Avocados

Avocados are the exception to the rule that fruits and vegetables are low in fat and calories. One-half of a California avocado has 150 calories, 89 percent of which come from fat. Ounce for ounce, Florida avocado varieties have about half the fat and two-thirds the calories of the varieties grown in California. Still, the majority of the fat is monounsaturated, and therefore may help lower cholesterol levels. Furthermore, avocados are rich in potassium, folacin, and fiber and contain a fair amount of iron and vitamin C.

Choose avocados that have no bruises or sunken spots. Many markets sell avocados while they're still hard and unripe, so you may have to allow them a few days at room temperature to soften; they are ripe when they yield to light pressure. Those that are not quite ready to eat can be ripened at room temperature. Store avocados that are already ripe in the refrigerator.

Beans

Fresh beans can be classified into two broad categories: those with edible pods, like snap beans, and those that are shelled, like lima beans. (Dried beans are covered on page 197.) The bulk of fresh beans are actually sold frozen or canned.

Snap beans, which are also called green beans or string beans, are either green or yellow, and are a good source of iron, folacin, and beta carotene (yellow beans are much lower in this nutrient than green, however) and contain a small amount of calcium as well. One cup cooked has 45 calories.

Despite their high fat content, 3½ ounces of avocado have less fat than a salad with 2 tablespoons of Italian dressing, a cup of potato salad made with mayonnaise, or a 3½-ounce hamburger made with lean ground beef.

Vegetables: Once Exotic, Now Familiar

Interest in vegetables has risen in the past few years, and many supermarkets and produce stands have begun stocking varieties that you wouldn't have found, or perhaps even heard of, ten years ago. They're no more nutritious than your old favorites, but they can add variety and interest to your diet. There are squashes of all descriptions, as well as uncommon newcomers such as daikon (Japanese radish) and jicama (the so-called Mexican potato), and salsify (used by American cooks of the last century and now undergoing a revival). The following guide sorts out some of the newer vegetables you are likely to see, most of which are not really new at all—just less familiar than broccoli or carrots in American markets.

For variety as well as nutrition and good taste, these vegetables are well worth trying. Many can be eaten raw; all are easy to cook. Some of the larger vegetables (spaghetti squash, for example) may come with a small label affixed that offers tips on cooking and handling. Like all vegetables, these are relatively low in calories and relatively high in vitamins, minerals, and fiber.

Bok choy (Chinese mustard cabbage). Large white stem, dark green leaves, mild flavor, shaped like a head of celery. Can be stir-fried, added to soups, or eaten raw in coleslaw or salads, like any cabbage. A half-cup serving (cooked) has 10 calories, some calcium, one-third of your daily requirement of vitamin C, and half your minimum daily requirement of beta carotene.

Celeriac (celery root). Bulbous white root, rough brown skin, celerylike flavor. Peel, then slice or julienne. Good raw if marinated in lemon juice or a flavorful dressing; also good in soups. A half-cup serving has 20 calories and also contains small amounts of beta carotene, iron, and calcium.

Chayote squash (mango squash or mirliton). Dark green. May be avocado-shaped or round. Zucchini-like flavor. Peel, then boil, bake, or stir-fry like any summer squash. The large seed is edible, too. Unpeeled halves can be stuffed with shrimp, ground meats, or rice and diced-vegetable combinations and then baked. A half-cup serving has 19 calories, plus small amounts of beta carotene, vitamin C, and potassium.

Daikon (Japanese radish). White carrot-shaped root. Crisp and spicy. Good raw in salads or sliced as a dipping vegetable. Can be added to soups, stews, or stir-fries. A half-cup serving has about 10 calories, with some vitamin C and potassium.

Fennel (finocchio, anise). Large bulb-shaped base (the edible part) with pale green, feathery tops. Common in Italian cooking. Mild licorice flavor. Trim, slice, and serve raw in salads or as a dipping vegetable. Add to soups and stir-fries. Also good grilled. A half-cup serving has about 15 calories, some beta carotene, and calcium.

Jerusalem artichoke (sunchoke, girasole). Small brown bulb with crisp white flesh. Nutty flavor. Not related to artichokes. Peel, slice, and serve raw in salads, or steam and substitute for potatoes as a side dish. A half-cup serving has 57 calories, plus some calcium, iron, and phosphorus.

Jicama (Mexican potato). Light brown skin; round but slightly flat; crisp, sweet, white flesh. Needs peeling. Good raw, served sliced and cold, in salads or with dips. Or steam or stir-fry quickly. Can be dressed with lemon juice and chili powder for an hors d'oeuvre. A half-cup serving has 25 calories and almost one-quarter of the RDA for vitamin C.

Salsify (oyster plant). A carrot-shaped root with black or white skin. Mild flavor, somewhat like asparagus. Steam whole, then peel and slice. Like potatoes, raw salsify darkens quickly when peeled. A good side dish or addition to soup. A half-cup serving has 35 calories, plus some calcium and iron.

Spaghetti squash. Yellow, football-shaped, with stringy but tender and flavorful yellow flesh. Halve and steam until tender, then use a fork to shred the pulp into "spaghetti." Serve plain, with pasta sauces, or with a small amount of olive oil and grated cheese. Cooked and cooled, it can be added to salads. A half-cup serving has 23 calories, some beta carotene, B vitamins, and potassium.

Fresh, Frozen, or Canned

Because it tastes better, many people prefer fresh produce. Nutritionally, too, fresh is better—in theory, that is, but not invariably. For maximum nutrition, fruits and vegetables should be harvested and eaten the same day. Still, even produce transported 1,000 miles or more and left in the bin for a day or two can be full of nutrients.

Fresh produce. To get the most from fresh produce, shop frequently and use fruits and vegetables as quickly as you can. Don't peel, slice, or chop anything until just before you are ready to cook and/or serve it. If you don't have to cut, don't. String beans, for example, retain more flavor and vitamins if cooked whole. Avoid buying precut produce such as cantaloupe. At least ask the manager how long cut fruits have been sitting around. Never soak fruits and vegetables, and wash them as little as is consistent with cleanliness. Choose a quick-cooking method (microwaving, for example, or steaming) over the long, slow boil that leaches out minerals and partially destroys vitamins. Always cook vegetables with a cover. No matter how careful you are, processing of any kind always destroys some nutrients.

If produce looks or feels wilted and pallid, or if you have inadvertently allowed the broccoli to sit in the crisper for a week, you'll be better off with a frozen or even a canned vegetable for dinner.

Frozen produce. Frozen food that has been scrupulously handled can be more nutritious than fresh that has sat in the grocery for days. Frozen fruits, in particular, may retain more vitamin C than fresh fruit that has been abused in transport or storage. Don't buy packages with ice crystals on the outside; this indicates that the food has thawed and refrozen. Pack frozen fruits and vegetables in a double bag and get them home fast. Your home freezer should stay at 0° F. If something begins to thaw, you can salvage it by cooking it as soon as possible.

Canned produce. Thanks to improved canning technology and the use of new types of lining, canned produce retains most of the food's vitamins and minerals. Canned beans, pumpkin, corn, pineapple, and beets, to name a few, are actually quite nutritious. But most canned vegetables also contain an unwanted extra: lots of sodium.

Some nutrient loss is inevitable whenever a food is prepared, whether commercially or at home. The extended heating process of commercial canning partially destroys certain vitamins, especially vitamin C and some of the B vitamins, as well as beta carotene. Minerals survive processing and heating better, though significant quantities end up in the canned liquid. Remember, however, that cooking vegetables at home also destroys some vitamins (microwaving is least destructive).

Once a can is sealed, there is little deterioration of nutrients, even after a couple of years, unless it is stored at high temperatures for long periods. To get the most nutrients from canned vegetables, don't overcook them; they're already cooked and need only to be heated. Use the liquid, juice, or syrup in the can whenever practicable, since these contain many nutrients. If you're trying to cut down on salt, rinse the canned vegetables, or look for specially labeled low-sodium canned goods.

Vegetables with high fiber are green peas, lima beans, parsnips, sweet peppers, broccoli, carrots, green beans, brussels sprouts, and sweet potatoes.

There are other bean varieties with edible pods that are similar nutritionally to snap beans. Chinese long beans, also called "yard-long" or "asparagus" beans, can measure up to eighteen inches long. They have a mild flavor. Italian green beans, also called Romano beans, are distinguished by broad flat, bright green pods. They are often available only in frozen form. Purple wax beans turn green when cooked.

Lima beans, fresh or frozen, are higher in protein, calories (one cup cooked has 170), iron, and fiber, and lower in beta carotene than edible-pod beans. They also contain a good amount of vitamin C, potassium, phosphorus, and magnesium.

Choose edible-pod beans that are brightly colored green, yellow, or purple depending on their variety. The beans should look young and tender and feel velvety. Avoid those that are bulging with seeds since these will be old and tough. The beans will keep for a few days wrapped in plastic in the refrigerator. Fresh lima beans are sold in their pods. Choose pods that are bright green and well filled. Avoid those that have brown spots or look old. Baby lima beans are usually more tender. Lima beans should be refrigerated and stored in their pods uncovered. They will keep three to five days.

Beets

While canned beets are most popular, fresh beets are crisper and more flavorful; they can be steamed, boiled, or baked. Never peel beets until after cooking and leave some of the stem on top for boiling. Beets contain more sugar than any other vegetable, but one cup (sliced) has only 60 calories. Beets are a good source of folacin, vitamin C, manganese, potassium, iron, and fiber.

Fresh beets are sometimes sold with their green tops attached. The greens are significantly more nutritious than the roots, supplying hefty amounts of beta carotene, vitamin C, calcium, and iron.

Choose beets that are firm and smooth with a deep red color. The greens, if attached, should be fresh-looking. Remove green tops before storing the roots. Beets keep about two weeks in the refrigerator.

Beet greens—which can be sold alone in bunches as well as part of the roots—should be in a refrigerated case as they may become bitter in warmer environment. Small, young leaves have the best flavor; the greens become tough as they mature. They should be green and moist-looking. Pass by greens that are heavily blemished or yellowed.

Broccoli

Broccoli is the nutritional leader of the cruciferous family of vegetables, the type that studies suggest may protect against colorectal, stomach, and respiratory cancers. One cup chopped and cooked contains 45 calories and provides you with 200 percent of the RDA for vitamin C, 90 percent of your minimum daily requirement of beta carotene, 43 percent of the RDA of folacin, 12 percent of phosphorus, 10 percent of thiamine, 9 percent of calcium, 9 percent of iron, and 6 percent of niacin. It is also rich in potassium and supplies 20 percent of your daily fiber requirements. Along with this rich supply of vitamins and minerals, it contains compounds called indoles and isothiocyantes, which various studies seem to indicate are effective in protecting against certain forms of cancer.

Choose crisp stalks and florets that do not show any yellow. Florets that are green, bluish-green, or purplish-green have more beta carotene and vitamin C than paler florets. The florets should be tightly closed and the stalks should look young and tender, not woody. Fresh broccoli will keep for a few days if wrapped in plastic and stored in the refrigerator.

Brussels sprouts

This vegetable looks like a miniature cabbage; indeed, it is a member of the cabbage family and like other cruciferous vegetables has cancer-protecting properties. Brussels sprouts are an excellent source of fiber and vitamin C. They are a good source of protein, beta carotene, folacin, potassium, and iron, and brussels sprouts also contain a small amount of calcium.

Choose tightly compact, firm heads with good color. Avoid those that are puffy and soft or those with a strong odor. Brussels sprouts kept in a plastic bag in the refrigerator will stay crisp and green. Use within a few days.

Cabbage

Cabbage can be eaten cooked or raw, although some people have trouble

Cooking: How to Preserve Nutrients

No matter how careful you are, cooking of any kind destroys some nutrients. The amount lost will depend on the freshness of the food (and how it was handled and stored before you bought it), how long you cook it and at what temperature, and how much surface area is exposed to water and air. Certain nutrients are more likely to be destroyed by heat than others—vitamin C, for instance, and B vitamins such as thiamine and riboflavin. Others, including most vitamins and some minerals, are likely to leach into cooking water. Here are a few guidelines to help you prepare foods so that they stay as nutritious as possible:

• Cook foods for the shortest time possible. Microwaving, steaming, and stir-frying are the quickest methods. Covering a pot or pan will help cut cooking time.

• Cook vegetables whole and unpeeled, as often as possible—or eat them raw. Avoid buying precut produce.

• Never soak fruits and vegetables.

• If you're boiling vegetables, use as little water as you can. Don't place them in the water until it's at a full boil. If you use the water from boiling or steaming to make soups and gravies, you'll consume any nutrients that leached away.

• Don't leave cooked foods standing at room temperature.

• Cook foods as close to serving time as possible.

Comparing Cooking Methods

Method	Comments	Examples (typical values)
Microwaving	Usually best at preserving nutrients in vegetables because it cooks so fast and requires no added water—provided you don't overcook.	Cabbage and broccoli lose only 10-20% of vitamin C when microwaved vs. 27-62% lost in boiling in lots of water.
	Little nutritional loss when reheating leftovers or cooking frozen foods.	Microwaved spinach loses only minimal amounts of folacin (a B vitamin) vs. 23% lost in boiling.
Steaming	Requires short cooking time and little water, so good at retaining nutrients.	Generally vegetables lose 50% less minerals during steaming than boiling.
		Carrots lose 17-30% vitamin C.
Boiling	To preserve nutrients: Use little water; place food in water only when it's at full boil; cover pot or pan; save water for soups and gravies.	Green beans lose 72% of vitamin C when french cut and boiled vs. 46% when cooked whole.
		Broccoli loses 25% of vitamin C when boiled for two minutes vs. 33% after eleven minutes.
		Unpeeled potatoes lose little vitamin C and folacin during boiling vs. up to 25% lost if peeled.
Baking/roasting	The higher the temperature and the longer the cooking time, the greater the vitamin loss.	Baked potato loses 60% of vitamin C if left to stand for one hour vs. only 20% lost if eaten right after cooking.
Frying	Conventional frying at high temperatures destroys heat-sensitive vitamins.	Most fried vegetables lose 25-85% of folacin.
	Stir-frying is quicker and should require less oil—thus it's less destructive.	French-fried potatoes lose up to 90% of vitamin C.

digesting it raw. Cabbage is a good source of fiber and vitamin C, and, like its relatives broccoli and cauliflower, has cancer-protecting potential. In fact, studies in animals fed a daily dose of indole compounds—substances in cruciferous vegetables that scientists now believe help protect against cancer —equal to the amount in a half a head of cabbage had less risk of breast and other forms of cancer. Other studies have found a lower incidence of colon and rectal cancer in people who eat cabbage frequently.

The tightly compact head of green cabbage may be most familiar, but there are other forms that are even more nutritious. Green cabbage is high in vitamin C, but red cabbage provides nearly 100 percent of the RDA for vitamin C in $1\frac{1}{2}$ cups uncooked. Savoy cabbage, which has crinkled, ruffly yellow leaves contains 20 percent of the daily recommended intake of beta carotene in a $1\frac{1}{2}$-cup serving. All three varieties of cabbage have just 25 calories per one-half cup and are a good source of fiber and folacin.

Choose heads that are tightly closed without signs of worm holes or bruises. The heads should be firm, not puffy, and feel heavy for their size. Unwashed cabbage will keep for a week to ten days—sometimes longer—if placed in a plastic bag and refrigerated.

Carrots

Long been rumored to have properties that can improve vision, carrots are, in fact, good for your eyes: they are rich in beta carotene, which the body converts to vitamin A—a crucial nutrient for the functioning of the retina. But vitamin A won't cure nearsightedness or farsightedness and can improve vision only if vision problems result from a vitamin A deficiency, which is a rare condition in this country. Still, beta

carotene is believed to be a protector against cancer and the soluble fiber in carrots may also help lower blood cholesterol levels. In one study, people who ate seven ounces of carrots a day for three weeks had, on average an 11 percent reduction in cholesterol levels.

One seven-inch carrot has about 30 calories and provides 12 milligrams of beta carotene (the deeper orange the color of the carrot, the more beta carotene it will contain). This root vegetable is also rich in potassium.

To retain maximum nutrients, scrub carrots but leave them unpeeled, unless the skin is very tough or blemished. Carrots contain more natural sugar than any other vegetable, except for beets, and thus they make a healthful addition to items such as quick breads, cakes, and muffins. Grated carrots can even be added to meatloaf to "stretch" the meat and make it juicier.

Choose carrots that are firm and well-shaped with good color. Avoid those that are cracked, shriveled, or rubbery. When buying carrots with their green tops still attached, make sure the greens are fresh-looking. Carrots keep well in the refrigerator. Green tops should be removed from carrots before storing. Otherwise, the greens will wilt and decay quickly; furthermore, moisture will be drawn away from the roots, turning them limp and rubbery.

Cauliflower

One of the cruciferous vegetables that may offer protection against some forms of cancer, cauliflower can be eaten cooked or raw, although some people have trouble digesting it uncooked. One cup of cauliflower diced and cooked is high in vitamin C, fiber, folacin, and potassium, and contains 30 calories. Frozen cauliflower has about a third less vitamin C and about half the potassium of fresh. Frozen cauliflower is

Carrots contain twice as much beta carotene as they did in 1950, according to the USDA, making them one of the best sources of this important antioxidant. Scientists are constantly improving food crops and developing new varieties. If current genetic research proceeds on track, the carotene content of carrots may double again by the year 2000.

not as flavorful as fresh; it looks and tastes watery, no matter how it's cooked.

Some markets sell a cauliflower-broccoli hybrid that looks like cauliflower but has a green curd. Less dense than white, this recently developed variety cooks more quickly and has a milder taste.

Choose white, firm, clean florets with no discoloration. The leaves should be green and fresh-looking. Store cauliflower wrapped in plastic in the vegetable bin of the refrigerator.

Celery

Because of its high water content, celery is nearly calorie free; one eight-inch stalk has just 6 calories. It is, however, low in nutrients, supplying just a small amount of potassium. Still, celery does contain some fiber, vitamin C, and folacin and makes a flavorful addition to soups and stews (celery leaves can also be used in making broth), or a healthful snack.

Choose bunches of celery that are tightly closed at the bottom. The stalks should be fresh-looking and free of bruises and growth cracks. The leaves should also look fresh. Avoid celery that is limp. Store celery in the refrigerator; wrapped in plastic, it will keep for about two weeks.

Corn

Corn on the cob is best in season (May through September), for that is when its flavor is at its peak. An ear of corn has just 85 calories and is a good source of fiber. Corn provides a small amount of protein, phosphorus, and potassium. Yellow corn also contains a small amount of beta carotene

Except for being lower in vitamin C, canned and frozen corn are about equal in nutritional value to fresh corn. However, frozen corn sometimes is packaged in a butter sauce that increases its fat

and sodium content. Canned corn has both salt and guar added, making it marginally higher in calories and sometimes substantially higher in sodium than fresh kernels. Despite its name, creamed corn contains no cream or dairy products, but it does have cornstarch and sugar, which adds calories.

Choose corn that has been picked that day and has been kept cold, or at least shaded from the sun. Do not buy corn that has already been husked. The husks should have a good green color and be free from decay where the silk ends. If possible, pull back the husk and look for well-formed, plump kernels. Eat the corn as soon as possible; the sugar in corn begins to turn to starch the moment it is picked. If you cannot eat the corn right away, store it in the coldest part of your refrigerator; cold temperatures retard the change from sugar to starch.

Cucumbers

Cucumbers are low in calories—six large slices have just 5 calories—but otherwise have little nutritional value. Their high water content, however, makes them particularly refreshing on a hot summer day. Full-sized cucumbers are usually waxed and should be peeled before eating; smaller-sized kirbys are usually not waxed and therefore do not need peeling.

Choose cucumbers that are slender and firm to the touch. Cucumbers should have a good green color and not be dull green or yellow. Avoid any overly large cucumbers and those with shriveled ends. Cucumbers will keep for about a week if they are stored in the refrigerator.

Eggplant

Eggplant comes in many colors—white, purple, purple-black, yellowish-white, red, and striped—but the most

Are "baby" vegetables nutritious?

The nutritional differences between "baby" vegetables and their regular counterparts are slight in most cases. One exception is baby carrots: ounce for ounce they may have only about one-tenth the beta carotene found in regular carrots. Baby vegetables are sometimes natural varieties, and sometimes ordinary vegetables harvested at tender ages. For example, the peeled, ready-to-use raw "baby" carrots, sold in plastic bags, are regular carrots harvested before maturity, then peeled and shaped.

Perhaps the most ubiquitous "baby" is the miniature corn often seen in Chinese dishes or in salad bars. Imported in cans from Asia, baby corn is somewhat less nutritious than regular corn since the water content is higher. Most people eat fresh baby vegetables only rarely, so their nutritional content is not a matter for concern. Some of the miniatures are expensive and hard to find. Ordinary vegetables are obviously a more practical source of daily nutrients.

common is the the dark purple, pear-shaped variety. Eggplant is a good source of fiber, potassium, and folacin. To get the most from its fiber content, do not peel eggplant before eating. One cup cooked has just 50 calories.

Like nearly all vegetables, eggplant contains virtually no fat. But according to one study, it absorbs more fat than any other vegetable. When researchers deep-fried a serving of eggplant, they found that it absorbed eighty-three grams of fat in just seventy seconds —four times as much as an equal portion of potatoes—adding more than 700 calories. Instead of frying, bake, broil or grill eggplant.

Choose eggplant that feels firm to the touch and is heavy for its size. Dark purple eggplant should have a clear, satiny color. Avoid any with soft spots or bruises. Small eggplants are often more tender. Eggplant will keep for about a week if refrigerated and wrapped in a plastic bag to prevent moisture loss.

Garlic

Garlic, a member of the onion family, has been used medicinally since the beginning of history. Ancient Egyptian, Greek, Roman, Chinese, and Indian physicians believed it cured a wide range of ills, including heart disease. Garlic and its relatives (onions, scallions, chives, leeks, and shallots) are not nutritional storehouses like potatoes, but they add savor to less flavorful foods and in one form or another are kitchen staples throughout the world.

Garlic's preventive and/or curative qualities have long been the subject of scientific investigation. No one really knows so far what the health benefits of garlic are, yet some findings have been interesting. Garlic (and onions) contains a substance that interferes with the formation of blood clots and in

addition may help reduce blood cholesterol. This might support its age-old reputation as a weapon against heart disease. Some studies also suggest that garlic has anticancer properties. For example, in one study, about 1,600 people in China, a third of whom had stomach cancer, were interviewed about their consumption of garlic and onions (including chives and scallions). Those who had eaten the most garlic and onions (fifty-three pounds a year) were 60 percent less likely to have stomach cancer than those who had consumed these foods rarely. Laboratory studies have also indicated that something in garlic can reduce the incidence of some tumors and inactivate some cancer-causing chemicals.

Nobody seems to know whether cooking destroys or reduces any medicinal properties garlic may have. But if it takes fifty-three pounds of garlic and onions annually to protect against cancer and if it must be eaten raw, that's more than most people would be capable of. Another problem is that large quantities of raw garlic may make the mouth burn or cause stomach distress.

Nevertheless, the National Cancer Institute, among other institutions, is currently studying the anticancer effects of garlic and many other foods. Promoters of garlic often point to studies showing that men in Greece, Italy, and other Mediterranean countries eat large amounts of garlic and have a lower heart-attack rate than in northern European countries. However, other dietary, lifestyle, and genetic factors could be at work here. The bottom line: eat as much garlic and onions (raw or cooked) as you find palatable.

Choose garlic bulbs that are plump and compact, free of damp or soft spots, and with the other skin taut and unbroken. The garlic should feel heavy and firm in your hand.

Greens

If iceberg lettuce is the only type of greens you eat, you are selecting the one weakling in a family of nutritional champions. Any other lettuce or leafy green vegetable would be a better choice. Most other greens are excellent sources of vitamin C and beta carotene, and good sources of iron, fiber, folacin, and calcium. As a general rule, the darker green a leaf vegetable is, the more nutritious. Romaine and loose-leaf lettuce thus have up to five times as much vitamin C and six times as much beta carotene as iceberg lettuce. What's more, greens—especially kale, collards, and others in the cabbage family—may help lower the risk of cancer. The iron in greens is not as easily assimilated by the body as iron from animal sources, but iron absorption is enhanced by vitamin C—by eating tomatoes or red peppers in your salad, for example.

NUTRITIONAL CONTENT OF
Raw Greens

Greens (3½ oz)	Calories	Beta Carotene (mg)	Vitamin C (mg)	Dietary Fiber (g)	Calcium (mg)	Iron (mg)	Comments
Iceberg or crisphead lettuce	13	0	4	0.9	19	0.5	The most popular kind of lettuce, but the least nutritious.
Butterhead, bibb, or Boston lettuce	13	0.6	8	1.5	35	0.2	Sweet and delicate taste.
Romaine or Cos lettuce	16	1.6	24	2.1	68	1.4	Strong taste. Used in Caesar salads.
Loose-leaf lettuce	18	1	18	2.1	68	1.4	Sweet and delicate taste.
Arugula or roquette	23	4.4	91	N/A	309	1.2	Strong and peppery. Spices up a salad.
Chicory or curly endive	23	2.4	24	1.6	100	0.9	Slightly bitter. Mix with milder greens. Radicchio is a red variety.
Escarole	17	1.2	7	N/A	52	0.8	An endive with broad leaves.
Spinach	22	4	28	2.4	100	2.7	Eat raw or cooked. High in folacin and potassium. Its iron is poorly absorbed by the body.
Watercress	11	2.8	43	3.3	120	0.2	Pungent. In cabbage family. Add to salads or sandwiches.
Beet greens	40	4.4	36	N/A	164	2.7	Eat cooked. High in potassium. Moderately high in sodium.
Dandelion greens	45	8.4	35	3.3	187	3.1	Pungent. Very nutritious. Use young leaves in salads; sauté tough leaves.
Turnip greens	27	4.6	60	3.9	190	1.1	Strong flavor. More nutritious than the root vegetable. Eat raw or cooked.
Swiss chard	19	2	30	N/A	51	1.8	Mild flavor. Steam or sauté.
Kale	50	5.3	120	6.6	135	1.7	Mild, cabbage-like taste. Cook or use in salad. Highly nutritious.
Collards	19	2	23	3.2	117	0.6	Strong flavor. In cabbage family; related to kale. Steam or sauté.

Choose greens with good color for their variety. Leaves should be fresh-looking. Avoid any greens with brown, rusty spots, torn, bruised leaves, or insect damage. Check the cut end of lettuce; it should be cream-colored, not brown. Wash and dry greens and store them in a plastic bag in the refrigerator. Do not store lettuce with apples, pears, or tomatoes because these fruits emit ethylene gas which can cause brown spotting on the leaves. Greens will keep a few days to a week.

Mushrooms

If you thought that mushrooms were just a tasty decoration, it should come as good news that they offer a significant amount of some vitamins and minerals. One cup of *Agaricus bisporus*, the common cultivated mushroom sold in supermarkets, has just 40 calories cooked and drained and provides you with 37 percent of the RDA for niacin, 28 percent of the riboflavin 18 percent of the iron, 14 percent of the folacin, and 10 percent of the vitamin C, and is high in potassium. Drained, canned mushrooms are less nutritious. The vitamins and minerals may be lost during processing or may seep out into the cooking liquids. Try to use the liquid in some part of your meal. But check the label on the can to make sure that salt and high-fat ingredients such as butter have not been added.

Increasingly, other mushroom varieties that offer a greater range of tastes and textures are becoming widely available. Shiitake mushrooms, for example, are intensely flavorful, with more calories but fewer minerals than *Agaricus bisporus*. Delicate oyster mushrooms, sproutlike enoki, and hearty portobellos are three other popular types.

Most varieties are available dried as well as fresh. Dried mushrooms have highly concentrated calories and minerals by weight, but because of their strong flavor they are used in much smaller quantities. You must soak them before using them in cooking.

Choose mushrooms with tightly closed caps. Even if the gills show, the mushrooms may still taste good, but avoid any that are pitted or spongy-looking. Store mushrooms in a paper bag in the refrigerator and use them as soon as possible.

Onions

Raw or cooked, onions can be used in a wide variety of dishes. They enhance the flavor of foods by irritating the membranes of the nose and mouth, and therefore are a good addition to low-sodium diets. Like garlic, an onion relative, onions may contain substances that can help protect against cancer and heart disease.

There are many varieties of onions. The most common is the yellow globe onion, which has a strong flavor and is used mostly for cooking. Spanish or Bermuda onions are milder and can be eaten raw or cooked. Sweet red Italian onions have a mellow flavor and are often eaten raw in sandwiches and salads. Shallots—a cross between garlic and onion—have a sweet flavor. Chives and scallions are immature onion plants; only the leaves of chives are used and scallions (which are sold with their green tops attached) are picked before the bulb has a chance to form.

A half-cup of chopped onions has 10 percent of the RDA for vitamin C and folacin and a fair amount of potassium. Scallions provide a good amount of beta carotene and vitamin C if their green tops are eaten. A half cup of chopped onions has about 75 calories; a half cup of chopped scallions has 13.

Choose onions that are firm and well-shaped with no soft or soggy spots. Their dry, paper-thin protective skin should be intact. Avoid onions that have sprouted. Scallions and chives should be green and fresh looking. Store onions in a cool dry place, or in the refrigerator. They will keep in either place for several weeks. Do not store onions with potatoes as they will draw moisture from the potatoes and rot very quickly. Store scallions and chives in the refrigerator vegetable bin and use within a few days.

Parsnips

This relative of the carrot has served as a good source of starch for 4,000 years but was largely replaced by the potato in the nineteenth century. Unjustly neglected today, it has a sweet, nutty flavor, particularly in the winter, when it is most abundant. Parsnips are a good source of vitamin C and folacin, and an excellent source of fiber; one cup of cooked slices has about 120 calories.

Choose small to medium, well-shaped parsnips; large ones can be tough and taste woody. Avoid those that are limp and shriveled. Wrapped in plastic, parsnips will stay fresh for several weeks in the refrigerator.

Peas

Most of the peas in this country are sold frozen, but finding fresh peas is well worth the search because the flavor is so much better. Fresh peas are tender and sweet. Some varieties, such as sugar snap and snow peas (or Chinese peas), can be eaten pods and all. Peas are very high in protein for a vegetable and provide a good amount of iron, potassium, beta carotene, phosphorus, folacin, and niacin. They contain 125 calories per cup, cooked. Snow peas supply nearly 100 percent of the RDA for vitamin C in 3½ ounces. They are high in protein, iron, and potassium, and also provide a small amount of calcium. One cup of cooked snow peas has 65 calories.

Choose uniformly green young pods that are well filled, and velvety to the touch. Pods that look as though they are about to explode or those that are yellow are overly mature and will taste tough and mealy. Snow peas should be bright green and look crisp and fresh. To prevent the sugar in the peas from converting to starch, store peas uncovered in their pods in the refrigerator. Eat them as soon as possible.

Peppers

The most popular variety of peppers is the bell, aptly named for its shape. This type can be either green, red, or yellow. While green peppers are a good source of beta carotene and vitamin C, red peppers are an even better source of these vitamins; one red pepper provides more than twice the RDA for vitamin C and 84 percent of the minimum recommended daily intake for beta carotene. Both shades are good sources of potassium and fiber and have just 20 calories per pepper. Hot peppers, such as cayenne, jalapeño, and chili, are also high in nutrients, but are usually not eaten in sufficient quantities to make any significant nutritional impact.

A common concern is that hot peppers cause ulcers, but there's no evidence that they do. Studies of areas where hot peppers are used extensively in cooking have found no higher incidence of stomach ulcers among their populations. Actually, evidence has shown that peppers may have some beneficial properties. Capsaicin—the chemical in peppers responsible for their "heat"—has been found to work as an anticoagulant, thus possibly helping to prevent heart attacks or strokes caused by a blood clot. Moreover, the high vitamin C and beta carotene content of peppers makes them valuable high-antioxidant foods.

Choose peppers that are firm and well

If you taste some food laced with hot peppers and find it intolerably hot, eat a bit of rice or bread, rather than have a drink of water. Water, or just about any other beverage, will only spread the fire. The one liquid that seems to work is milk. It contains a protein called casein, which literally wipes away capsaicin, the fiery compound in peppers.

shaped with good bright color. They should be thick fleshed and free of soft spots and wrinkled skin. Bell peppers should feel heavy for their size. Store peppers in a plastic bag in the refrigerator. They will keep for a week.

Potatoes

Potatoes have a reputation for being fattening, but this is not the case. One medium-sized baked potato with its skin has just 220 calories and is virtually fat free. Potatoes are bad for those watching their weight only when they are fried or served with high-calorie, high-fat toppings such as sour cream and butter. Potatoes are a good source of fiber, iron, phosphorus, vitamin B_6, and niacin, and a fair source of vitamin C. They are an excellent source of potassium; in fact, a half of a large baked potato with skin contains more potassium than a six-ounce glass of orange juice. New potatoes are not a different variety, but the young, small, thin-skinned potatoes of any variety that are harvested early. They are similarly nutritious.

To get the most nutrients from potatoes, you should eat the skin, since many nutrients are concentrated in or just below it. The only reason to avoid the skin is if the potato has a greenish tinge. That's chlorophyll, a sign that the potato has been exposed to too much light after harvest. It's also an indication that solanine (a naturally occurring toxin) may be present in increased amounts, especially in the skin. Eating such damaged potatoes may occasionally cause cramps, diarrhea, and fatigue. Potato sprouts contain lots of solanine, too. Although undamaged potatoes also contain some solanine, the concentration is very low in most American-grown varieties. You would have to eat about twelve pounds at one sitting to be affected adversely.

A 2½-ounce serving of french fries has nearly three times the calories and nearly twelve times the fat of a 2½-ounce baked potato.

Choose potatoes that have not sprouted and are virtually unblemished. Avoid those that have shriveled skin or are soft, wilted, or green. If a potato you have at home has seen better days, pare away all the green areas, including the skin, and gouge out all sprouts. But if it has become excessively soft or sprouted, discard it.

Don't store potatoes next to onions: the gasses given off by the onions accelerates the decay of the potatoes. Potatoes shouldn't be refrigerated because cold temperatures convert the starch to sugar and give the potatoes an undesirable sweet taste (however, the process can be reversed by leaving the potatoes at room temperature for a few days). Instead, store potatoes in a cool, dry, dark area in a burlap or brown paper bag. If stored properly, potatoes will keep for several months (new potatoes, several weeks) but it is best to buy potatoes in small amounts unless you plan to use them within a week or two.

Rutabagas

Often called yellow turnips, rutabagas are actually a different plant. One cup, cubed and cooked, provides more than half of your daily requirement for vitamin C, 13 percent of the RDA for folacin, and small amounts of beta carotene, calcium, iron, and potassium.

Choose rutabagas that are firm and feel heavy for their size. Do not refrigerate. Stored in a cool place, rutabagas will keep for several months.

Squash

Squash is broadly divided into two varieties: summer, which includes zucchini and pattypan; and winter, which includes acorn, butternut, buttercup, Hubbard, and pumpkin. One cup of summer squash sliced has just 35 calories and provides a small amount of potassium. At 80 calories, one cup of butternut squash, baked and cubed, provides nearly 9 milligrams of beta carotene, 52 percent of the RDA for vitamin C, 20 percent of the folacin, 11 percent of the calcium, and a good amount of potassium. Pumpkin is also a nutritious winter squash: a cup of canned pumpkin has 85 calories and is high in iron and beta carotene.

Choose summer squashes that have a rind soft enough to puncture with your fingernail. They should be free of bruises and soft spots. Small- to medium-sized summer squashes are best in flavor and texture. Winter squashes should have a smooth, hard rind and be free of soft spots. They should feel heavy for their size. Sum-mer squashes are very perishable. Store them in the refrigerator and use them as soon as possible. Winter squashes are more hardy; they will keep for several months if stored in a cool, dry area.

Sweet potatoes

Sweet potatoes either have a dry, light yellow flesh or a moist, deep yellow or orange flesh. The latter are sometimes called yams, but they are not true yams, which are grown in the tropics. One four-ounce sweet potato, baked and peeled, has 115 calories—about the same amount as a regular potato—and nearly 14 milligrams of beta carotene. Sweet potatoes are also an excellent source of vitamin C and fiber.

Nutrition All-Stars

When the National Cancer Institute and other groups recommend that you eat at least five vegetables and fruits a day, they're basing this on the fact that all produce is good for you (unless you drown it in butter or other fat). But some vegetables and fruits are better than others. In general, dark leafy greens, orange and yellow fruits, and members of the cabbage family are among the most nutrient dense. Some people may find such a recommendation too vague, however, and might be helped by more specific guidance. The following choices, in alphabetical order, are especially rich in antioxidants (vitamins C and E and beta carotene). Most are also rich sources of other nutrients —including folacin, fiber, and lesser known substances such as indoles and sulforaphane—that may reduce the risk of a variety of cancers and help keep you healthy in other ways. They also tend to be good sources of minerals such as copper, manganese, and even calcium. Legumes (beans), though technically vegetables, are not included because they are not good sources of antioxidants.

	Vitamin C (mg)	Beta Carotene (mg)	Vitamin E (mg)	Folacin (mcg)
Broccoli (½ cup cooked)	49	0.7	0.9	53
Cantaloupe (1 cup cubed)	68	3.1	0.3	27
Carrot (1 medium)	7	12.2	0.3	10
Kale (½ cup cooked)	27	2.9	3.7	9
Mango (1 medium)	57	4.8	2.3	31
Pumpkin (½ cup canned)	5	10.5	1.1	15
Red bell pepper (½ cup raw)	95	1.7	0.3	8
Spinach (½ cup cooked)	9	4.4	2.0	131
Strawberries (1 cup)	86	—	0.3	26
Sweet potato (1 medium, cooked)	28	14.9	5.5	26

Runners-up: Brussels sprouts, all citrus fruits, tomatoes, potatoes, other berries, other leafy greens (dandelion, turnip, and mustard greens, swiss chard, arugula), cauliflower, green pepper, asparagus, peas, beets, and winter squash.

Choose small- to medium-sized sweet potatoes with tapered ends, firm flesh, and smooth skin. Avoid those with shriveled or discolored ends. Sweet potatoes will keep in a cool room for about two weeks. Bake a few more than you need and save them for a healthy snack; they will keep for up to five days in the refrigerator.

Tomatoes

The best tasting fresh tomatoes are found during the summer months. But though out-of-season tomatoes are not as tasty, they aren't necessarily less nutritious. Many factors affect the nutrient content of a tomato, including its variety, soil conditions, when it was picked, and how it was handled, stored, and ripened. Supermarket tomatoes tend to be pale, hard, and tasteless because they're picked at the stage called "mature green" (still firm enough to ship, but only just at the point of turning red) and are then stored at low temperatures, which slows the ripening process. In addition, growers raise thicker-skinned varieties that can withstand the rigors of long-distance shipping.

To complete the ripening at their destination, supermarket tomatoes are gassed with ethylene, a plant hormone that is part of the natural maturing process. One U.S. Department of Agriculture study showed that artificial ripening of tomatoes picked at the mature green stage has only a small effect on their nutrients, however.s

A four-ounce tomato supplies about one-third of your daily RDA for vitamin C and one-seventh the minimum recommended amount of beta carotene, plus some B vitamins, iron, and fiber. Tomatoes contain a substance called lycopene, which is responsible for their red color. Lycopene enhances the body's absorption and utilization of beta carotene, so eat tomatoes in combination with high–beta carotene foods (such as carrots and dark leafy greens).

Sun-dried tomatoes are cropping up in more and more stores. These tomatoes are dehydrated to preserve them and intensify their flavor. Before being used, they are often reconstituted in liquid, primarily oil. It is better to buy them dehydrated and reconstitute them by soaking them in boiling water. They will taste fine, and you will avoid the extra calories and fat.

Choose tomatoes that are firm and plump and have a strong tomato fragrance. Avoid soft overripe tomatoes with blemishes, bruises, soft spots, or growth cracks. Don't buy tomatoes from a refrigerated case; the cold damages them. Store tomatoes in a warm location away from direct sunlight until ripe, then store in the refrigerator, where they will keep for about a week.

Turnips

Sold in bunches with their greens, early white turnips are marketed immediately after harvesting, so they are small and tender. Older ones are left in the field to mature until their skin toughens, making them easy to ship and store. One cup of boiled, cubed white turnips has 30 percent of the RDA of vitamin C and just 30 calories.

Turnip greens, sold atop the roots and also separately in bunches, are an excellent source of beta carotene, vitamin C, calcium, iron, and fiber.

Choose turnips that are small, firm, and fairly smooth. The greens, if attached, should be fresh looking and not wilted. Avoid those with obvious fibrous roots. Remove the green tops, and store turnips in the refrigerator crisper. Use them within a week. Turnip greens will keep for as long as three to five days if stored and refrigerated in a plastic bag.

DAIRY AND EGGS

Milk

Milk is a highly nutritious food that provides nearly all the substances essential for good health in people of all ages. It is particularly rich in high-quality protein, calcium, vitamin D, riboflavin, and other vitamins and minerals. One cup of milk on average supplies about 15 to 20 percent of an adult's daily protein needs, 25 percent of the vitamin D needed, as well as between 25 and 38 percent of the calcium needed.

Milk and milk products are primary dietary sources of calcium, which is essential for the growth and maintenance of bones and teeth. One cup of milk has about 300 milligrams of calcium. The RDA of calcium for children under age eleven is 800 milligrams; for teenagers and young adults, the RDA is 1,200 milligrams; and for most older adults, it is 800 milligrams. (Many experts think that optimal calcium intake levels are even higher, as explained on page 137.). To meet the calcium RDA and to get the other nutrients in milk, most pediatricians recommend that children and teenagers drink a quart a day (or an equivalent amount of yogurt or other dairy products).

Since, after menopause, women are particularly subject to osteoporosis (a gradual weakening of the bone structure, which puts them at greater risk for fractures), they must be sure to get extra calcium. The National Institutes of Health recommends that postmenopausal women consume 1,500 milligrams of calcium daily, or 1,000 milligrams if they take estrogen—amounts equivalent to three to four cups of milk (or three to four servings of yogurt or cheese).

Milk does have some drawbacks: whole milk contains a considerable amount of saturated fat and cholesterol, which can be harmful to the cardiovascular system. Skim and low-fat milk are as nutritious as whole milk, but contain much less fat and cholesterol than whole milk. Everyone over the age of two years should drink skim or 1 percent low-fat milk.

Two percent milk, despite its name, is not low in fat. Many people assume that only 2 percent of the calories come from fat, but the figure refers to the milk-fat percentage by *weight*. One cup of 2 percent milk has about 130 calories and five grams of fat—which calculates to about *35 percent* calories from fat. Whole milk derives about 50 percent of its calories from fat. So 2 percent milk is better, but not by much.

Skim and low-fat milk are lower in the fat-soluble vitamins A and D than whole milk. In the United States, they are therefore always fortified with vitamin A (usually in greater quantities than in whole milk) and almost always with vitamin D.

Caution on raw milk

Almost all milk is pasteurized these days; less than 1 percent of the 280 million glasses of milk drunk every day by Americans is raw milk. Yet this small percentage that escapes pasteurization is the subject of much debate among health food proponents, public health officials, and consumer groups. Milk is an excellent vehicle for bacterial infection, and in the nineteenth century it led to widespread outbreaks of disease. That's why pasteurization—a mild heating process that kills dangerous microorganisms in milk—is considered one of the greatest advances in food sanitation of all time.

Raw milk is still legally sold in some states, but that doesn't mean that

Chocolate milk made with 1 percent or skim milk is relatively low in fat. A cup of 1 percent chocolate milk contains three grams of fat. The chocolate syrup, though loaded with sugar, is low in fat—less than one gram per two-tablespoon serving. But because of the sugar, chocolate milk has about twice the calories of plain milk.

NUTRITIONAL CONTENT OF
Milk

Milk (8 fl oz)	Calories	Fat (g)	Fat Calories	Comments
Whole (3.5% fat)	150	8	60%	Usually fortified with vitamin D. High in saturated fat and cholesterol. Total fat content may vary from state to state. Best only for children under the age of two.
Low-fat (2% fat)	120	5	38%	Close in taste and texture to whole milk. Vitamins A and D almost always added. Too high in fat to be an acceptable choice for those on a low-fat diet.
Low-fat (1% fat)	100	3	27%	Low in fat; good choice for those on low-fat diets or those trying to restrict calories. Vitamins A and D almost always added.
Skim (nonfat)	80	trace	5%	Virtually fat free. Best choice for those on a low-fat diet. Should not be given to children under the age of two.
Buttermilk (1% fat)	100	2	18%	Tart and creamy. Low in fat and and cholesterol. Usually made from skim or low-fat milk. Easily digested; bacteria breaks down about 25 percent of lactose. Usually not fortified with vitamins A or D.
Dry (nonfat, reconstituted)	80	trace	5%	About as nutritious as fresh skim milk. Virtually fat- and cholesterol-free. Fortified with vitamins A and D. Thin consistency, flat taste; clumps in hot liquids.
Evaporated (canned, made from whole milk, undiluted)	340	20	53%	High in fat and cholesterol. Sterilized; long shelf life if can is turned over every few months. Can be used undiluted when specified in recipes, otherwise must be diluted. Slightly caramelized taste.
LactAid™ (lactase treated, 1% fat)	100	2	18%	Helps lactose intolerants digest milk. Contains lactase, which breaks down at least 70 percent of lactose in milk. Slightly sweet taste.
Goat's milk (whole)	168	10	54%	High in fat. Contains mostly the same proteins as cow's milk, but those allergic to cow's milk may be able to tolerate goat's milk.

it is safe to drink. In 1987, sixty-two Californians died from listerial bacteria in cheese made from unpasteurized milk; the same year, 16,000 Midwesterners were struck by salmonella poisoning after drinking improperly pasteurized milk.

Despite this, some people still believe that unpasteurized milk is more nutritious, since the heat of pasteurization destroys some nutrients, and that raw milk enhances resistance to disease. However, researchers have detected no nutritional advantages to raw milk. Current techniques of pasteurization heat milk for such brief periods that there is little effect on nutrients, only a nutritionally insignificant decrease in thiamine, vitamin B_{12}, and vitamin C. There's no evidence that raw milk enhances resistance to disease. It has been shown, however, that raw milk contains infectious bacteria and has been implicated in outbreaks of disease.

Combating lactose intolerance

Many people suffer from an enzyme deficiency that makes them unable to break down the lactose (milk sugar) in milk. While lactose intolerance most often affects Asians, African Americans, and other people who traditionally consume few milk products, a large portion of the general population may suffer from this condition as they grow older.

To avoid the discomfort of lactose intolerance—which includes cramps, gas, and diarrhea—sufferers can try consuming fermented milk products such as buttermilk or yogurt (the bacteria in these products help break down the lactose). Another option is to drink milk treated with lactase, the enzyme that breaks down lactose in the intestines. Lactase-treated milk is available in the dairy case of many supermarkets. (For more information on lactose intolerance, see page 370.)

Is goat's milk better?

Goat's milk (and the cheese made from it) is, for the most part, nutritionally similar to cow's milk; the calcium content of goat's milk is slightly, but not significantly, higher and its vitamin A content is higher, too, but so is the fat content. Cow's milk comes in low-fat versions, but goat's milk, so far, is sold only as whole milk. A cup of it has 165 calories and ten grams of fat, and more than half the calories come from fat.

Goat's milk contains a higher percentage of smaller fat globules, which in theory are more easily broken down by digestive enzymes, so some people think it is more digestible than cow's milk. But when cow's milk is homogenized, so that the cream does not rise to the top, the large fat globules in it are broken down. No human studies have shown that either homogenized cow's milk or goat's milk is more quickly digested than other kinds of milk. And the lactose levels are comparable, so if you are lactose intolerant, goat's milk is not the answer. However, some people who are allergic to cow's milk may be able to tolerate goat's milk.

If you like the tangy taste of goat's milk, just make sure it has been pasteurized. Raw goat's milk is subject to the same type of bacterial contamination as cow's milk.

Drugs and hormones in milk

Drugs given to cows can and do pass into milk, but the Food and Drug Administration (FDA) regulates drug use in dairy cattle, and millions of samples are tested each year to detect residues. In a recent survey, thirty-six of forty-nine samples collected in ten cities across the country showed low levels of a sulfa drug that is illegal in dairy animals. In twenty-five of the thirty-six positive samples, levels were so low that they were almost not detectable. The FDA, which took immediate corrective steps, cites this action as evidence of its vigilance. But some investigators believe FDA rules are not tough enough and insist that milk should be free of all antibiotic residues. Nevertheless, even the critics (such as the Center for Science in the Public Interest, an investigative and lobbying group in Washington, D.C.) conclude that you're better off drinking milk than not drinking it, and that the U.S. milk supply is safe.

Recently, much flurry has been raised by the FDA's approval of bovine growth hormone, also called bovine somatotropin (BST) used to treat cows so that they will produce more milk. The FDA says that milk from cows treated with BST is no different from

You can boost the calcium content of any dish by adding nonfat dry milk. Stir into soups, sauces, stews, and gravies, or add to casseroles, rice, and cereals.

milk from untreated cows; testing the milk from treated and untreated cows cannot reveal which is which. BST is a natural hormone, produced by cows themselves. Years of study have shown that milk from treated cows is safe. BST taken by mouth has no biological effect in humans. It's digested like any other protein. For that reason, the FDA won't require milk from treated cows to be labeled as such. The FDA's position is that such a label would be unnecessary and misleading. It's all just milk. And alternatively, it would certainly be misleading to label any milk as "BST-free" or "hormone-free," since all milk contains BST and other hormones. Even the label "from cows not treated with recombinant BST" could have misleading implications. However, a company could state that its milk came from untreated herds if it also said that such milk offered no health advantages.

Critics, however, say that there are potential health differences between milk from treated cows and milk from untreated cows. The milk of treated cows contains higher levels of a substance called insulin growth factor that could adversely affect human growth patterns. And cows treated with BST become more vulnerable to mastitis (udder infection): according to some data, they may be almost twice as likely to get mastitis. This would necessitate treatment with antibiotics, which might get into the milk. But the FDA says that as with BST, insulin growth factor is present in milk naturally. Again, increased levels from treated cows are within the normal range; the milk from treated and untreated cows can't be distinguished on this, or any, basis. And though there is some increase in mastitis, it's unclear how much. The incidence of mastitis also depends on proper sanitation and care

of herds. Furthermore, cows bred to produce more milk are also more likely to have mastitis—and they aren't regarded as a danger. A monitoring program is in place for detecting and managing any increase in mastitis. All milk is routinely tested for antibiotic residues, and dairy farmers are highly motivated to keep residues out of milk, since milk that fails the test cannot be sold and must be thrown out.

The economic impact is also an unknown. With recombinant BST, milk may be more plentiful and production costs may fall. But whether this will mean cheaper milk and lower taxes depends on consumer acceptance, future reduction of government price supports, and many other variables. But there's no *health* reason not to use milk that comes from treated herds. It's just like any other milk, and the scare talk about antibiotics is unrealistic.

Another concern about chemicals in milk is the presence of dioxin (a chemical by-product of chlorine bleaching and a suspected carcinogen) which is used in producing milk cartons. Low levels of dioxin have been detected in milk cartons and in some milk samples, according to an FDA report to Congress. But the human risk for cancer posed by detectable dioxin was estimated by the FDA to be less than one in a million, and the paper industry is in the process of eliminating dioxin altogether.

Cheese

Cheese is a concentrated form of milk, minus its liquid or whey. That makes it a mixed blessing—high in protein but also in saturated fat; usually full of calcium but also sodium; rich and creamy but loaded with cholesterol. About eight pounds of milk go into a pound of most types of cheese, with the result

NUTRITIONAL CONTENT OF
Cheese

	Calories	Fat (g)	Fat Calories	Calcium (mg)	Sodium (mg)
American, 1 oz	105	9	77%	190	400
Blue, 1 oz	100	8	72%	150	396
Camembert or brie, 1 oz	85	7	74%	60	200
Cheddar, 1 oz	115	9	70%	205	200
Cottage, creamed, ½ cup	108	5	42%	63	425
Cottage, dry curd, ½ cup	62	trace	7%	23	9
Cottage, low-fat, ½ cup	104	2	17%	78	459
Cream, 1 oz	100	10	90%	20	85
Feta, 1 oz	75	6	72%	140	315
Mozzarella, part skim, 1 oz	80	5	56%	207	150
Mozzarella, whole milk, 1 oz	80	6	68%	147	106
Muenster, 1 oz	105	9	77%	205	175
Neufchatel, 1 oz	74	7	85%	21	113
Parmesan, 1 oz	130	9	62%	390	528
Provolone, 1 oz	100	8	72%	214	248
Ricotta, part skim, ½ cup	170	10	53%	335	154
Ricotta, whole milk, ½ cup	216	16	66%	255	104
Swiss, 1 oz	105	8	69%	275	150

that just one ounce (an average slice) of cheese contains approximately as much fat and protein as a cup of milk. Some nutrients found in milk are lost when the whey is drained, in particular the B vitamins and some minerals. Also removed is most of the lactose (milk sugar); this makes cheese good for people who have difficulty digesting lactose. However, most of the calcium (except in cottage cheese and other soft cheeses), vitamin A, and phosphorus from the milk remain in the cheese.

Can cheese be low-fat?
Because almost all the fat from the milk is concentrated in it, cheese is a potent source of saturated fat and cholesterol—worse than most meats. The answer to a health-conscious cheese lover's prayers would seem to be cheeses labeled "light," "reduced-fat," or "part-skim." But these cheeses usually do not have significantly less fat than regular cheese, and truly low-fat products like hoop cheese and sapsago are hard-to-find and bland.

Dairy dates
Slightly soured milk won't make you sick, but spoiled cottage cheese, yogurt, or sour cream may contain molds which can make you sick. So pay attention to expiration dates. A "sell by" date indicates when the merchant should take the product off the shelf, but does not necessarily mean the food will have spoiled by then. A "use by" date indicates when the product may go bad. If there's only one date, and not the words "use by" or "sell by," assume it's a "use by" date.

Expired products may taste fine for another few days if they have been kept cold. Dairy products last longer and taste better when kept at 45° F. or below. If milk products are allowed to reach 50°, their life is halved. A twenty-minute trip by car on a hot day can raise the temperature of milk by 10°, so in the summer get dairy products home from the store quickly. Transport them in a cooler with ice if the trip is long or you aren't going straight home.

*Yogurt cheese is easy to
make at home. Follow
these simple instructions:*

*1. Line a medium-sized
strainer with dampened
cheesecloth—or use a
yogurt cheese funnel—
and place it over a bowl.*
*2. Place plain nonfat
yogurt in the strainer or
funnel and let it drain
uncovered in the refrigerator overnight.*
*3. What remains in the
funnel is yogurt cheese.
Discard the whey that has
drained into the bowl.*
*4. If you are not using the
cheese immediately,
place it in a tightly covered container and keep
refrigerated.*

*Each ounce of yogurt
yields one-half ounce of
yogurt cheese.*

Lately, however, a wide array of hard and soft cheeses labeled "low-fat" have come on the market. Many are stretching the truth, but some are made primarily with skim milk and a few are almost fat-free. The skim-milk products, and those made with partially hydrogenated soybean oil, may have only one gram of saturated fat per ounce. They may also be low in cholesterol. Manufacturers are paying some attention to sodium, too. The new cheeses may not be as tangy or creamy as you would hope, but some are quite tasty, or at least acceptable, especially when used in cooking. In choosing a low-fat cheese, keep the following points in mind:

•Read labels. Many cheeses claiming to be light and low-fat have almost as high a percentage of fat calories as regular Cheddar. Some brands contain five grams of fat per ounce, compared with nine grams of fat in regular Cheddar, which is a slight improvement. However, some brands of low-fat Swiss cheese contain three grams of fat per ounce (versus eight grams in regular Swiss) and there are nonfat versions of mozzarella and ricotta cheese available.

•Compare cheeses by considering the amount of fat: a low-fat cheese has three grams or less of fat per ounce; moderate fat content would be four to six grams per ounce; and high-fat, seven or more grams.

•Check the serving size. Some packaged slices weigh only two-thirds of an ounce, which makes them seem "lighter" than conventional one-ounce servings.

•Most low-fat cheeses don't melt as well as the regular kind. Shredding them before adding to casseroles and other baked dishes will definitely help. But if a true melted consistency is important to you, you might want to use regular cheese, but less of it.

**Another low-fat option:
yogurt cheese**

Yogurt cheese—yogurt drained so that the whey is removed—can be an excellent substitute for high-fat cheeses, sandwich spreads, dips, and desserts (See marginal at right.) If it is made from low-fat or nonfat yogurt, this cheese contains only a gram of fat or less per ounce.

What makes yogurt cheese special is that it picks up the flavor of anything it's mixed with. For example, two parts yogurt cheese can be blended with one part mayonnaise (real, imitation, or light) to make a sandwich spread that tastes like the real thing, but has much less fat and fewer calories, while adding a little calcium to boot. You can also use yogurt cheese as a substitute for butter, margarine, cream cheese, or sour cream. For a vegetable dip or topping, add herbs or spices like garlic and chives. For dessert, sweeten the yogurt cheese with honey, brown sugar, or frozen fruit-juice concentrate. Yogurt cheese can also be used to make a truly low-fat cheesecake.

Yogurt

Yogurt is merely milk—generally cow's milk in this country—curdled by the addition of bacteria. And like milk, yogurt is a nutritious food. One cup supplies 20 to 25 percent of your daily protein needs and 300 to 400 milligrams of calcium—about as much as a glass of milk—and is a good source of riboflavin, phosphorus, and potassium.

Yet, despite claims to the contrary, yogurt isn't necessarily a "diet food." The number of calories and amount of fat in it depend on which type of milk it is made from (whole, low-fat, or skim milk, to which may be added cream and nonfat milk solids) as well as the type and amount of sweetener (sucrose, fructose, corn syrup, honey, molasses, or some combination, or aspartame, an artificial sweetener) it may contain. A cup of yogurt can have 90 calories or nearly 400, no fat or 11 grams (supplying up to 45 percent of all calories). Plain yogurt has no sugar, but vanilla, coffee, and lemon varieties contain the equivalent of three and a half teaspoons of sugar, and fruit flavors up to seven teaspoons. And whereas a cup of yogurt made from skim milk has merely 4 milligrams of cholesterol, whole-milk brands contain about 30 milligrams. Flavored yogurts sweetened with aspartame contain fewer calories than other flavored yogurts —90 to 100 calories per cup, if the yogurt is nonfat.

If you are watching your weight or fat intake, steer away from highly sweetened, flavored yogurts and those made from whole milk. The various "styles" don't make a difference nutritionally. Sundae-style yogurt has the fruit on the bottom; Swiss- and French-style have yogurt and fruit already mixed (the Swiss-style is thicker because it contains a solidifying agent such as gelatin).

As for drinkable yogurt and frozen yogurt, look for the same things you look for in regular yogurt: low fat and low sugar. If you do, they'll be much better for you than a fast-food shake or an ice-cream sundae. You can also make your own shakes using low-fat yogurt and skim milk. And you can use plain low-fat yogurt on baked potatoes, fruit, and salads and in dips as a healthful alternative to sour cream, mayonnaise, and commercial dressings; in cakes and spreads in place of cream cheese; in shakes instead of ice cream. It even makes a good low-fat marinade for chicken.

Yogurt is especially appealing to many people who have difficulty digesting milk sugar (lactose). During the fermentation process, the bacteria convert much of the lactose into lactic acid, which accounts for yogurt's tangy taste (the more sour the yogurt, the less lactose it contains). So if you are lactose intolerant, you may not have a problem digesting yogurt.

Other benefits of yogurt are far more theoretical. Some people believe that the live bacteria in yogurt can lead to beneficial changes in the bacterial population of the intestines. Some doctors advise patients on antibiotics (which kill off some of the helpful bacterial along with the harmful in the digestive tract) to eat yogurt if they have diarrhea and stomach distress. One recent Finnish study did indeed find that yogurt could counter these side effects of antibiotics—but it used a yogurt with an exotic strain of bacteria. Most yogurts contain live cultures (the label will state this), though the amount varies greatly from brand to brand and most strains used here in commercial

NUTRITIONAL CONTENT OF
Yogurt

(8 oz)	Calories	Fat (g)	Calcium (mg)
Whole-milk			
plain	140-210	5-11	275-400
flavored	230-390	5-11	200-350
Low-fat			
plain	140-160	4	300-450
flavored	220-280	3	300-400
Nonfat			
plain	90-110	0	300-450
flavored	150	0	250-300
Low-fat yogurt drink			
flavored	180	2	250-400
Kefir, low-fat			
plain	110	3	300-550
fruit	150	3	250-530

yogurts do not survive to colonize the intestine. There is no convincing scientific evidence that yogurt can improve digestion or prevent infections in the digestive tract.

Yogurt has also been suggested as a preventive for vaginal yeast infections. One study indicated that eating a cup of yogurt containing active *Lactobacillus acidophilus* (a bacterium added to only a few brands) reduced the number of vaginal yeast infections. But the study was poorly designed, and other researchers doubt that yogurt can help.

Eggs

Most dietary guidelines limit egg intake to four a week for people with blood cholesterol levels of 200 mg/dl or below because eggs (more precisely yolks) are such a concentrated source of cholesterol—about 210 milligrams per large egg, according to the United States Department of Agriculture (USDA). However, if you eat a predominately vegetarian diet that contains only low-fat dairy products and small amounts of lean meat and fish, you could eat more than four eggs a week on a heart-healthy diet. People with elevated blood cholesterol levels may still need to limit their egg intake to one whole egg a week. (When considering egg intake, remember to count the eggs used in recipes and baked goods.)

Some chicken farmers claim that special breeding and feeding (some birds are being fed cholesterol-lowering fish oil, for instance) have enabled them to reduce their eggs' cholesterol content, but these claims have been largely undocumented, or, in some cases, fraudulent. Before you rush to the store for these "improved" eggs, keep in mind that 200, or even 175, milligrams of cholesterol still goes a long way toward the suggested daily allotment of 300 milligrams from all sources. Also, like any specialty item, "low-cholesterol" eggs have a premium price—as much as 30 percent higher than regular eggs.

In all other ways, an egg is an egg. A large whole egg contains five grams of fat, of which less than two grams are saturated (all of it in the yolk) and is an important source of vitamins B_{12}, riboflavin, folacin, iron, and phosphorus. There is no nutritional difference between "free range" or "organic" eggs and regular eggs. Similarly, there is no difference between brown eggs and white eggs in terms of nutrition or taste. Shell color depends on the breed of chicken, and no one breed of chicken is known to lay better eggs than another. And a pale egg yolk is just as nutritious as a dark one. The color depends on the amount of xanthophyll (a natural yellow pigment found in chicken feed) present in the yolk, not beta carotene as is sometimes claimed.

Egg substitutes

Anyone serious about cutting down on cholesterol should consider egg substi-

NUTRITIONAL CONTENT OF
Eggs and Egg Substitutes

	Calories	Fat (g)	Cholesterol (mg)	Sodium (mg)	Fat Calories
Whole egg	80	6	213	69	68%
Egg white	15	0	0	50	0%
Egg substitute, frozen (2 oz)	25-60	0-3	0	80-130	0-45%
Egg substitute, powdered (half packet)	60	4	7	124	60%
Egg substitute, powdered, no egg white (1½ tsp)	15	0	0	0	0%

tutes. Either frozen or powdered, these products usually have no cholesterol at all. But there's a trade-off: though most of the substitutes use egg whites, many also contain sodium—sometimes in the form of MSG (monosodium glutamate) and artificial coloring, flavoring, and preservatives. Brands that contain no egg white (just starch and leavening agents) are good for people with egg allergies; they can be used in baking but not scrambling.

One egg "substitute" is actual a liquid, whole egg product with only 45 milligrams of cholesterol per egg. The manufacturer figured out a fairly simple process for eliminating 80 percent of the cholesterol in an egg yolk. Separated yolks are mixed with a modified cornstarch and centrifuged (whirled), which causes much of the cholesterol to stick to the cornstarch, so that both can be removed. Then the yolks are remixed with the whites, ultra-pasteurized, and packaged in half-pint containers. Except for the cholesterol, all the nutrients are the same as in whole eggs, but some salt is added, so the sodium content of one of these liquid eggs is 120 milligrams.

How do "fake" eggs taste? Though they do resemble the real thing when cooked, taste varies from product to product. The liquid whole-egg product comes closest to the taste of regular whole eggs. It also depends on what they're used for: some will be better for omelets, some better in baking. It's largely a matter of personal choice. Cost is another factor. Most packages contain the equivalent of six to eight eggs at nearly double the price of a dozen eggs.

There's another, easier way to cut the cholesterol you get from eggs: substitute two whites for every whole egg. Egg whites are almost pure pure protein and contain no fat or cholesterol.

Omelets can be made using whites, nonfat dry milk, and skim milk, plus chopped vegetables and seasoning. Some recipes, such as soufflés and some cakes and muffins, call only for whites; chopped hard-cooked whites can also be used as a garnish for salads and vegetables. Cutting out all egg yolks may make some breads and other dishes dry and tasteless; in that case use two whites plus one whole egg instead of two eggs.

Egg safety
A few years back, the USDA warned everyone to avoid raw and soft-cooked eggs (which ruled out soft omelets, homemade hollandaise sauce, and Caesar salads) because salmonella bacteria were turning up in fresh Grade A eggs, particularly in the northeastern states. Salmonella can cause food poisoning, and it can be fatal among the very elderly or the very ill. Indeed the outbreaks of food poisoning from undercooked eggs have occurred mainly in nursing homes and hospitals. Proper cooking kills salmonella.

Now the USDA guidelines have been relaxed a bit: you still should avoid raw eggs, but you need not cook your eggs to the hard and rubbery stage. People in poor health, the very old, and pregnant women should perhaps continue to practice strict caution in preparing eggs. Others should follow these guidelines:

•You can safely eat a soft-boiled egg. Cooking an egg at 140°F. for $3\frac{1}{2}$ minutes pasteurizes it—that is, kills all bacteria. It's inconvenient if not impossible in most kitchens to test the temperature of a cooked egg. A sufficiently cooked egg white will be opaque but not hard-boiled and the yolk will have started to thicken (not thin and runny).

•Scrambled eggs and omelets are fine if cooked just past the runny, moist stage. They should be set, but they don't have to be rock hard.

•If you're frying eggs, "over easy" is best. Fry them for about three minutes on one side, then about one minute on the other. If you want your eggs sunny-side-up, cover the pan and cook for about four minutes.

•Cool hard-boiled eggs at room temperature, not in water unless you are going to eat them immediately. Plunging an egg into cold water will cause air pockets to develop under the shell, which may draw in bacteria. Refrigerate hard-boiled eggs and use within a week.

•It's okay to eat Caesar salads, hollandaise sauce, and other egg-based sauces in restaurants, provided pasteurized eggs are used. Most commercial egg products are pasteurized. Avoid raw eggs.

•Buy only government-inspected graded eggs. While it's no guarantee they won't have salmonella, at least they must be washed before marketing and kept under refrigeration.

•Handle eggs carefully. Store them in their original cartons in the coldest part of the refrigerator—not in an egg tray in the door. Discard any eggs with cracked shells. Wash your hands after handling raw eggs.

GRAINS AND LEGUMES

Whole Grains

Whole grains—except in the form of flour—are something of a mystery to many American cooks. While most people are familiar with rice as a side dish, or oatmeal as a breakfast cereal, other whole grains, such as cracked wheat and barley, are too often overlooked as potential main or side dishes.

Such foods as kasha or bulgur may sound a little too mysterious. And often only health food stores stock special grains.

Yet whole grains are high in complex carbohydrates, low in fat, and rich in protein and fiber, as well as some B vitamins. Many are also fairly good sources of calcium and iron. The average cup of cooked whole grains contains only about 200 calories and is as easy to prepare as rice or dried pasta.

Types and uses

Kasha is simply a term for roasted buckwheat kernels that are cooked like rice; bulgur is precooked wheat berries, which can also be handled much like rice. Mediterranean and Middle Eastern cuisines feature many famous whole-grain dishes: couscous, a delicious combination of cracked wheat berries (millet can be used, but the packaged product is usually ground semolina) with meat, vegetables, or even fruits; tabbouleh, a cold salad made of cracked wheat or bulgur, chopped tomatoes, mint, and parsley; and pilafs, cooked combinations of grains with meats or vegetables. There are endless adaptations of these dishes using everyday ingredients. Other whole grains, such as rye and oats, while not ready substitutes for rice or pasta, can be incorporated in bread, meat loaf, and other baked dishes. And one grain can, of course, be mixed with another.

Three unusual names on the chart on page 189 are amaranth (Greek, meaning "immortal grain"), triticale (the term combines *triticum* and *secale*, Latin words for "wheat" and "rye"), and quinoa (pronounced KEEN-wa, a Quechuan word meaning "the mother grain"). Amaranth and quinoa are native to South America. Both are high in protein, minerals, and vitamins; supermarkets and health food stores

Rice mixes

Preseasoned rice mixes are very high in sodium as well as price. They may also contain partially hydrogenated oils and usually require adding large amounts of fat in cooking (although in most mixes you can safely eliminate the added fat). Sugars, such as corn syrup and dextrose may also be ingredients. Flavoring ordinary rice yourself with herbs, defatted stock, and vegetables is an easy alternative that can keep the dish low in fat and sodium.

Grains

Grain (1 cup cooked)	Protein (g)	Fat (g)	Dietary Fiber (g)	Iron (mg)	Comments
Amaranth	15	7	4.5	11.8	High in protein, iron, and calcium. Native to South America; available in health food stores. Whole kernels sold pearled (polished). Good as side dish or cereal. Flour used in bread, tortillas, cookies, and cereal.
Barley	8	1	8.2	2.1	Available as "pot" or "Scotch" barley (whole kernels) or pearl barley (polished). Both good in soups and stews and for side dishes, puddings, and cereal. May lower blood cholesterol.
Buckwheat	12	2	11.4	3.8	Not a true grain but a seed. Roasted kernels can be cooked like rice as a side dish (kasha). Flour can be mixed with wheat for bread and pancakes. Distinctive, nutty flavor.
Millet	12	4	3.0	3.0	High in phosphorus and B vitamins. Used chiefly as animal feed in the United States but available in health food stores. Good as side dish or as a substitute for bread stuffings in poultry. Swells enormously in water.
Oats	16	6	2.7	4.2	Whole kernels (groats) take an hour to cook. Flattened rolled oats require less time. Oat flour (oatmeal processed in a blender) can be used in bread, pastry, meatloaf, and casseroles. May lower blood cholesterol.
Quinoa	16	7	4.6	6.6	High in protein, calcium, and iron. Good in puddings, soups, and stir-fries. Whole-grain version must be washed and strained. Flour can be used in combination or alone for baking. Native South American grain.
Rice, brown	5	1	4.8	1	Unpolished rice; retains the bran and germ that contain the majority of nutrients and fiber. Nutty flavor. Requires forty-five to fifty minutes of cooking time, but quick cooking versions are available.
Rice, white	4	trace	trace	1.8	Less nutritious than brown rice because the bran and germ have been removed. Usually enriched with iron and other nutrients.
Rye	12	2	11.4	4.6	Low-gluten content produces heavy bread. Cracked rye makes good cereal. Rolled rye from health food stores can be added to meat loaf and casseroles. Good in soups. Flour mixes well with wheat and/or oats.
Triticale	11	2	9.9	2.6	Wheat/rye hybrid; early man-made grain. Comes whole, cracked, and as flour. Flour low in gluten, best combined with wheat for bread making. Commercial brands of triticale bread available in supermarkets.
Whole wheat	10	2	9.6	3.5	Comes as whole berries or cracked. Whole berries need two to three hours of cooking, cracked about fifteen minutes. Both good for cereals, casseroles, and soups Bulgur (hulled, parboiled wheat) is good for tabbouleh salad and other cold side dishes. Sweet, nutty flavor.

carry them. Triticale, also high-protein, is a hybrid created about a century ago.

Whole grains contain natural oils in the bran and the germ (the outer parts, which are removed in refining) that can turn rancid, and they can also fall prey to insects and mold. This is why whole grains tend to be more costly, and one reason why most grains are refined in the first place—to increase their shelf life. Keep whole grains in tightly closed containers or plastic bags. You can store them at room temperature (in a dark, dry, cool place) for about one month, but they keep considerably longer in the refrigerator—at least four to five months.

Cereals

With more Americans concerned about fiber than ever, hot and cold cereals have become increasingly popular. While cereal grains are naturally high in fiber and low in fat, sodium, and sugar, this is not always true of the final products on supermarket shelves. Some brands have only a trace of fiber left, while others are as salty as potato chips or, if they are targeted toward children, as sugary as a candy bar.

Ready-to-eat cereals are grains (rice, wheat, corn, oats) that have been exploded into puffs, pressured into flakes, shredded and spun into little

Wild rice

One form of rice is not a grain but a grass seed (Zizania aquatica). It's native to North America and was once basic to the diet of the Chippewa and the Dakota tribes. Today, almost all wild rice is planted and grown in paddies. Nutty and rich in flavor, wild rice is more expensive than regular rice, but if you occasionally buy some as a treat, you're getting some nutritional extras. One cup cooked contains just 135 calories and is moderately high in protein (6.3 grams per cup), low in fat, and a good source of B vitamins.

Wheat Germ vs. Wheat Bran

For years people have been buying wheat germ to sprinkle on breakfast cereals, yogurt, and salads or add to baked goods and casseroles. Now, with the spotlight on fiber, wheat germ has been joined on supermarket shelves by wheat bran. Together, wheat germ and bran account for most of wheat's nutritional value. What are the differences between the two?

Wheat germ. This is the wheat kernel's embryo; it's what develops into a new stalk of grain if planted. It is often removed in milling because it contains a fair amount of fat (polyunsaturated), which tends to go rancid, thus increasing the risk of spoilage in stored whole-wheat flour, bread, and other products. One ounce provides 94 percent of the RDA for riboflavin, 77 percent of the RDA for vitamin E, 49 percent of the folacin, 32 percent of the zinc, 31 percent of the thiamine, and 17 percent of the iron.

It also has 100 calories, nine grams of protein, nearly four grams of dietary fiber, and three grams of fat. Defatted wheat germ is available, but it's lower in vitamin E; unlike regular wheat germ, it doesn't have to be stored in the refrigerator.

Wheat bran. This is the kernel's outer shell, usually sloughed off during milling. It contains a whopping twelve grams of dietary fiber per one-ounce serving. One ounce contains 49 percent of the RDA for magnesium, 35 percent of the phosphorus, 20 percent of the iron and niacin, and 18 percent of the vitamin B6. It also has 60 calories, five grams of protein, and one gram of fat.

Removing the germ and bran results in the familiar white flour used in most cooking and baking. This is made up chiefly of the third component of the kernel, the starchy endosperm, a source of energy and protein but with most other nutrients removed. While it's true that some of the nutrients (iron, niacin, thiamine, and riboflavin) lost in the milling process are replaced when white flour is enriched, the flour remains low in fiber as well as some trace nutrients (such as zinc and copper).

If you eat whole-wheat cereals and baked goods, you're already getting the germ and bran. Other whole-grain cereals and baked goods, including rye and oats, offer comparable nutritional riches. But even if you eat these, bottled wheat germ and bran are concentrated sources of these nutrients that are convenient to add to baked goods. You can sprinkle them on nearly everything, adding not only nutrients, but also flavor and texture.

biscuits, or perhaps extruded into some fanciful shape. Then the product is toasted. Next, in many cases, vitamins are sprayed on. Some cereals have many added ingredients: sugar, both brown and white, honey, molasses, corn syrup, and other sweeteners, as well as nuts, raisins, salt, and preservatives. Since the vitamins are added to the cereal, they are often also listed among the ingredients.

Nevertheless, if you keep your own concerns in mind—which probably include more fiber and less salt, sugar, and fat—you can find what you want in a cereal. Here are some guidelines for sorting out the nutritional information on the box, which can approach a legal document in complexity.

Check the ingredients list. A grain or grains should be listed first. The shorter the list, usually the less highly processed the cereal.

Watch serving sizes. Cereal manufacturers use one ounce as the standard serving size, but people usually eat more than that. Bear in mind that an ounce of puffed wheat or rice is about a cup (and supplies 50 calories), while an ounce of a dense cereal like granola may equal just one-quarter cup (and supplies about 125 calories).

Determine how much sugar is in it. If sugar—or any of its many forms such as corn syrup, honey, maltose, or dextrose—appears high on the ingredients list, or if there is more than one sweetener listed, you can be pretty sure that the cereal is high in added sugars. Another way to check, however, is to calculate the ratio of carbohydrates to protein; it should be about eight to one, or in others words, for every one gram of protein, there should be no more than eight grams of carbohydrates. If it is thirty grams of carbohydrates for every two grams of protein, you are probably getting lots of sugar.

Look for brands with a high fiber content. Some have seven to thirteen grams of fiber per serving (enough to supply one-third to one-half of your recommended intake), while many high-sugar cereals contain less than a gram.

Scrutinize the label for the fat content. Most cereals are low in fat, but check the ingredients list for the addition of oils, such as coconut or palm kernel. Granola cereals are almost always high in fat because they usually contain nuts, coconut, and coconut oil. You can keep the fat content low by using one percent or skim milk.

Don't count on cereals to supply protein. Most cereals, even the high-protein kind, provide only three to five grams of protein per ounce. Simply adding a cup of milk offers at lest twice as much protein as the cereal itself.

Ignore vitamin claims. Nearly all brands today are fortified with vitamins and minerals. If your diet is reasonably balanced, there's no need to eat a cereal fortified with 100 percent of the RDAs for vitamins and minerals. This is like taking a multivitamin pill with your cereal—a pill you pay a premium for.

Watch out for sodium. If you are trying to reduce your salt intake, look for a cereal containing little or no sodium, such as shredded or puffed wheat, or puffed rice. Most cold cereals have 200 to 300 milligrams or more of added sodium per serving.

Hot cereals

Hot cereals are usually made from unrefined grains—most notably oats and wheat. Unlike cold cereals, many hot cereals aren't fortified with vitamins and minerals and so contain only the nutrients found in the grain itself. These include fiber (both soluble and insoluble), B vitamins, vitamin E, iron, zinc, calcium, selenium, and magnesium. For an even more nutritious hot

Fresh or dried fruit makes a tasty, nutritious addition to cereal, but when fruit is added by the manufacturer, you may be getting more hype than fruit. One study found that the proportion of dried fruits by weight in cold cereals ranged from as little as 3 percent to 33 percent. To benefit from the added fiber and nutrients in fruit, you'd be better off adding your own.

cereal, just add some skim or low-fat milk and fruit.

While most hot cereals lack the sugar and salt that is often added to cold cereals, some are made from refined grains—such as cream of wheat and cream of rice—and therefore lacking in fiber and some vitamins. If the hot cereal is made from whole grains, that's probably an advantage, since all the grain's nutrients remain, while refined grains are fortified with only some of the nutrients removed during processing.

Oats and oat bran. Oats come in two forms: oatmeal and oat bran. Four varieties of oatmeal are available—steel-cut, rolled or old-fashioned, quick, and instant. The difference is in the cooking time (finer cuts cook more quickly) and texture, not in the nutritional value. The exception is instant oatmeal, which can be loaded with salt, sugar, and sometimes even fat.

Oat bran— simply the outer coating of the oat grain—has become popular because of its cholesterol-lowering abilities. The effective ingredient is the water-soluble fiber, which can be found not only in oat bran but in legumes and many vegetables and fruits. (Oatmeal contains the bran of the oat, and therefore soluble fiber, but not as much per serving as oat bran.)

Oat bran cannot, however, undo the effects of eating a three-egg omelet. Oats, like any cholesterol-lowering agent, are effective only in the context of a low-fat, low-cholesterol, high-fiber diet. And no one can say how much soluble fiber you need to eat each day to lower your blood cholesterol. In studies where cholesterol level reductions were dramatic, subjects ate a bowl of oatmeal and five oat bran muffins daily—not a diet most can stick to forever. Another study found that people who ate just two ounces of instant oats

per day reduced their cholesterol levels by an average of 12 milligrams per deciliter in only eight weeks. Recently researchers from the University of Minnesota reviewed all published studies on oats and cholesterol and concluded that consuming three grams of soluble fiber (the amount found in one-and-a-third cups of oat-bran cereal or three packets of instant oatmeal) daily does indeed have a modest effect. Cholesterol levels fell an average of 2 to 3 percent in all subjects; people with elevated cholesterol levels tended to have larger drops of 6 to 7 percent. And the more oats consumed, the greater the reduction.

However, it was soluble fiber, not any magical property of the oats, that produced the cholesterol-lowering response. If you begin to incorporate some oat bran into your heart-healthy diet and regularly eat fruits and vegetables high in soluble fiber, you should see results at your next cholesterol check—particularly if your cholesterol level was previously elevated.

If you want to add more oat bran to your diet, remember that plain oatmeal or oat bran is a better source of soluble fiber than processed foods. You can make your own oat flour by putting oatmeal through the blender. Use it for breading, baking, and thickening sauces, as you would any other flour. You can add oat bran to pancakes, baked goods, and even meat loaf. If you want to purchase oat-bran containing foods, be sure to check the ingredients list. Some oat bran products actually contain very little oat bran. A decent source of fiber will have at least three grams per serving—if the label doesn't list fiber, assume there's not much fiber. Oats should be the first ingredient listed, or at least be very high among the ingredients. Read the label for fat content, too. Some oat bran products contain saturated or hydrogenated oils that actually raise blood cholesterol and thus may cancel out any benefits the oats offer.

Wheat. Wheat berries and cracked wheat (bulgur) are sold in supermarkets and health food stores and make a nutritious, high-fiber breakfast cereal. Most of the fiber in wheat is insoluble, the type that can be helpful in preventing constipation and may protect against colon cancer. A few brand-name hot wheat cereals are sold nationally. Wheatena, which is made from toasted whole wheat, is made from the whole grain and therefore is high in nutrients and fiber. Cream of Wheat and Farina, on the other hand, are cereals that have been processed and have had the bran—and therefore the fiber and most of the nutrients—removed from them.

Rice. Most rice cereals are sold as baby cereals. These products are ordinarily made from white rice. There are brown rice cereals available—usually in health food stores—and these are higher in fiber. You can also use leftover brown or white rice. Reheat it in the microwave and stir in dried fruits, yogurt, and spices such as cinnamon and nutmeg, if desired.

Corn. The most familiar type of hot corn cereal—at least in the south—is hominy or grits. Unfortunately, turning corn into hominy involves removing the bran and germ of the corn, and therefore most of the nutrients and fiber. Cornmeal made into porridge or polenta, is a better choice; although most brands of cornmeal have been degermed to prevent them from deteriorating, some types of cornmeal retain the fiber-rich bran.

Other grains. Grains more commonly eaten at dinnertime can also be eaten for breakfast. You'll find whole-grain forms of barley, millet, kasha (buckwheat), and rye in health food stores. Multigrain hot cereals are also available.

Bread

Do you believe that bread is fattening, and that you must give it up if you're on a weight-loss diet? In fact, a slice of bread is no more "fattening" than an apple. The average slice of bread has 60 to 90 calories, and "diet" or "light" breads 35 to 40. Bread—which is made primarily from flour, water, yeast, and salt—is rich in complex carbohydrates, and a low-fat source of fiber, vitamins, and minerals, if you choose your loaf carefully. The choice of breads is wide these days, and it pays to do some label reading. What do you want in a bread, besides good taste and texture?

The answer is fiber, vitamins, and minerals. In general, the more fiber, the more nutrients. Bread ought to be a basic source of fiber in your diet—but it isn't always. That's because most breads are made of what's called "wheat flour." This isn't "whole wheat," but simply refined white flour, which has had most of the fiber-rich bran and germ mechanically removed. While most manufacturers replace the lost vitamins and some of the minerals (indeed sometimes with more than the grain had in the first place), they may not replace the fiber and the trace minerals. However, some white breads (made from refined wheat flour) actually have more fiber than so-called "six-grain" or even "twelve-grain" loaves. This is because manufacturers add fiber (from oat or wheat bran or soy flour) to some white breads, especially the diet breads, while some of the so-called multigrain breads are actually made chiefly from refined wheat flour and thus may have little fiber. A bread that claims it's made of triticale, wheat

Flour storage tips

Flour, both white and whole grain may be more susceptible to spoilage than you might think. If stored improperly or for too long, it can develop an off flavor or give unpredictable results in baking. Flour can absorb moisture from the air. The fat from the germ in whole-grain flours can go rancid.

White wheat flour, degermed cornmeal, potato flour, arrowroot, and tapioca can be stored at room temperature for six to twelve months in a tightly covered container. Whole-grain flour keeps for less than a month at room temperature. Stored in a tightly covered container in the freezer, it will stay fresh for up to a year.

bran, or pumpernickel may prove to have very little whole grain when you check the ingredients. Always check the label for fiber content—look for a bread with two or three grams per slice.

A guide to bread labels

"Diet" or *"light"* bread: usually just thinner, smaller slices.

"High fiber": this may be meaningless, but at least if the claim is made, the manufacturer is required to state the amount of fiber on the label.

"Low in fat": true of nearly all yeast breads, which generally have less than one gram of fat per slice.

"No cholesterol": true of most breads, unless large amounts of butter and eggs are used. Cholesterol is seldom an issue with bread.

"Oat bread": Usually just white bread with a small amount of oats added. Check the ingredients list to see how far down oats is listed.

"Unbleached" or *"unbromated"*: this means that the color of the wheat has not been lightened, though it does not mean it's whole wheat.

Quick breads

Quick breads are leavened with baking powder or baking soda instead of yeast; they're called quick because no rising time is required. (Muffins are a type of quick bread.) Store bought quick breads can be high in calories and fat, but you can make healthful quick breads at home, as follows:

•Substitute whole wheat flour, bran, oatmeal, or wheat germ for 25 percent of the white flour in recipes.

•Reduce the amount of sugar called for by 25 percent.

•Sweeten with dried fruits, such as apricots, which add beta carotene, or prunes, which add fiber and iron.

•Use canola, sunflower, or safflower oils—all highly unsaturated—instead of butter or margarine.

•For every two eggs, use one egg white and one whole egg. If just one egg is called for, use two egg whites.

NUTRITIONAL CONTENT OF
Breads

Bread	Calories	Protein (g)	Fat (g)	Comments
Whole wheat, 1-oz slice	70	3	1	Must be made from 100 percent whole-wheat flour. Good source of vitamins, minerals, and fiber. May contain sugar, honey, and molasses, which add calories. Bread labeled "wheat bread," "cracked wheat," or "sprouted wheat" usually contains white flour.
White, enriched, 1-oz slice	75	3	1	Made from white flour, which lacks the bran and germ of the wheat grain. Most of the lost nutrients are not replaced, even in "enriched" flour, which has only niacin, thiamine, riboflavin, and iron added. Fiber is reduced.
Rye, 1-oz slice	70	3	trace	Most rye breads contain mostly white flour. Look for rye flour, especially whole-rye flour, as a primary ingredient.
Pumpernickel, 1-oz slice	70	3	trace	Most American loaves are made from white and rye flour colored with caramel, so they have no advantage over white or rye bread.
Italian/French, 1-oz slice	80	3	trace	Loaves made at local bakeries are usually free of preservatives and they may contain little or no sugar or fat. Look for whole-grain varieties.
Bagel, plain	200	7	2	Usually made of high-protein flour and little or no fat, making it dense. Egg bagels contain added fat and cholesterol.
Pita	165	6	1	Often made just of flour, salt, and water. May have sweeteners and additives.
Croissant	235	5	12	Contains butter and sugar. High in saturated fat, cholesterol, and calories.
English muffin	140	5	1	Has no nutritional advantage over white bread.

"Wheat bread": this is white bread; "wheat flour" or "enriched wheat flour" (not whole-wheat flour) is the first ingredient. Just because a bread is brown in color does not mean it is truly whole wheat. Some brands use large amounts of burned sugar syrup to give them a dark brown color.

"Whole-wheat bread": this contains the whole grain, including the fiber-rich bran and germ. Consumers must read the label: some whole-wheat breads, while still made of nutrient-rich flour, can be heavily laced with honey and brown sugar or molasses. "Whole-wheat flour" should be the first ingredient and the only type of flour listed.

Pasta

Pasta, meaning "paste" in Italian, is rich in complex carbohydrates, high in protein, virtually fat-free and sodium-free, and contains no cholesterol (unless you pour on cheese, cream, butter, and salt). Pasta also provides good amounts of B vitamins and iron. And despite its reputation, pasta is not especially fattening. In fact, a main-course plateful of spaghetti with simple tomato, vegetable, or fish sauce usually contains fewer calories than a steak or a tuna salad sandwich.

Types of pasta

Pasta is a simple product made essentially of flour and water. The flour is usually semolina, a high-protein variety milled from hard, golden durum wheat, which produces a truly fine pasta with a mellow flavor and sturdy texture. If the pasta will be shaped as noodles, eggs are mixed in, adding small amounts of protein, fat, and cholesterol. Whole-wheat pasta is formed from unprocessed whole-wheat flour containing bran and germ; it has a

brownish color, a nutty taste, and additional protein and fiber. Varieties touted as "high protein" have fewer carbohydrates and more protein because they contain wheat germ, yeast, or other protein rich ingredients. Other high-protein varieties substitute soy flour for some of the semolina. Vegetable powder or juice, such as that made from spinach or tomatoes, may also be added to basic pasta; while this enhances the taste, it improves the nutritional content only slightly.

Despite the growing popularity of fresh pasta in supermarkets and specialty stores, pasta is one food for which fresh doesn't necessarily mean best. A good commercial dried pasta made from durum wheat can be just as tasty as fresh store-bought pasta or pasta made at home from all-purpose flour— and it's often more nutritious.

Noodles that are an integral part of the national cuisine in Asian countries are becoming increasingly popular here. They are not technically pasta; they don't conform to government standards for macaroni or noodles, and may be labeled "alimentary paste," "imitation noodles" or Asian noodles.

Bean thread noodles (which may be called *fen si*, or *harusame*) turn clear when cooked. They are nearly pure starch and contain almost no protein, vitamins, or minerals (other than iron).

Buckwheat noodles (called *soba* or *qiao mian*) are high in protein. They are served hot in broth or cold with a dipping sauce.

Rice noodles (called *sha he fen* or *sa ho fun*) are boiled or stirfried for use in salad or soups, or used to make dumplings. Like bean thread noodles, they are almost pure starch and contain little protein.

Wheat noodles, made with or without eggs, are popular in Asian cuisine. Among other things, they are used in

Some people rinse pasta to wash away starch. Don't do it. Rinsing pasta only increases the loss of nutrients—and cools off the pasta.

soups and lo mein and chow mein dishes, topped with sesame sauce, and used to make egg rolls, wontons, and dumplings. Asian wheat noodles are similar nutritionally to Western-style wheat pasta, except that the sodium content may be higher.

Toppings for pasta

The most popular topping for pasta by far is tomato sauce, or meat and tomato sauce, usually from a jar or a can when one is pressed for time. Yet many canned or bottled sauces are fairly high in sodium and fat. Some brands can contain up to 800 milligrams of sodium per half-cup serving—a large portion of your daily allowance—and get up to 47 percent of their calories from fat. They may also contain significant amounts of sugar or corn syrup. As with all prepared foods, it is important to check the labels.

Homemade sauce: easy and better

A good tomato sauce need not simmer all afternoon to be flavorful. You can make your own in very little more time than it takes to boil the pasta. Buy canned tomato purée, tomato paste,

Whole-wheat pasta is an excellent source of dietary fiber, providing 13 grams in two cups cooked. The same serving size of regular pasta has about 2 grams.

NUTRITIONAL CONTENT OF

Pasta

Average main-course servings of pasta are about four ounces uncooked, which cooks up to two cups cooked; side-dish or appetizer servings are about two to three ounces dry. Because of absorption of water, four ounces of dry spaghetti weighs ten ounces when cooked al dente and thirteen ounces when cooked to a softer consistency.

Pasta (4 oz dry)	Calories	Protein (g)	Fat (g)	Comments
Regular spaghetti, shell, or other types of pasta	380	14	2	Domestic and imported brands and vegetable-enriched varieties (such as spinach) have approximately the same nutritional value.
Egg noodles	400	14	4	Slightly higher in fat and cholesterol due to eggs.
Whole wheat	400	15-20	2	Higher amounts of fiber and trace minerals.
Soy wheat	400	25	3	High in protein; available at many health food stores.
High-protein (or "light")	420	20-30	2	Almost 50 percent more protein (from wheat germ or yeast) than regular pasta.
Fresh pasta	328	13	3	Made with whole eggs, so contains 83 milligrams of cholesterol per serving.
Corn pasta	407	9	2	Wheat free, so good for people who are allergic to wheat.
Buckwheat noodles (soba)	383	16	1	Made of buckwheat and wheat flour, or just buckwheat flour. Rich in protein
Asian wheat noodles (Udon and somen)	406	13	1	Nutritionally similar to regular pasta, except may be higher in sodium. Udon are thick and chewy; somen are very thin and fine.

NUTRITIONAL CONTENT OF
Dried Beans and Peas

Type (1/2 cup cooked)	Calories	Fat (g)	Fiber (g)	Iron (mg)	Calcium (mg)
Black	113	<1	6	2	24
Black-eyed peas	100	<1	5	2	21
Chickpeas	134	2	4	2	40
Fava	93	<1	5	1	31
Kidney	112	<1	7	3	25
Lentils	115	<1	5	3	19
Lima	108	<1	4	2	16
Mung	107	<1	3	1	27
Navy	129	<1	7	2	64
Pinto	117	<1	6	2	41
Soybeans	149	8	5	4	88
Split peas	116	<1	3	1	13
White	125	<1	5	3	81

and/or crushed tomatoes with no salt added; all are virtually fat-free. (If good fresh tomatoes are available, simply chop them up and cook to taste.) Cook some minced onion in a small amount of beef or chicken stock, then add the canned tomato product, and—if you wish—a small amount of very lean ground beef. Season with black pepper, plenty of garlic, and such characteristically Italian herbs as basil, oregano, and rosemary.

If you're cooking without salt, you can add flavor with other combinations, too: experiment with a touch of curry, cumin, or chili powder.

Other low-fat sauces

There's no law that says spaghetti has to be topped with a tomato sauce. You can make delicious sauces with fresh vegetables simmered in stock until crisp-tender. Herbs and spices will improve the flavor. For a meat sauce, add chunks of skinless white-meat turkey or chicken, then toss with the pasta. A "cream" sauce can be made by puréeing white kidney (cannelli) beans in a blender with some chicken stock and Italian spices. A tablespoon of grated Parmesan cheese per serving

adds a lot of flavor, with only about 25 calories and two grams of fat.

Top Asian noodles with stir-fried vegetables seasoned with soy sauce, ginger, and hot peppers.

Dried Beans and Peas

Dried beans and peas belong to the family *Leguminosae,* or legumes (that is, they are seeds from pods), and exist in hundreds of varieties. Dried beans are an inexpensive source of many nutrients—perhaps the best nutritional value, pound for pound, in the market. They are rich in B vitamins, calcium, iron, zinc, and potassium, and are a boon to any diet (especially a diabetic, low-fat, or weight-loss diet). As a source of fiber, they are second only to wheat bran, containing about nine grams of fiber per cup (cooked), nearly half the minimum amount of fiber you should eat each day. The fiber they contain is largely soluble, the kind that may lower blood cholesterol. Beans themselves contain no cholesterol and little fat, except for soybeans, which are high in unsaturated fat.

Though many people think that

Tofu tips

Often used in Asian cooking, tofu—a high-protein soybean curd used in everything from soup and salad to dessert—has become a popular staple in this country. That's good news: tofu is low in fat, cholesterol, and sodium, and is inexpensive. But unfortunately, tofu is often sold in open markets or the vegetable section of a store, sitting out in a tray of water, unrefrigerated—inviting coliform bacteria to grow. High levels of bacteria can cause gastrointestinal tract ailments including nausea, vomiting, and diarrhea.

To lower your risk, choose dated fresh-looking products sold in sealed, refrigerated packages. Even properly packaged products, though, may not be microbe free. To be completely safe, heat the tofu for two minutes in boiling water before using it.

beans are starchy and fattening, they are actually are much lower in calories than meat; one cup of cooked dried beans or peas has only 200 to 300 calories. Beans provide nearly as much protein as meat. (One cup of cooked beans will provide you with twelve to twenty-five grams of protein, which is 25 to 50 percent of the RDA). To be sure, this protein has insufficient amounts of one or more essential amino acids, but that can easily be completed if you eat some bread, rice, dairy product, or a small amount of meat the same day. The protein in soybeans, however, is complete protein.

Research has turned up more good news about these legumes. Not only are beans free of cholesterol and almost free of saturated fat, but they contain soluble fiber—the type that may actually lower cholesterol levels. In addition, beans are a boon to diabetics. Because beans are digested slowly, they cause a gentle rise in blood sugar, thus requiring less insulin than most carbohydrate-rich foods. Some evidence suggests that soybeans—and products made from them such as soy milk and tofu—contain several chemical compound that may have anticancer activity. These include isoflavones and phytosterols—which occur in other plants but are especially concentrated in soybeans. Isoflavones may slightly decrease estrogen production in premenopausal women, and so may play a role in breast cancer prevention.

Dried beans, like such staples as rice and pasta, are the cook's friend. If you don't want to start from scratch, canned beans are as nutritious as dried, except that the canned ones have extra sodium and a little less of the B vitamin folacin. (If you're watching sodium, rinse the canned beans.) On the other hand, if you prefer to start from scratch, soaking and cooking are easy,

Sprouted alfalfa, mung beans, lentils, peas, soybeans, and wheat are more nutritious than their unsprouted counterparts. Beta carotene, vitamin C, and most B vitamins are all synthesized as the sprouts grow.

Meatless Meats

Many meat substitutes, or analogues, as they've come to be called, are made with traditional soy products like tofu, a soybean curd; tempeh, cooked and fermented soybeans; or miso, a fermented soy paste. Others are based on modern laboratory-produced soy derivatives. You can buy meatless beef, meatless turkey, and meatless chicken—some meatless meats even have a smoked taste.

Ounce for ounce, these products contain as much protein as meat. Most of the oil (largely polyunsaturated) is removed from soy protein concentrates and isolated soy protein, so they are virtually fat-free. Another advantage of isolated soy protein is that it contains much less of the carbohydrates that may cause flatulence.

Unfortunately, in most meatless meats, soy protein is not all you're getting. Processors generally add oils and fats (some partially hydrogenated) to soy protein concentrates and isolated soy protein to fake the look and taste of beef, bacon, ham, tuna, or even luncheon meats. Some soy-based products have as much fat as lean ground beef, but less saturated fat and no cholesterol. They may also contain artificial colorings and flavorings—even a jolt of sodium in the form of MSG (monosodium glutamate), soy sauce, or salt. Vitamins and minerals may be added, too, but compared to meat, many of these products remain notably deficient in iron, zinc, and other trace minerals.

You can concoct your own meat analogue at home, using cooked soybeans or other high-protein legumes (chick-peas, lentils, pinto beans) and adding chopped onion, celery, herbs, perhaps cooked barley or rice, and salt to taste. These can be shaped into patties and browned in a nonstick pan.

If you would rather try a commercial product, remember that no meat substitute will completely mimic the taste and texture of meat. And as with all prepared foods, it's worthwhile reading the labels. Some meatless products are as high in fat as real hot dogs; many are also high in sodium. In some cases, you'll be at least as well off nutritionally with lean meat—except for its cholesterol content.

requiring time, but not labor. Cooked beans will keep five days refrigerated and up to six months frozen. Thus they can be prepared in large batches.

Either way, beans and peas are infinitely adaptable. For a semivegetarian main-dish casserole, combine them with small amounts of lean ground beef, diced ham, or chicken, season them to taste, and bake them in a slow oven. Add them to vegetable soups, or make bean soups. Combine them with other vegetables, such as fresh or canned tomatoes, eggplant, or squash. Use them cold in salads, combined with pasta and/or greens. Serve them hot or cold as a side dish. Other possibilities: mash or purée beans or chickpeas and mix them with seasonings for such middle-Eastern specialties as hummus (a good dip for raw vegetables) and for Southwestern dishes such as tacos and tostadas. Kidney, black, and pinto beans are typical in Mexican dishes. Puréed mung beans or lentils, called dal, are a staple of Pakistani and Indian cooking.

A common problem with beans is flatulence, due mainly to the presence of certain complex sugars that cannot be digested and that cause gas and bloating. To reduce gas significantly, discard the water after soaking, then boil the beans in a large quantity of water, and then discard the water again (don't use the water as a soup base). This method can eliminate more than half of the gas-producing complex sugars in the beans.

When purchased dried, beans have a long shelf life, but need to be rinsed and soaked before cooking. Dried peas and beans may contain small pebbles, bits of soil, or other debris, so its always a good idea to wash them under running water and to look at them by the handful so that you can easily find and remove any foreign material.

Beef: Cooking Tips

Though conventional wisdom says that fatty beef tastes better and is more tender than lean, taste tests suggest that lean beef can be just as flavorful and tender, if it is prepared correctly.

- Trim all external fat before cooking.
- Reduce normal cooking times by 20 percent when using lean beef, since it cooks faster and becomes tough when overcooked. Don't be deceived by the redness of the meat: lean pieces cooked to a medium degree may look rare. Use a meat thermometer to measure doneness. Or, use the finger test: the meat is done when it gives a little when pressed.
- Broil meat so that the fat can drip off. Drain fat well when sautéing ground beef for chili or spaghetti sauce.
- To seal in the juices, sear meat in a skillet or roasting pan before cooking it.

MEAT AND POULTRY

Beef

Beef consumption has dropped 28 percent in the last twenty years, a decline best explained in two words: fat and cholesterol, both linked to an increased risk of heart disease. But today's beef isn't as fatty as meat from years past. Ranchers are crossbreeding leaner, larger cattle with traditional breeds. In addition, cattle are being fed more grass and less corn and being sent to market younger so they will develop less fat. And meatpackers and retailers are trimming more external fat, often leaving only one-tenth of an inch, down from three-fourths of an inch just a decade or so ago.

But beef's fat content is widely variable, and only the leanest pieces are as low in fat as broiled fish or skinless chicken. Despite the industry's efforts to promote lean beef, it's often hard to

---

Red meat and cancer
A recent study has added weight to the theory that a high intake of fat, particularly from red meat, increases the risk of advanced prostate cancer. The study followed almost 48,000 male health professionals (age forty to seventy-five) with no previous history of cancer. The researchers found that the men who ate the most fat had a 79 percent higher risk of advanced prostate cancer than those who ate the least fat. And men who ate the most red meat had a 164 percent higher risk than those with the lowest intake.

Fats from dairy products, fish, and vegetable oils did not increase the risk. Only advanced—not all—prostate cancer was linked to fat intake.

Do these results mean that you should give up red meat? It's still too early, and indeed may never make sense, to make this recommendation. Rather, eat red meat only occasionally and choose lean cuts.

NUTRITIONAL CONTENT OF
Beef

(3½ oz trimmed and cooked)	Calories	Fat (g)	Saturated fat (g)	Cholesterol (mg)
Arm, choice	219	9	3	101
Arm, prime ††	261	13	5	101
Blade roast, choice	265	15	6	106
Blade roast, prime ††	318	21	8	106
Blade roast, select	238	12	5	106
Bottom round, choice	193	8	3	78
Bottom round, prime ††	249	13	5	96
Bottom round, select	171	5	2	78
Brisket, half point, all grades	212	9	3	95
Brisket, whole, all grades	218	10	4	93
Eye of round, choice	175	6	2	69
Eye of round, prime ††	198	8	3	69
Eye of round, select	155	4	1	69
Flank, choice	237	13	6	71
Porterhouse steak, choice †	218	11	4	80
Rib eye, choice	225	12	5	80
Ribs, whole, choice †	237	14	6	77
Ribs, whole, prime †	280	19	8	81
Ribs, whole, select †	206	10	4	77
Round, select †	172	5	2	78
Round, choice †	191	7	3	78
Shank crosscuts, choice †	201	6	2	78
Short ribs, choice †	295	18	8	93
Sirloin, choice	200	8	3	89
Sirloin, prime ††	237	12	5	89
T-Bone steak, choice †	214	10	4	80
Tenderloin, choice	212	10	4	84
Tenderloin, prime †	232	12	5	84
Tenderloin, select	200	9	3	84
Tip round, choice	180	6	2	81
Tip round, prime †	213	10	4	81
Tip round, select	170	5	2	81
Top loin, choice	209	10	4	76
Top loin, prime †	245	14	5	76
Top loin, select	184	7	3	76
Top round, choice	207	6	2	90
Top round, prime †	215	9	3	84
Top round, select	190	4	1	90

All cuts are completely trimmed of external fat unless otherwise noted. Cuts marked with † are trimmed to ¼ inch; cuts marked with †† are trimmed to ½ inch. Further trimming of those cuts would lower the calorie, fat, and saturated fat content.

recognize a low-fat piece of beef. One way to tell fatty beef from lean is to look at it. If the beef is marblized—that is, there are interior streaks or specks of fat—it is fatty. A better way is to consider grade and cut. The best grade, "prime," is the fattiest, followed by "choice" and "select." "Select." "Select" has, on average, 5 to 20 percent less fat than "choice" beef of the same cut, and 40 percent less fat than "prime." Even if they have to sacrifice a little taste, many people would opt for the leanness of "select" meat. And "select" meat is also less expensive than other grades.

Still, "choice" beef can be low in fat, if you select the right cuts. Top round, eye round, London broil, and sirloin tip are leaner cuts, while brisket, rib roast, and short ribs are among the fattiest cuts. And as the chart at lower right shows, the best way to cut the fat content of meat is still with a knife — trim all external fat before cooking.

How about hamburgers?

Evaluating the fat content of packaged hamburger meat can be even more difficult than judging full cuts. The packages may carry seemingly helpful labels such as "75 percent lean," "lean," or "extra lean," but this terminology can be misleading. Beef labeled "75 percent lean" is 25 percent fat *by weight*—which is a lot of fat. Thus a patty made from this meat would derive more than 70 percent of its total calories from fat, since, ounce for ounce, fat has more than twice as many calories as lean meat. And while a steak or other cut of beef labeled "lean" must have no more than 10 percent fat by weight, and "extra lean" no more than 5 percent, these standards don't apply when the meat is ground. Ground beef labeled "lean" or even "extra lean" can have as much as 22 percent fat by weight, with this fat supply-ing about 70 percent of total calories.

Still, there is a way to get a burger you can trust. While hamburgers have acquired a bad name among health-conscious people, they are a good source of protein, and even a fast-food burger has a fair amount of B vitamins, iron, and zinc. The trick is to create your own home-cooked burger made from carefully selected ground beef. (See the marginal on this page.) Go easy on the fatty toppings; adding cheese and mayonnaise to a hamburger more than doubles the calories and significantly increases the fat content.

Proper storage and handling

Raw and undercooked beef can contain a bacterium called *E. coli*. This bacterium normally inhabits the intestines and feces of humans and other animals without harm to the host. If these fecal bacteria contaminate food and are eaten, however, diarrhea may result. This strain, designated *E. coli* 0157:H7, can cause bloody diarrhea and abdominal cramps, as well as the more serious hemolytic uremic syndrome (HUS), which affects the kidneys and the blood clotting system. There's no cure for the disease, which has to run its course; hospitalization is usually necessary. Most people can expect to recover completely, though HUS is sometimes fatal, especially for kids. Ground meats are most dangerous because grinding equipment may be a source of contaminants and because ground meat offers microorganisms more surfaces on which to multiply. Steaks, roasts, and other whole cuts pose much less of a risk.

Keeping beef cold can inhibit the multiplication of *E. coli*, but proper cooking is essential to eliminate the risk. Heat above 155°F. kills *E. coli*. Follow these guidelines:

•Cook ground meat until well-done:

The Wellness burger

You can still enjoy hamburgers on a low-fat diet if you follow these steps:

1. Go to a store that has a butcher, choose a very lean cut of round, then ask him to trim all the fat and grind the meat for you. This will result in a burger with only 20 percent of its calories coming from fat.

2. Use three ounces of meat for each patty.

3. To make the lean beef less dry, mix it with tomato juice, chopped onion, or Worcestershire sauce before cooking.

4. Broil or panbroil your burger instead of frying it.

5. If you like cooked onions and mushrooms for a garnish, simmer them in stock (or water and wine) instead of sautéing them in butter.

6. Place the burger on a whole-wheat bun (or whole-wheat bread). Add a slice of tomato and some lettuce.

This hamburger will have 315 calories, 7 grams of fat, 34 grams of protein, 72 milligrams of cholesterol, and 415 milligrams of sodium.

the center should look gray or brown, and the juices should run clear, not pink or red. In restaurants, check small children's portions before they eat.

•Don't depend on the sniff test. Meat contaminated with *E. coli* does not smell bad.

•At home, keep utensils and working surfaces clean. Wash them, and your hands, thoroughly with soap and warm water after you've finished.

•Thaw beef in the refrigerator, and cook it right away. Don't let the meat sit outside the refrigerator.

•If you buy packaged prebrowned hamburger, make sure it is thoroughly cooked before you use it.

•Don't eat steak tartare or other raw-meat dishes.

Hormones: should you worry?

Every so often, reports appear in the media about the hormones—natural sex steroids estradiol (estrogen), progesterone, and testosterone, and two synthetic ones—used in the raising of 70 to 90 percent of American cattle to make the animals gain weight faster. Numerous studies have shown that this concern has not been warranted.

The FDA says hormone-treated beef is safe to eat. At the prescribed dosages used in feedlots, these hormones have been certified safe. There is virtually no evidence to the contrary. The residues left in meat are so minuscule that a pound of beef contains about 15,000 times less hormone than is produced each day by an average man—and several million times less than what's produced by a pregnant woman. And don't forget that many foods naturally contain estrogen: milk contains five times more estrogen by weight than hormone-treated beef, and wheat germ 1,700 times more.

The claim that hormones pose health risks may be based on an experience with a synthetic estrogen called diethylstilbestrol (DES). Banned as a carcinogen in Europe and the United States, black-market DES was injected into calves in Italy. The treated veal was used for baby food in 1981, and it was claimed—but never scientifically proven—that babies of both sexes who ate the veal grew breasts, and girls began to menstruate.

Hormones used in American beef today are chemically quite different from DES. And the way cattle today receive the hormones is far safer. Instead of injecting these substances into muscle tissue that may be eaten, feedlot operators implant time-release hormone pellets behind animals' ears, which are not used for human food.

American consumer groups have by and large supported the FDA's stand on hormones. However, some groups, including the Center for Science in the Public Interest, are concerned about the potential misuse of hormones in cattle. If the hormone pellet is placed not behind the ear but in a part of the animal that is used for ground beef—the neck or breast, for example—as a 1986 study by the USDA showed sometimes happens, a consumer might get more hormone that is proven safe.

You may wonder why the hormones are used at all, if questions of safety remain. Hormone implants save U.S. cattlemen about 650 million dollars per year, and part of these savings are passed on to consumers. A one-dollar hormone pellet behind the ear means the animal will consume about four fewer bushels of corn (a twenty-dollar savings) and reach market weight eighteen days sooner (15 percent faster than if untreated). It will be more docile and it will gain approximately fifty pounds more lean muscle tissue than an untreated animal. So not only do we save money and resources, but we also get leaner meat. If you still feel concerned about hormone treatment, you don't have to give up beef. There are several types of certified untreated beef on the market—at a premium price. From the evidence now available, though, you don't need to switch to untreated beef.

Poultry

Chicken and other poultry provide high-quality protein for people who are turning away from beef, lamb, and pork, which can be high in saturated fat. In fact, a small portion of cooked poultry (three to four ounces without bones or skin) provides about half the daily adult protein requirement and has half to one-third the calories and fat of a similar portion of steak. Moreover, the fat in chicken is highly monounsaturated—much closer to peanut oil than to the fat in beef and other red meats.

Poultry is also a good source of B vitamins, but has less iron than red meat. The cholesterol content of poultry is similar to that of beef, since all animal products have 20 to 25 milligrams of cholesterol per ounce. A 3½-ounce serving of chicken breast (with or without skin) has about 75 milligrams of cholesterol. That's 25 percent of the recommended maximum daily intake of 300 milligrams and only slightly less than a similar serving of beef.

Chicken. When shopping for chicken, look for plump, firm meat with no off odor or slimy texture. The skin may be white or yellow, depending on what the bird was fed, but skin color has no relation to quality or nutrition. Choose white meat over dark; dark meat has far more fat and a little more cholesterol.

Any cooking method except deep-frying is fine: roasting, poaching, braising, broiling, or pan-broiling (stir-frying, too, if minimal fat is used). It's okay to cook the chicken in the skin, since there's some evidence that the meat won't absorb fat from the skin during cooking—just don't eat the skin. But if you remove all skin from poultry pieces before cooking, the pan juices will be relatively fat-free. If you prefer fried chicken, don't bread it, since the coating will absorb fat.

Turkey. Skinless turkey breast is one of the leanest meats—a 3½-ounce portion has less than a gram of fat, which contributes only 5 percent of its 135 calories. Like chicken, turkey is now available in parts—breasts (with bones or without), drumsticks, and cutlets, for example—so you can have the benefits of turkey without having to wrestle with a sixteen-pound bird that takes hours to cook.

If you opt for the traditional whole bird, avoid self-basting turkeys since the basting solutions contain, for the most part, fat—usually highly saturated coconut oil or partially hydrogenated soy or corn oil—water, and sodium. The water and the sodium help keep the bird juicy; the fat is used mostly for flavoring. Butter is an ingredient in some basting solutions. Baste the turkey yourself to keep it juicy. Instead of using turkey drippings —which are a concentrated source of fat—try basting with defatted chicken or turkey stock. Or skim the fat from the drippings before you baste. To make a low-fat gravy, you can use a gravy separator, which looks like a measuring cup with the spout at the bottom. This utensil makes it easy to separate the fat from the flavorful juices and discard it.

Turkey cold cuts. Turkey cold cuts are another poultry option. Unfortunately, these are often high in fat and always loaded with sodium, which serves as a

Low-fat gravy

To make a low-fat gravy for roast chicken or turkey, remove the bird from the cooking pan, then drain all juices into a fat skimmer, preferably one with a spout set close to the bottom. Rinse out the pan. Let the drippings sit until the fat rises. Remove the small amount of fat in the spout with a paper towel, and pour out the clear broth. You can also pour the drippings into a jar and use a bulb baster to remove the fat (or else simply skim the fat from the juices in the roast pan—there'll be some fat left, but considerably less). Proceed with the gravy recipe. Clear juices can be thickened with flour if you add a small amount at a time. Have some precooked broth on hand to enrich the sauce.

Poultry

Poultry (3½ oz edible portion)	Calories	Fat (g)	Fat Calories	Cholesterol (mg)	Sodium (mg)
Broiler-fryer chicken					
light meat, with skin, roasted	222	11	45%	84	75
dark meat, with skin, roasted	253	16	57%	91	87
light meat, with skin, batter dipped, fried	277	15	49%	84	287
light meat, no skin, roasted	173	5	26%	85	77
dark meat, no skin, roasted	205	10	44%	93	93
Roasting chicken					
light meat, no skin, roasted	153	4	24%	75	51
dark meat, no skin, roasted	178	9	46%	75	95
Capon					
flesh and skin, roasted	229	12	47%	86	49
Turkey					
light meat, with skin, roasted	197	8	37%	76	63
dark meat, with skin, roasted	221	12	49%	89	76
light meat, no skin, roasted	157	3	17%	69	64
breast meat, no skin, roasted	135	1	7%	83	52
dark meat, no skin, roasted	187	7	34%	85	79
ground, dark and light meat, with skin	233	14	54%	65	111
Turkey cold cuts					
Pastrami	141	6	38%	53	1,045
Ham	128	5	35%	65	933
Barbecued breast slices	128	4	28%	65	1,050
Bologna	199	15	68%	99	878
Salami	196	14	64%	82	1,004
Smoked breast	123	4	29%	65	747
Duck					
flesh and skin, roasted	337	28	75%	84	59
flesh, no skin, roasted	201	11	49%	89	65
Goose					
flesh and skin, roasted	305	22	65%	91	70
flesh, no skin, roasted	238	13	50%	96	76

Many new fast-food chains are specializing in roasted, or rotisserie) chicken rather than fried. Roasted chicken is often only slightly lower in fat than fried. The most important thing is to remove the skin, which can reduce the fat content of roasted or fried chicken by one-third to one-half. And order white meat, not dark.

preservative. Many are made from high-fat dark meat, and some brands contain high-cholesterol organ meats, such as the heart and gizzard. One brand of turkey bologna (advertised as "80 percent fat-free" by weight) gets 77 percent of its calories from fat and has 1,100 milligrams of sodium in just one three-ounce serving.

Look for cold cuts that have one gram or less of fat per ounce (at least 95 percent fat-free by weight). In many cases, turkey pastrami, ham, and breast slices fill this bill. Turkey bologna and salami tend to be nearly as rich in fat as their beef counterparts. Turkey "breast" cold cuts are low in fat, but don't think you're getting only sliced turkey; the meat has been processed and filled with additives such as modified food starch. The fat content of turkey roll depends on whether it is made primarily from dark or light meat; it contains gelatin, sugar, and other fillers and flavorings.

You're better off with sliced fresh turkey from the deli counter.

When buying turkey cold cuts, be sure to check ingredients lists carefully for sodium and sugar. Sodium comes in many forms besides salt. As a basic rule of thumb, any ingredient that has sodium as part of its name is going to be a source of sodium, including monosodium glutamate—MSG—a popular additive in turkey products. Kosher turkeys have been heavily salted and then rinsed, so sodium levels vary. Products that are barbecue-flavor and smoked are not only likely to be high in sodium, but may contain nitrites (a potential carcinogen) as well. Sugar also comes in many forms: dextrose, corn syrup, and honey are just a few of the types of sugar used in turkey cold cuts. There is no reason to choose sweetened turkey.

Duck and goose. These birds are bred today to have more meat and less fat and bones, but they are still high in saturated fat. Except for special occasions, avoid duck and goose. When you do choose to have them, be sure to roast them so that some of the fat melts away. And, as with chicken and turkey, don't eat the skin.

Proper storage and handling

All fresh poultry, even kosher or organic poultry, is much more prone to contamination by salmonella and campylobacter bacteria—which can cause food poisoning—than other meats. But these organisms can be killed by heat, and their growth inhibited by refrigeration. Keep the following points in mind:

•Always cook poultry thoroughly. Juices should run clear, not pink. White meat should register 170° F. on a meat thermometer, dark meat 180° F.

•Thaw frozen poultry in the refrigerator, never at room temperature. Use a microwave for thawing only if you plan to cook it right away or re-refrigerate until cooking.

•When trimming or preparing raw poultry, don't let it touch other foods, especially salad greens or any food that will be served raw or undercooked.

•After washing and preparing raw poultry, wash the cutting board, kitchen counter, knives, and other utensils—and your hands—thoroughly with soap and hot water.

•Make sure the raw poultry and fluids from the packaging don't come in contact with other foods in the grocery bag or in the refrigerator.

•Always refrigerate raw poultry immediately in a loose wrapping. Don't keep it refrigerated for more than two or three days. Cooked poultry can be safely refrigerated for up to four days.

•Marinate chicken pieces in the refrigerator, since chicken can spoil if it sits out for even three hours on a warm day. If you plan to serve the marinade as a sauce, boil it thoroughly.

Pork

Because so many pork products—especially bacon, sausage, spareribs, and hot dogs—are high in fat, pork has a dubious reputation. But, in fact, fresh pork, on average, is 31 percent leaner than it was a decade ago, thanks to changes in the breeding and feeding of hogs. Other advantages of pork include: the fat in pork is slightly less saturated than that in beef; and pork is an excellent source of B vitamins (it's the leading food source of thiamin), zinc, iron, and high-quality protein.

Since the fat in pork is less saturated than that of beef, it turns rancid faster. Fresh pork will keep for two to three days in the refrigerator depending on the size of the cut (smaller cuts spoil

A safe turkey stuffing

When stuffing a whole turkey, it's important to guard against salmonella poisoning. Remember that the bacteria present in raw poultry can get into the stuffing and multiply. To prevent contamination, follow these steps:

•Stuff the bird loosely (tightly packed stuffing cooks more slowly.) Don't stuff the bird until you are ready to roast it.

•Consider cooking the stuffing separately—it's easier. Flavor the cavity with a little chopped onion, celery, and herbs.

•After cooking, check the stuffing temperature with a thermometer. You should get a reading of 165 degrees.

•Remove the cooked stuffing from the turkey and serve it separately. Don't allow a stuffed bird to sit around the kitchen for hours. Refrigerate leftovers as soon as you can. Remember that rice stuffings are high in starch and should be handled just like bread stuffings.

more quickly). Cooked pork will keep in the refrigerator for four to five days.

Getting the most from pork
To keep pork lean and flavorful, try the following:

•Choose lean cuts, such as tenderloin, center loin, fresh pork leg, or lean ham. Fattier cuts of pork (such as ribs, loin blade, and shoulder) and pork-based meats (sausage, bacon, ribs, etc.)—still the most popular fare—are hard to justify on a heart-healthy diet.

•If you're trying to minimize your salt intake, avoid all cured pork products such as bacon, ham, and cold cuts.

•Trim all visible fat from pork before cooking.

•Limit portion sizes—say, three to five ounces at a meal—so that your cholesterol intake won't exceed 300 milligrams a day from all sources. Meat can go a long way in dishes such as kabobs, sautés, and stir-fries.

•To keep lean meat moist and flavorful, marinate it in fruit juice, honey, or sherry. Experiment with seasonings such as thyme, ginger, rosemary, mint, garlic, fennel seed, or oregano.

How about hot dogs?
Hot dogs, like all sausages, are by definition high in fat. Not so, according to the makers of the dozen or so "light" franks now on the market. But don't take their word for it: a close reading of the labels shows that most of the new franks are only slightly leaner than the standard wieners.

The "light" dogs are made of beef,

The iridescent film that appears on some cooked hams in harmless. Ham has a high fat and water content and these substances ooze out and react with the nitrites used in curing, causing a reflection like oil on a puddle.

NUTRITIONAL CONTENT OF
Pork

(3½ oz cooked)	Calories	Fat (g)	Saturated fat (g)	Cholesterol (mg)
Bacon*	576	49	17	85
Blade loin	247	15	5	93
Boston butt, fresh	273	16	6	116
Canadian bacon*	185	8	3	58
Center loin	199	9	3	79
Center rib, boneless	214	10	4	83
Country-style ribs	234	14	5	86
Ground pork	297	21	8	94
Ham, canned, extra lean*	136	5	2	30
Ham, cured, extra lean	145	6	2	53
Ham, cured, lean*	157	6	2	55
Ham, fresh, butt half	206	8	3	96
Ham, fresh, shank half	215	11	4	92
Loin, whole	187	8	3	77
Picnic shoulder, fresh	228	13	4	95
Sirloin	216	10	4	86
Spareribs	397	30	11	121
Tenderloin	164	5	2	79
Top loin	194	7	3	78

Contains over 1,000 milligrams of sodium

pork, turkey, chicken, or tofu. A few are genuinely low in fat; one is even fat-free. But most still contain nine to twelve grams of fat, which account for 70 to 80 percent of the calories, compared to twelve or seventeen grams of fat in conventional franks (80 to 85 percent of the calories). The processors accomplish this reduction by adding water and milk protein, vegetable protein, and/or beef stock. Bear in mind:

•Franks made from chicken or turkey aren't necessarily low in fat, since they often contain the dark meat and the skin, both high in fat. They contain 20 to 50 milligrams of cholesterol—as much as or more than beef or pork franks.

•Ignore claims such as "80 percent fat-free/20 percent fat," seen on the label of one brand of "light" franks, for instance. That means 20 percent fat by weight—the eleven grams of fat in each of these franks supplies 76 percent of the calories, and that's the number that matters most.

•Tofu hot dogs (made from soybeans) may not be particularly lean—five to nine grams of fat per dog—but at least the fat they contain is primarily unsaturated. There's no cholesterol and less sodium.

•Some people worry that hot dogs contain animal by-products, such as pork stomach, snout, heart, spleen, lips, and cartilage. Few brands actually do. If by-products are used, they must be listed on the label.

•Low-fat hot dogs, not surprisingly, don't have the taste and texture of regular franks. But once you put them in a bun and top them with mustard, ketchup, or sauerkraut you may not notice the difference.

Cooking pork

Food scientists now say that it is no longer necessary to cook pork until the well-done stage; "medium" is okay. Trichinosis has indeed been virtually eliminated in the United States; most hogs are not fed raw scraps that may carry the parasite. Moreover, most hogs are raised on sanitary lots. As a result, it's estimated that only about one in 1,000 hogs are now infected with the parasite that causes trichinosis. In any case, researchers have discovered that the parasite is destroyed at 137°F. To allow for a margin of safety, the USDA's Food Safety and Inspection Service recommends cooking pork to an internal temperature of 160°F. (instead of 170°F., or "well-done"), which leaves the meat juicy and with traces of pink. Freezing the meat for a three-weeks will also destroy the parasite.

The leaner the meat, the more quickly it will cook—so don't overcook it. When microwaving pork, cover the meat so that heating is even; and if the meat has bones, make sure the meat near the bones is fully cooked.

Wild Game

Most people lack the opportunity—or the desire—to make venison, buffalo meat, and game birds a regular part of their diet. And thus, the nutritional values of game may seem beside the point. Yet "wild" meat, usually farm-raised, is appearing more and more often in restaurants and markets, especially in the West; and you can order venison, quail, and other game by mail. Many people still hunt and serve wild game in season.

In fact, game is better for you than most other meats. Wild animals usually don't get fat, and when they do the meat is only slightly marbled. Thus game is generally lower in fat than beef or pork. A 3½-ounce serving of bison steak contains only about two grams of

Fat isn't the only problem with hot dogs—light or not, they are usually very high in sodium (400 to 650 milligrams). Only a few of the new franks are lower in sodium.

fat, compared with thirteen grams in a similar serving of chuck roast (prime grade). The calorie count is less, too (135 for the buffalo, 205 for the beef). Since cholesterol is found in all animal tissue, lean or fat, beef and buffalo have about the same amount (62 milligrams), which doesn't crowd the recommended daily limit of 300 milligrams. Like all meats, wild game is rich in vitamins and minerals.

Farm-raised game is meatier and more tender than wild game, but slightly higher in fat—though less than beef or pork. It is usually available year round in frozen form.

Cooking tips

•The low fat content is one reason that venison and other game steaks are chewy. If you're cooking a tender cut, you might braise it in a liquid so it doesn't dry out. Chops can be marinated and then broiled. Marinated also helps tame the "gamey taste," which comes from the animal's "wild"

diet—tree bark, leaves, and weeds. Try olive oil mixed with vinegar or citrus juice, plus mustard and herbs. (The gamey taste may be less noticeable in farm-raised game.)

•Most chefs recommend low cooking temperatures for game, since high heat tends to toughen it. Boar, rabbit, and game birds should be cooked through. However, avoid overcooking, which tends to toughen game, especially buffalo and venison.

•Use ground buffalo meat for meat loaves and chili; use buffalo strips for stir-fry dishes with vegetables; try a venison stew or kebabs; barbecue wild boar. Wild rabbit can be stewed or roasted, or substituted for chicken in many recipes. Simmered in a liquid for an hour or two, with vegetables and spices added, venison makes a good stew.

•When cooking partridge or pheasant, as with any poultry, it's a good idea to remove the skin, since that's where much of the fat is.

NUTRITIONAL CONTENT OF
Wild Game

(3½ oz cooked) (mg)	Calories	Fat (g)	Saturated fat (g)	Cholesterol
Antelope, roasted	150	3	1	126
Bear, simmered	259	13	N	N
Bison, roasted	143	2	1	82
Buffalo, roasted	188	6	3	58
Caribou, roasted	167	4	2	109
Deer, roasted	158	3	1	112
Elk, roasted	146	2	1	73
Moose, roasted	134	1	1	78
Rabbit, roasted	154	6	2	64
Rabbit, stewed	173	4	1	123
Water buffalo, roasted	131	2	1	61
Wild boar, roasted	160	4	1	N

N=Not Available

S E A F O O D

Fish

Like meat and poultry, fish is an excellent source of protein. But unlike these other animal foods, most types of fish are relatively low in calories, fat, and cholesterol. While a four-ounce serving of trimmed, broiled sirloin has 241 calories, ten grams of fat, and 102 milligrams of cholesterol, the same size serving of broiled snapper has just 146 calories, two grams of fat, and 54 milligrams of cholesterol.

Fish also supply certain vitamins —particularly the B vitamins thiamine, riboflavin, and niacin—and are a good source of potassium. Higher-fat fish, such as salmon, tuna, sardines, and mackerel, are rich in vitamins A and D, and saltwater fish are the best natural source of iodine.

Fish and heart disease

Not only does fish tend to have less fat than meat, but the fat in fish is highly polyunsaturated and so preferable to the fat in meat, which is mostly saturated. (It is saturated fat that raises blood cholesterol levels.) Moreover, fish fat contains special polyunsaturated fatty acids known as omega-3s, which have anti-clotting properties and thus may protect against heart attacks and perhaps high blood pressure. They may also help control inflammatory responses in the body, including arthritis and psoriasis.

Eating even small amounts of fish appears to significantly reduce the risk of fatal heart attack. In one of the most recent studies confirming this benefit, 2,000 men in Wales, all of whom had previously suffered a heart attack, were divided into three groups, each of which was told to follow a different commonly recommended type of "heart-healthy" diet: one group was advised to eat more fish, one to eat more fiber, and one to eat less saturated fat. After two years, the fish group, which ate an average of about ten ounces of fish a week, had a 29 percent lower mortality rate (from all causes, but entirely attributable to a reduction in deaths from heart disease) compared to the other groups.

The study did not allow for a fair judgment about the benefits of either a high-fiber regimen or a low-fat diet, since the subjects in those two groups did not alter their fat and fiber intake substantially. What the study suggested, though, was that it may be easier for many people to add modest amounts of fish to their diet than to dramatically cut down on fat or substantially boost their fiber intake.

A guide to fat content

Researchers have found that the higher the fat content of fish, the greater the cardiovascular benefits. As a rule, darker fish contain more oil than light fish. The highest fat content is found in deepwater fish like tuna, which need the fat as insulation against cold water. Herring, mackerel, salmon, and sardines are also fatty, containing between 5 and 20 percent fat by weight. Moderately fatty fish that have between 2 and 5 percent fat include bass, bluefish, halibut, ocean perch, pollock, rockfish, and smelt. Lean fish—less than 2 percent fat—include flatfish like flounder and sole. Although lean fish have less fat, a greater percentage of the fat they do contain is in the form of omega-3 as compared to fatty fish.

Is fresh fish safe?

Many people worry about eating fish because of the potential hazards of contaminants of various kinds from pol-

Good sources of omega-3 fatty acids

Albacore tuna, canned
Anchovies
Bass, freshwater
Bass, striped
Butterfish
Carp
Catfish
Halibut
Herring
Mackerel
Mullet
Ocean perch
Orange roughy
Pompano
Sablefish
Salmon
Sardines
Shad
Smelt
Swordfish
Tilefish
Trout, rainbow
Tuna, fresh
Whitefish

Fish: Cooking Tips

- Fish can be baked, poached, steamed, broiled, stir-fried with a small amount of vegetable oil, or microwaved. These cooking methods allow you to retain the moistness of the fish without having to add much fat.

- Fish ceases to become a low-fat food when it is cooked with butter or topped with a high-fat cream sauce. Try adding flavor without fat by marinating the fish in lemon or lime juice or wine; using herbs and spices (bay leaf, curry powder, dry mustard, fennel, green pepper, marjoram, paprika and tarragon all enhance the flavor of fish); or making a cream sauce from low-fat or nonfat yogurt. Always marinate fish under refrigeration.

- For maximum flavor, it is important not to overcook fish. The best way to judge cooking time is to cook fresh or thawed fish ten minutes for every inch of thickness. Cook frozen fish twenty minutes for every inch of thickness. (These guidelines do not apply when microwaving fish.) Fish is cooked when it has just turned opaque and the flesh barely flakes when it is separated with a fork.

Fish is a low-fat, low-sodium food, unless it's the deep-fried kind from the supermarket's freezer. Fat supplies half the calories in most frozen deep-fried fish, and a single serving contains 350 to 900 milligrams of sodium. There are some healthier frozen fish products on the market with only about four grams of fat per serving. But read nutrition labels carefully.

luted waters. Fish (and shellfish) are among the most perishable of commodities—even when properly refrigerated they don't last as long as chicken or beef. Even fish from the purest water has to be handled carefully. Complicating matters is the fact that lakes, rivers, and oceans, here and all over the world are polluted with sewage, industrial waste, and heavy metals such as mercury and lead, as well as other contaminants. The U.S. government at many levels, does inspect fish (fresh and canned) and makes rules about where fish may be harvested, but funds are always short, and consumer groups have long complained that a lot more vigilance and money are needed.

Any fish may carry some bacteria and viruses—and fish from sewage-polluted waters may carry large doses of them. Many varieties of fish commonly contain the larvae of tapeworms and roundworms. Cooking will kill all such parasites and the microorganisms. Of course, if bacteria reach a certain level, the fish will be unfit for consumption no matter how long it is cooked. And cooking won't eliminate heavy metals or industrial pollutants that are probable carcinogens or may cause birth defects.

According to a recent report form the National Academy of Sciences, fish are more susceptible to chemical contamination than food animals raised on land because, for one thing, they feed not just on plants, but also on other animals, and they filter gallons of water through their bodies daily. The potential health effects of long-term consumption of these chemicals is not obvious and dramatic (as is, for example, food poisoning from eating contaminated food). It may be that the consumption of small amounts of chemicals raises the risk of cancer or of birth defects only slightly. As the Academy admitted, "the current state of knowledge on these subjects must be regarded as quite tentative." Nevertheless, the Academy concluded that fish (and shellfish)—if cooked—are safe and wholesome, and that Americans should be eating them.

Guide to safe fish

A few simple precautions can allow you to eat fish with less worry. The key to safety is variety—don't eat the same fish every day, week after week. This protects you against repeated doses of pollutants, if any are present. Keep in mind these other safety guidelines:

- Eat fish no more than three times a week. Three servings of fish is plenty to get the benefits of omega-3 fatty acids.

•Saltwater fish caught in the open ocean are less likely to be polluted than lake fish.

•Farm-raised fish may or may not have been raised in pure water; it depends on the locality. Check the source with your fish merchant.

•When you catch fish, be sure you are fishing in waters that are not polluted. When you buy your fishing license, you often will be given information on polluted waters in the area. If it is not provided, ask for this information or check with the local health department about it. And throw the big ones back. The younger and smaller the fish, the lower the level of toxic residues.

•Before cooking fish, trim off fatty areas—usually in the back and belly and in any dark meat just under the skin—since this is where toxic residues may accumulate. Discard the skin, too. You'll still get omega-3s from the fish flesh. When possible, broil fish, since this cooking method tends to reduce residues.

•Don't eat raw fish. Even when it is extremely fresh, raw fish—as used in sushi, sashimi, ceviche, and other dishes—may be a source of parasites as well as bacteria and viruses. Marinating the fish in lemon or lime juice won't kill all bacteria and parasites. It's true that a well-trained sushi chef may know how to purchase and handle fish so as to minimize the risk of illness and parasitic infection, but while sushi chefs ar licensed in Japan, there's no way to check their credentials in the United States.

•If you decide to take a chance on raw fish, the FDA recommend that the fish first be frozen to destroy parasites. The temperature must be −4° F, and the fish must stay frozen for at least three days. Keep in mind, though, that freezing doesn't kill bacteria, and so pregnant and nursing women, the very old, the very young, and anyone coping with a serious illness should take no chanced with raw fish.

Selecting fresh fish
To choose the best-quality fish:

•Buy fish from a reputable fish dealer. Not all stores sell seafood that is reliably fresh.

•In the market, fish should be refrigerated or stored on a thick layers of ice. Whole, dressed fish can be directly on the ice, but fish fillets and steaks should be placed on a metal tray or on plastic wrap so that they do not come into direct contact with the ice.

•Beware of stacked fillets on ice; the topmost layer may not be cold enough.

•Fresh fish smells mild, sweetish, and clean. Do not buy any fish that has a fishy, sour, or ammonia-like odor.

•Avoid fish filets that look bruised or brown.

•When buying whole fish, look for

NUTRITIONAL CONTENT OF
Cooked Fish

Fish (3½ oz)	Calories	Protein (g)	Fat (g)	Fat Calories	Cholesterol (mg)
Cod	105	23	1	9%	55
Haddock	112	24	1	8%	74
Halibut	140	27	3	19%	41
Herring	203	23	12	53%	77
Mackerel	262	24	18	62%	75
Mullet	150	25	5	30%	63
Ocean perch	121	24	2	15%	54
Perch	117	25	1	8%	115
Pike	113	25	1	8%	50
Pollock	113	24	1	8%	96
Rockfish	121	24	2	15%	44
Salmon, Coho	185	27	8	39%	49
Salmon, sockeye	216	27	11	46%	87
Sea bass	124	24	4	29%	53
Smelt	124	23	3	22%	90
Snapper	128	26	2	14%	47
Swordfish	155	25	5	29%	50
Trout, rainbow	151	26	4	24%	73
Tuna, fresh	184	30	6	29%	49

bright, clear, unsunken eyes; moist, shiny skin; and bright red or pink gills. The flesh should feel firm and spring back when you touch it. Fish fillets and steaks should be moist and firm.

• Be cautious about prewrapped fish in the supermarket. It may not be fresh. At least ask when it was packaged.

• Frozen fish—which can be as fresh as fresh fish if it was flash-frozen soon after being caught—should be solidly frozen when purchased. Avoid any frozen fish that has ice crystals or that is discolored.

• Beware of seafood salads or any cooked seafood product displayed right next to raw fish. Bacteria from raw fish can contaminate the cooked.

• Refrigerate fresh fish immediately and use it as soon as possible; fish can spoil within a day or two.

Shellfish

Shellfish is divided into two categories: mollusks and crustaceans. Mollusks are surrounded either wholly or partially by a hard shell. Common types include clams, oysters, scallops, and mussels. Crustaceans have segmented bodies and are covered with a thin shell. The most common type of crustaceans are lobster, shrimp, crab, and crayfish. Any of these shellfish is low in calories and is an excellent source of protein, iron, and the trace minerals zinc and copper. Most types also contribute a significant amount of B vitamins and iodine to the diet and are not particularly high in sodium.

Cholesterol and fat content
One of the popular misconceptions about shellfish is that it is high in cholesterol. This misunderstanding arose from traditional methods of food analysis that identified certain fats in

Discard the greenish tomalley, or liver, in lobsters or the "mustard" (hepatopancreas) in blue crabs. If the shellfish have lived in contaminated water, these body parts may have high concentrations of PCBs (polychlorinated biphenyls, a class of chemicals that are toxic) and cadmium (a toxic element).

shellfish that are similar to cholesterol as the true cholesterol. Newer analytical methods indicate that the cholesterol content of most shellfish is lower than that of canned tuna or broiled chicken breast. Though shrimp and crayfish have about twice as much cholesterol as meat, they contain much less fat than meat, and their fat is largely unsaturated and contains heart-healthy omega-3 fatty acids. Foods high in saturated fat are more responsible for raising blood cholesterol levels than foods high in dietary cholesterol. Shellfish are a low-fat food, unless, of course, they are breaded and fried or served in a butter sauce.

Shopping for and storing shellfish
The following tips will help you in selecting high-quality shellfish as well as give you guidelines for safe storage of shellfish:

• Buy shellfish only from licensed stores and markets.

• Be sure the seller is storing the shellfish properly. Shellfish should be kept cold: surrounded by ice but not in direct contact with it.

• Clams, oysters, and mussels that are still in their shells must be sold alive. Buy only those with tightly closed shells, or those that snap shut when they are touched. Lobsters and crabs are also often sold alive. Buy the ones that are lively and feel heavy for their size.

• When buying shucked clams, oysters, and mussels, choose those that are plump, free of broken shell, and in a clear liquid.

• Make sure that all frozen shellfish has been kept solidly frozen. Avoid those that have begun to thaw, or those that contain ice crystals or show any sign of discoloration.

• Refrigerate shellfish immediately after purchase.

A Shellfish Substitute

Surimi—you may never have heard of it, but if you like shellfish, you probably have eaten it. For centuries the Japanese have been making these "kneaded foods" from fish paste, which is flavored, textured, and then artfully shaped into over 2,000 products—from fish balls to fish sausage and hot dogs. Surimi is becoming a booming industry in this country, too, as substitutes for expensive crabmeat, shrimp, lobster, and scallops. In supermarkets it may be labeled "sea legs" or "imitation crab meat," but on restaurant menus there's often no indication that the shellfish dishes are actually made from surimi.

What is surimi?

Most American surimi is made from Alaskan pollack, a lean, white-fleshed fish. After the skin and bones are removed, the fish is ground up and then repeatedly washed and strained, which removes blood, pigment, the fishy odor, as well as some fat, niacin, and potassium. Sugar and/or sorbitol is added to this white, odorless, flavorless protein concentrate to decrease damage from freezing; this is followed by salt, starch, and sometimes MSG (monosodium glutamate), which are added to enhance the flavor and texture. The pulp is flavored either naturally (with real shellfish or liquid from boiled shells) or artificially. Finally, coloring may be added, and then the pulp is shaped like crab legs or lobster tails, for instance.

Telling the difference

Surimi can be a fraud if you get it when you have ordered and paid for real crab salad or lobster Newburg. The Food and Drug Administration (FDA) insists that surimi products be labeled "imitation" if they resemble any actual type of seafood and are nutritionally inferior to it. The ingredients must always be listed—for instance, "crab-flavored minced pollack." That doesn't stop manufacturers from burying this information in tiny print and picturing real lobster or crab on packages. However, even a magnifying glass won't help you in restaurants and at sushi bars and deli counters, where the surimi is removed from its package, added to various dishes, and often served as real shellfish.

The bottom line is that, unless you are on a sodium-restricted diet, surimi is a good way to add low-cholesterol fish protein to your diet.

Surimi: pluses and minuses

Advantages:
- Low cholesterol (up to 75 percent less than shellfish).
- Rich in high-quality protein.
- Readily available.
- Cooked, so it's not as perishable as fresh fish.
- Good ratings for taste and texture when used in salads, casseroles, soups, and with sauces.

Disadvantages:
- High sodium (up to ten times more than real shellfish).
- Has virtually no omega-3 fatty acids.
- About 25 percent more calories than comparable shellfish.
- Reduced niacin and potassium.
- Gelatin-like texture.
- Not good when eaten alone.

Nearly all shrimp (95 percent) sold in the United States has been frozen without significantly affecting its taste or nutritional content.

- Keep live shellfish alive until you are ready to cook them. Clams, mussels, and oysters should be stored in a well-ventilated area of your refrigerator, not in tightly closed plastic bags or containers. Lobsters and crabs also need ventilation and should be stored covered with damp paper towels. Discard any shellfish that has died during storage (the shell is open, and remains open even when tapped).

- Fresh, uncooked shellfish spoils quickly. Keep refrigerated and use it within a day or two of purchase.

Caution on raw shellfish

Cherrystone clams and raw oysters are a favorite with many people. And while most Americans are aware that eating raw shellfish from contaminated waters could make them sick, many have assumed that if they heeded periodic health prohibitions regarding the eating of raw clams and oysters, they

NUTRITIONAL CONTENT OF **Shellfish**				
(3½ oz cooked)	Calories	Fat (g)	Saturated fat (g)	Cholesterol (mg)
Clams	148	2	<1	67
Crab, blue	102	2	<1	100
Crab, king	97	2	<1	53
Crawfish	114	1	<1	178
Lobster, northern	98	1	<1	72
Mussels	172	5	1	56
Oysters, eastern	137	5	1	109
Scallops	112	1	<1	53
Shrimp	99	1	<1	195

could enjoy them worry free the rest of the time. Unfortunately, this is no longer the case.

Eating raw or undercooked shellfish is a high-risk venture for several reasons. Most shellfish are harvested from estuaries that may be contaminated by untreated sewage. Clams and oysters live by filtering fifteen to twenty gallons of water per day, so they become concentrated sources of bacteria (such as salmonella and campylobacter) and viruses (such as hepatitis A and the Norwalk virus) if they live in polluted waters. Eating raw shellfish may also carry the risk of poisoning by red plankton ("red tide"), which the shellfish consume in the late summer and early fall.

In addition the Food and Drug Administration (FDA) estimates that 5 to 10 percent of all raw shellfish are contaminated by disease-causing vibrio bacteria, a natural part of the marine environment that has nothing to do with pollution. Most people who eat vibrio-contaminated shellfish do not get sick—or only mildly. Normally, the bacteria are destroyed in the digestive tract or neutralized by the immune system. But people with certain chronic diseases (liver, kidney, or gastrointesti-

nal disease, as well as diabetes and alcoholism) or impaired immunity (from AIDS or cancer, for instance) face a high risk of serious vibrio-related illness. This ranges from gastroenteritis (symptoms include nausea, fever, abdominal cramps, and vomiting) to potentially fatal blood poisoning.

Inadequately cooked shellfish, too, can be a source of infection. Steamed clams, for example, are typically cooked just to the instant of opening, about one minute, so the clam never gets hot enough inside to inactivate any virus present. Mussels, clams, and oysters should be steamed for about five minutes, until they are heated through—to a temperature of 140°F.

Despite the risks, many people will be unable to give up eating raw shellfish. If you decide to take a chance on raw oysters or clams, you can reduce, but not eliminate, your risk by heeding the following tips. Buy shellfish only from reputable markets and ask the dealer to show you the tag certifying that the shellfish were harvested from state-approved waters. In restaurants, you can inquire about the origin of shellfish (though the waiter is hardly likely or able to tell you whether they're from polluted beds. Stick to the old rule about eating oysters only in months that contain the letter "r." In late spring and summer (May through August), the bacterial count is likely to be higher because the water is warmer. Also the shellfish are more likely to consume red plankton during these months. Don't be led into false security by reports that hot sauce or alcohol kill bacteria in shellfish; they don't. And as with raw fish, pregnant and nursing women, the very old, the very young, and anyone coping with a serious illness should not eat raw shellfish at all.

Canned Fish

To most Americans, "fish" means canned tuna—we eat nearly three pounds of it per person each year. But tuna isn't the only type of canned fish available; salmon and sardines also come conveniently packaged. And like fresh fish, canned fish has many nutri-

tional assets. It provides as much protein as meats and is rich in niacin, potassium, and, if bones are eaten, calcium. Canned salmon, sardines, and solid white albacore tuna are also good sources of omega-3 fatty acids.

Fresh from the sea, fish is low in calories. But when fish is canned, processors often add fat in the form of vegetable oil. This added oil usually doubles the calories in the fish and adds up to ten times more fat. Only 15 percent of the calories in water-pack tuna come from fat, compared to over 60 percent in oil-pack tuna. Another reason that water packed is preferred is that draining the oil can remove the valuable omega-3 fatty acids: one study found that while draining the water from water-pack tuna was found to remove only about 3 percent of the omega-3s, draining vegetable oil removed 15 to 25 percent because these fatty acids are oil-soluble. Still, if you prefer the taste of oil-pack tuna, you

---

NUTRITIONAL CONTENT OF
Canned Fish

Fish (3 oz)	Calories	Protein (g)	Fat (g)	Cholesterol (mg)	Calcium (mg)	Sodium (mg)	Comments
Tuna							
in oil	200-250	19-21	15-19	40-60	10	300-500	High in B vitamins, especially
oil drained	140-200	22-24	8-12	40-60	10	250-450	niacin. Solid white tuna is slightly
in water	90-110	21	1	40-60	10	300-500	lower in fat and calories than chunk
low salt	90-110	21	1	40-60	10	200	white or chunk light.
no salt added	90-110	21	1	40-60	10	40	
Salmon (with bones)							
pink (humpback)	120	17	5	35	150-200	350-450	The redder the fish, the fattier and
red (sockeye)	160	17	8	35	150-200	350-450	moister. Rich in vitamin B_{12}, lots of
							added sodium. Lower in calcium if
							bones are not eaten.
Sardines (with skin and bones)							
in oil	250-350	16	20-30	85-100	250-350	400-600	Higher in cholesterol and fat than
oil drained	175-250	20	9-18	85-100	300-400	400-600	tuna or salmon. Rich in iron and
in water	200	16	16	85-100	250-350	400-600	vitamin D. Skinless and boneless
no salt added	200	16	16	85-100	250-350	100	sardines have no calcium and
in tomato sauce	200	15	15	75-90	250-350	700	reduced nutrients.

should be sure to drain the oil; this eliminates about a third of the total calories and half the fat.

Salt is more of a problem: processors usually add four to ten times the amount of sodium naturally in saltwater fish. Fortunately, "low-salt" and "no salt added" varieties are available. "Low-salt" tuna, for example, usually has about 50 percent less added sodium, leaving about 200 milligrams in three ounces. Tuna marked "no salt added" contains 90 percent less sodium than regular cans, so it is good for people on sodium-restricted diets. To avoid paying a premium price for low- or no-salt tuna, rinse regular water-pack tuna, which removes most of the sodium.

FATS AND OILS

Vegetable Oils

A tablespoon of oil here and there may not seem like a big deal, but vegetable oils account in large part for a major shift in American eating habits in recent years. These oils are simply fat in liquid form. While we have cut back on animal fats, the amount of vegetable oil we eat is rising—in our cooking oils, margarines, baked goods, fried foods, mayonnaise, and salad dressings—thus boosting our *total* fat consumption as a result. All vegetable oils contain 120 calories and 13.5 grams of fat per tablespoon.

Nutritionists agree that we should increase the ratio of unsaturated/ saturated fats in our diet to help lower blood cholesterol levels and thus reduce the risk of heart disease. High polyunsaturated vegetable oils—such as safflower, sunflower, and soybean—used to be considered the most healthful oils, but in recent years nutritionists

have focused on the possible negative effects of these oils. Polyunsaturated fats lower total cholesterol levels, but large amounts also lower HDL ("good") cholesterol. Highly monounsaturated oils, such as olive and canola, do not lower HDL as much as polyunsaturated oils.

No vegetable oil is 100 percent unsaturated. Corn, soybean, safflower, and other kinds of oil all contain some saturated fatty acids. In fact, coconut and palm kernel oil actually contain a higher percentage of saturated fatty acids than animal fats do.

Despite these substantial variations, many shoppers do not know which type of vegetable oil is in the cooking or salad oil they buy. According to a survey by the National Sunflower Association, price and brand loyalty were found to be key considerations, rather than the type of oil. Shoppers also reported that they were attracted to their brand because of its "low cholesterol" content. They were apparently unaware that no vegetable product contains cholesterol, which is found only in animal products.

Consumers are even less aware of the type of "invisible" oil in processed foods such as crackers, cakes, frozen dinners, snack foods—even nondairy creamers. These often contain highly saturated coconut or palm kernel oil.

The chart on page 217 lists the breakdown of fatty acids in various oils. The higher the ratio of unsaturated/saturated fatty acids, the more healthful the oil. This doesn't mean that you should merely add unsaturated oils to your diet. The trick is to cut down on *all* fats. But when you do eat fat, try to make it as unsaturated as possible.

Choosing and using oils
•There's no evidence that cold-pressed oils are purer or more healthful

Keeping canned fish low fat

The ways canned fish are traditionally prepared eliminate them as low-fat, low-calorie foods. Tuna, for instance, is fairly tasteless so people tend to add a lot of mayonnaise (90 percent fat) to their tuna salads and sandwiches. Here are some alternate fixings you can use with canned fish:

•Cut the mayonnaise in half and dilute it with lemon or lime juice.

•Add finely diced apples, celery, and carrots and leave out the dressing.

•Use low-fat yogurt and lemon juice as a dressing, with a little mustard if you like.

Vegetable Oils: A Fat Breakdown

Oils, least to most saturated	FATTY ACID CONTENT				Comments
	Poly-unsaturated (%)	Mono-unsaturated (%)	Saturated (%)	Unsaturated/ Saturated Fat Ratio	
Canola	32%	62%	6%	15.7:1	Best fatty acid ratio.
Safflower	75%	12%	9%	9.6:1	Highest in polyunsatu-rates.
Sunflower	66%	20%	10%	8.6:1	Sometimes used in place of olive oil, but blander.
Corn	59%	24%	13%	6.4:1	Heavy taste. Often used for deep frying.
Soybean	59%	23%	14%	5.9:1	Most commonly used oil—in baked goods, salad dressings, margarine, mayonnaise.
Olive	9%	72%	14%	5.8:1	Highest in monounsatu-rated fat. Expensive.
Peanut	32%	46%	17%	4.6:1	More pronounced flavor than safflower oil.
Sesame seed	40%	40%	18%	4.4:1	Used in Asian and Mid-dle Eastern cooking. Flavorful.
Cottonseed	52%	18%	26%	2.7:1	Higher in saturated fat. Used in processed foods and salad dressings.
Palm kernel	2%	10%	80%	0.2:1	Palm and coconut oils are the only vegetable oils high in saturated fat. Used in baked goods and candies.
Coconut	2%	6%	87%	0.1:1	

Note: These percentages do not add up to 100% because other fatlike substances make up the total composition.

than any other. "Cold-pressed" means that the oil has been pressed out of the seeds by a mechanical press prior to cooking, as is the case with most olive oil. In hot pressing, seeds are crushed and cooked, then pressed to extract more of the oil. In solvent extraction, the most efficient and common method, seeds or nuts are cooked and then the fat is extracted with a chemi-cal solvent, which is then removed; no residues remain in the oil. Claims that cold-pressed oils contain more vitamin E have not been supported by most studies. You may prefer olive oil or other cold-pressed oils for their strong flavor: solvent extraction results in a blander flavor—an advantage for those who prefer this.

•Read labels on store-bought foods and avoid those containing coconut or palm kernel oil, which have a long shelf life but are highly saturated. Also avoid foods with hydrogenated oils, since hydrogenation makes the fat more satu-rated and changes their structure in other subtle ways.

•Heat cooking oil before adding

food. The food will sit in the oil for a shorter time and absorb less of it.

• Stir-fry vegetables and meat (cut up in small pieces). Using this method, you can cook food faster and with very little oil.

• Use a spray-on vegetable oil, such as Pam, which can coat a pan with a mere quarter teaspoon of oil.

• Make your own salad dressing, using two parts canola or olive oil to one part vinegar or lemon juice. Add fresh or dried herbs or mustard.

Butter and Margarine

A bewildering array of margarine products and substitute butters—semisoft spreads, squeezable liquids, even powders—has expanded what used to be a small corner of the dairy section in the supermarket. Three out of four Americans today use margarine regularly, often because they think it is better for them than butter. However, recent reports have suggested that the hydrogenated oils in margarine—called trans fats—can raise total cholesterol levels and lower HDL ("good") cholesterol levels, this increasing the risk of heart disease (see page 109).

If you're trying to follow a "heart-healthy" diet, you should limit your use of butter and stick margarines, since most of their calories come from saturated fat. Butter also contains a fair amount of cholesterol. And both butter and stick margarine contain 100 calories and 11 grams of fat per tablespoon Of course, if your diet is sensibly low in fat and cholesterol, a daily pat of either won't hurt you. If you eat lots of margarine (and also many processed foods that contain hydrogenated oils) cut back. If you want to forgo both butter and margarine, try a little olive oil on bread, and put just jam or jelly on your morning toast. On vegetables, use herb mixtures or lemon juice instead of butter or margarine. When cooking or baking, use liquid vegetable oil whenever possible.

There are many butter substitutes on the market, and even "light" butters. Here are some of your options:

Margarines. Stick margarines contain hydrogenated oils; the more solid the margarine, the more hydrogenated oils it contains, and therefore the more trans fatty acids it has.

Vegetable-oil spreads. These contain less than the 80 percent fat by weight required in a margarine and are no better or worse than margarine.

Diet or reduced-calorie margarines. One way to cut fat is to use a "diet" margarine. Though all of its calories still come from fat, it is diluted with water, so it has half the fat and calories of regular margarine per tablespoon. "Squeeze" or liquid margarines are even better.

Butter-margarine blends. These are anywhere from 15 percent to 40 percent butter. Thus they contain some of butter's cholesterol and saturated fat.

Light butters. These are made from butter and water and have half the fat and cholesterol of regular butter. These products are fine for toast and vegetables, but can't be used in cooking.

Sprinkle-on powders. Made from carbohydrates, these powders are virtually fat- and cholesterol-free. They melt well on hot, moist foods like baked potatoes. But they won't do for spreading on toast, in recipes, or for sautéing.

Choosing a margarine or spread

How much saturated fat a margarine or spread contains depends both on which vegetable oil it contains and how it was made. When shopping for a margarine or spread, let the label be your guide:

• Most margarine products tell how much saturated and polyunsaturated

Ghee—clarified butter with a rich nutty flavor—is not a healthier substitute for butter. Used predominantly in Indian cuisine, ghee is made by simmering butter over low heat so that its water boils away and the tiny amount of milk solids coagulates (and is then strained away). This leaves a clear oil, which is pure fat. Because of the water loss, ghee is a more concentrated source of fat than butter: one tablespoon has about 13 grams of fat and 117 calories, versus 11 grams and 100 calories in butter.

fats they contain. Look for one with at least twice as much polyunsaturated as saturated fat. If a brand doesn't give you a breakdown of fats, be suspicious.

•Although all the oils commonly used in margarines are high in polyunsaturated fat and low in saturated fat, they vary substantially. Those lowest in saturated fat are safflower, sunflower, and corn oil, in that order.

•If a hydrogenated or partially hydrogenated oil is listed first, the product is likely to be more saturated. To make oil solid and prolong its shelf life, manufacturers add hydrogen molecules—a process called hydrogenation. It transforms good unsaturated vegetable oil into a more saturated kind.

•The softer or more fluid a margarine is, the less saturated it is likely to be. For this reason, *liquid or tub margarines are almost always better than stick margarines.* One sign of a high polyunsaturate content is a liquid oil as the first ingredient, rather than a partially hydrogenated oil.

•Watch the sodium content, which tends to be relatively high. Salted margarine is just as undesirable as salted butter. Unsalted varieties are available.

SNACKS AND DESSERTS

Snack Foods

Salty, crunchy foods are second only to sweets as America's favorite snacks. Popcorn, pretzels, and even potato chips can all be healthful foods, provided you choose them carefully (or, in some cases, make your own) and eat them in reasonable amounts. After all, they are little more than corn, wheat, or potatoes—low-fat sources of complex carbohydrates and fiber plus some protein, vitamins, and minerals.

Yet these staples can become problem foods when, during processing, they are fried in oil and coated with salt or sometimes sugar. In addition, chips and prepopped popcorn frequently contain highly saturated palm or coconut oil, or a hydrogenated oil (hydrogenation makes vegetable oils more saturated, thus giving them a longer shelf life). Most of these snacks are, however, cholesterol-free.

Healthful chips, popcorn, and pretzels

•If you are trying to cut calories, stick to plain, unbuttered popcorn. By substituting one cup of plain popcorn for a one-ounce bag of potato chips, you save 135 calories and ten grams of fat. You would have to eat two quarts of plain popcorn to get the calories in twenty potato chips.

•Make your own popcorn. Prepopped corn and packaged kernels meant to be popped in microwave ovens are expensive and usually coated with oil and salt. You can eliminate all oil by heating plain kernels in a hot-air popper or in a special microwave popper. Otherwise, brush the pan with a small amount of highly unsaturated oil (such as safflower, sunflower, or canola oil). Use only a sprinkling of salt, or substitute herbs or spices.

•If you like cheese popcorn, make your own by using grated parmesan cheese. Commercial cheese popcorns are very high in fat and calories.

•Buy unsalted pretzels—an excellent low-fat snack food.

•Make your own potato chips. See the recipe on this page.

•Don't buy a large bag of potato chips if you are likely to finish it in a sitting or two. Even a relatively small eight-ounce bag of chips has fifty to eighty grams of fat—as much as most people should eat in an entire day.

The lightweight chip

Here's a recipe that takes potato chips out of the junk-food category.

Ingredients:

One large baking potato (about ¾ pound)

Vegetable oil cooking spray (or, if you prefer, a teaspoon of bottled oil)

Paprika

Preheat the oven to 400°F. Scrub the potato well and slice it thinly. Lightly coat a large baking sheet with cooking spray (or oil the sheet with a small amount of oil on a paper towel). Arrange the slices in one layer, overlapping them slightly if necessary, then spray the slices lightly with cooking spray (or brush with remaining oil). Sprinkle with paprika. Bake thirty minutes, turning once, then reduce the heat to 300°F. Bake another fifteen to twenty minutes, or until the chips are crisp and brown.

Snack Foods

	Calories	Fat (g)	Sodium (mg)	Comments
Popcorn (1 cup)				Excellent snack food—low in calories, high in fiber and iron. Plain popcorn is nearly fat-free, but if you add oil and/or butter, about half the calories will come from fat. Limit the amount of salt you add.
plain, air-popped	30	trace	0	
popped in oil, with salt	40	2	100-300	
sugar-coated	140	1	0	
cheddar cheese	100	6	170-200	
Potato chips (15 chips)	150-170	10	130-300	One ounce of chips has most of the nutrients in a small potato (high fiber, potassium, niacin, vitamin E). However, about 60 percent of calories come from oil (fat), which is usually hydrogenated. BBQ and bacon-flavored chips are especially high in sodium.
unsalted	150-170	10	0	
"light"	130-140	6-7	100	
Pretzels (1 oz, 5 medium/2 large)	110	1	400-650	Good low-fat snack food, but usually highly salted. Made from wheat flour enriched with iron, niacin, thiamine, and riboflavin; whole wheat varieties are also available.
unsalted	110	1	30	
Tortilla and other corn chips (1 oz)	150-160	7-9	160-260	About 60 percent of calories come from fat. Taco-flavored chips are highest in sodium. Look for unsalted varieties.
Cheese puffs or twists (1 oz)	160	10	300-350	Made from corn meal, with a small amount of cheese. High in fat and sodium.

• Try the new low-fat and fat-free potato chips and tortilla chips on the market. These contain one to four grams of fat and 100 calories per ounce. There are also reduced-fat potato chips that have about a third less fat than regular potato chips.

• Avoid commercial dips, which are high in fat (from whole milk, cream cheese, coconut oil, and/or hydrogenated vegetable oil), calories, and sodium. They have, on average, three times more calories and ten times more fat than homemade dips using low-fat yogurt or low-fat cottage cheese.

Nuts

Though nuts do differ, they have a lot in common, too. Ounce for ounce, they are packed with protein and fat, though the fat is largely unsaturated. Nuts, of course, contain no cholesterol, which is found only in animal products. They are a significant source of vitamin E and fiber. They also contain calcium, zinc, magnesium, potassium, iron, and B vitamins.

But, alas, nuts are high in fat and calories: most have over 160 calories per ounce, and who stops at an ounce? Weight-conscious people usually try to avoid nuts: a handful of roasted peanuts can pack as many calories as a piece of cake.

Some possible, but unproven, benefits of nuts made headlines recently. One study suggested eating nuts regularly might reduce the risk of heart attack. Of 26,274 Seventh Day Adventists in the study, those who ate nuts (mostly peanuts and almonds) more than four times a week had half as many heart attacks as those who ate them less than once a week. Researchers

NUTRITIONAL CONTENT OF
Nuts

	Serving Size	Calories	Protein (g)	Fat (g)	Comments
Almonds, raw	1 oz	165	6	15	Best ratio of nutrients to calories; good source of calcium, riboflavin, vitamin E. Primarily monounsaturated fat. Often blanched to remove dark skin.
Brazil nuts, raw	1 oz	185	4	19	High in fat, calories, and calcium.
Cashews, dry roasted	1 oz	165	4	13	Usually roasted, but raw cashews are less greasy and have slightly less fat and calories.
Chestnuts, fresh, roasted	1 oz	69	1	trace	Always cooked (roasted or boiled) or dried. More carbohydrates and less protein, fat, and calories than other nuts.
Coconut, dried, sweetened, shredded	1/4 cup	118	1	8	Low in protein, high in sugar. Fresh coconut contains fewer calories. Fat is mostly saturated.
Hazelnuts (filberts), raw	1 oz	180	4	18	High in fat, though primarily unsaturated.Often ground and used in baked goods.
Macadamia nuts, roasted in oil	1 oz	205	2	22	High in fat and calories, low in protein.
Peanuts roasted	1 oz	180	7	15	Good nutritional value—highest in protein, high in calcium, niacin, and vitamin E. Primarily monounsaturated fat.
roasted	1 oz	170	7	14	
partially defatted	1 oz	145	10	10	
raw	1 oz	160	7	14	
Peanut butter	2 tbsp	190	10	16	Fat is primarily monounsaturated, but some commercial brands contain hydrogenated oils, which can increase the amount of saturated fat. Some brands also contain sugar.
Pecans, raw	1 oz	190	2	19	High in fat and calories and low in protein.
Pistachios, dry roasted	1 oz	165	6	14	Avoid those dyed with red artificial coloring. High in iron. Fat is primarily monounsaturated.
Walnuts, English, raw	1 oz	170	7	16	High in fat and calories. Fat is primarily polyunsaturated.

Chestnuts are a good source of vitamin C, supplying about half the RDA per 3/4 cup serving.

theorized that healthful monounsaturated fats in nuts were responsible. But most experts thought it was too early to recommend a handful of nuts along with a daily aspirin as a way to ward off heart attacks. Seventh Day Adventists are a special group when it comes to health habits: they don't smoke, and most follow a vegetarian or semivegetarian diet. Thus their risk of heart attack is much lower than in the general population. Since they eat little or no meat, they can afford to consume more vegetable fats. Nuts are certainly not the whole story in their lowered heart attack rate.

Nuts come in many varieties, and are processed in many different ways.

Raw nuts. Nuts come with or without shells—except cashews, which are always sold shelled. (The shells contain a caustic oil, related to urushiol, which produces the poison ivy rash.) Shelled raw nuts become rancid quickly if not refrigerated or vacuum-packed. If you shell your own nuts, you know that no fat or salt has been added. If you want to roast or toast them in the oven, this improves the flavor. You need not add fat.

Roasted nuts. This is a euphemism: roasted nuts are actually fried in oil, usually highly saturated coconut oil. This adds a few calories. Salt is usually also added—with a heavy hand. A cup of salted peanuts has 1,000 milligrams of sodium, about one-third the suggested daily intake.

Dry-roasted nuts. Dry-roasted nuts are not cooked in oil, but because nuts are so high in fat to begin with, dry-roasted are not significantly lower in fat than regular roasted (fried) nuts. They may be heavily salted and contain other ingredients such as sugar, honey, and preservatives.

Defatted or "lite" peanuts. These have been processed to remove some of their oils and they are somewhat lower in fat and calories. But these nuts may be hard to find.

How can you eat nuts without going overboard? Instead of using nuts as a snack, when you'll be tempted to eat large amounts, use them as part of a meal. Chopped nuts make tasty additions to fruit or vegetable salads, yogurt, home baked breads and muffins, pancakes, casseroles, and pilafs. Nuts are good with meats, too: try cashews or peanuts in chicken dishes, for example. And take advantage of chestnuts, which have fewer calories and less fat than other nuts. Puréed chestnuts can be served as a side dish instead of potatoes, or as an ingredient in stuffings. Sweetened and flavored with vanilla, they make a nutritious dessert. Nut butters (peanut butter, for example) have the same nutritional advantages and disadvantages of nuts. But used sparingly they can be healthy snacks or flavorings.

Caution on peanuts

Peanuts can be the source of another health hazard—aflatoxin, a common mold that grows on peanuts as well as on corn and other crops. If ingested in large amounts, it is known to be a factor in liver cancer. Although it is impossible to produce a peanut crop completely free of aflatoxin, this does not mean that peanuts and peanut butter on the market are likely to be unsafe. The Food and Drug Administration has set a maximum permissible level at twenty parts per billion, and the United States Department of Agriculture inspects peanut shipments for any sign of the mold and will ban any crop with detectable contamination. In addition, most American food processors have established rigorous programs to monitor the presence of aflatoxin, and most peanut products fall considerably below

All of the calories in cotton candy, hard candy, and jelly beans come from sugar.

Beware of "Healthy Snacks"

A lot of food companies try to take the guilt out of snacking by offering products that appear to have a healthy image. Below is a sample of a few snacks that sound promising, but often don't deliver. This doesn't mean you should rule out all of the following products—just don't be lulled into a false sense of security by a healthy-sounding name. Always read labels.

Bran muffins. Bakery or deli bran muffins will contain fiber if they contain bran. The question is how much. Most store-bought muffins have far more hydrogenated oils, sugar, and eggs than oat or wheat bran. Check the ingredients list: if bran is close to the bottom, you're being rooked. Look for whole-wheat flour as the main ingredient, not "wheat flour" (that is, refined white flour). If the muffin weighs heavily in your hand (some are 5 ounces or more) and has a sticky surface, it is likely to have as many calories and fat as any cupcake.

Carrot cakes. Carrots are healthful (rich in beta carotene and fiber), but carrot cakes are surprisingly rich in drawbacks. They are almost inevitably dense and moist, usually signs of a high-fat content. A typical cake may contain more than a cup of oil, which has nearly 2,000 calories by itself, or about 200 calories per slice—all fat calories—before adding the other ingredients. You'll find that nearly all store-bought carrot cakes also contain a variety of sugars, refined flour, eggs, and shortening, plus cream cheese and more sugar in the frosting. In the interest of health, you'll almost always be better off with apple pie, even though it may be loaded with sugar.

Banana cakes and breads. Most commercial banana cakes offer few, if any, advantages over chocolate cake. For instance, the list of ingredients in one widely sold banana cake begins with sugar, continues with partially hydrogenated vegetable shortening (partly saturated, in effect), and then flour. Only then comes the alibi for it all, bananas. Like carrot cakes, banana cakes usually get 40 to 50 percent of their calories from fat. Store-bought banana breads may be as full of fat as cakes. Look for flour first among the ingredients and shortening toward the bottom. You'll be better off, however, making your own banana bread, which requires less fat and sugar.

Granola bars. When granola bars first arrived on the market, they were a mixture of rolled oats, dried fruit, nuts, seeds, honey, some sugar, and a variety of oils but they contained both protein and carbohydrates in sufficient quantity to be better for you than most candy bars. Over the years, the ingredients of granola bars have changed so that now many granola bars commonly contain candy ingredients such as caramel, chocolate, and marshmallow afloat in increasing amounts of saturated oils and sweeteners. As a result, granola bars are practically nothing more than fat and sugar. The small amount of oats and nuts remaining give them a nutritional edge over candy bars, but it is slight.

Blue corn chips. These are high in fat and have no nutritional advantage over regular corn chips. Blue corn turns pale gray, brown, or lavender when processed. There are thousands of varieties of corn, some of which are not yellow or white, and they may vary slightly in nutritional content. For instance, some blue corn may be somewhat higher in protein than some yellow corn. But the fat content of tortilla chips comes overwhelmingly from the vegetable oil they're fried in, not the small amount of fat naturally in the corn (about one gram per ounce). One ounce of corn chips typically contains six to nine grams of fat—supplying 50 percent or more of their 130 to 150 calories. Chips labeled "organic" are no lower in fat and no more healthful than other chips. Read the nutrition data on the label; if none is listed, assume that the fat content is at the high end of the range.

---

the allowable twenty parts per billion; in practice most are voluntarily keeping the level of aflatoxin down to less than two parts per billion.

Thus, commercial peanut butter and commercially packaged, roasted and dry-roasted peanuts are likely to be safe. Another protective factor: added salt helps protect against mold. However, you should take the following precautions when buying and using peanuts and freshly ground peanut butter:

- Keep an eye on the peanuts you buy in the shell. Discard any peanuts that are discolored, shriveled, or moldy-looking.

- Peanut butter that is ground for you in a store may not be as safe as commercial brands. Peanuts that sit around after they have passed inspection have a chance of picking up mold. Also, freshly ground peanut butter won't contain any added salt, so it needs refrigeration.

- If peanut butter from any source becomes moldy, don't just skim off the mold, as you might cut the mold off cheese to salvage the good part. Throw the whole jar out.

Try this cracker fat test: if a cracker makes your fingers feel greasy, or leaves a greasy mark when rubbed on a paper napkin, it's too fatty.

Crackers

Ounce for ounce, some popular crackers contain as much fat and sodium as the cheese you put on them. About 60 percent of the calories in some crackers come from fat, for instance. Others have virtually no fat or sodium and instead pack healthy amounts of fiber.

How can you navigate between these two extremes? It's not easy. The serving sizes listed on nutrition labels can vary greatly, making it difficult to compare crackers. The large flatbreads usually count one cracker as a serving size, and the smaller crackers allow up to eight crackers or about half an ounce. Make allowances for what you really eat. Most cracker snackers don't stop with just one.

Another problem is that crackers claiming to be whole wheat actually may not be. Bread can't be labeled "whole wheat" unless it is made from 100 percent whole-wheat flour, but crackers are not required to abide by this ruling. So the whole-wheat—or rye, rice, or multi-grain—cracker you think you're buying may not contain much besides refined white flour. And terms like "stoned wheat" don't mean whole wheat. Stoned wheat is just "stone-ground" white flour. The only way to tell is to read the ingredients list. "Whole wheat" should be the first and only flour listed.

What about fat? Many crackers have as high a fat content as cookies. Check the label; crackers that get more than 30 percent of their calories from fat are too fatty. Many cracker boxes these days bear a "no cholesterol" banner—but few crackers, unless made with butter, ever contained any cholesterol in the first place. However, many crackers do contain partially hydrogenated fats, which may raise blood cholesterol levels almost as much as saturated fats.

As for sodium, a single serving of crackers hardly ever contains more than 200 milligrams of sodium, which isn't a lot unless you're on a very restricted diet. But if you eat them with a salty dip or cheese, or if you eat half a box, the sodium can really add up.

Crackers, even at their best, are hardly a "health food," but they can offer one great nutritional plus, and that's fiber. When selecting a brand, try to pick one with whole grains (check the ingredients), or one with a nutritional label that lists fiber content. Look for at least two grams of fiber per half-ounce serving. The flatbreads are often high in fiber. Try the fat-free crackers. Some may be quite tasty, but if you can't quite learn to love them, at least try to find a brand with no more than two grams of fat per half-ounce serving.

While there's a plethora of new names and notions on the cracker shelf at the supermarket, don't forget old favorites like melba toast, Ry-Krisp, matzo, and rice cakes. A low-fat or nonfat cracker that's also high in fiber can indeed be a healthful snack.

Cookies

While it's true that no one has yet invented a cookie that is good for you, some cookie manufacturers are taking steps in the right direction. Cookies aren't much more than flour, sugar, and fat, but usually the overwhelming emphasis is on fat. While in the average cookie, about 40 percent of the calories come from fat, in some brands 60 percent are fat calories. But some manufacturers are making low-fat and fat-free cookies and others have rewritten their recipes to exclude palm and coconut oils—two highly saturated fats. The trick is to find a type of cookie with a less-than-average fat content (primarily unsaturated)—plus, if possible, reduced sugar and moderate-to-high fiber. When reading labels, keep an eye on the listed serving size, which may include anything from one to three cookies.

Here's what to look for in a cookie:

Fat. Vegetable oil, butter, and lard are the main fats in cookies. Butter and animal fats are the least desirable because they are highly saturated and contain cholesterol. Palm oil is as saturated as animal fats, and coconut oil even more saturated, but, like all vegetable products, they are both cholesterol-free. Hydrogenated or partially hydrogenated vegetable oils may also be very saturated. Your best bets are brands that contain plain, unhydrogenated vegetable oil, such as soybean or corn. However, such oils aren't any lower in calories than other fats, just less saturated.

Remember, in addition, that chocolate is packed with lots of fat, which is mostly saturated. All nuts and peanut butter are also concentrated sources of fat, though the fat they contain is mostly unsaturated.

NUTRITIONAL CONTENT OF
Crackers

Crispbreads and matzo-type crackers are lowest in both calories and fats, but even a matzo-like cracker will hit the fat jackpot if spread with Camembert or topped with cheddar. The crackers below are listed in order of fat content—from lowest to highest.

	Crackers per Ounce	Calories	Fat (g)	Sodium (mg)
Rice Cakes	3	105	trace	105
Crispbread, rye, lite	3	120	trace	80
Matzo	1	110	trace	3
Crispbread, no salt	5	70	trace	3
Crispbread, fiber, with sesame	5	100	trace	335
Crispbread, rye	5	100	trace	325
Ry Krisp, original	4	80	trace	224
Melba Toast, wheat, unsalted	10	112	trace	7
Crispbread	3	140	1	125
Zwieback	4	125	2	72
Stoned Wheat Thins	4	130	2	110
Ry Krisp, sesame	4	120	3	296
Saltines	10	130	3	400
Graham	4	120	3	230
Crispbread, fiber plus	3	105	3	138
Table water crackers	9	112	5	68
Triscuits	7	125	5	180
Waverly Wafers	8	145	6	384
Round, snack type	9	160	9	291
Goldfish, original	60	150	10	250

If you want to skip the fat but satisfy your urge for a sweet morsel, you'll find plenty of low-fat or even nonfat cookies on your supermarket shelf. Most rely on nonfat milk, a little fruit, and plenty of sugar. The fat-free tend to taste aggressively sweet; some of the low-fat variety have a better flavor and texture. And three types of classic cookies have always been low in fat—ginger snaps, graham crackers, and fruit bars.

Sugar. Whether it goes by the name brown sugar, molasses, fructose, corn syrup, dextrose, syrup, or sugar, it's sugar. And its calories are deficient in nutrients. Many brands of cookies include several sugars scattered throughout their ingredients lists; when these are added together sugar may constitute the cookies' main ingredient. Some cookies labeled "natural" are sweetened with dried fruits (which are a source of fiber) or fruit juice, which may contribute a few nutrients, but neither of these are lower in calories than refined sugar. And many of these "natural" cookies are loaded with fat.

The bottom line

Cookies fall into the same category as whipped cream for some people: they would rather eat just a little of the "real" thing once in a while than settle for ersatz frequently. If you enjoy cookies as an occasional treat, you needn't be too concerned about their nutritional benefits or shortcomings. But if you can't open a bag without eating at least six of them—which means consuming as much as thirty grams of fat and 480 calories or more in many popular brands—you might think twice about your choice of sweets: four ounces (two scoops) of premium ice cream have about eighteen grams of fat and 265 calories—and regular ice cream, ice milk, and frozen yogurt far less. You could even have a serving of graham crackers with your ice cream and consume fewer calories and less fat than you would on a cookie binge. And even low-fat and fat-free cookies add up to lots of calories if you consume the whole bag.

NUTRITIONAL CONTENT OF
Frozen Desserts*

	Calories	Fat (g)	Fat Calories
Ice cream, 1/2 cup			
standard	135	7	47%
premium	175	12	62%
Ice milk, 1/2 cup	92	3	29%
Frozen yogurt, 1/2 cup	125	3	22%
Frozen tofu, 1/2 cup			
light	90	trace	0%
regular	230	14	55%
Sherbet, 1/2 cup	135	2	13%
Sorbet, 1/2 cup	100	0	0%
Polydextrose product, 1/2 cup	50	0	0%
Fruit and juice bar	70	0	0%

All values on this chart may vary widely from brand to brand depending on the amount of sugar, milk solids (including fat), and air in the products.

Frozen Desserts

Open the door of the ice cream section of your supermarket and you may get a glimpse of the future: foods made with fat replacers. There are now dozens of new ice-cream clones with the taste and texture of "real" ice cream, but with less than half the calories and little or no fat. These new low-fat desserts are really an improvement—they're basically sweetened skim milk. We're not talking about watery, old-fashioned ice milk. These frozen desserts use new ingredients and technologies to approximate (some fairly successfully, others not) the creamy texture of ice cream.

Here are some guidelines to the new frozen desserts:

• Most are made of skim milk instead of whole milk and cream. They are generally called something like "gourmet ice milk" or "frozen dairy dessert." (To be "ice cream," according to the law, a product must contain at least 10 percent milk fat by weight.) Some list water as the first ingredient.

•In an attempt to match the texture of ice cream, the new frozen desserts use an array of ingredients, from Simplesse (a fat substitute made from proteins of egg whites and milk) and maltodextrin (a starch-based product) to polydextrose (a derivative of cornstarch) and a variety of natural gums (such as guar and cellulose).

•Frozen desserts made from skim milk and/or nonfat milk solids may actually contain more calcium than ice creams, since the lack of fat leaves more room for other nutrients.

•Some frozen desserts are made from tofu and are dairy-free: they thus contain no lactose (milk sugar, which some people have trouble digesting) or cholesterol. Still, some of the tofu products are high in fat, though the fat is largely unsaturated.

•Frozen yogurt may or may not be low-fat, depending on whether it's made from whole milk and cream or skim milk. Lactose intolerants may find that frozen yogurt, like regular yogurt, causes fewer symptoms than ice cream—provided that it contains a sufficient amount of active cultures.

•Within a product line, different flavors can vary by a few grams of fat per serving, especially if nuts or chocolate chips are added. A chocolate coating also adds a fair amount of fat.

•Some frozen desserts are fruit based. Sherbets usually contain some dairy products as well as fruit, while sorbets, fruit ices, and fruit-juice bars usually do not contain dairy products. Most are fat- and cholesterol-free.

•Most frozen desserts contain little cholesterol or, if they're nondairy, none at all. Ice cream contains the most: about 30 milligrams per half cup—as much as in a glass of whole milk. Dense premium brands have about 50 milligrams of cholesterol per half cup.

•Look for a product with four grams of fat or less per four-ounce serving. For comparison, standard ice cream has about eight grams of fat per four-ounce serving, premium brands about seventeen grams.

•Check the serving size used to determine the nutritional content. Some sneaky manufacturers have reduced the standard serving from four to three ounces. In some cases, a product may be "lighter" than another (even if both are made by the same company) only because its serving size is 25 percent smaller. Of course, even a four-ounce serving is unrealistic—who eats just one scoop?

CONVENIENCE FOODS

Frozen Dinners

Most of us succumb now and again to the convenience of frozen dinners. Fortunately, there's been a shift in style in the supermarket freezer department from old standbys like Salisbury steak with french fries to frozen entrées aimed at health-conscious, weight-conscious shoppers.

Not all entrées labeled "lean" or "lite" are better than conventional TV dinners. Most have fewer calories (250 to 400 calories per serving) than the conventional frozen dishes (400 to 700 calories) but often less food. And they can still be loaded with fat, salt, sugar, flavor enhancers, and starchy fillers. Few packages list fiber, cholesterol, and the breakdown of saturated/ polyunsaturated fat, and many don't list vitamin and mineral content. Skip brands that don't have any nutritional labeling beyond the ingredients, or write to the company for nutritional information.

Here's what to look for in a healthful frozen dinner or entree:

Milk chocolate is lower in fat than semisweet chocolate: 30 percent of its calories are from fat compared to 45 percent in semisweet.

Less than 850 milligrams of sodium. That's about a third of the recommended daily maximum for most people. If you're on a sodium-restricted diet, even that amount will be too much. Like so many processed foods, most frozen meals—even those low in fat and calories—are sabotaged by an unacceptable amount of sodium (sometimes containing over 2,000 milligrams per serving) in an attempt to hype the flavor.

Less than ten grams of fat. In a 300-calorie serving, that means fat contributes less than 30 percent of the calories. (Since each gram of fat has 9 calories, to compute the percentage of calories that comes from fat, multiply the number of grams of fat by nine and divide this figure by the total number of calories.) Look for primarily unsaturated fat. Fish and poultry are usually low in fat, unless they are deep-fried: fat supplies half the calories in most deep-fried frozen fish. Similarly, pasta entrées are basically low-fat, provided you keep away from the cream and butter sauces. Even vegetarian dishes can be overwhelmed by oil and high-fat ingredients.

Little or no added sugar. Sugar in its variety of forms (sucrose, dextrose, high fructose, corn syrup, honey, molasses, etc.) shouldn't rank high in the ingredients list (ingredients are listed by weight). Any of these sugars adds unnecessary—and unwanted—calories to your chicken, pasta, vegetables, or other frozen dishes.

Little or no cholesterol. Since few brands list cholesterol, just remember that three ounces of red meat or chicken have about 25 percent of the recommended daily maximum. Fish has less, and vegetarian dishes, including tofu, contain no cholesterol.

Few additives. Some brands don't use any additives. Check the ingredients list—the word "natural" doesn't tell you anything.

Even the best of these frozen dishes don't make completely balanced meals. Most are low in such vital nutrients as calcium, vitamins A and C, and fiber. So supplement them with a salad or vegetable side dish, whole-grain bread, low-fat dairy products, and fruit for dessert. These will also make the meal more filling. A small green salad, a slice of bread, a glass of skim milk, and a pear will add only about 300 calories to your low-calorie meal.

Of course, you can make your own frozen entrées for those days when you can't face cooking from scratch. Not only will they usually be less expensive but you will have full control over what goes into them.

Soups

We think of soup as comforting, nourishing, and sometimes downright medicinal. Canned or packaged varieties are easy to prepare, and dieters often resort to a cupful to stave off hunger. But even at their best, commercially available soups are seldom meals by themselves. Many are about 90 percent water, which helps account for their relatively low calorie count. Considering the average size of a serving, and then figuring only 10 percent of that as potentially nutritious, the outlook can be pretty dismal. A single serving usually provides less than 10 percent of the daily RDA of vitamins, protein, and minerals.

The exceptions to this 90-percent-water rule are those nutritious soups made with beans, lentils, or peas (all excellent sources of fiber and protein), and chunky vegetable soups made with carrots, whole tomato pieces, and cauliflower, for instance.

Sodium. This is one nutrient that soups don't lack. Except for specially marked low-sodium varieties, almost all packaged soups contain 600 to more than 1,000 milligrams of sodium per eight-ounce serving. If you finish the whole serving, as many people do, and eat it with other high-sodium foods, you can consume the recommended daily maximum of sodium (2,000 to 3,000 milligrams) in one meal.

Fat. Most vegetable or noodle soups are low in fat. Creamy varieties, however, are generally rich (as much as 60 percent of their calories come from fat), as are the condensed types made with whole milk rather than water. Thus, milk-based New England clam chowders tend to be much higher in fat than tomato-based Manhattan chowders. When reading the labels, look out for palm, palm kernel, and coconut oils, chicken or beef fat, and butter—all highly saturated.

One way to defat soup is to chill it in its can so that the fat congeals on top; then remove this layer. If you are preparing a milk-based soup, use low-fat or skim milk instead of whole milk. To add spice without adding extra salt, experiment with cayenne pepper, cloves, dill, basil, oregano, or garlic.

Many vegetable or bean soups contain meat stock, so if you're a vegetarian, read ingredients lists carefully.

Condiments

Sandwich ingredients—beef, ham, cheese, and bread—have all come under nutritional scrutiny. But what about mayonnaise, mustard, ketchup, and other condiments? The two danger points here are sodium and, in one important case, fat. You can buy low-sodium mustard and Worcestershire sauce and "lite" versions of mayonnaise and even ketchup. Less familiar condiments such as chutney and horseradish, are flavorful alternatives with few nutritional drawbacks, except that a few brands may contain large amounts of salt.

Mayonnaise. "Hold the mayo" is definitely the way to go: the only high-fat condiment, mayonnaise is an emulsion of oil, egg yolk, and vinegar; the regular version is almost 100 percent fat. However, since it is made with liquid vegetable oil (usually soybean), mayo is not particularly high in saturated fat. Despite its egg content, it contains only a small amount of cholesterol—about five milligrams per tablespoon. Thus a mayonnaise that is "cholesterol-free" is not an improvement.

Homemade mayonnaise is not nutritionally superior to store-bought. A standard recipe calls for two egg yolks and one cup of oil. And since it is made with raw eggs and without preservatives, homemade mayonnaise may be a source of food poisoning due to salmonella.

"Light" or "reduced-calorie" mayonnaise has 40 to 50 calories and four to five grams of fat per tablespoon. "Fat-free" mayonnaise has 12 to 20 calories and less than half a gram of fat. According to federal standards, mayonnaise must contain at least 65 percent oil by weight; thus products containing less are usually called salad dressing or imitation mayonnaise. The fat-free varieties are made primarily of thickeners, such as cellulose, maltodextrin, gums, and starch, all of which are safe; some list water as the first ingredient. They contain no oil and usually use egg white instead of yolk. Fat-free mayo may not taste as rich as regular mayo, but usually has a similar texture. Fat-free brands often contain extra sodium (100 to 210 milligrams per tablespoon) probably to make up for lost flavor.

The worst sodium offender among condiments is soy sauce, which may contain more than 1,000 milligrams of sodium per tablespoon. Although "light" versions have 30 to 40 percent less sodium, one tablespoon can still contain approximately 600 milligrams of sodium.

If your palate demands real mayonnaise, use a teaspoonful rather than a tablespoonful on a sandwich, or blend the mayo with plain low-fat yogurt. Flavor yogurt with a little mustard, lemon juice, and pepper to add to the mayonnaise in chicken or tuna salad. Tartar sauce and the "secret sauce" used on fast-food hamburgers are both mayonnaise-based: substitute a light mayo or plain low-fat yogurt with a little chopped pickle mixed in. And although it's not usually suggested as a low-fat substitute, even sour cream is a better choice than mayonnaise when you're making a dip: a tablespoon of sour cream has only about 25 calories and 2.5 grams of fat—just one-quarter the calories and fat in mayonnaise. Even better, use plain low-fat yogurt.

Ketchup. Although it consists mainly of tomatoes, the average ketchup is 20 percent sweetener and contains up to 180 milligrams of sodium per tablespoon. Even the national-brand "lite" ketchup has a fairly high sodium level, although a dietetic brand labeled "low-sodium" contains practically no sodium at all. Other substitutes for the ketchup lover with a sodium problem include tomato paste or purée, or low-sodium or homemade spaghetti sauce (for use in recipes). Worcestershire, steak sauce, and pickle relish, most chili sauces, barbecue sauces, and cocktail sauces have even *more* sodium than ketchup.

Salsa. A combination of chopped tomatoes, hot peppers, onions, lemon or lime juice, and herbs and spices, such as garlic and cilantro, salsa is fast becoming a popular condiment in this country. It's most commonly served with tortilla chips, but salsa makes a good low-fat topping for baked potatoes or burgers, a zesty sandwich spread, or even a good salad dressing.

All types of salsa are fat-free, but bottled salsa may be high in sodium. Check nutritional labels.

Mustard. The natural pungency of mustard somewhat limits the amount you use, but even a tablespoonful can pack a major sodium wallop. If you need to watch your sodium intake, buy a no-salt-added mustard; dilute the mustard with some plain low-fat yogurt; or mix your own from dry mustard powder (you'll find basic directions on the package). Vary the strength, texture, and flavor by using water, vinegar, or milk as the liquid.

Chutney. Usually served with Indian food (but equally good with cheese, plain meats, and poultry), sweet-and-spicy chutneys are fruit- or vegetable-based relishes. All contain negligible fat; however, some are very high in sodium. Look for chutneys made from apples, tomatoes, cranberries, and other fruits at health food stores or specialty markets. If you can't find a salt-free chutney, choose one that has salt at the bottom—not the top—of the ingredients list. Or substitute apple, cranberry, or other fruit sauces, which are low in sodium and are virtually fat-free.

Horseradish. Though its pungency complements meat, poultry, and vegetables, prepared horseradish is not often used as a condiment. And while it is usually made with salt, its sodium content is fairly low. Combine it with low-sodium mustard for an eye-opening sandwich spread, blend it with plain low-fat yogurt to make a less biting sauce, or stir it into applesauce for a traditional Austrian accompaniment to beef. Powdered horseradish can be mixed with water or other condiments to make a tasty sauce.

Tartar sauce has three-quarters of the calories in mayonnaise, plus two to three times the sodium.

EXERCISE

The benefits of exercise have become increasingly clear: it can improve your cardiovascular fitness and muscular endurance, which translates into an increase in energy; it can dramatically reduce the risk of coronary artery disease; it may also help lower blood pressure and cholesterol levels, and aid in weight control; and it appears to give self-esteem a measurable boost, and in general to improve your sense of well-being. You can derive these benefits at any age, and, indeed, exercise—or at least staying physically active—appears to be increasingly important the older we get. Many of the problems commonly associated with aging—increased body fat, decreased muscular strength and flexibility, loss of bone mass, lower metabolism, and slower reaction times—are often signs of inactivity that can be minimized or even prevented by exercise.

Moreover, a growing number of physicians, physiologists, and other researchers affirm that more moderate forms of exercise are sufficient to improve fitness and health. Acknowledging this recent emphasis on "taking it easy," the following chapters explain the basic components of fitness, present guidelines for exercising safely, and contain entries covering a complete range of exercise activities.

Part 3

The Elements of Fitness

Now that the fitness boom has been underway for a decade or more, what have we learned? Throughout the United States, millions of Americans have been taking advantage of health clubs, tennis courts, jogging tracks, swimming pools, home exercise equipment and all manner of road races and triathlons. Every day an estimated 50 million people are making choices about an activity, a program, or a piece of equipment in an effort to obtain benefits ranging from more vigor and alertness to a lowered risk of heart disease and premature mortality. Yet for all the surge in enthusiasm over exercise, probably just as many people have fallen by the wayside. Part of the reason is that plenty of them pushed too hard and too fast. In the 1980s, high-impact aerobic classes and high-mileage training dominated the fitness landscape, and at times it seemed as if you had to be in almost perfect shape even to begin an exercise program. But as exercise programs have proliferated, research on them has gained in sophistication, and studies conducted over the past ten years are redefining the standards of what makes physical activity beneficial.

Four components

Running, cycling, and other aerobic activities have been given the most emphasis during the past decade because they enhance cardiorespiratory endurance—the aspect of fitness that provides the most impressive health benefits. Aerobic exercise, which is covered in detail starting on page 248, will continue to be the cornerstone of fitness programs. Yet many people in long-term aerobic programs may lose muscle mass and flexibility, particularly in their upper bodies.

Also, keep in mind that exercising to build fitness is not the same thing as working out to improve athletic performance. For example, Olympic weight lifters have extraordinary muscular strength—they can heft tremendous weights, but they do it only in single efforts; football players typically have great muscular endurance but less cardiovascular endurance than runners or other long-distance athletes; yet while runners may build exceptional cardiorespiratory endurance, they commonly neglect their upper-body strength. To be truly fit, you should develop all of the elements of fitness, not just one or two.

Physical fitness, as experts in the field have long emphasized, actually has four components.

Cardiorespiratory endurance is reflected in the sustained ability of the heart and blood vessels to carry oxygen to your body's cells.

Muscular fitness consists of both strength and endurance. *Muscular strength* is the force a muscle produces in one effort—a lift, a jump, a heave—as when you swing a mallet to ring a carnival bell. *Muscular endurance* refers to the ability to perform *repeated* muscular contractions in quick succession, as in doing twenty push-ups or situps in a minute. Although muscular endurance requires strength, it is not a single all-out effort.

Flexibility refers to the ability of your joints to move freely and without discomfort through their full range of motion.

Body composition refers to how much of your weight is lean mass (muscle and bone) and how much is fat.

Each of these components can be measurably improved with appropriate types of exercise. Recently, there has been an increasing emphasis on exercising to enhance muscular fitness and flexibility. Consider this: while a decade ago a very small proportion of women worked out with weights, a recent Gallup survey found that 15 percent of women who exercise regularly include some kind of weight training. The new interest in strengthening muscles is also evident in the growing number of low-impact aerobics classes that utilize light weights.

Two keys: variety and moderation

No longer is fitness synonymous with exhaustive workouts, running marathons, or "going for the burn." Being active is the key to becoming and staying fit, and you can achieve this—enjoyably—by being active in a variety of pursuits. Jogging and aerobics classes, the premier exercise activities of the 1980s, continue to attract participants. But as the nation and its fitness habits mature, people have been shifting to all manner of activities, from fitness walking to ballroom dancing. Two classic low-impact activities, swimming and cycling, continue to gain in popularity. At the same time, others are choosing new types of sports and recreations, from mountain biking to in-line skating. Step-aerobics is one innovative form of exercise that has turned up at health clubs: it's like low-impact aerobic dance, except that participants step up and down on low platforms, often holding light weights. Exercisers are also cross training—combining different (usually complementary) types of exercise to create a more rounded, less boring program.

Moreover, the notion that exercise training should be painful or exhausting has lost its validity. Starting in the 1980s, researchers began to pay more attention to what they call "moderate exercise," and found that expending just 1,000 calories a week in moderate exercise and daily activities can provide fitness and health benefits. And as long as the calories are expended, almost any activity will do—even activities like bowling, golf, or active housework offer some health benefits for people who have been sedentary.

One additional reason for this move toward gentler exercise is the rising incidence of injuries associated with some popular activities, particularly aerobic dance and running. Moderate workouts not only reduce the risk of injuries, but, equally important, they are also accessible to people who are intimidated by—or who have given up on—highly strenuous regimens.

Moderate exercise doesn't mean that it's best to do as little as possible. The most significant health benefits that exercise can provide—lower blood pressure, greater cardiorespiratory improvements, a sense of well-being, more energy, among others—come only from sustained, regular workouts. But a long-term study conducted by the University of Minnesota showed that a moderate level of activity does have clear-cut advantages over a sedentary lifestyle. The subjects in the study were men at high risk for heart disease, and researchers found that those who engaged daily in such activities as gardening, dancing, home exercise and other so-called moderate exercise activities reduced the risk of a fatal heart attack by as much as one third over a seven-year period. In this study—a reevaluation of data from an earlier long-term study of almost 13,000 middle-aged men at risk for heart disease—benefits appeared to stabilize at about an hour's worth of physical

Strength training for everyone

To provide a "well-rounded program," the American College of Sports Medicine has altered its exercise guide-lines to include strength training along with aerobic exercise for healthy adults. But the emphasis isn't on lifting heavy weights to build hulking muscles. Rather, the College recommends resistance training of moderate intensity at least twice a week, in workouts that can take as little as 15 minutes per session. The "resistance" can be provided by bar-bells or weight machines. You can also use your own body weight as resistance, as in calisthenics such as push-ups or sit-ups. (See pages 284-285 for a sample routine.)

A New Exercise Prescription

Recently, federal health authorities and fitness experts published new relaxed guidelines about how much exercise people need to stay healthy. Every adult should accumulate at least thirty minutes of moderate physical activity over the course of most days. Previously they had recommended that Americans work out strenuously for at least twenty minutes three to five times a week in order to strengthen their heart and lungs. Did the experts throw in the towel when they lowered the official guidelines?

It had become clear that progress was not being made in getting Americans to follow the old recommendation. Only about 22 percent of us are active enough, and more than half are completely sedentary or barely active, according to federal surveys, and those statistics haven't changed for the past two decades. There is an "epidemic of physical inactivity," concluded the Centers for Disease Control and Prevention, the American College of Sports Medicine, and the President's Council on Physical Fitness and Sports. And, they said, inactivity has as detrimental an effect on the nation's health as smoking and high cholesterol levels. It increases the risk of coronary artery disease, non–insulin-dependent diabetes, osteoporosis, colon cancer, and other disorders.

Ironically, the old guidelines may have been counterproductive, since many people apparently were turned off by "regimented physical activity that required wearing funny clothes and sweating," in the words of one expert.

But there were other good reasons, besides practicality, to relax the guidelines. As science has learned more about exercise, fewer and fewer of the old hard-and-fast rules apply. Though strenuous exercise (such as jogging or cycling) provides the most benefits, more moderate exercise and even everyday physical activities (gardening, house cleaning, walking to work, or climbing a flight or two of stairs) can also keep you healthy, as we've reported previously.

And not only can you work out less strenuously, but you don't need to do all the exercise in a single, continuous session, as had been recommended. You can break up your activities, as long as they add up to at least thirty minutes on most days: walk part of the way to work, get off the elevator and walk the last two flights of stairs, use your coffee break for a ten-minute walk. If you are now sedentary, start by adding a few minutes of increased activity into your day and work up to thirty minutes. All you have to do are the normal things, like walking, but just do them a little longer and a little faster.

activity daily: that is, gardening for over an hour didn't result in better health.

Another potential benefit provided by less-than-strenuous exercise is for women over forty who are concerned about osteoporosis. Any type of weight-bearing exercise that places stress on the bones can help maintain or increase bone mass. Walking, dancing, or a modest weight-training program are often recommended.

If you're basically sedentary and feel you can't face a program of vigorous, sweaty exercise, then include at least thirty minutes of some enjoyable and/or useful activity in each day, as recommended in the box above. It's the first step toward a longer, healthier life.

It's never too late

More and more studies are showing that exercise may inhibit, arrest, or even reverse many of the declines associated with aging. According to a long-term study of thousands of Harvard graduates aged forty-five to eighty-four, men middle-aged and older who take up moderately vigorous activities such as tennis, swimming, jogging or brisk walking have up to a 41 percent reduction in coronary artery disease. In effect, the exercisers in the study could expect to live nine or ten months longer, on average, than those who remained sedentary. Men who were

How Fit Are You?

A twelve-minute running test, developed by Dr. Kenneth Cooper of the Aerobic Center in Dallas, Texas provides an easy and reliable way to evaluate your aerobic fitness. Thousands of men and women in the Air Force have used this test. While not as accurate as traditional treadmill tests, the running test is an excellent way for you to measure your fitness progress periodically.

If you are a man over forty years old, or a woman over fifty, and you have not been exercising regularly, don't take this or any other test requiring maximum physical exertion without first checking with your physician.

The test calls for running as far as you can in twelve minutes and then comparing the distance with the chart below. Run on an indoor or outdoor track—at a health club or high school, for instance—where you can compute the distance you've run. If a track isn't handy, run on any level terrain and later check your distance on a car odometer (although less precise, this will provide an adequate guide). If you can't run for the whole twelve minutes, walk part of the time. Stop if any unusual symptoms occur, such as chest discomfort or pain in the knees or ankles. Use this chart to evaluate your results.

Miles Covered in Twelve Minutes

Fitness Category	AGE (YEARS)				
	20-29	30-39	40-49	50-59	60+
Very Poor					
men	<1.22	<1.18	<1.14	<1.03	<0.87
women	<0.96	<0.94	<0.88	<0.84	<0.78
Poor					
men	1.22-1.31	1.18-1.30	1.14-1.24	1.03-1.16	0.87-1.02
women	0.96-1.11	0.95-1.05	0.88-0.98	0.84-0.93	0.78-0.86
Fair					
men	1.32-1.49	1.31-1.45	1.25-1.39	1.17-1.30	1.03-1.20
women	1.12-1.22	1.06-1.18	0.99-1.11	0.94-1.05	0.87-0.98
Good					
men	1.50-1.64	1.46-1.56	1.40-1.53	1.31-1.44	1.21-1.32
women	1.23-1.34	1.19-1.29	1.12-1.24	1.06-1.18	0.99-1.09
Excellent					
men	1.65-1.76	1.57-1.69	1.54-1.65	1.45-1.58	1.33-1.55
women	1.35-1.45	1.30-1.39	1.25-1.34	1.19-1.30	1.10-1.18
Superior					
men	>1.77	>1.70	>1.66	>1.59	>1.56
women	>1.46	>1.40	>1.35	>1.31	>1.19

Chart is from the The Aerobics Program for Total Well-Being *by Kenneth H. Cooper, M.D., M.P.H., Copyright © 1982 by Kenneth H. Cooper, M.D., M.P.H. Used by permission of Bantam Books, a division of Bantam Doubleday Dell Publishing Group, Inc.*

Don't be dismayed if your results are less than "good." Dr. Cooper estimates that 80 percent of all Americans fall in the "very poor," "poor," or "fair" categories. If running isn't your usual form of exercise, however, it's possible that you are in better shape than this test reflects. If you are a swimmer or cyclist, for instance, this test may not be as good a gauge of your level of fitness as it is for someone who walks or runs regularly. If your initial test results are not up to par, you can improve them by undertaking a regular aerobic conditioning program.

at highest risk and began to exercise probably gained more time, while others may have gained less.

Another study, published in the *Journal of the American Medical Association,* found that an eight-week weight-training program allowed frail eighty-six- to ninety-six-year-olds to build muscle mass and become more mobile and self-sufficient. And comparisons of the mental agility of younger people and healthy older people who exercise at about the same level show that the elders react about as fast as their juniors and significantly faster than their sedentary peers.

As this message sinks in, we're likely to see more people in their sixties, seventies, and eighties starting or continuing to exercise. Older people who start exercising have to take more time and work at a lower intensity to build cardiorespiratory function and muscle strength and endurance. But it doesn't matter if you never really exercised before—the benefits will still accrue.

Maintaining fitness

The beneficial effects of exercise are transitory, so when you stop, you start to lose the benefits in as little as two weeks—an effect called "detraining." Studies suggest that how quickly this occurs depends as much on how fit you are and whether or not you have been on a long-term exercise program as on how long you have been sedentary. It also depends in part on which type of exercise you were doing. Most research has focused on the effects of detraining on aerobic fitness. For instance, in a small study of well-trained athletes who discontinued their workouts for three months as part of the experiment, researchers at Washington University School of Medicine in St. Louis and the University of Texas at Austin found that physical fitness (as measured by endurance, changes in maximal heart rate, and other criteria) declined rapidly in the first twelve days, and then continued to decline, but not as quickly. However, even after three months of not exercising, these people were still measurably fitter than people who had never exercised. By contrast, in another study in which sedentary people undertook an eight-week cycling regimen and then stopped for eight weeks, the subjects lost all their aerobic gains and returned to their pretraining fitness levels.

Other studies show, however, that when people merely cut back on exercise, they are often able to avoid or postpone the effects of detraining for at least several months. If you get sidelined by an injury, illness, or some other circumstance that forces you to discontinue your exercise program, remember that although you may lose some ground, you won't sacrifice all your gains. Also, you can gradually build yourself up once again. The detraining effect depends on how fit you are to begin with and what type of exercise you usually do. If it's lack of time that's forcing you to cut back on exercise, don't give it up entirely—try shorter but more intense workouts twice a week. Any exercise you do will allow you to postpone the detraining effect and reduce the amount of time you need to retrain.

Even if you have been sedentary most of your life, it's not too late to start benefiting from exercise. "Sedentary men who become more active might reduce their risk of death by 24 percent"—that is one of the findings of a study of nearly 17,000 Harvard alumni directed by Dr. Ralph S. Paffenbarger, Jr.

A Workout Guide

People who have been relatively inactive often take up exercise enthusiastically—so much so that it's easy for them to be carried away by the joy of the moment and to forget, or skip, certain measures that can reduce risk of injury. And even veteran exercisers may neglect certain basic precautions that can help minimize aches and pains. The following eleven pages contain guidelines and tips that can protect you from injury and will make exercise itself more enjoyable.

Eight basic tips

1. Whatever activity you pursue, don't overdo it. Studies show that the most common cause of injury is exercising too aggressively—the "too much, too soon" syndrome. Even if you consider yourself in good shape, start any new exercise at a relatively low intensity and gradually increase your level of exertion over a number of weeks. In an exercise class, don't feel constrained to do any set number of repetitions or lift a predetermined amount of weight. You don't have to keep up with an instructor or other exercisers. If a class includes an exercise that is too difficult for you, substitute something easier.

2. "No pain, no gain" is a myth. Exercise should require some effort, but discomfort isn't necessary. If you are in an exercise class, beware of any instructor who says that exercise must hurt (or "burn") to do any good. Indeed, pain is a warning sign you are foolish to ignore. If you have continuing pain during an exercise, stop and don't do it again unless you can do so painlessly. (If the pain occurs in the chest or neck area, you should see a doctor immediately.)

General muscle soreness that comes after exercise is another matter: it usually indicates that you are not warming up sufficiently or that you are working too long or too hard. Sore muscles need not make you stop exercising, but they should make you slow down. (For more information on assessing exercise-related aches and pains, see page 409.)

3. Use adequate footwear. Wearing improper or worn-out shoes places added stress on your hips, knees, ankles, and feet—the sites of up to 90 percent of all sports injuries. Choose a shoe suitable for your activity (see page 242) and replace shoes before you wear them out—with frequent use, athletic shoes can lose one-third or more of their shock-absorbing ability in a matter of months.

4. Control your movements— if you can't, slow down. Rapid, jerky movement can set the stage for injury. Flailing your arms or legs can overstress joints. Instead, as you move your limbs, keep the muscles contracted and move them as if you are pushing against some resistance—for instance, squeezing a beach ball or pushing a weight.

5. Watch your form and posture. In most activities, stress can result from poor form, whether it's landing on the balls of your feet (instead of your heels) when running, or constantly cycling in the highest gears. Keep your back aligned (abdominal muscles contracted, buttocks tucked in, and knees aligned over feet). This is particularly important when jumping or reaching overhead.

6. Don't bounce while stretching. "Ballistic" stretching, in which you stretch to your limit and perform quick, pulsing movements, actually shortens muscles and increases the chance of muscle tears and soreness. Instead, do "static" stretches, which call for gradually stretching through a muscle's full range of movement until you feel resistance. This gradually loosens muscles without straining them.

7. Avoid high-impact aerobics. Surveys have found that most aerobics instructors and many students suffer injuries to their shins, calves, lower back, ankles, and knees because of the repetitive, jarring movements of some aerobics routines. Fortunately, there's a less stressful form called low-impact aerobics, which substitutes marching or gliding movements for the jolting, up-and-down motion of typical aerobics (see page 249). A well-designed low-impact aerobics routine can easily raise your heart rate enough to provide cardiovascular benefits. Working out more strenuously than that isn't necessary and may cause injury.

8. Warm up and cool down. Even the best exercise routine can become risky if you don't take the time to do this properly (see below).

The right way to warm up

If you think that stretching is the smart way to start your workout, you're wrong. Stretching cold muscles can injure them. Whether you're running, playing a sport, doing calisthenics, or lifting weights, it's essential to warm up first, then stretch. Warming up prepares you for exercise by gradually increasing your heart rate and blood flow, raising the temperature of muscles and connective tissue, and improving muscle function. It may also decrease the chance of a sports injury. Sudden exertion without a gradual warm-up can lead to abnormal heart rate and inadequate blood flow to the heart along with changes in blood pressure, all of which can be dangerous, especially for older exercisers.

Before you begin

The American College of Sports Medicine recommends that healthy women over fifty years old, and men over forty, who wish to start a vigorous exercise program should first consult a physician. Your doctor may recommend that you take an exercise stress test (see page 511).

Younger people should also see a physician if two or more risk factors for heart disease (such as recurrent chest pain, high blood pressure or cholesterol levels, smoking, or obesity) are present. And at any age, you should consult with a physician first if you have cardiovascular, lung, or joint-muscle conditions (or symptoms suggestive of these conditions).

Keys to Maintaining Exercise

Despite the best of intentions, half of all people who take up new exercise programs drop by the wayside within six months. Here are six ways to bolster your perseverance:

Set realistic exercise goals. Adopting a plan beyond your capacities is a sure route to failure, especially if you are a perfectionist. Set definite goals rather than hazy ones ("I'll cycle ten miles this week," not "I really should get more exercise this week."). Even more important, set exercise goals that you know you can achieve.

Record your progress. Before you start, evaluate your condition. For each workout, weigh yourself, monitor your heart rate, and record both your time and achievements (such as the distance covered).

Start slow and easy. If you haven't exercised regularly in some time, working out ten minutes three times a week is just plain easier to stick to than forty-five minutes four times a week. So is starting with a moderate level of intensity, one that leaves you feeling good afterward. Gradually lengthen your workouts and step up the pace.

Seek convenience. Have you found a convenient time slot? A convenient location for your workout? If the gym, track, or pool you use isn't nearby, or if you frequently can't find parking space, you may use this as an excuse and stop going.

Find a support group. A workout partner can help keep you motivated. One recent study found that 55 percent of women who exercised with a partner stuck with a twelve-month program versus only 31 percent of those who went it alone.

Add variety. Performing one type of exercise day in, day out, can become boring; instead, try swimming one day, riding a bike the day after, and jogging the next. Indeed, there are many activities you can choose from to stay motivated and maintain or even enhance fitness benefits.

There are two techniques for warming up. The generic type—such as jogging in place or stationary cycling—is a full-body warm-up not necessarily geared to the particular activity you're about to perform. Because they use the large muscle groups, general warm-ups are most effective for elevating deep muscle temperature. You should always perform a general warm-up before you stretch or work with weights.

Specific warm-ups are slightly less vigorous rehearsals of the sport or exercise you're about to perform. A tennis player, for instance, would warm up by lightly hitting balls. Specific warm-ups are particularly effective in preparing both physically and psychologically for activities involving skill and coordination.

Warm-up tips

•A five- to ten-minute warm-up is usually enough to raise your body temperature. However, if you exercise in warm weather, you may not have to warm up as much, and in the cold, you may need a longer warm-up. A light sweat is a good indication that you have warmed up sufficiently.

•After exercise, cool down. Slow down gradually and take an extra lap around the track or pool; pedal the last quarter mile slowly; or stretch gently for five to ten minutes. Not only can this reduce muscle stiffness, but it can also prevent the abrupt drop in blood pressure that occurs when you suddenly halt vigorous activity. Never stand still immediately after vigorous exercise.

•In cold weather, try warming up before going outdoors; also, wind up cooling down indoors. Many exercisers find that when it's cold outside, they stretch more fully in the comfort of their homes.

The need for fluid replacement

When you exercise intensely, indoors or out, you need to replace fluids lost through sweating. This is particularly important in hot weather, when you can easily lose more than a quart of water in an hour. At the very least, neglecting to compensate for fluid loss can cause lethargy and nausea, interfering with your performance. In endurance activities like marathon running, long-distance cycling, strenuous hiking, or cross-country skiing, water loss can be severe, potentially producing heat exhaustion or heat stroke.

•In hot weather, drink at least sixteen to twenty ounces of fluid two hours before exercising and another eight ounces fifteen to thirty minutes before. While you exercise, drink four to eight ounces every ten to twenty minutes.

•After exercising, drink enough to replace the fluid you've sweated off. In hot weather, weigh yourself before and after your workout; drink one pint for each pound lost and eat normally.

•While heat buildup may be slower when you exercise in cold weather or in water, you still lose fluid from sweating. Therefore, it's important to replace fluids just as regularly when you swim or work out in the cold as you do in the heat.

Sports drinks vs. plain water. What should you drink when working out for long periods? Most exercise physiologists have recommended water as the ideal replacement fluid, and have consistently cautioned that beverages containing more than 2.5 percent sugar would slow the rate at which fluids leave your stomach and thus hamper performance. However, during the past decade researchers have found that drinks containing up to 10 percent sugar are usually as well absorbed as water.

Myth: Beer is a good post-exercise drink.

Fact: *It may taste good when you're thirsty, but beer is not a good way to get the fluid you need after prolonged exercise. Alcohol is a diuretic, so that rather than replenishing the water you've lost in perspiration, beer can promote dehydration.*

Some people say that beer gives them a quick shot of carbohydrates (the basic fuel for muscles) and potassium. But there's no pressing need for these nutrients immediately after a workout.

Ironically, even if you needed these nutrients, beer isn't a very good source. Compare beer to orange juice. The beer has 13 grams of carbohydrates, versus 39 in orange juice. And while the beer has just 89 milligrams of potassium, the orange juice has a whopping 700 milligrams.

Moreover, when consumed during a strenuous endurance event, sugared beverages may help your body conserve its carbohydrate stores, maintain normal blood sugar levels, and thus delay fatigue. Many people also find sugared (and slightly salty) drinks more palatable than water and thus easier to drink in large quantities. However, fruit juices and soft drinks contain more than 10 percent sugar, so they should be diluted. Most of us prefer cold fluids, but there's no other advantage to them; cold beverages will rarely cause cramping or a "stitch." Carbonated beverages are fine, too, unless they make you bloated. Alcoholic beverages are poor choices: they promote dehydration, hamper coordination, and impair performance.

Specially formulated "sports drinks" such as Gatorade and Exceed supply the optimal amount of carbohydrates—6 to 9 percent carbohydrate concentration—for endurance exercise. But, in fact, they are nutritionally similar to diluted juice or soft drinks, only more expensive. Sports drinks promise to replace the electrolytes (sodium and potassium) lost in sweating. Except under the most extreme circumstances, there is no need to replace them by consuming special drinks or mineral supplements (your normal diet should do the trick). In any case, sports drinks actually contain only a little potassium. Still, many athletes prefer the convenience and taste of sports drinks. In the end, it's a matter of personal preferences.

For some people, caffeine may reduce the perceived effort during exercise, which could be a boon. In others, it may cause jitteriness that interferes with their performance. More important, caffeine combined with prolonged exertion can sometimes boost heart rate and blood pressure excessively. If caffeinated beverages help you with mental performance, they may also help you with physical endeavors. But if you're not accustomed to caffeine, be careful, since you may have a reaction. Remember, too, that caffeine is a diuretic and thus may increase urination, so increase your intake of other fluids.

The most important thing is to drink, period—even if you don't feel thirsty. Thirst is satisfied long before you have replenished lost fluids. Because of the strain and excitement of physical activity, it's possible to lose two quarts of water before you notice your fluid loss. If fluid replacement after prolonged exercise is left totally up to your thirst, it can take several days to reestablish your body's fluid balance.

Exercise and pregnancy

Proper exercise during pregnancy can have many benefits. For a woman who enjoyed working out before becoming pregnant, it can be important psychologically to continue with a regular exercise program. Moderate exercise during pregnancy can help prevent excessive weight gain and help speed recovery after birth.

Which kind of exercise, and how much, is safe to perform during pregnancy? Medical experts say that your exercise program must be geared to your level of fitness, medical history (particularly any problems during past pregnancies), the stage of development of the fetus, and maternal complicating factors. Therefore, it's important to consult your physician.

Generally, you should not take up new exercise programs during pregnancy. Stick with your usual exercise routine, but cut back on the intensity. Remember that pregnancy puts extra demands on your heart and lungs. Your oxygen consumption and heart rate goes up. As pregnancy advances, breathing becomes harder work because each breath must displace the enlarging uterus downward.

For exercise to be effective, it should be regular. Try to exercise no less than

Sports bras

According to one university study, 56 percent of women experience breast discomfort while exercising. The researchers suggested that large-breasted women in particular might benefit from sports bras. The problem is, many so-called sports bras aren't any better than regular models. Here are points to keep in mind when shopping for a sports bra:

•Sports bras come in two types: those that compress the breasts and those that encapsulate each breast. Try on both types to find which is best for you.

•Simulate the motions of your activity when trying on the bra.

•Choose a bra with seamless cups or with seams that don't cross a nipple; avoid models with hooks, fasteners, or rough seams that may chafe.

•Bands at top and bottom should be slightly elastic and wide enough to control bouncing and prevent the bra from riding up. Be sure the straps don't dig into your shoulders.

three times a week in half-hour sessions. The best exercise is an activity you enjoy. Walking and swimming are particularly good for pregnant women who have been relatively sedentary. Warming up and cooling down are especially important during pregnancy, but stretch carefully because muscles and joints are looser than usual. Cool down with leisurely walking, which helps return blood to your heart from your lower extremities.

What to avoid. Avoid bouncing, jarring, twisting, and any activity that puts your abdomen in jeopardy. Contact sports are too risky, as is any activity that requires rapid stops and starts, since your center of gravity has changed and it is easier to lose your balance. In addition, take the following precautions:

•If you feel very tired or experience discomfort, stop and rest. You should not exercise so intensely that you are unable to talk. You should recover your pre-exercise heart rate within fifteen minutes of your exercise session.

•Don't exercise while lying on your back after the fourth month. This can block the blood supply to the uterus and depress the fetal heart rate. If you need to rest during an exercise session, lie down on your side, not on your back.

•Don't exercise vigorously in hot, humid weather, and always drink plenty of water before and after exercising. This avoids the dehydration and elevated body temperature that could injure the fetus.

•Remember that your muscles and connective tissues are gradually undergoing hormonal changes that will relax them. This will facilitate the baby's birth, but it also makes you more susceptible to strains and sprains. Wear properly fitting shoes that support your feet in whichever activity you choose.

Exercise and kids

Parents shouldn't assume that schools are taking care of their kids' "physical education." On average, schools are offering fewer gym classes; only 36 percent have required daily gym classes, according to the President's Council on Physical Fitness and Sports. More important, few gym programs are effective in promoting cardiovascular fitness. Instead of aerobic activities, gym classes tend to stress competitive sports, which involve only a limited number of students who have the required abilities. All kids, though, can participate in aerobic exercise, since it requires minimal hand-eye coordination and little athletic talent. Aerobic activities are also likely to become lifelong habits. Running, for example, can be a good aerobic activity for children. Long-distance running poses an increased risk of injury for prepubescents, but if a running program is gradual and well supervised, and if the child wears good running shoes and warms up properly, the risks should be minimal. Swimming, cycling, brisk walking, and hiking are other good aerobic options that can easily be shared as family activities.

Exercise should be fun for children: the adage "no pain, no gain" is even more dangerous for kids than for adults. For example, weight lifting that calls for hefting as much weight as possible may be hazardous for youngsters. If a child over nine wishes to begin a weight-lifting program, make sure he or she works with a trained supervisor who allows only slow lifts that can be repeated twelve to fifteen times. Indeed, a child who wants to engage in any type of strenuous after-school exercise or sports program should be supervised by a qualified person—and should also have a physical exam beforehand.

Aging and exercise

Adults of any age should basically follow the same safety guidelines for exercise. However, as you get older, it's especially important to start a workout slowly: begin with five to ten minutes of exercise at a comfortable level of exertion and increase your effort gradually. Also, there is no need to exceed 70 percent of your maximum heart rate, and 50 to 60 percent is sufficient if you are starting out or find more exertion too strenuous.

The Right Footwear

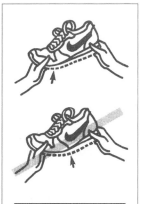

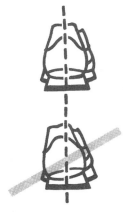

Running shoes should bend at the ball of the foot; shoes that bend at mid-foot offer no support. A mid-sole that is too soft will feel very good in the store, but can cause the foot to turn inward.

Make sure the uppers are correctly attached to the soles—they should be perpendicular to the heels, not slanted, when examined from the back.

Athletic shoes

Specialized athletic shoes have proliferated during the last decade. But do you really need different shoes for running, aerobics, tennis, calisthenics, even walking?

With all the types and models available, it's helpful to realize that there are two basic kinds of athletic shoes—running shoes and tennis-type shoes. Active people generally need both kinds, and athletes may require other specialized shoes for their sport as well.

Running shoes. These are good for activities that primarily involve forward movement. These light weight shoes have a durable, deeply patterned outer-sole; a thick heel wedge to tilt the body forward; a firm, shock-absorbent mid-sole; and a breathable upper.

A study at Tulane University found that all running shoes lose about 30 percent of their shock absorbability after 500 miles of use, regardless of the brand, price, or construction. If shoes can't be repaired, replace them (see page 267).

Tennis-type shoes. Good for any activity that primarily involves side-to-side movement, such as tennis, squash, and other racquet sports. These are heavier and stiffer than running shoes, and they usually have a herringbone outer-sole and a reinforcement under the toes for stop-and-go action.

Aerobics shoes. Because aerobic dance calls for multidirectional, high-stress movement, these shoes combine the features of running and tennis-type shoes. You can use tennis-type shoes in aerobics classes, but not running shoes.

Walking shoes. Shoes for everyday walking should have a rigid shank for support. Rubber heels are a must—they absorb shock and are replaceable. Shoes specially designed for long treks may have curved soles to facilitate the rocking motion of walking and extended heel counters at the backs.

Cross-training shoes. If you engage in a variety of activities and don't want to purchase shoes for each type, cross-training shoes combine characteristics of many types of shoes, including cushioning and heel support for walking and jogging, and ankle support and added stability for lifting weights or playing a stop-and-start game like basketball.

Can insoles protect your feet?

Special insoles that can be inserted in shoes are often claimed by manufacturers to provide better shock absorption than the soles built into athletic shoes. (These flat insoles shouldn't be confused with orthotic devices that are molded foot supports designed to correct abnormal foot motion and alignment.) But based on a number of studies, most experts don't think that these insoles significantly increase the shock-absorbing ability of good athletic shoes. Your best bet is to concentrate on choosing shoes that provide sufficient cushioning by themselves. The material used in conventional insoles (ethylene vinyl acetate, or EVA) wears out after about 600 miles of running—by which time it's probably time to replace the shoes. Of course, if you have chronic or recurrent pain, you should consult a podiatrist or orthopedist to see whether you might benefit from an orthotic device.

A better reason to buy replacement insoles is that they may make your athletic shoes more comfortable. And if you stand for long periods in shoes that have no built-in cushioning, insoles may provide additional comfort.

If you decide to buy insoles, try different brands to see which ones feel most comfortable. Be sure to try them in the shoes they'll be worn in. Also bear in mind that some insoles may make feet feel overheated.

Sports-specific socks

For people who take their athletics seriously, there are socks designed for specific sports, including tennis, cycling, running, skiing, aerobics—even for walking and golf. These differ according to where protective padding is placed (ball, toes, instep, heel, arch, or shin), how thick the padding is, and which materials are used. Nearly all of these are made of Orlon, polypropylene, or other synthetic materials that draw (or "wick") away perspiration.

Do you really need such sports-specific socks? They do provide extra cushioning and can help decrease foot abrasion. But the sock is less important than the appropriate athletic shoe, since the shoe can make up for many shortcomings of a sock. Thus, good shoes and all-purpose socks that wick away moisture will do the trick for most people.

Exercising Outdoors

Exercising in different conditions can be exhilarating, whether you are hiking in the heat of summer, cross-country skiing on a crisp winter day, or heading out for an evening run. Yet it's important to be aware of potential hazards associated with these conditions and how to sidestep them. As the following guidelines show, the trick is to combine a few simple precautions with the right gear.

Being active in heat and humidity

Drinking plenty of fluids is the most important step to minimize the effects of hot and humid weather. At the very least, neglecting to compensate for fluid loss can cause lethargy and nausea, interfering with your performance. In endurance activities like brisk walking, running, strenuous hiking, cycling and cross-country skiing, water loss can be severe, potentially producing heat exhaustion or heat stroke. The former condition is a result of dehydration and is signaled by such symptoms as headache, nausea, loss of coordination and sometimes chills. Heat stroke is far more serious, since it involves a failure of the body's cooling mechanism and can result in neurological damage or death.

However, replacing the fluid lost through sweating is only one of several measures you should take to exercise safely in the heat. Under humid conditions, sweat doesn't evaporate as readily and so contributes much less to cooling the body.

Dress for the heat. Your exercise clothing should be light-colored, loose-fitting and made of lightweight, absorbent material such as cotton. As this material becomes sweat-soaked, it actually provides a cooling effect. Changing to dry clothing during a workout or when playing a game like tennis makes little sense for proper temperature regulation in hot weather.

Use common sense. Try to exercise in the early morning or late afternoon or early evening to avoid the worst of the heat. And during very hot spells, consider alternatives like swimming or exercising indoors in an air-conditioned space.

Take time to adjust. Most cases of heat illness occur among exercisers during their first exposure to hot weather, before their bodies have become acclimatized to heat—a gradual physiological adjustment that allows the body to lose unwanted body heat more efficiently during exercise. The best way to acclimatize is to increase your exercise time gradually in hot weather over a period of several days. The average person needs seven to fourteen days to acclimatize fully.

Cold-weather workouts

Cold weather doesn't have to mean the end of outdoor exercise for most people. Running, cycling, or walking in winter can be as much fun as skiing. They're also good ways to get you outside in the sunlight and thus help you avoid wintertime blues. All you have to do is make allowances for the weather. (If you regularly exercise in the cold, you may also notice some gradual acclimatization—for instance, shivering starts at a lower skin temperature, and heat loss through the skin decreases. As with heat acclimatization, the process usually takes about two weeks of frequent exposure.)

Most of us bundle up when we go outdoors in the winter, perhaps as a carry-over from childhood, but one of the most common errors people make when exercising in cold weather is wearing too much clothing. Even a moderate amount of brisk walking or other aerobic exercise can make you feel that it's 30° warmer than it really is. So when you're about to run on a 25° day, dress for about 55°.

Here are some other guidelines for dressing right:

Don't overdress. Dress so that you are slightly chilled when your first go outdoors. As you start exercising, you'll warm up.

Zip up. Zippers make clothes adaptable: when you get too hot, you can unzip them halfway to let in air and can remove a garment easily. In general, it's best to start opening zippers or removing layers *as soon as you start to sweat.* Zippers on sports apparel often have small fabric loops so you can pull them open without having to take off your gloves; if they don't, you can tie string to the zippers.

Choose the right fabrics. Traditionally people were told to stay with cotton and wool rather than synthetics for greater absorbency and warmth. But a new generation of manmade materials gives you more choices. It's not necessary to buy fancy new clothes to enjoy the benefits of exercise, but if you're in the market for such garments, you should consider these innovative synthetics, as described below.

Use a three-part system of layering. Layers should be lose in order to trap the body heat and act as insulation. The first thin layer removes perspiration from the skin, the second provides warmth, and the third protects against wind and rain. Layering also allows for fine tuning—a layer or two can be removed to lower body temperature during strenuous exertion. When you remove a garment, tie it around your waist or put it in a day pack.

First layer: Start with thermal underwear made of a fabric (such as polypropylene, Capilene, or Thermax) that "wicks" away perspiration—that is, it stays dry by drawing moisture away from your skin to the next layer of clothing. This is essential, since wet clothes transfer heat away from you. Wool is a good insulator, but many people find it itchy. Cotton holds moisture next to your skin, making you feel cold and clammy; silk feels warm and soft, but it also retains moisture.

Middle layers: Next add a synthetic pile or fleece jacket, or a wool or synthetic sweater. Manmade materials such as Thinsulate provide warmth without bulk. Keep legs warm with wind-resistant pants or spandex tights (worn over thermal long johns when it's really cold). If you'll be working up a heavy sweat, you might skip this layer.

Outer layer: A jacket that's waterproof, wind-resistant, and yet breathable (so that moisture isn't trapped inside) is optimal. Synthetics like Gore-Tex fit the bill. An ordinary windbreaker is okay for a short workout in dry weather.

Mittens or gloves. Mittens are warmer than gloves since they keep fingers together and have less surface area from which heat can escape. In very cold weather, the added warmth from mittens is worth the loss in dexterity. You can also wear inner liners made of polypropylene or another material that draws sweat from your skin with a second layer over them. Waterproof gloves or mitten are recommended.

Head-wear. Oddly enough, one way to keep your feet warm is to wear a hat, since you lose so much heat through your head. Wear a wool or synthetic cap or a hood. Another option is a cap that folds down into a face mask in case the wind starts gusting or it begins to snow (make sure it doesn't obscure your vision or hearing).

Shoes. Wear shoes that offer good traction and shock absorption, especially when running on hard, frozen ground. Shoes should have a little extra space inside to trap warm air and, when it's really cold, let you wear an extra pair of socks.

Myth: Hot drinks keep you warm in the cold.

Fact: Hot drinks taste good and may have a psychological benefit, but they don't do anything to boost body temperature. According to research conducted at the U.S. Army Research Institute of Environmental Medicine at Natick, Mass., you would have to drink a quart of hot liquid (130°) at a time to generate any body heat, but it would be hard to keep down that much hot fluid. Hot liquids can dilate blood vessels in the skin, which may make you feel warmer, but actually leads to a small (and harmless) amount of heat loss. The important thing is to keep your fluid intake up when you're out in the cold—hot or cold drinks, as you prefer.

Heading outdoors

Warm up and stretch. It's a good idea to warm up first (such as jogging in place) and stretch indoors, and then perhaps stretch again outside. When you've finished exercising, cool down and stretch indoors.

Drink as much water in the cold as in the heat. This is crucial. It's easy to become dehydrated in cold weather because of the water you lose from sweating and breathing (you have to warm and moisten the cold air you inhale), and because of your stepped-up urine production. And dehydration hinders your body's ability to regulate its temperature. Drink fluids before, during, and after your workout. Skip alcohol and caffeine; both types of beverages dehydrate you. Drinking alcohol may offer the illusion of warmth but actually robs you of heat by dilating surface blood vessels in the skin.

Compensate for the wind. The wind can penetrate clothes and remove the insulating layer of warm air around the body. When the temperature is 20°F, a fifteen-mph wind makes it feel like −5° (this is the wind-chill factor). Fast motion, as in cycling or skiing, has the same effect as the wind since it increases air movement past the body. Compensate for a strong wind by running or riding against it on your way out, then with it behind you on the way back—you'll do the most work before you're tired and sweaty.

Be on the defensive. Shorter daylight hours, poor visibility, plus the risk of skidding cars call for careful running, walking, and cycling.

Keep moving. If you stop exercising for any reason and remain outdoors, put on extra clothes before you start to feel cold. To stay warm, try to keep moving.

Snow and ice. Though some joggers manage to run in even the worst weather without injury, exercising on snow or ice is not worth the risk. One exception: some people are able to run reasonably well on hard, packed snow, provided they slow their pace, take smaller steps, and wear shoes with good traction. Wet snow and ice, however, are extremely treacherous, so in such weather you're better off exercising indoors.

Wear sunglasses and sunscreen. Snow-covered ground on clear days can reflect the sun and thus burn your face and obscure your vision, especially at high altitudes. (See pages 301-304 for tips on choosing these products.)

When to come in from the cold

Breathing cold air is not harmful to healthy people; you can't "freeze your lungs." However, it can be risky for those who suffer from angina, asthma, or high blood pressure—they should check with a doctor before exercising in the cold. For such people, wearing a ski mask or scarf pulled loosely in front of the face may help warm up inhaled air.

Frostbite and hypothermia. These are the two main dangers of exercising in the cold. Dressing properly and taking other precautions described here are your best safeguards. Be on guard for the numbness and white discoloration of frostbite—particularly on your hands, ears, toes, and face.

Cyclists and runners have also reported cases of penile frostbite, so consider wearing an extra pair of shorts. Hypothermia, which involves a dangerous drop in body temperature, is mostly a risk when you're outside in very cold weather for many hours, especially if you're wet, injured, and/or not moving around enough to stay warm.

Safeguards at night

If you exercise at night, as many do when winter days grow shorter, dress in bright colors. Reflective clothing should be part of every exerciser's attire, since even people who avoid nighttime cycling or jogging occasionally find themselves out later than planned. *Night cycling is fifteen to twenty times more dangerous than cycling during daylight hours.* A National Safety Council study found that 54 percent of all pedestrian fatalities occur at night, and a report from Florida shows that half of all cyclists killed on that state's roads are night riders, even though they make up only 3 to 5 percent of the bike-riding population.

Wearing light-colored clothing isn't enough. A study by the National Highway Traffic Safety Administration found that at night a pedestrian in white shirt and jeans is visible at a distance of only a little more than 200 feet, usually not enough space to allow a driver to swerve or stop. So it's essential to adopt additional safety measures, such as these:

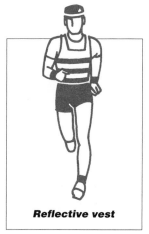

Reflective vest

For running and walking at night

•Wear fluorescent or reflective material as vests, headbands, wrist and ankle bands, belts, or as patches stuck on cuffs, waist, or shoes.

•Run or walk against the traffic. That way you can see oncoming cars. If you know you're approaching a blind curve, switch to the other side.

•Use lights. There are battery-operated flashing devices that clip to belts or strap onto legs. Carrying a flashlight helps. In a National Highway Traffic Safety Administration study, a pedestrian with a flashlight was visible to drivers 600 feet farther off than one wearing reflective material.

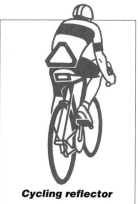

Cycling reflector

For cycling at night

•Get a headlight and taillight, preferably halogen (brighter than incandescent) and powered by a generator or rechargeable batteries. Test them before buying. A good headlight should be visible 500 feet away and light up potholes and other hazards. The red taillight should be visible from 600 feet.

•Wear reflective Day-Glo clothing and patches. The most visible way to wear a reflective stripe is horizontally, across the full width of your back. Stick patches on your helmet, chest, upper arms, seat, shoes, and saddlebags or wear the special reflector for cyclists—a triangle of fluorescent fabric edged with reflective tape.

•Wear the same kinds of lights recommended for runners.

•Try a reflective spacer, a horizontal rod attached at a right angle to the rear wheel and topped with a flag or disk, to keep traffic at bay.

•Make sure your bike is equipped with front, side, rear, and pedal reflectors, which are now required by law on new bikes. They aren't enough, but they help.

•Use a rearview mirror to check for passing cars. You can also use your shadow as a gauge. Passing on the left, a car throws your shadow to the right. If your shadow stays straight in front of you, the car is on your tail: be ready to pull over.

•Ride with the traffic. Drivers expect you to follow the same rules they do.

Other nighttime safety tips

•Don't look directly at approaching headlights; they'll blind you temporarily.

•Stay off high-speed roads.

•Don't wear headphones—you may not hear a car approaching.

Exercising in bad air

Polluted air contains a variety of noxious gases, including carbon monoxide, sulfur dioxide, ozone, and nitrogen oxides—as well as particulate matter, which is visible as soot or smoke. Because exercise makes you breathe faster and more deeply, it can dramatically increase the adverse effects air pollutants have on the respiratory and cardiovascular systems. In addition, joggers and cyclists often breathe through the mouth, bypassing the nasal passages (which help filter out water-soluble compounds such as sulfur dioxide). Many studies agree that endurance athletes who work out strenuously are most likely to exhibit pollution-related symptoms, such as coughing, throat irritation, headaches, shortness of breath, and tightness in the chest. Those with pulmonary disorders may develop inflamed and dangerously constricted airways.

What ozone can do to you. Ozone, a colorless gas formed when sunlight acts on car and industrial emissions, is one of the more dangerous components of urban smog. Concentrations are highest on sunny afternoons with little wind, particularly in valleys. Ozone irritates the airways and can injure cells by producing compounds known as free radicals. Endurance athletes exercising strenuously for at least thirty to sixty minutes when ozone levels are high (as they are in Los Angeles for at least one hour a day during half the year) tend to perform poorly because of impaired lung function and suffer a variety of pollution-related symptoms. Shorter or less intense exercise in lower levels of ozone generally has few or no ill effects. However, people vary in how much they react to ozone. Some studies have suggested that, over time, healthy people can adapt to repeated exposure to a given level of ozone (though it's not known whether they will suffer long-term damage).

Other pollutants, such as sulfur dioxide, are less likely to cause problems in healthy exercisers under average conditions. But asthmatics may have trouble breathing after exercising for even ten minutes in low levels of sulfur dioxide. Carbon monoxide does not directly cause respiratory problems, but it does interfere with oxygen transport in the blood, which means that the heart must work harder to deliver oxygen to the working muscles, and can thus interfere with athletic performance. More important, for people with coronary disease, exercise in highly polluted air can lead to irregular heart rhythm or angina.

You can't avoid air pollution completely in most urban and many suburban areas, but there are ways to minimize the risks when exercising:

•Schedule your outdoor workouts in the early morning, if possible, when there's less car exhaust and the sun is weaker. After sunset is the second-best time, but may not be a safe option.

•If you do exercise during rush hour, choose areas with little traffic. Open, windy areas are preferable, since air currents can disperse pollutants.

•Breathe through your nose, not mouth. This should reduce the amount of pollutants reaching your lungs.

•If there's an air-pollution alert, exercise indoors.

•If you have asthma or heart disease, consult your doctor about exercise options.

•A gas mask isn't the solution. Though a carbon-filtered mask removes most ozone and some other pollutants from the air, it may be uncomfortable, make breathing difficult, and cause chafing.

The so-called antioxidant nutrients (such as vitamin C and E and beta carotene) help fight against the free radicals created by ozone and other pollutants and thus may prevent or repair long-term lung and cellular damage. This is one reason why scientists recommend a high intake of antioxidant-rich foods.

Aerobic Activities

One of the truly pleasant aspects of exercising is that you have plenty of options. You can choose to do something as simple as walking, you can take up one or more recreational sports, or you can perform a specific routine in an exercise class or at home. In fact, variety is one of the keys to staying fit. For one thing, no single exercise adequately builds all aspects of fitness equally well. And having more than one activity to turn to keeps exercise from getting monotonous. Studies also show that people tend to stick with activities that are accessible and enjoyable.

The activities that follow provide aerobic exercise—that is, exercise that utilizes oxygen for energy production for long periods, and so can work your heart and lungs to promote cardiovascular fitness. In addition, these activities help make muscles stronger and more limber. Most of these are outdoor activities, but if exercising outdoors is not convenient, there are machines that allow you to perform most outdoor activities indoors. You can also take up these activities at any age and continue them for a lifetime. This section spells out the benefits of each activity and basic techniques for performing it effectively and safely.

Aerobic exercise guidelines

The American College of Sports Medicine has made the following recommendations in designing an exercise program:

How often, how long. If you are below average in cardiovascular fitness, you should aim at *three exercise sessions per week, for twenty minutes per session,* preferably on alternate days. After six to eight weeks, if you wish to continue improving your cardiovascular fitness, you can increase the frequency and duration of your sessions. This is also necessary if you want to lose body fat. The optimal schedule is *four weekly sessions of forty minutes each* (not including the warm-up and cool-down). Exercising more than this will not improve your fitness significantly, and it can increase your risk of injury if you are exercising at a high intensity.

How hard. To achieve an aerobic training effect, the American College of Sports Medicine suggests that you exercise at a level of intensity called your *target heart rate.* The easiest way to calculate this rate is to subtract your age from 220—a person's theoretical maximum heart rate—then take 60 percent and 90 percent of that number (multiply the number by 0.6 and by 0.9). The results are the upper and lower end of your target heart rate zone. While you exercise, your heart rate per minute should fall somewhere between these two numbers: for example, a forty-year-old has a target heart rate of 108 to 162 beats per minute. (If you take medication for your heart or blood pressure, your target heart rate may be lower than determined by this calculation.)

• A schedule of low- to moderate-intensity exercise is best for most people, especially those who aren't in peak condition.

• If one of these three factors is low, compensate by increasing the others. For example, if you exercise only for short periods, increase the frequency of the activity. Or increase the intensity of the exercise, but only do this gradually.

Aerobic Movement

A popular form of exercise, especially among women, aerobic dance and movement uses a wide variety of dance forms—folk, modern, jazz, ballet, and disco—and combines them with body movements such as skipping, walking, running, jumping, and toe-touching in order to tone muscles and develop cardiovascular fitness. Learning aerobic dance routines is important, but the emphasis is on exercising the heart and lungs, not giving a command performance.

Here is how a typical aerobic movement class might be divided:
- four to five minutes of stretching done to music;
- five minutes of slow aerobic movement to further stretch and limber the body;
- fifteen to thirty minutes of routines done at low, medium, or high intensity—the heart of the class;
- five minutes of slow aerobic movement to cool down.

Benefits of aerobics

Overall, aerobic movement promotes fitness through enjoyable exercise, and that is exactly what irritates its critics, who contend that it is more fun than fitness. Yet a number of studies support proponents' claims that aerobic movement builds cardiovascular fitness and develops leg muscles, and contributes to muscular endurance and flexibility. Low-intensity routines, however, are not always strenuous enough to improve cardiovascular efficiency, especially in fit, young individuals. And most controlled studies have found no evidence that aerobic dance is better than any other type of aerobic exercise at taking off pounds or inches. For those trying to lose weight, one reason aerobic dance may not prove effective appears to be the relatively short time devoted to strenuous activity— only twenty to thirty minutes out of a fifty-minute class. Most participants take only two or three classes per week. Significant weight loss, however, requires workouts of thirty to sixty minutes four to six times per week. (Weight loss also depends upon body size and caloric intake.)

Tips and techniques

Like all forms of cardiovascular training, aerobic movement must be performed three to five times per week to develop cardiovascular fitness. Research has also shown that it takes at least three months for training benefits from aerobic movement to become significant.

During the first two weeks, the heart rate should be monitored after each aerobic routine or about every five minutes and should usually not exceed the lower end of your training rate (that is, 60 percent of your maximum heart rate); if it does, modify the workout to make it less strenuous—for example, by lowering your jumps, pumping your arms less vigorously, or reducing the number of steps you take per beat of music.

Softening your workout

Along with the fun and fitness benefits of aerobic movement, the repetitive, jarring motions can sometimes be traumatic to your body. Exercising too often or too long, improperly warming up, wearing shoes that don't give enough support, and working out on a surface that is too hard are possible causes of injury. In fact,

Setting your own pace

Don't let pulse taking and various computations make exercise frustrating. Once you've gained some experience, you may no longer need to take your pulse—you'll simply know how it "feels" to work out at your training heart rate. And if you find doing so too strenuous at first, then do less.

Although exercising at your target heart rate is a proven recommendation for increasing your fitness level, researchers are still learning about how little a person "can get away with" and still become fitter. We do know that, compared to being sedentary, significant health benefits occur with less intense exercise— such as simply taking a brisk walk for thirty minutes.

Interval Training

Exercising at a moderate pace for twenty to thirty minutes (preceded by warming up and followed by cooling down) three to five times a week is the accepted standard for boosting your body's ability to utilize oxygen and enhancing your cardiovascular system. Recent research suggests, however, that you may be able to get in shape faster with interval training—spurts of intense exertion alternating with lower-intensity recovery periods.

Benefits

Researchers at the Human Performance Laboratory at the University of Miami studied the question by having female students participate in thirty-five minute aerobic dance sessions (not including warm-up and cool-down periods) three times a week for twelve weeks. They found that interval training—three to five minutes of intense exercise alternating with up to three minutes of brisk walking or mild running—produced greater gains (18 percent) in aerobic capacity than did steady-speed dance sessions (8 percent). Both groups also lost body fat (but not weight, necessarily, since the exercise increased their muscle mass).

Researchers theorize that the recovery periods in interval training may make it easier for participants to maintain the intensity of the workout, knowing that a low-intensity period is coming up, while those attempting to work at a steady speed may gradually slow down as the workout continues. Another advantage is that interval training is less monotonous than steady-pace exercise.

How to train

Interval training can be applied to nearly any exercise. Alternate fifteen seconds to three minutes of high-intensity running, cycling, hiking, swimming, rowing, or aerobic dancing with low-intensity intervals of the same length. During the intense bouts, your heart rate should reach 80 percent of its maximum (85 to 90 percent if you are in excellent condition). (Since this puts markedly increased stress on your heart as well as on your joints and muscles, consult your doctor about interval training if you are forty-five or over, are out of shape, or have a medical condition or previous injury that restricts your ability to exercise.) During the recovery periods, don't let your heart rate drop below 60 percent of its maximum. You can also use the computerized exercise bikes, specially programmed for interval training, found in many gyms.

If you have less than twenty minutes to exercise, it appears that only interval training will give you a significant cardiovascular workout—but don't necessarily expect maximum conditioning. If you're after all the benefits of aerobic exercise, twenty- to forty-minute workouts are still recommended.

Step aerobics

Also called bench stepping or step training, step aerobics involves stepping onto and off a small platform in a routine that gives you a cardiovascular workout while it tones your legs and buttocks. In one study at San Diego State University, researchers found that working at a rate of 120 steps per minute while pumping the arms was as exerting as running at seven miles per hour, but that impact forces were low—similar to those created by walking at three miles per hour.

If you plan to purchase a bench and work out at home, take a few classes to learn the necessary coordination and technique. Beginners should use a four-inch step, increasing the height eventually to eight to twelve inches. Your knee should not flex beyond 90° as you step up, or you risk strain and possible injury. Always place your sole flat on the center of the platform. Land back on the floor with the ball of your foot, then bring your heel down smoothly.

---

according to two studies published in *The Physician and Sportsmedicine,* 76 percent of aerobics instructors who responded to a questionnaire and 43 percent of their students sustained injuries from this activity. Their shins seemed most vulnerable, with calf, lower back, foot, ankle, and knee problems also reported.

Fortunately, low-impact aerobic exercises—which were initially designed for people recovering from an injury and for older people—have gained general popularity as a way of achieving the benefits of aerobic exercise without subjecting the body to excessive stress. In low-impact aerobics, at least one foot is almost always kept on the floor, and the exerciser's arms are constantly busy—swinging as well as doing biceps curls, triceps extensions, and overhead arm presses. It is important that the movements be strenuous enough to raise the heart rate sufficiently; otherwise, the exercises will not truly be aerobic.

Any kind of exercise, of course, requires reasonable caution. The side-to-side movements in low-impact aerobics, for example, could injure the feet or legs if overdone. And arm movements have to be done carefully, especially if you are using hand weights, which can be dangerous. Also, the floor shouldn't be too hard, and your shoes should be well padded.

Rating an aerobics class

It's important that an exercise class be fun and that you like the teacher, but that's not enough. You will get only a fraction of the potential health benefits from a poorly run class—and you are more likely to injure yourself or drop out. In deciding on a class, consider the following factors:

The routine. Many exercise professionals recommend mixing aerobics with stretching and strengthening calisthenics. The level of the class—beginning, intermediate, or advanced—must be correct for you. The class should start with a warm-up of gentle stretching and end with a cooling-down period, each at least five minutes. At least twenty minutes worth of the exercises should be designed to get your heart to its training rate. If there are calisthenic exercises, they should work all the major muscle groups, starting with the large muscles in the legs and ending with the smaller muscles in the arms.

The workout room. The temperature shouldn't be too hot or too cold, and the ventilation should be good. A suspended wooden floor with carpeting is safest; harder floors must be covered with thick carpet. For calisthenics, there should be mats. And you should be able to move around without bumping into people.

The instructor. The most difficult—and perhaps most important—judgment you will have to make concerns the qualifications of the instructor. Being an athlete or dancer doesn't qualify a person to teach a class, though many athletes and dancers, with suitable training, make excellent instructors. There is no single organization that provides nationwide standards for instructors, and until legal standards are adopted, it is difficult to recommend any one program. American College of Sports Medicine certification is currently one of the best.

Even if a teacher is certified, you should ask about the requirements of the particular program that he or she was enrolled in. One sign of an instructor's in-depth

---

Hand and Ankle Weights: Pros and Cons

Studies show that using small weights (one to five pounds) during aerobic exercise can increase oxygen consumption, heart rate, and the number of calories burned during exercise—but usually only by 5 to 10 percent, depending on the amount and location of the weights. That's much less than the claims made by most proponents of the weights. Similar increases in energy output can easily be achieved by exercising a little longer or harder. Anyone thinking of using hand or ankle weights should first consider the following:

•The weights can increase the chance of injury during exercise, particularly traditional aerobic dance or running. Ankle weights, in particular, add to stress on the legs and feet. Unless you have complete control over them,, using weights can lead to muscle sprains and damage to the ligaments and tendons.

•People with high blood pressure or heart disease should avoid exercising with weights, especially hand weights, because they tax the cardiovascular system.

Lifting light hand weights rapidly while standing in place can be a part of your warm-up routine; it helps raise your heart rate and tone your upper body. Moreover, hand weights may be suitable for individuals who are unable to perform running or jumping movements and wish to increase the work of the heart and upper body while walking. They should start with light weights (one pound) and, with elbows bent, briskly swing the arms from the shoulder.

For most people, however, the drawbacks of wearing weights during aerobic exercise outnumber any possible advantages. Even if you are aerobically fit and fully able to control your weight-bound movements, hand and, especially, ankle weights are not recommended for aerobics classes or other activities that involve running or jumping.

Is ballroom dancing good exercise?

At the competitive level, ballroom dancing can elevate your heart rate just as much as running or cross-country skiing. And one study showed that even beginning dance students can derive health benefits. During a twenty-minute aerobic section consisting of the cha-cha, a polka, two swing dances (the jitterbug and the lindy), a Viennese waltz, and a samba, the great majority of the subjects (age eighteen to thirty-five) got their heart rates up to near maximum training rates, particularly in the polka, swing dancing, and the waltz. As for caloric expenditure, even moderate ballroom dancing can burn between 250 and 300 calories per hour, and fast, vigorous dancing burns upward of 400 calories per hour.

involvement is a degree in an exercise-related field such as exercise physiology. Instructors may also receive excellent training from seminars and courses offered at local fitness workshops. (If you are taking an exercise class as part of a rehabilitation program after an illness, you should ask a health professional for a specific recommendation or referral.)

Still, the best way to judge an instructor is not by educational degrees or training certificates but by watching a class. Or, better yet, see if you can try a class before signing up. Notice whether the instructor tells participants how to avoid injuries and reminds them to check their pulse rates so that they reach—but don't exceed—their recommended training heart rates. Also, the instructor should not be a drill sergeant, but should let you work at your own speed. Finally, the instructor should watch the exercisers and actually instruct them—not be too busy looking at his or her own performance.

Cross-Country Skiing

A down-to-earth combination of skiing and hiking, cross-country skiing can provide a more complete workout than running or cycling, since it emphasizes muscles in both the upper and lower body. It can also help develop coordination. Done correctly, it's the best aerobic exercise there is.

You can ski fancy, or you can ski plain. All you need is some equipment (rentable), warm clothing, and some snow-covered, open terrain. Urbanites and suburbanites can go to a park or the nearest open field or golf course. Most people don't need more than one lesson before starting out. Cross-country skiing can be much less expensive than downhill, and poses a lower risk of serious injury. It's a wonderful activity for loners or for families. Age is no barrier. New, easy-to-use short skis and a relatively new technique called "skating" can add to the fun.

Cross-country skiing can offer a variety of outdoor experiences. "Back-country skiing" is hiking in the wild on skis. But now, in this country and Canada, there are hundreds of resorts with groomed trails (no rocks or obstructions), a choice of terrains, and a wide range of accommodations. Instruction and rental equipment are usually available, too.

Equipment. Skis are shorter and simpler than they used to be, designed to get you going without preliminaries. If you're a beginner, rent equipment until you decide what suits you best.

Traditional cross-country skis are narrower and longer than downhill skis—the old rule was that they should be as long as the distance between the wrist of your upstretched arm and the ground. With long skis, you can cross almost any terrain without sinking into the snow. However, the trend is toward shorter, more maneuverable skis.

Short skis—about twenty-seven inches shorter than regular ones—are more responsive, easier to learn to use, easier to balance on, easier to transport, and roughly comparable in price. They are also increasingly popular on groomed trails.

Waxed vs. waxless: Waxless skis require less fuss and provide more control on downhill inclines. Once you've become proficient, you may want the better overall performance and speed afforded by waxable skis. You have to learn how to match the wax to the type of snow and to change it as snow conditions change.

Poles: Whether you're renting or buying, you'll need advice on what pole length is best suited to your height, skiing ability, and type of skiing. Poles should be lightweight and easy to handle; be sure they have a comfortable grip and strong, adjustable strap. Tip: when trying out your poles, wear the gloves you'll wear while skiing.

Boots and bindings: The boots typically resemble high-top hiking boots. Try the boots on while wearing the socks you'll use for skiing. The binding usually attaches to the front of the boot only, leaving the heel free to move as you take the long strides typical of good form. Make sure you understand how the boot snaps into the binding and how you can get in and out of it.

If you do decide to buy equipment, expect to pay from $200 to $300 for a basic package of skis, poles, boots, and bindings.

Technique. Your first time out, use the skis like snowshoes and tramp across the snow utilizing the poles for balance. But as soon as you feel comfortable, you'll want to get in the swing of things.

You may also enjoy a relatively new technique called skating. It can be done in an open field, but a trail especially groomed for skating is better, since the snow must be packed. You push off on one foot, riding the glide as long as possible, then push off with the other foot. You can do double poling (both down at once) or alternate poling—or use no poles at all. Once you master the technique, you can almost fly. Complications: you will definitely need waxed skis and longer poles. Also, it's not regarded as "good form" to skate over tracks groomed for classic cross-country skiing. Some resorts have special snow trails for skating, but some discourage it.

Clothing. Dress in layers that you can peel off, since this activity generates lots of heat. You could start off in jeans, long cotton underwear, a couple of shirts, and a wool sweater, but cotton and wool may leave you wet and cold. Veterans of the sport know the advantages of garments made of newer synthetic fabrics that protect against the elements while allowing moisture (perspiration) to escape. Don't forget a hat and lightweight insulated mittens or gloves.

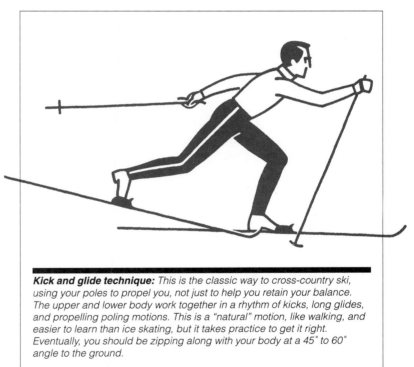

Kick and glide technique: *This is the classic way to cross-country ski, using your poles to propel you, not just to help you retain your balance. The upper and lower body work together in a rhythm of kicks, long glides, and propelling poling motions. This is a "natural" motion, like walking, and easier to learn than ice skating, but it takes practice to get it right. Eventually, you should be zipping along with your body at a 45° to 60° angle to the ground.*

Water. You'll need to drink plenty, because this is a sweaty sport. Thirst may not be a reliable gauge—drink before, during, and after. For all-day treks, bring along a light backpack or "fanny" pack to hold water, food, and an extra sweater for rest stops.

Getting ready. If you are over forty or not in good shape, check with your doctor before you begin skiing. Gradually build up the amount of time you spend at it. Otherwise you run the risk of overuse strains (such as tendinitis) of the shoulder, knee, and arm. To prepare for a season of cross-country skiing, it's best to alternate activities that primarily strengthen the upper body (rowing or swimming) with those emphasizing the lower body (skating, in-line skating, biking, running, or brisk walking) to promote overall muscle tone. Or you can use a cross-country ski machine (see page 252).

Cross Training

(see page 252).

More and more people these days alternate the types of sport or exercise they do, and biathlons (two sports) and triathlons (three sports) are catching up to marathons in popularity. This combination of activities is called cross training—working out regularly at more than one physical activity. Not only is it a way to avoid the boredom of day-in, day-out routine exercise, but it can also provide good overall conditioning, while reducing the risk of injury.

The advantages of variety

Cross training allows you to exercise more muscle groups than a single activity would. For instance, cycling builds your lower body, and swimming works your upper body, so alternating them can help give you the benefits of both while you build aerobic endurance. Similarly, running strengthens the hamstring muscles (located at the rear of the thigh) far more than the quadriceps (at the front of the thigh), a muscle imbalance that may be a factor in some injuries. But by combining cycling, which strengthens the quadriceps, with running, you can work complementary muscle groups in your legs and thus achieve better muscle balance.

Overtraining at one sport or activity continually stresses the same muscles and joints, thus increasing the risk of injury. If instead of running every day, you alternate it with swimming every other day, you'll give your leg muscles and joints a needed rest between runs. And if you do hurt your knee while running, you won't have to stop exercising—you can keep on swimming to maintain your aerobic capacity. Or if you pull a shoulder muscle playing tennis, you can give it a rest while you continue to cycle.

Some sports-medicine specialists believe that cross training may also reduce the risk of injury by moderating the "addiction" to a single sport that can result in overtraining. However, competitive cross trainers may fall prey to certain overuse injuries, due to insufficient muscle rest and an unbalanced training schedule.

If you're serious about one particular sport, don't expect cross training to help improve your performance. The plain fact is, you've got to run to become an outstanding runner or swimmer to win swimming meets. Several studies of the cross trainers who make the headlines—the triathletes who run a marathon, bike a century (one hundred miles), and swim over two miles all in one day, in heroic events like the Hawaii Ironman triathlon—show that however qualified they may be to take on three events, triathletes don't approach the competitive levels in individual events achieved by single-sport specialists. But in terms of overall fitness, top-class triathletes are some of the best-conditioned athletes in the world.

Tips for cross training

If you decide to take up cross training, start slowly, as you would any exercise pro-

---

Myth: Women don't tolerate the heat as well as men when exercising.

Fact: Women and men who are equally fit are likely to tolerate exercise in the heat equally well. Women do tend to sweat less than men, but this doesn't appear to affect their ability to cope with the heat or their physical performance. Furthermore, while some studies have suggested that it may take women longer to start sweating during certain phases of the menstrual cycle, most researchers have not found significant differences in heat regulation during the different phases of the cycle. Overall, sex is far less important than cardiovascular fitness when it comes to the way a person responds to heat.

gram. The best method is to pair sports that train different parts of your body: swimming with cycling, rowing with running. Instead of three or more forty-minute cycling sessions per week, cycle for twenty minutes and spend the other twenty running, or swim one day and play tennis the next. If you belong to a health club that has a track, a pool, weight-training machines, and stationary bikes, you'll find cross training a snap.

Cycling

Cycling is one of the best forms of exercise around: it gives the heart and circulatory system an outstanding aerobic workout; it can burn between four and seven hundred calories per hour; and it conditions not only your legs but, if you ride a touring bike with drop handle bars, your upper back and shoulders as well. For injured runners, cycling is ideal, since it develops aerobic capacity while imposing far less stress on joints than running. You can also choose to ride indoors on an exercise bike—one of the most convenient forms of aerobic conditioning—or to ride outdoors, which offers considerably more variety and mobility than practically any other form of exercise.

To get the most from cycling for fitness, you need to consider both your location and your bike. If you ride in stop-and-go traffic in a suburb or a city, gaining any aerobic benefit will be difficult. Similarly, riding in the country over hilly terrain may be too strenuous for beginners. When you begin cycling, it's best if you can ride on paved roadway that ranges from level to gently rolling; this allows you to ride in low to moderate gears at a good, even pace without straining. Then, as you get stronger, you can increase your cadence—the rate at which you pedal—and also try climbing long hills.

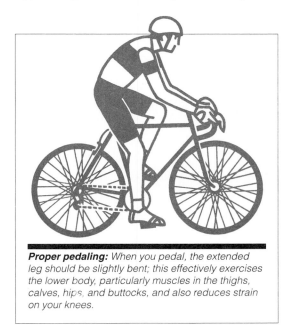

Proper pedaling: *When you pedal, the extended leg should be slightly bent; this effectively exercises the lower body, particularly muscles in the thighs, calves, hips, and buttocks, and also reduces strain on your knees.*

To ride for any significant distance, especially if you will be tackling hills, you should acquire a bike that has at least ten to twelve speeds. The introduction of mountain bikes—also called all-terrain bikes, or ATBs—has extended the enjoyment of biking by letting cyclists traverse routes that were once inaccessible to them. Such bikes have smaller, heavier frame sizes than conventional racing bikes, and wider, knobby tires, as well as upright handlebars. There are also "hybrids"—models with ATB-type features, but lighter in weight. ATBs and hybrids have become so popular that they make up the bulk of bicycle sales in most parts of the United States. Because these bikes allow better maneuverability and a more upright position than touring or racing bicycles, and because they usually have a minimum of eighteen speeds, many cyclists have adopted them for city riding as well.

Fitting Your Bike

For optimal cycling efficiency and comfort, it is crucial that your bike be fitted properly to your body proportions; otherwise, you may suffer discomfort and even injury. If you purchase a new bike at a reputable cycle shop, the sales personnel will help you make the proper measurements and adjustments. Here are some tips to help you select the right bike or alter the one you already own.

•Your first consideration is the frame size, which cannot be adjusted. A bicycle with a top tube is best; it is sturdier than one with no top tube and is likely to have a more efficient braking system. To find the right frame size, straddle the bike over the top tube and stand flat-footed in front of the seat, or saddle. With a touring or race bike, there should be a one- to two-inch clearance between the top tube and your crotch. Because a smaller frame size is preferable on an all-terrain or mountain bike, you should allow a clearance of at least three to five inches on these bikes.

•On a touring bike, drop handlebars should be about as wide as your shoulders or slightly narrower. The handlebars should be at the same level as the seat or slightly lower. Some cyclists with neck or back problems may prefer upright handlebars, which are also standard on all-terrain bikes. While you can easily rotate the handlebars, the length of the stem—which connects the handlebars to the frame—can be changed only by replacing the stem. To check stem length, stand alongside the bike, put your elbow at the tip of the saddle, and reach for the handlebars. Your fingertips should just reach them or come within half an inch. If not, the handlebar stem is too long.

•To determine the appropriate seat height, have someone hold the bike steady while you sit in a comfortable riding position with your hands on the handlebars. Pedal backwards so that one of your feet is at the bottom of the down stroke; in that position, your knee should be slightly bent, while the thigh of your other leg should be about parallel to the top tube. If you adjust the seat, adjust the handlebars, too.

After a long uphill climb on a bike, don't coast downhill without pedaling. As you climb up the hill, lactic acid builds up in your muscles and can contribute to muscle soreness; by pedaling lightly but constantly while coasting downhill (even if there's little resistance), you can help remove the lactic acid.

Racing and touring models are still popular, however. These bikes typically have sturdy but lightweight frames and are usually equipped with drop handlebars that can help alleviate stress on your back.

Prices for bikes vary depending upon their construction, weight, quality of components, and workmanship; well-made bikes start at around $300. Whatever type of bike you choose, it's important that the frame fit you properly; otherwise you can develop muscle soreness in your neck, lower back, and legs (see above).

Tips on pedaling and form

Many inexperienced cyclists think that the higher the gear you ride in, the better the workout. But, in fact, riding in very high gear, which increases the force you need for pedaling, can lead to overuse injuries such as biker's knee (a generic term usually referring to pain around or under the kneecap). Pushing hard on the pedals also puts a lot of stress on the sole of the foot, and may interfere with blood circulation in leg muscles. But pedaling fast at a very low gear (one with low resistance) may not be preferable since your muscles have to contract quickly, which can lead to muscle soreness.

•Studies have found that the optimal cadence for most cyclists is 60 to 80 rpm (revolutions per minute), though racers cycle in the range of 80 to 100 rpm and, when they sprint, even faster. Optimal cadence does vary somewhat from person to person, depending on training level, speed, and the use of accessories like toe clips.

•Save high gears for level terrain, and the highest gears for riding downhill or with a good tail wind. Use very low gears if you're climbing steep grades, carrying heavy gear, or if you have a knee problem that's aggravated by strenuous cycling.

You can better maintain a constant pedaling effort if your riding posture is both comfortable and efficient. When you ride, bend from the waist but don't slouch; your back should be slightly curved, not hunched (see illustration on page 255).

•Don't ride in the racing "drop" position (with your hands on the curved parts of the handlebars) for any extended period of time. Although this position does make you a bit more aerodynamic and thus makes your pedaling more efficient, it may cramp your hands and shoulders. Instead, switch hand positions frequently to the tops of the handlebars.

•Keep your arms relaxed, and don't lock your elbows. This technique helps you to absorb bumps from the road better. Also, when you see bumps ahead in the road, raise your buttocks slightly off the seat—this will prevent painful bouncing.

•Wear shoes with rigid soles. These allow for more efficient pedaling, since they transmit more power to the pedals.

Cycling Helmets

Experts from the American Academy of Pediatrics, the National Safety Council, the Bicycle Federation of America are unconditionally in favor of helmets. Reasons for not wearing helmets are usually based on aesthetics or comfort. But such objections don't hold up considering the attractive lightweight designs now approved by the American National Standards Institute (ANSI) or the Snell Memorial Foundation, whose test standards are accepted nationwide.

Choosing a helmet
Helmets keep getting lighter. Conventional helmets with a hard outer shell and an energy-absorbing interior made of polystyrene foam liner weigh a pound or less. Ultralight models weigh as little as seven ounces; they are made of very dense foam and have no outer shell, which makes them cool and comfortable. However, such helmets may be less able to withstand daily wear and tear than helmets with hard outer shells. And some research suggests that, in the event of a head-first crash, the foam may grip or stick to the ground temporarily, increasing the risk of serious neck injuries. In contrast, a helmet with a hard shell slides along the pavement.

Fortunately, there are also many thin-shell foam models, which combine the best aspects of foam and hard-shell designs. The smooth protective covering should reduce the helmet's grip on the ground in case of a crash.

Whichever style you choose, check for the ANSI approval sticker. This tells you that the helmet meets reasonable laboratory standards for absorbing severe blows. An ANSI sticker

should be adequate for most cyclists. A Snell sticker means the helmet meets even stricter standards (though it has not been proven this makes the helmet any safer).

Helmets should be replaced every five years. The plastics used in both their inner and outer layers deteriorate under the stress of weather and hard knocks. If you have an accident, send your helmet to the manufacturer for inspection—many manufacturers will replace damaged helmets free of charge. Or replace it yourself. A good helmet may cost from forty to seventy dollars.

Shopping tips
When you buy a helmet, look for the same features for yourself and your children:

Shock absorbency. The liner is as important as the shell. A good liner should be at least half an inch thick and made from crushable expanded polystyrene (the foam used for picnic coolers and packing material). Although it is stiff, it will give under impact, absorbing the shock of a collision or fall.

Comfort and fit. You (and your child) are less likely to wear an uncomfortable helmet. Sponge-rubber or fabric pads should hold the helmet firmly to your head. The helmet should allow for good ventilation, which is crucial on summer days.

Impenetrability. A rigid outer shell can stand up to abrasion and collision with sharp, hard objects like car doors and handles. The usual materials are polycarbonate or fiberglass.

Security. A snug-fitting chin strap, fastened with a D-ring or buckle, will keep the helmet from flying off.

Helmets—a must
Helmets should be a must for everyone—and especially children. In a nationwide survey undertaken by the U.S. Consumer Product Safety Commission, 71 percent of the injured riders were under age fifteen. Moreover, 50 percent of the injuries suffered by children under age ten involved the head or face, compared with 19 percent for riders age ten or older. (About 62 percent of all bicycle-related deaths in the U.S. involve head injuries.)

According to two recent case-control studies, wearing a helmet decreases the risk of head injury by 63 to 85 percent. Yet based on the CPSC survey findings, an estimated 76 percent of all riders (who number about 67 million) never or almost never wear helmets. Helmet use was lowest for children ages eleven to fourteen.

Defensive riding

When you ride outdoors, road conditions, traffic, and weather can pose potential hazards. Bicycling is generally a safe activity, but more than 1,000 people die annually in the United States because of cycling accidents. Here are steps you can take to improve cycling safety:

- Always wear a helmet: this is the most important precaution a cyclist can take.
- When cycling at night or when visibility is poor, wear brightly colored, reflective clothing—in fact, this is good advice at any time—and use your headlight if you have one.
- Don't wear headphones. They can block out most of the street sounds you need to hear to ride defensively. That's why wearing headphones while cycling is a misdemeanor in some municipalities.
- Don't wear a heavy backpack. It can throw you off balance. Carry necessities in baskets, handlebar or seat bags, fanny packs, or panniers (side pouches made especially for bicycles).
- Use hand signals. This will allow the drivers of the cars around you to predict your actions.
- Learn to change gears without taking your eyes off the road so that you won't swerve into traffic.
- Watch out for storm drains, cattle guards (for country riders), and railroad tracks. They're all slippery when wet. And if you don't cross them at the right angle, your front tire may get caught, causing you to be thrown off your bike.
- Don't ride side by side with another cyclist.

Braking

- For most road conditions, use both brakes; using one or the other alone can be hazardous. Remember that each of the two hand brakes has a specific function. The front brake (the left lever) has the power to stop you more quickly than the back (the right lever) and, given enough pressure, can throw you over the handlebars. The back brake, with strong pressure, may cause the bicycle to skid.
- Brake with your hand at the end of the lever. This will allow you to exert optimal pressure.
- Don't brake abruptly when it starts to rain, since roads are especially slippery.
- On long, steep downhills, as well as in wet weather, it is safest to "feather" the brakes—that is, gently tap the brakes, applying intermittent pressure.
- For a quick stop, as you firmly press the brakes, slide your buttocks to the very back of the saddle. This will keep the rear of the bike down so that you don't flip over the handlebars. Be careful not to jam the brakes, however, or you may lose control of the bike.

Bicycle touring

As growing numbers of long-distance cyclists are discovering, bicycling allows you to combine an excellent form of exercise with a wonderful way to travel—to see the world up close, meet new people, and enjoy the flora, fauna, and geology of whichever area you choose to tour.

Any reasonably healthy person with some experience in ordinary cycling can, after a few weeks of conditioning exercises, be prepared to tour. Cycling a few miles a day several times a week will build up your speed and endurance. Increase

Biking indoors

A stationary exercise bike is an excellent conditioning tool. Not only is it convenient, but it also allows you to vary the intensity of your workout by simply adjusting the resistance of the metal flywheel at the front. The two keys for choosing a good exercise bike are a heavy flywheel, which ensures smooth pedaling, and a comfortable seat. In the long run, a more expensive bike is a better investment than a bottom-of-the-line model. A wobbly bike that's hard to pedal will only make you quickly give up your exercise program.

Some models have an ergometer, which calculates your work output in watts or calories (though you should still monitor your heart rate). Recumbent models let you sit back in a chairlike seat with your feet in front of you; this puts less strain on your back, neck, and shoulders.

your goals 5 to 10 percent each week until you can comfortably cover the average daily distance anticipated on your bicycle-touring itinerary. When road workouts are not practical, a reasonable alternative is the stationary bicycle, which should be ridden several times a week for thirty to forty-five minutes. Precede every workout with warm-up exercises and conclude with cool-downs.

Tips for touring

Saddle soreness often waylays the best-prepared touring cyclist. To minimize discomfort on long rides, ride on an anatomically comfortable, padded bicycle seat, and wear shorts that do not bunch up or have seams where you sit. Take great care to set the seat and handlebars to your particular body proportions. The seat should be level, or only slightly tilted up or down, and at a height that permits your legs to be slightly bent at the bottom of the down stroke when your feet are positioned properly on the pedals, thereby lessening the strain on knee joints. Drop bars, which offer three grip positions for your hands, allow you to change your upper-body position frequently, thus minimizing back and neck strain.

Footgear. Select a cycling shoe with a stiff sole that spreads the pressure of the pedal across the length of the foot. Shoes should also be comfortable for walking, have plenty of toe room, and soft, well-ventilated uppers. For maximum riding efficiency, equip pedals with toe clips that hold shoes firmly in place.

Gloves. These decrease pressure on the hands, which can cause numbness in riders who do not relax their grip. Gloves also reduce scrapes in case of falls. They should be padded, well ventilated, and made of a fast-drying material.

Helmets. A cycling helmet is a must (see page 257). Your helmet should also offer good peripheral vision, ventilation, light reflectance, and a visor. Shatterproof, tinted goggles or sunglasses to protect eyes from stones or other debris thrown up from the road and to reduce sun glare are another piece of safety gear no touring cyclist should fail to wear.

Lastly, riders should equip themselves with some means of carrying essentials, such as a bag (pannier) or carrying rack. Properly distributed over the front and rear wheels, racks will permit you to carry comfortably thirty to thirty-five pounds of clothing, a water bottle, food, bike and tire repair tools, first-aid equipment, maps, flashlights, camera gear, and sunscreen.

For your first long-distance trip, consider joining an organized tour with an experienced leader. Chances are you'll have more fun, and should you need it, there will be moral and mechanical support in the event of a breakdown. Your local bike shop and biking magazines can steer you to a list of congenial tours and touring organizations.

Ice Skating

Ice skating is an exhilarating winter activity that can be enjoyed by young and old alike. It is an excellent aerobic sport that markedly increases flexibility and uses more muscle groups than running. The stroking motion over the ice strengthens the calves, quadriceps, buttocks, and abdomen, while the back, neck, and shoulders are worked to control the position of the upper body. Surprisingly, despite the potential for falls, skating is also relatively safe, having one of the lowest injury

Adapting your own bike

If you already have a conventional bicycle, you can convert it into an indoor exercise bike—one that you know will be comfortable—and you will pay far less than you would for a good store-bought stationary bike. One option is to purchase a device outfitted with rollers that supports your bike while allowing you to pedal; you can adjust the rollers as well as the gears on your bike to control the resistance. You can also buy a wind-load simulator, which is a round, cage-like device that simulates the wind resistance of actual outdoor bicycling. You put your regular bike on a frame with the simulator; then the harder you pedal, the greater the resistance, just as if you were pedaling into the wind.

rates of any sport. And with indoor rinks, it is possible to skate year round under nearly ideal, controlled conditions.

Most indoor rinks also rent skates, sharpen dull blades, and provide instruction for those whose legs are still a bit shaky—though skating is not a hard sport to learn. Most people find that within their first few hours on the ice, they have mastered enough of the basics to both enjoy the sport and reap the principal benefits from it. Older people learning to skate for the first time or starting again after a long hiatus should take care in developing their skills. This applies especially to postmenopausal women, who may be at greater risk of incurring bone fractures. They should learn under the supervision of a careful instructor, and they should wear protective padding until they improve their sense of balance.

Equipment

Good skates are important. While beginning skaters often complain of weak ankles, their wobbliness is more likely due to loose, poorly fitted skates or worn-out skates that no longer offer support, rather than to inherent muscle weakness. A good pair of ice skates costs at least $100. So before rushing out and buying a pair, or attempting to salvage grandpa's rusted classics from the basement, you may want to experiment with rental skates until you've developed a feel for the sport.

Skate boots should hug your feet, especially around the ankle, and fit snugly without bunching up your toes. (Be sure to try on skates with the socks you will wear skating; thin socks made from Orlon or other synthetics that "wick" away moisture from skin are best.) Arch and toe areas should have padded support, and the tongue should be well padded. Blades should be good-quality tempered steel and be kept sharpened at all times: dull, rusty blades will not only slow you down, they'll make you fall. Lace your skates so that the toe area is loose enough for your toes to move freely, but so that the area across the instep of your foot is tight and the top of the boot is snug enough to provide support and comfort.

Slacks and sweaters that are warm without being bulky are good choices for skating apparel. But since most skating injuries involve the hands—scrapped or sprained while shielding against falls—the most important piece of clothing the skater should wear is a good pair of gloves.

Beginning technique

While the skating motion does not exactly resemble walking, skating does become a simple matter of transferring the body weight from one foot to the other in a rhythmic fashion. The trick is in learning to glide. As you gain confidence on the ice, lower your center of gravity over the foot you glide forward on, gracefully "squatting" into each stride. With practice and perhaps a few lessons from a good instructor, you'll soon be zooming around the rink, taking sometimes as few as two strides to glide from one end of the ice to the other.

A thorough loosening of stiff muscles before skating will help prevent injury and greatly increase your enjoyment of the sport. Pay particular attention to stretching your Achilles tendons and the muscles of your calves. While it may not be possible for you to skate often enough to maintain a high level of fitness, ice skating—as a supplementary aerobic exercise—can provide a refreshing change of pace for a runner or cyclist—or a family outing—during inclement winter weather.

Wind chill

Ice skaters, as well as skiers and runners, can create their own wind chill. Skating at ten miles per hour in 20°F weather is the equivalent of standing still at 4°. If you move into the wind, it is even colder. Therefore, when possible, run or skate away from the wind. If you must face into the wind on a cold day, be sure to cover exposed flesh, including earlobes and nose, and be on the lookout for frostbite.

In-Line Skating

Probably no recreational exercise has so quickly gained in popularity as skating on streamlined skates that are a cross between roller skates and ice skates. They're called in-line skates because they have three to five donut-shaped wheels in a single row, rather than the two parallel pairs of wheels on conventional roller skates. They're sometimes called Rollerblades, but that's actually the trade name of the leading manufacturer of these skates. Whatever skate you use, conventional or in-line, it's easy to get a good workout, particularly if you've ever ice skated.

Vigorous roller skaters can burn 600 calories or more per hour and get a substantial aerobic workout, which helps strengthen the cardiovascular system. Roller skating, like ice skating, also strengthens hip and leg muscles as well as back and arm muscles, depending on how much you swing your arms. As far as injuries go, there is good and bad news: roller skating is a low-impact sport that's far less likely to lead to overuse injuries than, say, jogging. But the chance of hurting yourself in a fall or crash is much greater—though you can protect yourself somewhat.

Unlike the relatively heavy leather boot of regular skates, the boot of the in-line skate is usually made of lightweight plastic or nylon. Some plastic models have a support system resembling that of a ski boot: there's a hinged upper cuff for forward flexibility, yet good lateral support to prevent twisting at the ankle. Because of this lateral stiffness, you must rely more on your leg muscles to make turns than you would with regular skates.

You can go faster with in-line skates, since their smooth narrow polyurethane wheels create less friction against the ground than conventional wide wheels; they're also easier to maneuver. And while most conventional skates have a brake at the front, in-line models usually have rear braking devices. Because in-line skating uses many of the same muscles—and a similar technique—as cross-country skiing and ice skating, many skiers, ice skaters, and hockey players do it as part of their training regimen. Skating is also a good sport to alternate with other sports, such as running, cycling, or swimming, for a more varied exercise schedule.

Getting started—safely

In-line skates tend to be more expensive than conventional models—about $100 up to $300 a pair—so it's wise to rent them first to see if you really like them. Make sure that you also rent (and later buy) elbow and knee guards as well as wrist protectors to prevent the most common types of skating injuries—especially if you're inexperienced. It's also important to wear a lightweight bike helmet.

•When it comes to purchasing skates, you can choose boots with four wheels, which provide good balance and traction and are perfectly suited for all skaters. More experienced skaters often opt for five-wheeled models, which afford a smoother ride on rough pavement, making it easier to maintain speed, but lack the side-to-side turning ability of four-wheel models.

•*The injury rate is highest for people skating for the first time.* Though you may teach yourself in-line skating—especially if you've ever ice skated or roller skated—you might consider taking a few lessons in an indoor rink at first, in order to learn proper technique and how to fall safely. (You'll be taught, for instance, not to use your arms to cushion your fall, since this only increases your risk of injury, but to roll onto your shoulders.)

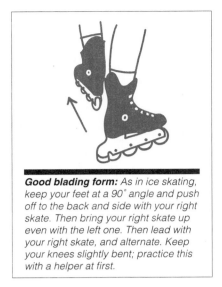

Good blading form: *As in ice skating, keep your feet at a 90° angle and push off to the back and side with your right skate. Then bring your right skate up even with the left one. Then lead with your right skate, and alternate. Keep your knees slightly bent; practice this with a helper at first.*

•Learning how to slow down and stop is the most important element in skating—it takes some practice, so go slow until you master it.

•For safety's sake, skate in an area free of traffic, crowds, debris, and surface irregularities. Start on flat surfaces: one recent study found that three out of four injuries occurred on sloped surfaces. Avoid surfaces with sand, water, gravel, dirt, snow, or ice. And don't skate at night. In addition to your having difficulty seeing and avoiding obstacles, it will be difficult for motorists to see you.

•When you're first getting used to in-line skates, start by balancing on a grassy surface (you can try holding onto a friend who's not wearing skates). Your weight should rest on the balls of your feet. Practice transferring your weight from one foot to the other, since you propel yourself by alternately pushing off toward the sides (see illustration). Keep your weight forward and your knees slightly bent. If you lose your balance, crouch a bit, which will lower your center of gravity.

Jumping Rope

As aerobic exercise became a byword in the 1980s, rope jumping came into its own—a sport for all seasons and both sexes. The only equipment it requires is a rope, and it's easy to learn. You can jump rope almost anywhere, any time. Like running, cycling, and swimming, it helps builds endurance and provides aerobic benefits. You may have heard claims that ten minutes of rope skipping equals thirty minutes of jogging. That's not true, but jumping rope can be just as strenuous as jogging. Nor is it true that jumping rope provides a full-body workout—the range of motion is too limited. But it's still a good cardiovascular workout with these benefits:

•It's a good calorie-burner. If you weigh 150 pounds and jump at a beginning rate of seventy skips per minute, you'll burn 11 calories a minute. This is equivalent to running at a speed of approximately six miles per hour or cycling at thirteen miles per hour.

•It's lower in impact and less hard on the knees than running, since you should jump no more than an inch off the ground.

•It's a good "fall-back" activity for people who usually exercise outdoors. If the weather is terrible, you can jump rope instead of jogging, walking, or playing tennis outdoors.

Getting started

If you've been relatively sedentary and are just starting to jump rope, start out at about seventy rope-turns a minute, which allows you to double-hop each jump. There are two basic ways to jump: on one foot at a time or both feet together. As you get accustomed to double-hopping at a moderate pace, gradually increase the pace. Another way to vary your routine is to go from a front swing to a back swing. You can jump in place or move around the area. Try jumping while you're watching television or listening to music.

If you are increasing speed and intensity, monitor your heart rate by stopping for ten seconds to check your pulse (multiply by six to get your rate per minute), since jumping rope can elevate your heart rate very quickly. Slow down if you get winded or too tired. As with any extended exercise, it's wise to start with a five-minute warm-up and end with a cool-down period.

Another tip: when you turn the rope, use your wrists and forearms. Don't turn from the shoulders. And remember your feet: don't jump on your toes. Let your heel help absorb the impact and keep your knees slightly bent. Your knees may not be taking a beating, but your feet and calves may be. It's not a good idea to jump rope every day. Do other exercises on alternate days—cycling, walking, swimming.

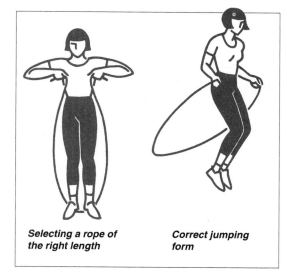

Selecting a rope of the right length

Correct jumping form

Does table tennis provide a workout?

For average players, a swift game of singles table tennis burns about 350 to 450 calories per hour, about the same as brisk walking, doubles tennis, or cycling at six to eight miles per hour. It also helps improve agility and coordination, and its stroking action may increase flexibility and strength in the upper body. The key to making table tennis a workout is to keep moving. Try to keep the ball in play constantly; try not to pause between points. Also, push yourself; reach, bend, and stretch for every shot. It helps if you can play with someone who is slightly above your own skill level.

Equipment

Besides a pair of good supportive shoes (the kind designed for aerobic dance is best), you'll need a rope. Make sure the handles fit comfortably in your hands, and be sure the rope turns easily at the handle—those with ball bearings work well. Cotton ropes are cheap and probably the best; synthetics and rope made of plastic beads are all right, too, though they may sting more if the rope hits your leg.

Check the rope's length. Stand on the center of the rope and pull the handles up the sides of your body: they should come just up to your armpits (see illustration above). Some ropes come with instructions for adjusting the length.

It is best to jump on the kind of wood floor you'll find at a gym or health club, but a lawn or a mat works well, too. Carpets are fine, but a thick one may throw your timing off. Concrete is too hard and may increase the risk of injury, but if your shoes are good enough you should be able to jump anywhere.

Racquet Sports

More than thirty million Americans play a racquet sport regularly. Chasing a ball around a squash, tennis, or racquetball court is an excellent way to develop agility and coordination, but can it promote cardiovascular fitness? In the past, the stop-and-go nature of these activities led many researchers to believe that the aerobic benefits were few and far between. Yet studies that looked at tennis players, for instance, found them to be a fit bunch—lean and aerobically well conditioned. Could it be that these sports attract people who are already fit? Such questions have prompted researchers to look more closely at the physiological effects of racquet sports and conclude that racquet sports can indeed produce aerobic benefits similar to those of running, but these depend completely on which game you choose and how you play it.

The aerobic benefits derived from a racquet sport depend upon how long you play, how skillful you are, how hard you push yourself, how long the ball is in play, and how quickly you retrieve the ball. Two basic requirements: to get an aerobic workout from any racquet sport, you must play vigorously enough to raise your heart to its training rate for twenty minutes at least three times a week. And you should play with an opponent who is at your level of skill and fitness so that you'll have extended volleys.

Tennis

As exercise, tennis is less demanding aerobically than squash or racquetball: just watch a recreational tennis player sometime and estimate how much of the time he is inactive. Some studies have shown that tennis players reach their optimum exercise heart rates and maintain them despite the stop-and-go action, while other studies have found that tennis players hardly give their hearts a workout at all. One thing is sure: doubles tennis generally does little to promote cardiovascular fitness. In recreational doubles, your heart rate stays relatively low, and your caloric expenditure is much less (averaging 300 calories per hour for doubles versus 450 per hour for singles). After all, you're covering only half the court in doubles and the ball is in play less. Competitive tennis is another matter: professional tennis players can burn over 600 calories per hour during a match.

If tennis is your game, stick to singles. You can also turn the game into a better workout by trying the following techniques:

•Run as hard, as far, and as constantly as you can. Run to get behind the ball, which will increase the power of your shot. Sprint to the net for volleying shots. Run down every ball, even the wide ones you think you can't reach. And after a point, run after the ball to retrieve it.

•Exaggerate bending, reaching, and stretching. Put all of your torso into forehand and backhand shots; bend at the knees and then rise up to meet low shots; and stretch high for serves and overhead slams. These full-body strokes may also help prevent tennis elbow, the foremost injury of tennis players (see page 419).

•Play shadow tennis. Developed by former Davis Cup captain Dennis Ralston, shadow tennis is like shadow boxing; you play against an imaginary opponent, without actually hitting the ball. Work out a sequence of strokes that mixes up lobs and volleys and forces you to race around the court. Keep moving, bending, and reaching as you would in a game. Begin playing shadow tennis for one-minute stints and work up to five minutes. This not only conditions you but also makes an excellent pregame warm-up.

Squash and racquetball

Both of these games are usually faster paced than recreational tennis because the courts are contained by walls; this keeps the ball in play and minimizes the time between points. Thus, studies show that players can maintain a heart rate more than high enough for aerobic conditioning, and burn 600 to 850 calories per hour, with racquetball being slightly less demanding than squash. One study at the University of Manitoba in Canada looked at the effects on aerobic capacity in novice racquetball players. The men in the study, who played for an hour three times a week, had a

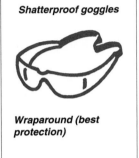

Shatterproof goggles

Wraparound (best protection)

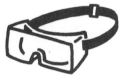

Protectors for people wearing glasses

Conventional type (poor protection at sides)

Open-type empty frame (poor protection)

significant increase in maximum oxygen consumption (a measure of aerobic fitness) as well as a decrease in percentage of body fat. The women in the study, however, showed no significant improvement in fitness level; the researchers suggested that the reason for this was that they played only twice a week.

If you're used to leisurely tennis, the additional aerobic demands of squash or racquetball may well leave you feeling winded at first. You can prepare yourself by cycling, running, or jumping rope several times a week.

You should also purchase—and use—a pair of eye protectors. Because of its speed (up to 140 miles per hour), a racquetball or squash ball can seriously damage an eye. Or, in the heat of the game, it is all too easy to get hit with an opponent's racquet, particularly a squash racquet (which has a long neck). Get protectors with plastic shields over the eyes. Some models are simply empty frames, and racquetballs have been known to squeeze through these frames. Regular eyeglasses, even those with shatterproof lenses, are no protection.

Rowing

Among the very fittest of all athletes are members of the Olympic rowing teams. They use more muscles—not only the arms, but also the legs, abdomen, and torso—and burn more calories than anyone else except cross-country skiers. They get all the aerobic benefits of running in a workout that also effectively builds muscular strength and endurance. At the same time, rowing is a relatively stress-free exercise. The joint and muscle problems that can trouble runners are not evident among people who row regularly, and rowing also puts little strain on the back; indeed, sports physicians often prescribe it for people with lower back and disk problems. (Rowing can, however, aggravate some types of back conditions, so check with your physician if you have back trouble. People with heart trouble should also approach rowing cautiously, since it sends up the heart rate rapidly.)

Rowing machines
You can spend up to $2,000 for a rowing machine, but a satisfactory model can be purchased for $300 to $400. A good machine will mimic a real scull. The machine will have two handles (oars) rigged with adjustable (usually hydraulic) pistons to provide variable resistance as you pull against the handles. It will have a

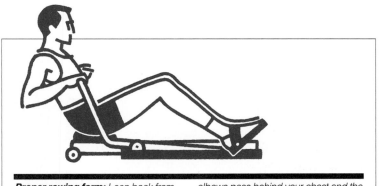

Proper rowing form: Lean back from your hips, pushing back with your legs and torso. Bend your arms until your elbows pass behind your chest and the handles are an inch from your stomach. Keep your back straight throughout.

comfortable padded or contoured seat that slides on rollers or ball bearings back along the stationary frame. It will usually have footrests that rotate as you push backward with your legs and straps to hold your feet firmly in position.

The fanciest machines have ergometers that read out your speed, distance, and even calories burned during your workout. Some larger models have a flywheel instead of hydraulic pistons to provide resistance, on the theory that a flywheel more closely resembles the feel of a real scull because it has a continuous momentum that approximates gliding. Less fancy but often first rate are the lightweight machines that are easy to fold up and store in a closet or put out of the way. At the least, any machine you get should sit solidly on the floor, not wobble or "jump" as you row. Its seat and oars should move smoothly and not stick. Some machines have a single bar to pull back on instead of two handles; either one of these designs is acceptable.

Whether you use a rowing machine or a real shell, you can begin your workouts by performing sets of strokes with the sliding seat in different positions—a routine that helps establish your sense of rhythm and also warms up the right muscles. Row for two minutes using a quarter of the slide on each stroke, then another two or three minutes using three quarters of the slide, before going on to use the full slide. And make sure your legs, not your back, power the rowing motion.

Running

For overall fitness, running is one of the easiest and least expensive activities. Running is *the* aerobic sport, and the one by which every other aerobic fitness program is measured. Running for half an hour three or four days a week will provide excellent fitness benefits very rapidly. It quickly increases the fitness of the cardiovascular system—as shown by decreased heart rate and blood pressure. Running is also good as part of a weight-reduction program, since a runner can burn an impressive 400 calories in half an hour.

One great advantage of running over other sports is that it is accessible to virtually everyone. People of any age can run, it can be done almost anyplace, and it requires a relatively small outlay of money—well-fitting running shoes will be your chief expense. You can pass up all the costly clothes and other paraphernalia.

Because Americans are obsessed with speed and distance, many people think that the best way to run is fast and far. They start off at full speed, and when they find they can't sustain it for more than a mile, they quit. Actually, you get a far greater fitness benefit from running at a moderate pace for thirty minutes than by gunning it for fifteen. And there is no need to become obsessed about piling up mileage day after day. Dr. Kenneth Cooper, president of the Aerobics Center in Dallas, Texas, recommends running four times a week; that is sufficient for building and maintaining aerobic fitness.

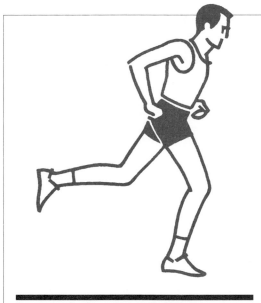

Proper running form: Stand tall with head up, eyes ahead, back straight, chest high, hips forward, arms and hands relaxed. Land on your heels to put less strain on feet and legs.

Guidelines for running
The best way for people who are out of shape to start a running program is to walk; otherwise, your muscles and tendons become sore and still.

•At a brisk pace, walk nonstop for thirty to forty-five minutes three days a

The Right Running Shoes

A study at Tulane University found that all running shoes, regardless of brand, price, or type of construction, lose about 30 percent of their ability to absorb shocks after around 500 miles of use. So if you have been experiencing aches and pains and suspect that running or another type of exercise might be the cause of this, check your shoes—you may need a new pair.

Before you discard your old shoes, however, take a good look at them. The signs of wear tell a lot about your running form, and may help explain any knee or leg pain you feel after a run. Using these clues to help select your next pair of shoes, may even prevent injuries.

Normally, when you run or walk fast, the outer part of your heel strikes the ground first, so that's where you see the most wear on your sole. Your foot then rolls inward and your weight is transferred to the inner side of the foot, causing wear on the middle of the sole in the area below the toes. The illustration at left shows areas of normal wear; the more wear, the darker the shading.

Too much rolling inward (pronation) or outward (supination) can put added strain on the feet, hips, lower legs, knees, or ankles. Many runners overpronate—that is, their feet roll too far inward—and your shoes may indicate to what extent you are doing this. When checking the signs of wear on your old shoes, here's what to look for:

Outer-sole. People who roll their feet outward (for instance, those with high arches) tend to wear down the outer side of the heel, while people who roll inward (such as those with flat feet) show more wear on the inner side. Such signs of wear are usually accompanied by damage inside the shoe, thus further reducing shock absorption and increasing stress on the lower leg and foot.

Mid-sole. This shock-absorbing layer between the outer-sole and insole can usually be seen from the side of the shoe. If one side is more compressed than the other, the mid-sole may absorb shock poorly, which could lead to foot instability and an ankle sprain or stress fracture. Rolling inward on your feet may severely compress the inside edge of the mid-soles. If your mid-soles are excessively or unevenly worn, look for firmer ones in your next shoes—and be sure to replace your shoes more frequently.

Heel counter. This rigid section at the back of the shoe stabilizes the heel. Look at the shoe from behind—does the counter bulge or lean to one side? Runners who roll their feet outward tend to force an outward bend on the counter, thus destabilizing the heel.

Upper. If both sides of the shoe extend beyond the sole, the shoe may have been too small for you. If the upper portion hangs over the sole on one side, the basic shape of the shoe (called the last) may be wrong for your foot. People who roll inward when they run need extra support on the shoe's inner side, which can be provided, in part, by a straight last. (To find a straight last, look at the soles—left and right soles should be almost indistinguishable.) In contrast, if you have high arches and your foot rolls outward, a curved last will conform better to the shape of your foot and give better support. If there's a hole or tear over the big toe, the shoe was probably too small. There should be one-half inch of space between your longest toe and the tip of the shoe when you put all your weight on that foot.

Shopping tips

• If you have an old pair of running shoes, take them with you when you shop for a new pair; a knowledgeable salesperson can evaluate the wear pattern to help you choose a suitable shoe. Run around in the store. Remember to wear your running socks.

• Examine new shoes carefully. Make sure they are the same length and width. Put the shoes side by side on a flat surface and look at them from behind: the uppers should be perpendicular to the sole; they should not lean to one side.

• Hold onto the front and back of the shoe and try to bend it. It should bend where the foot bends—at the ball; if the shoe bends at midfoot, it will offer little support. It shouldn't bend too easily or be too stiff. Also, hold the heel and try to move the counter: it shouldn't move from side to side.

• In general, if your foot rolls outward significantly when you run (supination), you're probably better off with a shoe with a strong heel counter, a substantial yet somewhat soft midsole, a curved last, and a flexible sole. If your foot rolls inward (pronation), you might benefit from a shoe with a good arch support, a straight last, and a less flexible sole, especially along the inside edge.

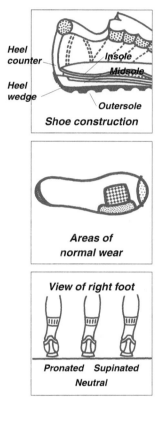

Heel counter / Insole / Midsole / Heel wedge / Outersole

Shoe construction

Areas of normal wear

View of right foot

Pronated   Supinated
Neutral

week. As you get fitter, run for a few minutes, then walk briskly for a few more, and repeat for half an hour, increasing the running and decreasing the walking gradually until you are running steadily for half an hour.

•As you improve, don't be tempted to run too quickly: this is more likely to lead to injury than to fitness. Stay well within your target heart rate zone (see page 248). If you are running at a good pace and still have enough breath to carry on a conversation, you are probably training at the proper intensity.

•Run for time, not mileage. If you aim to run three miles at each session, you will probably run the same course again and again, and you may also try to run it as fast as possible. If you run for a set period of time, though, you can be creative about your route and maintain a reasonable pace.

Some precautions

If you want to increase your distance and running time, keep in mind that running more than twenty miles a week does not greatly increase your aerobic fitness, but it does increase your chance of injury. Running places harsh stresses on the legs and feet. Avoid hard surfaces and excessive downhill running—and whenever you experience a recurring pain, take heed.

Many injuries occur because muscles are tight and joints are not prepared for stress. So before running, warm up the muscles by walking briskly and jogging slowly for ten to fifteen minutes. Then stretch, which is a crucial part of running because running tends to stiffen the muscles at the back of the leg.

It is also extremely important to know how to stop. If you stop running abruptly, you may faint or even suffer heart rhythm abnormalities because your blood pressure may drop sharply. The way to stop is gradually—cool down by slowing your pace and then walking briskly for five to ten minutes or so. If you do feel faint, don't remain standing—lie flat on your back.

If running has a drawback, it is the lack of a workout for the upper body—your arms and shoulders will not be strengthened by running. But running regularly can give you the discipline and confidence to undertake a broad program of exercise. And after a running program has gotten you into shape, you'll find that you get more enjoyment out of tennis, hiking, volleyball, and other recreations.

Swimming

Swimming calls into play nearly all the major muscle groups; it works out more than two-thirds of the body's total muscle mass, and so it places a vigorous demand on the heart and lungs, making it one of the very best aerobic exercises. It develops muscle strength and endurance and improves posture and flexibility. It does all this at the same time that the body is supported by water—and so stress is taken off the bones and joints. The buoyancy factor makes it especially good for people who are overweight, or who have leg or lower back problems. But it is good exercise for people of all ages and at all levels of proficiency.

The best stroke for achieving all the benefits of swimming is the forward crawl. The breast stroke and side stroke—which have long periods of gliding—will not achieve an aerobic effect (though they can be made more strenuous by reducing the glide phase). The breast stroke and side stroke can be used, however, as a change of

Running downhill

Contrary to popular belief, running downhill is much riskier for the joints and muscles in your feet and legs than running uphill. As you go down a hill, you speed up, your stride lengthens, and thus your impact with the ground increases. While jogging on a level surface causes your foot to strike the ground with a force equal to at least three times your body weight, running downhill can double the impact.

Because your muscles simultaneously tense up and elongate—known as "eccentric muscle contraction"—when you run downhill, there's an increased risk of muscle soreness later. Your distorted gait can also leave you with "runner's knee," a pain behind the kneecap.

To avoid injury, never run straight down a steep hill. Walk down it. Or run down in a zigzag pattern, leaning slightly forward and keeping your knees bent.

pace between laps of the crawl, as can the back stroke. Synchronized swimming may look aerobic, but it is too stately to be aerobically beneficial.

Swimming and target heart rate

For reasons that physiologists don't yet understand, studies have shown that people have a lower maximum heart rate when swimming than when running. So if swimming is your means of training, this difference—averaging thirteen beats per minute—must be subtracted from the age-related maximum heart rate (220 minus your age). Thus, a forty-year-old swimmer would subtract forty *plus* thirteen from 220 and get a maximum rate of 167, and then take 60 to 80 percent of that to get a training range of 100 to 134 beats per minute.

A swimmer's heart rate may be lower because of the body's horizontal position, which helps to distribute blood more uniformly. Also, the cool water leads to a more rapid dissipation of heat, so the heart may not have to work as hard to keep body temperature stable. And swimming depends primarily on arm movements and thus involves smaller muscle groups than does running and cycling, which depend on the large leg muscles.

Techniques for swimming faster, longer, easier

Though the crawl is a standard stroke, swimming is a very personal thing. You may have your own way of kicking or breathing, while somebody else does things very differently. One nice thing about the crawl is the room for individual variation it allows. But one problem among those who swim for fun and fitness is fatigue—that is, becoming breathless and discouraged after only a few laps. Check out your stroke by comparing it with the drawings on page 270 and then making corrections, if need be. It might also be worth asking a qualified swimming instructor for further advice.

Better breathing. Breathe only once every two or three strokes. Keep your head low, with the water between your hairline and the top of your head. To inhale, turn your head just far enough to breathe—you need not lift your mouth out of the water. As you take a breath to your right, your left arm should be fully extended, entering the water in front of you, and your right arm extended to the back. If you breathe toward the arm that's out ahead of you, you'll waste energy and your hips will tend to sink, slowing you down.

Tips: Learn to breathe on alternate sides. This will reduce shoulder tension. Begin exhaling as soon as your face is in the water. Don't try to hold your breath.

Efficient kicking. Keep your legs close together and your knees straight. Kick from your hips, not your knees. Your kicking foot should just break the surface of the water, and your toes should be pointed. *Tip: Kicking your feet out of the water will slow you down.*

Stronger stroking. Stroking is not a matter of pulling straight back. Think of your arms as propeller blades, not paddlewheels, and use your hands to trace an "S" pattern through the water. Keep your hands at an angle, just as a propeller blade is at an angle. Your hand should enter the water in front of your shoulder with the palm facing out. Then rotate your palm inward as you sweep under your head, and back outward again as your arm moves toward your hips.

The position of your arm as it rises out of the water during the recovery phase is important. Holding the arm straight will pull your hips out of position. Your

Will swimming help you lose weight?

Researchers have suggested that swimmers tend to lose less weight than would be expected from an equivalent expenditure of energy during other aerobic activity. But studies have had inconsistent results—some found that swimmers lost weight (and body fat), others that they gained a few pounds, and some that they had no change in weight. And often, if the swimmers gained weight, it was lean body mass (muscle), not fat. If your main reason for swimming is to lose weight, it's only common sense that you should also try to cut down on calories. In addition, though, make sure you swim fast. Many overweight people don't swim fast enough or long enough. At a slow pace, twenty lengths of the pool may burn only 50 calories more than just staying afloat—hardly enough to make you lose weight.

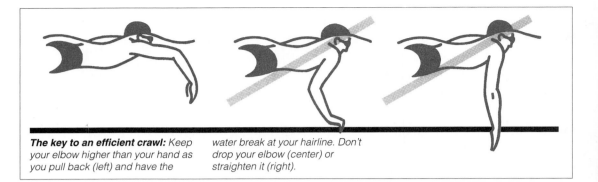

The key to an efficient crawl: *Keep your elbow higher than your hand as you pull back (left) and have the* water break at your hairline. Don't drop your elbow (center) or straighten it (right).

Choosing swimming goggles

To get a tight seal and comfortable fit, it's essential to try goggles on. Some are made to fit on the outside of the eye socket, others within it. Choose the type that feels most comfortable to you. Some goggles have a one-piece frame with no nosepiece—this may not suit a person with a wide nose bridge. But if you choose a pair with a nosepiece, make sure it does not pinch. Here are some other things to keep in mind:

•For a better seal, buy goggles with polyvinyl gaskets.

•Buy clear lenses for indoor use, tinted for outdoor use. If you'll be out in the sun, try to find lenses treated against ultra-violet rays, or have them treated by an optician. Some models have snap-out lenses, so you can change from clear to tinted.

•Buy a model with double straps, which are usually more comfortable. They are usually made of rubber.

elbow should be bent high (see illustration above). *Tip: As you pull each arm out of the water to prepare for a new stroke, keep your elbow high, but your hand close to the surface. That saves energy.*

Better body position. Don't hold your body at an angle in the water, and don't keep your head high and your back arched, as shown below. This increases drag 20 to 35 percent and will wear you out. Keep your body in a streamlined position to reduce drag. As you stroke, roll at least 45° to each side, and bring your shoulder out of the water; this will keep your hips and feet from being pulled out of line.

Tip: Move your shoulders, hips, and legs as a unit to reduce drag.

Starting a program

You can begin a swimming program easily and build to a more rigorous workout in several steps. You will want to start out with four laps of twenty-five yards each, with a rest between each lap, and gradually add laps and decrease rest intervals. Eventually you will want to swim continuously thirty to forty minutes at least three days a week. As with all exercises, your goal is to reach a level of exertion that causes your heart to pump for twenty to thirty minutes at your target heart rate.

Taking your pulse while you are swimming can be tricky. Once you are going at cruising speed, stop between laps and take your pulse for ten seconds; multiply by six to get your heart rate, and adjust your swimming accordingly. If you are counting calories, remember, it is the intensity and duration of your swimming that largely determines how many calories you burn. A 150-pound swimmer doing a brisk forward crawl will often burn as much as 11 calories per minute.

You shouldn't train in water that is too warm, since your body will have to work harder to throw off the heat generated by the exercise. Most pools used by swim teams are 70° to 73°F, but at that temperature you need to keep moving to stay warm.

Swimmers are subject to some minor vexations. Chlorine will make your hair dry and brittle, so it is wise to wear a bathing cap in the pool. A shower after swimming in a pool or the ocean is a must. Both chlorine and salt dry out the skin. If your skin does get dry, rub moisturizing lotion into it while it is still wet.

Infection of the ear canal is another common problem for swimmers. This can sometimes be prevented by the use of alcohol or glycerin drops after a swim. If you do get an infected ear, have it treated by a physician (see page 347).

Goggles will reduce the risk of eye problems due to chlorine, salt, sand, and microorganisms—and also make it easier to see. It may take some effort to find goggles that fit properly, but it's worth the trouble (see marginal at left).

Should babies learn to swim?

Water programs designed to give babies and toddlers a head start in learning to swim and in water safety are enjoying increasing popularity around the country. Such programs should be well supervised. Perhaps the greatest risk is the misconception that children who learn to swim as toddlers are "drownproof." Children who can paddle around a pool will not necessarily be able to swim if they fall into the water. According to the American Academy of Pediatrics, the only way to keep children safe around the water is to supervise them. Children in boats need properly fitted flotation jackets, whether they can swim or not.

Particular attention should be paid to pool cleanliness. If a child defecates in a pool, the stool should be removed and all swimmers should leave the pool for thirty minutes or so to give the chlorine time to kill any parasites. In addition, the American Academy of Pediatrics has proposed the following guidelines:

- A qualified instructor trained in infant CPR should be in charge.
- Each infant should be "taught" one on one by the parent or other supervisor.
- Forced total submersion is prohibited.
- All participants must shower immediately before class.
- Any child with diarrhea should be excluded until recovery.
- All children must wear training pants or plastic pants.

Open-water swimming

Surf swimming can be a great pleasure and good exercise as well, and in summertime, many people also swim in lakes, ponds, and rivers. If you're accustomed to a pool, you'll need to approach the great outdoors with somewhat more caution. About 7,000 people drown each year, most of them in lakes, rivers, and oceans rather than pools. Most of these drownings are alcohol related, so to be safe in the water keep your outing alcohol free. In addition, take the following measures:

- Don't swim alone. Stick to areas where there's a lifeguard if possible, or at the very least, go with someone who is a capable swimmer.
- Keep children under constant observation.
- Test yourself in shallow water before swimming out. The water may be colder or rougher than it looks, or there may be currents. Locate any steep drop-offs. Discover how far out you can go and still touch bottom. Check with the lifeguard, if there is one, about water conditions.
- If you want to do long-distance swimming, swim along parallel to the shore or riverbank, and not too far out.
- Backwash from waves (undertow) is of less concern for swimmers than underwater rip currents (water moving swiftly seaward, usually not more than ten or twenty feet wide). These are hard to spot and may exist even in calm-looking waters. A break in the wave pattern or discoloration (usually caused by sand) can help you spot rip currents. If you get caught in one, however, *don't struggle.* Swim with it, but angle toward the shore or bank. Or just ride the current seaward, and as soon as possible turn and swim to shore outside the current.
- Avoid weedy areas. If you do get tangled up, don't struggle. Tread water, and try to move with the current. You'll soon break free.
- If you get into any situation you're afraid you can't handle, call for help.

Finally, don't swim in waters that have not been tested for safety by the local board of health. Contamination isn't always visible to the naked eye.

Women can swim a given distance at about 30 percent lower energy cost than men, probably because women have more total body fat and that provides greater buoyancy. Also, the distribution of body fat in women allows their legs to float, making them more horizontal, and therefore more streamlined, as they move through the water.

Walking

An ideal activity for anyone who wants to get into shape, walking is accessible and convenient—you need no equipment other than comfortable shoes—and it's easy on your knees, ankles, and back. It is pleasurable, alone or with a companion. Few devotees ever get tired of it and quit. And while it's not injury-proof, the injury rate is very low. Walking is also versatile: you can vary the style, setting, and intensity of your workouts—you can even race-walk. All of this makes it an appropriate and adaptable choice for long-term exercise, even for those who are already in good physical condition.

Briskly walking at 3.5 to 4 miles an hour burns nearly as many calories as running at a moderate pace, and confers similar fitness benefits. (A woman of average size can walk comfortably at this pace, while the average-sized man can walk at 4.5 to 5 miles per hour.) As an adjunct to a low-fat diet, walking is also a good way to lose weight. In a recent national survey of people who were trying to lose weight, government researchers found that walking was more common by far than any other weight-loss activity.

Slower walking (two miles per hour) may confer some health benefits and can be advantageous for older people, cardiac patients, or people recuperating from an illness. Walking at speeds of five miles an hour can burn as many calories as moderate jogging, but even slow walking can burn 60 to 80 calories per mile.

Still, walking by itself is not enough to prevent disease. It must be combined with other good habits, such as avoiding cigarettes, controlling blood pressure, and following a prudent diet. It's important to remember, too, that in order to get the maximum benefits from exercise, it must become a long-term habit. *Walking represents a particularly effective way to develop a lifelong program of exercise.*

Tips and techniques for a walking program

If you're inactive but healthy, start with mile-long walks at a pace of three miles per hour five times a week. Over the course of a month, gradually increase your distance to three miles at a pace of four miles per hour five times a week. If you are unable to walk that fast, walk a little farther. Once your fit-

---

How Fast Do You Walk?

Many people have no idea what their pace is as they're walking. One way to measure your speed is to use a pedometer. Or you can walk on a measured track. Here is another way to get a rough estimate of your speed: count how many steps you take per minute and compare the results with this table.

WALKING SPEED CONVERSION TABLE

Steps per minute	Minutes per mile	Miles per hour
70	30	2
90	24	2.5
105	20	3
120	17	3.5
140	15	4
160	13	4.5
175	12	5
190	11	5.5
210+	less than 10	more than 6

This table is based on 2.5-foot-long stride. If your stride is closer to 3-feet long, here's an easy way to estimate your walking speed: count how many steps you take in a minute and divide this number by 30. Thus, if you are taking about 105 steps per minute, you are covering about 3.5 miles per hour.

ness has improved, it's easy to vary your walking routine—for fun and for greater fitness benefits.

Walk up and down hills. Combine hill walking with your regular flat-terrain walking as a form of interval training. You can vary the intensity of your workouts by brisk walking on level ground, then take to the hills, and finish again by walking on the flats. When walking uphill, try leaning forward slightly—it's easier on your leg muscles. Walking downhill, contrary to what you might think, can be harder on your body than walking uphill, because the downhill road can jar your joints, especially the knees, and cause muscle soreness. It may be tempting to speed downhill, but in fact it's a good idea to slow your pace slightly and take shorter steps. That way, you're less likely to end up with sore knees.

Walking uphill, by the way, burns more calories. If you weigh 150 pounds, walking at 3.5 miles an hour on flat terrain burns about 300 calories per hour. At the same pace on a gentle incline (a 4 percent grade), you burn almost 400 calories per hour. On a slightly steeper incline (an 8 percent grade), you burn nearly 500. If you're walking on a treadmill, you can elevate the grade mechanically. As you intensify your workout, do so gradually.

Choose varied terrains. Walking on grass or a gravel trail burns more calories than walking on a track. And walking on soft sand increases caloric expenditure by almost 50 percent, provided you can maintain the same pace.

Let your elbows do some walking. By swinging your arms, you'll burn 5 to 10 percent more calories and get an upper-body workout as well. Move your arms in opposition to your legs—swing your right arm forward as you step forward with your left leg. This arm movement helps counterbalance the motion of your legs. As you increase your pace, switch to pumping your arms: bend your elbows at a 90° angle and pump from the shoulder instead of the elbow joint. (This is similar to the arm position in racewalking—see page 274.) Keep your wrists straight. To reduce fatigue, keep your hands unclenched. Swing your arms in a small arc: your elbow should come forward to about the middle of your chest and as far back as your buttock.

Try striding. Lengthen your stride, swing your arms freely with increasing vigor, and aim for a faster pace (about 4.5 miles per hour)—this is called striding. As your pace increases, your feet will land closer to an imaginary center line stretching in front of you.

Take up waterwalking. Waterwalking started as rehabilitative therapy for people with injuries, and soon was recognized as a boon for everybody. You can waterwalk anywhere—along a lakeshore or beach or in a pool—without getting your hair wet or even knowing how to swim. You can even keep your hat on. If you walk at a steady pace, you can burn 300 to 500 calories per hour. Deep water provides more resistance, but you may do better in waist-high water since you won't tire so easily. Shallow water is okay, too—just walk faster and longer. Because of the water's resistance, you don't have to walk as fast in water as you would on land to burn the same number of calories. Walking two miles per hour in thigh-high water is the equivalent of walking three miles per hour on land. If you take a friend along, waterwalking can be a sociable activity.

Use hand weights—with care. Hand weights can boost your caloric expenditure, but they remain controversial (see page 251). They may alter your arm swing and thus lead to muscle soreness or even injury. They're generally not recommended for peo-

Stair climbing

Walking up several flights of stairs every day is great exercise, since your legs lift the entire weight of your body at every step. It burns extra calories, and provides an extra workout for your leg muscles. If you work or live on a high floor of a building, get off a few floors below and walk up the last flights.

You can also use stair-climbing machines, which are now found in most health clubs. It's easy to get a strenuous workout on one of these—in fact, beginners should be careful not to overexert themselves, since blood pressure and heart rate may rise quickly. Start with short steps and a slow pace. Put your entire foot on the pedal, not just the ball of your foot, and try to keep your knees aligned over your toes. For an intense workout, don't lean on the railing or front monitor, since that will reduce your energy expenditure.

ple with high blood pressure or heart disease. If you want to use them, start with one-pound weights and increase the weight gradually. The weights shouldn't add up to more than 10 percent of your body weight. Ankle weights are not recommended, as they increase the chance of injury.

Racewalking: stepping up the pace

Racewalking, a great calorie burner, turns walking into a sport. The object of racewalking is to move your body ahead as quickly as possible without running and to avoid the up/down motions of regular walking. You accomplish this with a forward-thrusting hip-swivel, which is meant to propel you more efficiently than the normal side-to-side swing of the hips. Here's how to start:

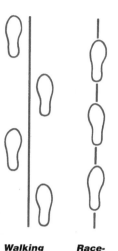

Walking   **Race-walking**

• Think of racewalking as walking a tightrope. In normal walking, your feet make parallel tracks, but in racewalking you put one foot down in front of the other, almost in a straight line. Because of anatomical differences, this form may not be completely achievable for everyone, but come as close to it as you can.

• Swing your hip forward as you step forward—it's the hips and legs that act as the propulsive force.

• Your feet should stay close to the ground, with no wasted motion. Each foot should strike the ground solidly on the back of the heel with toes pointed up slightly. Two rules of competitive racewalking are that one foot must always be on the ground, and your legs must be straight at one point in the cycle.

• Use long strides. Your motion should be fluid, efficient, and smooth.

• Bend your arms at a 90° angle, keeping your wrists straight. Pump your arms rhythmically—from the shoulder, not the elbow—with your leg motion. When you pump back, your hand should come about six inches behind the hip, while on the swing forward the wrist should be near the center of your chest. Keep your hands above your hips. The vigorous arm pumping counterbalances your leg/hip motion, allows for a quick pace, and provides a good workout for your upper body.

• Keep your torso, shoulders, and neck relaxed, and your head in line with your back. Don't bend from the waist—this can lead to back strain. Some racewalkers angle their whole bodies slightly forward when they're in motion.

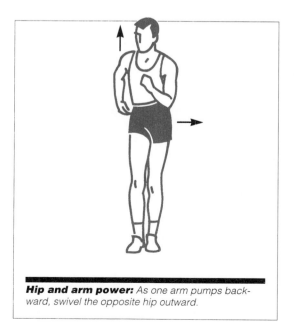

Hip and arm power: As one arm pumps backward, swivel the opposite hip outward.

Since technique is important, you will need practice. If there's an experienced racewalker around who can give you pointers, so much the better. Start with the leg movement first, build up some speed, and then incorporate the arm motion. See what a difference it makes to have your arms in the proper 90° angle position instead of hanging at your side. Your pace should quicken automatically as you learn to use your arms. Start slowly and increase your pace gradually. Try interval walking—racewalk for a few minutes, then do normal brisk walking. Pause occasionally to check your heart rate.

Hiking

Hiking along a rough but level trail expends about 50 percent more energy than walking on a paved road. Caloric expenditure and aerobic benefit increase dramatically when you hike uphill: ascending a 14° slope requires nearly four times as much effort as walking on a level surface. Hence, the caloric expenditure during a day-long hike can be considerable. A 150-pound person hiking at a normal pace for eight hours over varied terrain will use up about 3,500 calories — a thousand more than a good runner expends during a marathon. Of course, even a one-hour hike can provide a good aerobic workout. There are psychological benefits as well. Passing through beautiful scenery relaxes the mind, eases stress, and stimulates creativity.

Footwear. For light hiking on smooth trails, several manufacturers make low-cut trail shoes that weigh only a bit more than running shoes but provide better support. Sturdy leather Oxford-style shoes with a treaded rubber sole are also appropriate. For trails that are at all rough or steep, or in wet weather, ankle-high boots are best. The lightest ones are made of nylon, canvas, or breathable waterproof fabric reinforced with leather. Boots with all-leather uppers are heavier—high-top off-trail boots may weight over five pounds—but offer better support and durability in rough terrain.

Try on several models of the boot style you prefer, starting with a half-size larger than your street shoes. A laced boot should be snug across the ball of your foot and around the ankle, but with a half inch between your toes and the boot front.

Clothing and supplies. In fair weather, wear loose cotton pants and a long-sleeved cotton shirt. Since temperatures can vary abruptly even in summer, take along extra clothes that you can add in layers if you get cold.

Other basic articles for day-long hikes include a small first-aid kit (with bandages for blisters), insect repellent, a knife, a flashlight, and matches. A container of water, iced tea, or juice is essential to avoid dehydration. Carry your gear in a day pack with wide shoulder straps. Choose a size that you can load loosely; it will be more comfortable to carry than a tightly stuffed pack.

Hiking tips. Walk upright and relaxed. Your arms should swing easily, but keep shoulders, hips, and feet straight. If you are carrying a pack, lean forward slightly so that the combined weight is centered over your feet. Maintain a steady pace, even uphill; if the slope is extreme, though, pause briefly before each step, resting your weight a second on your back foot. Walk around, not on, roots, rocks, and logs, and take your time with hills—these are the spots where injuries occur. Novice hikers should take five-minute rest stops every half hour. Use the time to drink water and stretch.

Boosting the benefits. Any recreational hike will work your heart and lungs and burn off calories. But for those who want to combine the pleasures of a jaunt through the woods with the benefits of vigorous exercise, try sustained sprint-walking: on smooth stretches, alternate 100 yards of hiking with 100 yards of easy jogging. If you are going to retrace a route, hike at a leisurely pace going in, then double your pace returning. If your pack is light, add some smooth stones to increase its weight. Every seven pounds will burn off about 30 calories per hour.

Strength and Flexibility

Developing strong, flexible muscles is important for everyone, not just for athletes and body builders. Well-conditioned muscles and joints help you perform better physically, assist you in maintaining good posture, and may help prevent injuries and chronic lower-back pain.

In the 1970s and '80s, strengthening muscles was something that largely concerned only bodybuilders and was done out of vanity. But recently more and more fitness experts have been recommending strength training for health reasons—for women as well as men, the elderly as well as younger people. The American College of Sports Medicine has altered its exercise guidelines, recommending a "well-rounded" program that includes strength training along with aerobic exercise.

Benefits of strength training

Many of the declines associated with aging are the consequence of inactivity. Strength training, like aerobic exercise, can help prevent or delay many of these declines by providing the following benefits:

Quality of life. Most people start losing muscle tissue (and gain body fat) in their thirties, particularly if they are inactive. Maintaining muscle strength can have obvious benefits in your daily activities—when lifting grocery bags, gardening, or shoveling snow, for example—and give you increased stamina and self-confidence.

Strong bones. Like any exercise that puts stress on your bones, strength training may increase bone density and thus help delay or minimize osteoporosis, the loss of bone mass that makes many older people (especially postmenopausal women) vulnerable to fractures.

Injury prevention. Many musculoskeletal injuries, especially those related to exercise (such as runner's knee or shin splints), are caused in part by muscle weakness and imbalances as well as joint instability, and these conditions may be corrected by strength training.

Reduced back pain. Exercise is essential for maintaining a strong back and protecting it from injury. Lower back pain often results from weakness of back muscles as well as abdominal muscles (which help support the back). Poor posture can also contribute to back problems, and strength training may help improve posture.

Improved athletic performance. Strong muscles can help power your golf swing, for instance, or tennis serve.

Balanced fitness. Aerobic fitness is still the key to good health, but it may not be enough. Studies have found that over time people who only jog, for instance, typically lose muscle mass in the upper body. Strength training may counter this.

It's also never too late to start. Strength training can help the elderly remain active and independent. A study at Tufts University last year found that an eight-week weight-training program allowed frail ninety-year-olds to build muscle mass and thus become, as the researchers pointed out, more mobile and self-sufficient.

The following pages show you the correct way to perform basic strengthening exercises, offer guidelines on how to start a weight-training program, and show you how to test and improve your flexibility. (If you are forty-five or over, or if you have hypertension or a cardiovascular condition, it's important to consult your doctor before beginning any strengthening routines, particularly lifting weights.)

Basic Calisthenics

You can increase both the strength and endurance of your muscles with exercises that apply resistance to normal body motion. The resistance, or load, should be sufficient so that muscles contract at tensions close to maximum. You can use adjustable weights or your own body weight, but adjustable weights allow you to progressively increase the resistance as the muscles develop (see page 280). But for most people, calisthenics—such as sit-ups and push-ups—are quite effective and usually more convenient. This is the most basic type of resistance exercise, since you lift your own body weight: all you need is a padded surface to exercise on. You can also buy a slant board (for sit-ups), a chinning bar, or other inexpensive equipment to vary your routine.

Toning the abdominals

A trim waist and a flat stomach are goals that many of us yearn to achieve. Even in people who are not overweight, a few extra pounds often seem to accumulate around the midsection. Are there specific exercises that can help? Aerobics classes, for example, often begin with side bends and waist twists, which teachers and students believe will reduce their waistlines. And there are a hundred gadgets on the market that promise that if you bend at the waist often enough, you can flatten your abdomen, eliminate your "love handles," or whittle inches from your middle.

The truth may sound discouraging at first: there's no way to spot reduce. Exercising small muscle groups, such as those at the waist, won't burn the fat around those muscles. Moreover, limited exercise of this sort using only specific muscles burns fewer calories than exercising large muscles in dynamic activity. If you're really interested in shedding some fat, you have to perform aerobic exercises such as cycling, running, or brisk walking.

But fat may not be what worries you. Poor muscle tone can contribute to a flabby look, and exercise can improve muscle strength and firmness. *However, side bends and waist twists are not effective for strengthening abdominal muscles.* Neither exercise puts a great enough load on the muscles to promote toning. In side bends, gravity does most of the work. Bends and twists can stretch torso muscles, but they won't strengthen them significantly.

Sit-ups, though, can strengthen and tone three sets of abdominal muscles—the *rectus abdominus* (the long muscle running vertically down the abdomen) and the external and internal obliques (the diagonal muscles that form the letter V across the lower abdomen)—which are all otherwise hard to exercise. Even more important, sit-ups can prevent or alleviate back problems, since strong abdominal muscles provide better support for the back. Strengthening these muscles will also give you more power for running, tennis, and other activities that involve the torso.

Sit-ups to avoid. These benefits occur only when sit-ups are done correctly. *Here are some variations that are not recommended:*

• The old-fashioned straight-leg sit-ups, in which you come all the way up to a

Muscle is denser than fat, so if you lose fat tissue but add muscle, your weight may climb. However, you will probably look like you have lost weight, since muscles are firmer and more pleasing to the eye than fat, and, even though your weight may go up, your waistline may actually shrink. Furthermore, most people will not gain more than two or three pounds of muscle from body-shaping workouts.

vertical position, are a waste of effort and potentially dangerous. Keeping your legs flat on the floor arches the lower back, which overextends it and places it under stress. Also, there's no need to sit up fully, since the abdominal muscles work only during the first part of the movement. After that the hip flexor muscles (the ones that bend your leg at the hip) take over, and the shift to these muscles can pull the hip out of alignment and arch the lower back, which can cause back strain.

•Alternating bent-leg sit-ups, in which you hold one leg straight out, produce an asymmetric pull on the pelvis, so they aren't recommended.

•Using a slant board can increase the resistance of sit-ups, but many people may find sit-ups too difficult if the slant board is set at a steep angle. Moreover, because the feet are hooked under the bar of the board, leg and hip muscles can end up doing much of the work.

•Another difficult maneuver is to keep the legs straight up as you curl towards them, which keeps the abdominal muscles continually contracted. If you want to raise your legs, lean them against a wall for support, which allows the abdominal muscles to relax during the rest phase of the exercise.

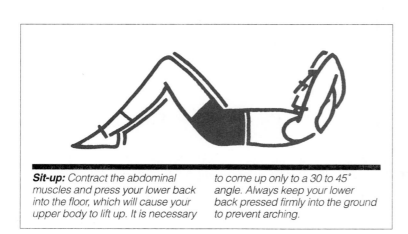

Sit-up: Contract the abdominal muscles and press your lower back into the floor, which will cause your upper body to lift up. It is necessary to come up only to a 30 to 45° angle. Always keep your lower back pressed firmly into the ground to prevent arching.

The best sit-up

The safest, most effective way to do a sit-up is to lie on your back, keeping your knees bent and feet on the floor. This works all the abdominal muscles as a group. Cross your arms behind your head with your hands placed on the opposite shoulders; this lets your arms support your head. Holding your hands behind the head or neck tends to jerk the neck and put pressure on it, possibly causing injury. It also makes you work your arms, not your abdomen.

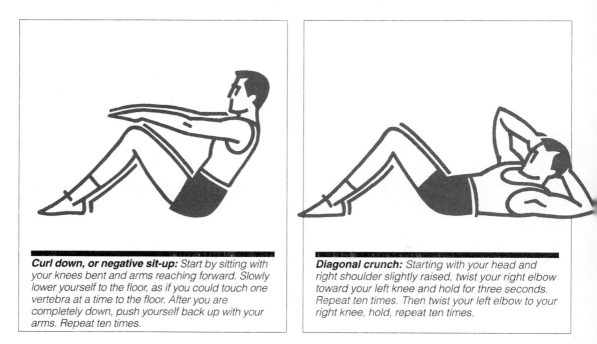

Curl down, or negative sit-up: Start by sitting with your knees bent and arms reaching forward. Slowly lower yourself to the floor, as if you could touch one vertebra at a time to the floor. After you are completely down, push yourself back up with your arms. Repeat ten times.

Diagonal crunch: Starting with your head and right shoulder slightly raised, twist your right elbow toward your left knee and hold for three seconds. Repeat ten times. Then twist your left elbow to your right knee, hold, repeat ten times.

For easier sit-ups, put your hands at your sides or folded across the chest. As the hands are brought closer to the head, the exercise becomes more difficult due to a shift in the center of gravity. If you still find this too taxing, try a *curl down*, or negative sit-up, which eases the load on your muscles because you are moving in the direction of gravity.

Beginners should start with three sets of five sit-ups with a rest between sets and gradually work up to three sets of fifteen repetitions. Those in good shape can start with sets of ten. Do these at least three times a week.

If you want to tone the muscles that shape the sides of your waist, try *diagonal crunches.* However, stop if you feel any discomfort in the lower back.

Sit-ups by themselves won't improve your posture, and bad posture can lead to back pain. To maximize the beneficial effects of sit-ups on posture, try tightening the abdominal muscles for a few seconds while standing several times a day.

Push-ups

Push-ups put off a lot of people—especially women—in part, because of their association with military basic training and a tough, macho image. In this age of Nautilus machines, push-ups may also seem old-fashioned. Yet the push-up remains one of the best upper-body exercises around, one that can be done anywhere, requires no equipment, and is easily adapted to any level of proficiency. Women in particular will find push-ups useful for strengthening their upper arm and shoulder muscles, which tend to be underdeveloped.

The standard push-up works muscles in the shoulders (deltoids), backs of upper arms (triceps), and chest (pectorals). The beauty of the push-up is that it also exercises muscles in the abdomen, hips, and back, which are tensed to keep the body stiff while it moves up and down. Aligning the body like this and contracting opposing muscle groups also helps promote good posture.

Standard push-up: Place your hands slightly wider than shoulder width, feet close together, knees locked, and arms perpendicular to the floor. Most important, hold your body in a straight line—from shoulders to ankles—throughout. Try to touch your chest to the floor for a second, but don't rest there. Go slowly. Inhaling on the way up and exhaling on the way down makes the exercise easier. Do 3 or 4 sets of as many repetitions as you can, but don't strain.

Modified push-ups

Don't give up if your arm muscles are not strong enough to lift your body at first. There are modified push-ups that let you slowly build up your muscles. By keeping your knees on the floor, for example, you will have less body weight to lift. Still, avoid the common mistake of arching your lower back and moving only your chest up and down. Always keep your torso straight and lift your body from the knees to insure that your arms receive the maximum workout and you do not strain your back.

Let-downs. The U.S. Army has been using an updated form of push-up called the "let-down" for recruits who can't manage the traditional version. It is part of the Army's "negative strength training" program that allows you to strengthen muscles without overwhelming them. The rationale behind the let-down is that it's easier to hold your body up than to lift it up. You begin in the "up" position of the standard push-up, with your arms fully extended and body straight. Slowly lower your body a few inches at a time, keeping your body aligned, until your chest is almost on the floor; this should take ten to fifteen seconds. Relax; then, using your knees, return to the starting position and repeat. In a short time, you should be able to repeat this exercise for ten to fifteen minutes.

When the let-down becomes too easy for you, move on to the standard push-up. Once proficient at that, you can increase the difficulty with various advanced push-ups. Placing your hands close together on the floor with elbows flared out emphasizes the arm (triceps) muscles. In contrast, keeping your hands far apart works the chest (pectoral) muscles more. You can also try keeping your feet on a chair or a step as you do push-ups, which places more weight on the arms. In addition to targeting specific muscle groups, a variety of push-ups also helps prevent boredom.

Strength Training with Weights

Despite the stereotype of a weight lifter—muscle-bound, hefting and grunting—training with weights can be used by everyone, not just those interested in becoming body builders. Weight training doesn't necessarily mean lifting massive weights in order to build bulging muscles. Such "power lifting" has nothing to do with fitness—and, in fact, may be injurious. Weight training, as generally recommended, calls for working out against moderate resistance in order to tone muscles and build muscle endurance. The resistance can be provided by free weights (dumbbells or barbells) or weight machines—but also thick elastic bands or even cans of tomatoes.

Not just for men
Women tend to have less muscle mass—especially in the upper body—than men because of hormonal differences, because they are smaller than men, and because of the type of activities they generally engage in. However, women who work out can gain strength at the same rate as men.

In the past many women neglected strength training because they did not want to look muscle-bound. They needn't worry. A moderate training program won't create obvious muscle bulk in men or women, but instead a firmer, trimmer physique. ("Bulking up" requires heavier weights and much more time—perhaps several hours a day.) Women have even more to gain from weight training because they are more prone to osteoporosis than men, and weight-bearing exercise may help delay this disease (see page 429).

Making muscles strong
When a muscle contracts against a resistance (usually a weight) with sufficient force, the muscle cells adapt to the strain by synthesizing protein—and thus increasing in size and strength. Tendons and ligaments (tissue connecting muscles and/or bones) are also strengthened when placed under tension. In addition, strength training can help enhance nerve activity and muscle fibers in ways that improve physical performance.

There are two basic types of muscular fitness—muscle endurance and strength. Most workouts build both to some degree, though you can emphasize one or the other, as follows:

Light resistance, many repetitions. Lifting light-to-moderate weights (50 to 75 percent of the maximum amount you can lift) many times primarily builds muscle endurance—that is, the ability to contract a muscle repeatedly in quick succession, as in lifting a suitcase twenty times in a minute or two. To a lesser extent, this also builds muscle strength and increases muscle size. This type of training can actually enhance oxygen utilization by muscle cells and make muscles work more efficiently. It can thus help improve performance in endurance activities such as brisk walking or cycling. Circuit training (that is lifting light weights or using weight machines without stopping between sets, for at least twenty minutes per session), when done regularly (at least twice a week), can also have some of the same effects as aerobic exercise: reducing elevated blood pressure, raising beneficial HDL cholesterol, and improving the body's ability to utilize blood sugar.

Heavy resistance, few repetitions. Lifting a heavy weight (more than 75 percent of your maximal lift) a few times, in contrast, primarily increases muscle strength (and size). Strength is the force a muscle produces in one all-out effort—as when you swing a mallet to ring a carnival bell. This type of training can be useful—for instance, when preparing for an activity that requires explosive strength, such as a jump. However, anyone with high blood pressure or heart disease should avoid exercising with heavy resistance.

Free weights and machines

Weight-training exercises use both free weights and machines. Free weights are barbells (long bars with adjustable weights at each end) and dumbbells (shortened barbells, ordinarily used in pairs, one in each hand). The advantage of free weights is that they allow movement in any direction and so lend themselves to an enormous variety of exercise routines; and they are relatively inexpensive. Their disadvantage is that they do not isolate muscles as clearly as machines do; and the stress that they provide is not nearly as uniform over the full range of motion as that provided by some machines.

Comparing Equipment

FREE WEIGHTS

Advantages:
- Relatively inexpensive (as little as $100 for a basic set of barbells and dumbbells).
- Can be used at home.
- Versatile—you can work virtually any muscle from any angle.
- Can help improve balance and coordination.

Disadvantages:
- Adjusting weights can take time.
- Weights can slip or be dropped, causing injury.
- Safely lifting heavy weights requires a "spotter."

MACHINES

Advantages:
- Easy to use—machines guide your movements, and the weight load can be quickly adjusted.
- Muscles are isolated more efficiently than with free weights.
- Newer machines tax muscles consistently through their full range of movement.
- Safe—weights are held in place in stacks.

Disadvantages:
- Expensive and bulky; using them usually requires joining a health club.
- A variety of machines is necessary for a good workout.
- Some machines won't "fit" all body sizes.

Machines can isolate muscle groups very efficiently by maintaining your body in a particular position and by making you move a weight along a predetermined path. And isokinetic machines such as those by Nautilus are also designed to provide variable resistance through the full range of motion, so that as you move a limb, the resistance stays at or close to maximum. Nautilus machines, for example, provide variable resistance with a special cam device.

The most advanced isokinetic machines—many of them hydraulic or pneumatic—work on the principle of accommodating resistance: that is, the harder you push them, the harder they push back, ensuring the absolute maximum resistance at every point along a muscle's range of movement. Such machines can isolate muscles most efficiently and tax them to the maximum.

Weight-training tips

A typical workout with weights includes a warm-up of five to ten minutes followed by an exercise routine that leaves the muscles thoroughly exhausted. Your exact exercise routine should be formulated with an exercise specialist in a gym, who will tell you just how to position yourself, how to lift so as to prevent strain or injury, which weights or machines to use, and how many repetitions and sets to do. If you continue to work out with a trainer or a friend, he or she will keep your routines interesting, give you emotional support, and help see to it, through proper "spotting" techniques, that you do not injure yourself.

A good exercise routine for overall fitness works out different parts of the body (see page 284). It will consist of about a dozen exercises—six for the upper body, six for the lower body. Above all, it will be scheduled so that you give each muscle a full day's rest before you exercise it again. If you exercise the same muscle two days in a row, it won't recuperate; it will become weaker, not stronger. Therefore, you should either exercise different muscles on successive days (upper body one day, lower body the next, for example) or space workouts at least two days apart.

Stretching

In addition to just making you feel good, stretching promotes flexibility—the ability to use muscles and joints through their full range of movement. Whether you are a cyclist, runner, tennis player, or walker, being flexible is an essential part of your overall fitness. Research has suggested that good muscle elasticity lends agility, a potential for greater speed, and—since it keeps your muscles from tightening up quickly—a reduced chance of injury to muscles, tendons, and ligaments. So stretching is an excellent activity to do before and after a workout.

At the same time, stretching is not just for joggers, ballet dancers, and athletes. More than anyone, sedentary people need the relief from muscle tension and stiffness that stretching provides. Stretching, when done the right way and regularly, feels good. Improper or excessive stretching, however, may actually increase the likelihood of injury. So the trick is to stretch correctly and in moderation.

The three basic types of stretching
Ballistic stretching, which is done by many beginners, is generally the type to avoid. It involves stretching to your limit and performing repetitive, bouncing move-

If you are interested in using machines at a gym or health club, make sure that there is a sufficient variety to give you a full workout. You should be able to perform four to six exercises for the lower body and six to eight for the upper body. Machines should be arranged to that you can work larger muscles before smaller ones, since this is the desirable sequence for the most efficient workout.

ments, usually quickly. This may do more harm than good, actually shortening muscles (because of a protective relax contraction) and increasing the risk of tiny muscle tears, soreness, and injury.

In contrast to ballistic stretching, there are two types that are highly recommended because they are slow and gentle:

Static stretching calls for gradually stretching through a muscle's full range of movement until you feel resistance or the beginning of discomfort. You hold the maximum position for ten to thirty seconds, relax, then repeat this several times. In static toe touches, for instance, you roll down slowly (with knees bent) towards your toes and hang in the down position without bouncing. Then slowly roll up. A basic routine of static stretches is shown on pages 286-287.

Proprioceptive neuromuscular facilitation stretching is more complicated. One type is called *contract-relax stretching,* illustrated above. In this stretch, you first contract a muscle against a resistance, usually provided by another person, then relax into a static extension of the muscle. Because it brings the opposing muscle into play, contract-relax stretching is a good way to increase muscle flexibility.

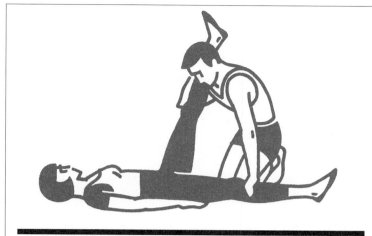

Contract-relax stretching: To stretch your hamstrings (the muscles behind the thighs), lie on your back with one leg extended upward. While your partner kneels under the raised leg, push it down against his shoulder for five to ten seconds, which contracts the hamstring muscles. Then stretch the leg toward your head, which tenses the quadriceps (the opposing muscles) and relaxes the hamstrings.

It's never too late to get flexible. In a study that compared the joint stiffness of a group of twenty young men (age fifteen to nineteen) and a group of twenty elderly men (age sixty-three to eighty-eight), it was found that both groups could reverse joint stiffness with equal ease. A number of other studies have shown that virtually anyone, regardless of age, can improve flexibility by stretching.

Strength Training: A Basic Workout

To start a weight-training routine, a personal trainer can be a great help. If this is not an option, however, you can design your own program.

On these two pages you'll find a basic twenty- to thirty-minute weight-training routine designed to work most major muscle groups. (You can get a similar workout with weight machines, if you belong to a gym that has them.) This routine uses "free weights"—small dumbbells and ankle weights, which are not costly. You can start with a pair of two- or three-pound weights, a pair of five- or ten-pound weights, and a pair of light ankle weights. Barbells have removable metal disks to adjust their weight—which can be an advantage, for as you become stronger, you'll want to increase the weight you are using. *Although working with light weights is very safe, if you're thirty-five or older or have heart disease or another medical condition, you should check with your doctor before starting any exercise program.*

Try to work out three times a week; on alternate days you can do your aerobic exercise. If you want to strength-train every day, divide your workout—for example, work your lower body one day, then the upper body the next. It is important to give muscles at least a day to recover between workouts to reduce the chance of soreness or injury. If you do the same exercises every day, your muscles may not be able to rebuild and could become chronically fatigued; this may not only prevent strength gains, but also lead to injury. If you wait too long between workouts—a week, for example—muscles may not maintain their strength gains.

1. Warm up before each workout —for instance, run or walk in place for a few minutes. Then do some gentle stretches.

2. Start with light weights, ones you can lift comfortably eight to fifteen times. This is called a set; do three sets of each exercise. Once that becomes easy, you can gradually increase the weight; you may have to reduce the number of repetitions at first and then gradually increase them. This is called progressive resistance training. Lifting the weights should not be effortless. The goal is to tax your muscles somewhat. If you're aiming for twelve repetitions, you should be able to do twelve but not easily do the thirteenth if you try. (With a buildable barbell set you can easily adjust the weight.)

But don't overdo it: if you can't repeat an exercise ten times, the weight is too heavy. However, if you feel you could do more, it's too light.

3. Rest between sets for one or two minutes (longer for heavier weights) to allow muscles to recover somewhat. You needn't rest before starting an exercise that stresses a different muscle group.

4. Work slowly and smoothly through the entire range of the muscles. This gives them a steady stress, thus reducing the chance of injury and subsequent soreness. Lowering the weight in a slow, controlled manner is also important. Don't jerk the weight around. If you lift too quickly, the momentum of the weight will do much of the work, not your muscles. If you lower a weight too quickly, you won't adequately stress the muscle. Don't "lock" (fully straighten) your knees or elbows when these are involved in an exercise—for instance, don't lock your elbow when doing biceps curls (see illustration)—since that puts excess stress on the joint.

5. Exhale while you lift and inhale when you bring the weight down. Breathe evenly: holding your breath when lifting can raise blood pressure precipitously.

6. If you feel any pain during a particular exercise, stop immediately. Continue only if the pain subsides, but first reduce the amount of weight you're lifting; make sure you were doing the maneuver properly. A mild burning sensation is acceptable, but pain is a warning that you're causing damage. Soreness the next day is normal when first starting to exercise or increasing the amount of weight you lift.

7. Isolate the muscle group that you're working. That is, try to move only the muscles that are involved. Avoid arching your back when lifting a weight.

8. Work large muscle groups first, such as those in the legs, chest, and back, which require heavier loads. It is best to exercise these before cumulative fatigue sets in. If you work small muscles in the arms first and tire them, you may not be able to perform the exercises for larger muscle groups in the chest or back that require arm movement.

9. Design a balanced workout. Don't overemphasize one part of the body, such as the chest or arms. Work all major muscle groups: shoulder, upper back, chest, abdomen, lower back, upper and lower legs, and arms.

10. Pair your exercises. Each muscle group has an opposing one (or antagonist) with which it works, so it is important to work both—for example, the quadriceps and hamstrings (on the front and back of the thigh), or the biceps and triceps (on the front and back of the upper arm). An imbalance in strength between opposing muscles increases the risk of injury.

11. Cool down after the workout. Repeat part of your warm-up and stretching routine to help muscles recover. Stopping abruptly may produce lightheadedness or fainting.

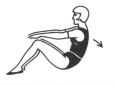

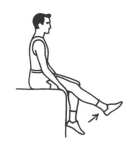

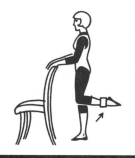

Curl down, or negative sit-up, for midsection (abdominals). Start by sitting with your knees bent, feet flat, and arms reaching forward. Slowly lower yourself to the floor to a count of ten. Push yourself back up with your arms, and repeat.

Knee extensions (quadriceps). Sit on a desk or stool with light weights on your ankles. Slowly straighten one leg, extending the knee almost completely; keep your back straight and foot flexed. Hold for five seconds, then lower slowly. Repeat, then switch legs.

Backward leg lifts (hamstrings). Attach a light weight to your ankle and hold onto something for support. Slowly lift your heel toward your buttocks, then slowly lower it to the floor. Repeat, then use other foot.

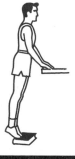

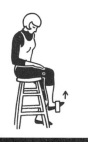

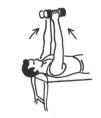

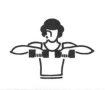

Heel raises and dips, for calf muscles (gastrocnemius and soleus). Standing with the balls of your feet on a thick book or step, slowly rise on your toes, then lower your heels as low as you can. Repeat. Use your hands for balance, not support.

Toe raises, for shin muscles (tibialis anterior). Sit on a stool or desk with a light weight on your foot. Slowly raise the ball of the foot and then lower; repeat. Switch legs.

Bench fly, for chest (pectorals). Lying on a bench, hold weights straight up over your chest, with elbows slightly bent. Slowly lower your arms in a semicircular arc until they are level with your chest, or slightly lower. Then reverse the movement, bringing weights over your chest. Repeat.

Upright row, for upper back (trapezius), shoulders, and arms. Standing with your feet shoulder-width apart and knees slightly bent, hold dumbbells side by side at thigh level (palms toward thighs). Slowly lift them straight up in front of you to your collarbone, until elbows are just above shoulder height. Lower, and repeat.

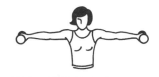

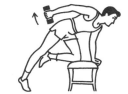

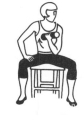

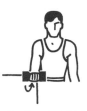

Lateral raise, for shoulders (deltoids). Standing with your feet shoulder-width apart and knees slightly bent, hold dumbbells at your sides at thigh level. Slowly lift the weights out to the sides to shoulder level; keep elbows slightly bent. Slowly lower, and repeat.

Single-arm fly (triceps). Supporting one knee and hand on a bench or chair, hold a weight at the side of your chest, keeping your arm bent so that your elbow is far behind you. Without moving the elbow, extend the weight behind you. Return to starting position; repeat. Switch arms.

Curls (biceps). Sit leaning forward with your legs slightly spread and one hand on your thigh. Keeping the other elbow on the other thigh, hold a weight so that your forearm is horizontal. Slowly curl the weight up and in toward your chest; lower and repeat. Switch arms.

Wrist curls (forearm flexors). Holding a light weight, lay your forearm on a table with your hand over the edge, palm up. Slowly curl up the weight, then lower it as far as possible; repeat. Then reverse the maneuver: turn your palm downward and repeat the curl. Switch arms and repeat.

A Basic Stretching Routine

Stretching should always be *preceded* by a brief (five- to ten-minute) warm-up, such as jogging in place, riding a stationary bicycle, or performing less-vigorous rehearsals of the sport or exercise you're about to perform. Warming up prepares you for exercise by gradually increasing your heart rate and blood flow and by raising temperature of muscles (and ligaments and tendons), all vital for elasticity and optimal functioning of muscles and connective tissue. Stretching while muscles are cold may sprain or tear them. Sudden exertion without a gradual warm-up can lead to abnormal heart rate and blood flow and changes in blood pressure, which can be dangerous, especially for older exercisers.

Eleven tips for a stretching program

1. Try to stretch at least three times a week to maintain flexibility. If you are recovering from an injury or disability, your doctor or physical therapist may tell you to stretch more often—perhaps several times a day.

2. An optimal session should last ten to twenty minutes, with each stretch held at least ten seconds, working up to twenty to thirty seconds. That will maintain flexibility, but to significantly increase your flexibility, stretches should be held for one to two minutes.

3. Stretch before exercising or playing a sport to limber up muscles and help prevent muscle strain and perhaps injury.

4. Stretch major muscle groups as well as the specific muscles required for your sport or activity.

5. Do not stretch until it hurts. If there's any pain, stop. At worst, any discomfort should be mild and brief.

6. Don't bounce. Stretching should be gradual and relaxed.

7. Focus on the muscles you want to stretch, and try to minimize the movement of other body parts.

8. Don't hold your breath during a stretch.

9. Stretch after exercise to prevent muscles from tightening up.

10. Remember, always warm up first.

11. Consider taking up yoga, since one of its benefits is to enhance flexibility.

What stretching can't do

Stretching before a workout, it used to be assumed, decreases the risk of injury, because tightness makes muscles (along with ligaments and tendons) susceptible to pulls and tears if they are forced beyond their normal range. But a few years ago, a study from McMaster University in Ontario found that runners who said they never stretched before running were no likelier to be injured than those who said they always stretched. Even more surprising, those who *only sometimes* stretched had the highest risk for injury. These results raised some questions about the conventional wisdom of stretching before exercise.

Since it depended solely on a questionnaire, with only very general questions about stretching, this Canadian study was hardly definitive. Moreover, the runners, especially those who stretched only occasionally, may not have been stretching correctly—and some types of stretching are ineffectual or perhaps even counterproductive. Also, paradoxically, injury-prone athletes are more likely to stretch, which may skew the results. Though there's a good theory why stretching should be protective and countless anecdotal reports that it is, studies on the link between stretching and injury prevention have yielded contradictory results. One thing is clear, though: cold muscles are more likely to tear than warmer ones, so warming-up is an important way to prevent injuries.

Stretching *after* a workout cannot head off the delayed-onset muscle soreness—the kind that generally occurs the day after unaccustomed strenuous exercise. This doesn't mean you should forgo stretching after a workout: it does promote flexibility and can keep your muscles from tightening up quickly.

Stretching: mind/body workouts

Stretching may affect your mind as well as body. When done in a slow and focused manner, an extended stretching routine can be an excellent relaxation method and stress reducer. For many Western practitioners, this is one of the attractions of yoga.

Among the numerous studies on this subject was a recent one in the *Journal of the Royal Society of Medicine,* in which researchers found that a stretching-and-breathing routine was as effective as other means of relaxation, but at the same time increased the subjects' perception of mental and physical energy and alertness. Two studies in the *Journal of Behavioral Therapy and Experimental Psychiatry* showed that stretching could help tense people reduce anxiety and muscle tension, as well as lower blood pressure and breathing rate.

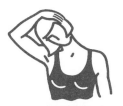

Neck stretch. Tilt head to right, keeping shoulders down. Place right hand on left side of head. Gently pull head toward right shoulder for ten to thirty seconds. Switch sides and repeat.

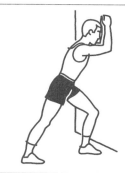

Calf stretch (for gastrocnemius and soleus muscles). Stand two to three feet from a wall, with feet perpendicular to wall, and lean against it for ten to thirty seconds. Keep feet parallel to each other; make sure rear heel stays on floor. Switch legs and repeat. Variation: keep rear knee slightly bent during stretch.

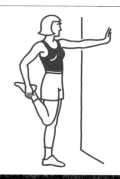

Thigh stretch (for quadriceps). Placing left hand against wall for balance, grab right ankle with right hand and pull heel gently toward buttocks for ten to thirty seconds. Do not arch back. Switch sides and repeat.

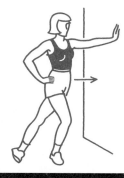

Outer thigh stretch (for iliotibial band). Placing left hand against wall for balance, place left foot behind and beyond right foot. Bend left ankle and lean into wall. Hold for ten to thirty seconds, then switch and repeat.

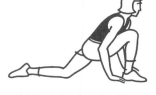

Butterfly stretch (for adductor muscles in groin). Sit on floor, bringing heels together near groin and holding feet together. Have a partner gently push your legs down; hold for five seconds. Try to bring your knees upward as partner provides resistance. Relax, then have partner gently push down again for a greater stretch. Repeat. You can do the first part without a partner, simply by lowering your knees as far as possible.

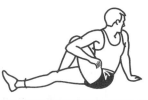

Hip stretch (for hip flexor). From a kneeling position, bring right foot forward until knee is directly over ankle; keep right foot straight. Rest left knee on floor behind you. Leaning into front knee, lower pelvis and front of left hip toward floor to create an easy stretch. Hold for ten to thirty seconds, then switch legs and repeat.

Spinal twist (for back and sides). Sit with right leg straight out, and left knee bent, with left foot placed on the outside of right knee. Bend right elbow and place it on outside of upper left thigh, just above knee, to keep that leg stationary. Place left hand behind you, slowly turn head to look over left shoulder, and twist upper body toward left arm. Hold for ten to thirty seconds. Switch sides and repeat.

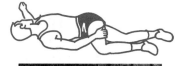

Crossover stretch (for lower back). Lying on back, bend left knee at 90° and stretch arms out to sides. Place right hand on left thigh and pull that bent knee over right leg. Keeping head on floor, turn to look toward outstretched left arm. Pull bent left knee toward floor; keep shoulders flat on floor. Hold for ten to thirty seconds, then switch sides and repeat.

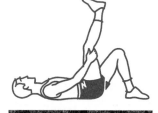

Thigh stretch (for hamstrings). Lie on back with both knees bent. Grasp behind the right thigh with both hands and pull toward chest. Slowly straighten leg, keeping foot relaxed. Hold for ten to thirty seconds, then lower leg, switch legs, and repeat.

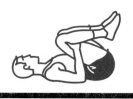

Lumbar stretch (for lower back). Lying on back, clasp one hand under each knee. Gently pull both knees toward chest, keeping lower back on floor. Hold for ten to thirty seconds, relax, then repeat.

Correcting Common Mistakes

Not all strengthening and stretching exercises performed in classes or in videotaped workouts are good for you. Some are just ineffective; others are hazardous because they are so often performed incorrectly. And even good exercises can be risky if you overdo them, especially if you're out of shape, have muscle or joint problems, or simply haven't warmed up. Realizing this shouldn't scare you off exercise. But it should tell you that you can't just walk into a fitness class or turn on an exercise tape, turn off your mind, and follow orders.

To help you take an active role in selecting exercises and deciding how to do them, here is a list of some of the most commonly done high-risk exercises, along with safer alternatives. The general categories of problems are: overflexing a joint (such as the knee or elbow), overarching the back or neck, sudden twisting or flexing, bouncing while stretching, and poor body alignment.

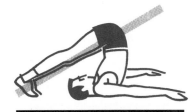

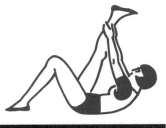

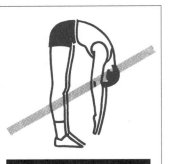

Double leg lifts can strain your lower back since raising both legs causes your back to arch. Leg scissors present similar risks.

Raised-leg crunches are a safe way to strengthen abdominal muscles. Keep one leg bent with the foot on the floor; raise the other leg straight up. Raise your upper back and reach toward the lifted ankle.

Locked-knee toe touches can over-stress the back, knees, and hamstring muscles, especially when done quickly with a bouncing movement.

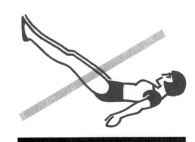

Yoga plow can compress disks in your neck area. A shoulder stand (or bicycling position in which you rest on your shoulders and upper back) can do similar damage.

Fold-up stretch is a safer way to stretch your upper and lower back. Just sit back on your heels and press your chest to your thighs, reaching forward with your hands.

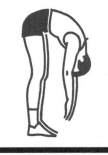

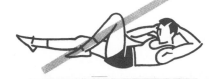

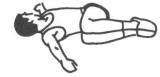

Alternating bent-leg sit-ups, in which you pump your legs and hold one straight out, put an asymmetric pull on the pelvis, which can strain the lower back. Also, in your effort to keep both legs off the floor, you may arch your back.

Knee rolls strengthen oblique abdominal muscles safely. Lie on your back, knees up toward your chest, arms out flat. Slowly lower your knees to the right side, keeping your lower back on the floor; hold for a few seconds. Slowly return to starting position. Repeat to the left.

Bent-knee hang-downs call for rolling down slowly with your knees slightly bent and abdominal muscles tight until you feel your hamstring and back muscles start to stretch. Hang over for ten to twenty seconds. Don't use force, don't try to reach the floor, and don't bounce.

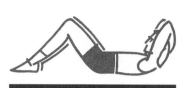

Straight-leg sit-ups arch the back and strain it. Also, there's no need to sit up fully. The abdominal muscles work only during the first part of the movement. After that, the hip flexors take over, and the shift to these muscles can further arch the back.

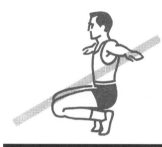

Full squats, like deep-knee bends or squat thrusts, greatly increase stress on the knees.

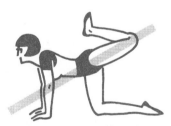

Donkey kicks, in which you rapidly lift your leg as high as possible while on all fours, arch the back and also contort the shoulders and neck.

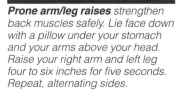

Swan stretches—lying on your stomach and lifting your chest and legs—put your back in jeopardy.

Bent-leg sit-ups are the safest, most effective way to strengthen abdominal muscles. Keep your knees bent and come up only thirty to forty-five degrees. Always keep your lower back pressed to the ground. Cross your arms over your chest or behind your head.

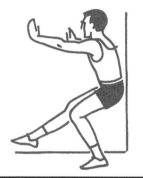

Partial squats strengthen the muscles on the front of your thigh. Squat no more than one-quarter way down: hold on to the wall for support as you extend one leg forward.

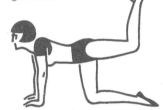

Rear-thigh lifts safely work your buttock muscles. Bring your thigh only parallel to your torso. Keep your back straight, and move your leg in a slow, controlled manner.

Prone arm/leg raises strengthen back muscles safely. Lie face down with a pillow under your stomach and your arms above your head. Raise your right arm and left leg four to six inches for five seconds. Repeat, alternating sides.

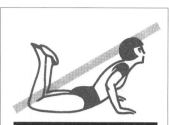

Arched push-ups are sloppy push-ups in which you lower your hips and pelvis to the floor. Like any exercise that arches the back, these can injure the disks in the lower spine. And they do little for arm and shoulder muscles.

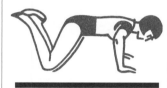

Straight-back push-ups give your shoulders and arms the maximum workout without straining your back. Hold your torso in a straight line and slowly lower your chest to the ground by bending your elbows.

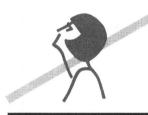

Three-hundred-and-sixty-degree head rolls, in which you vigorously roll your head around or bend your head back, may injure the disks in your neck.

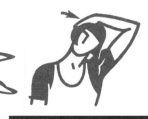

Side neck stretches use the weight of your hand to pull your head gently to the side and then forward. Also pull it diagonally.

Part 4

Self-Care

Many of the common health problems that affect your well-being—from an aching back to a sunburn—often don't require expert medical attention, but can be prevented or treated effectively on your own. The chapters that follow spell out self-care measures for a wide variety of concerns, complaints, and disorders. Throughout, the focus is on what options are available and which remedies work (and which don't). For the most part, the guidelines are intended for individuals with no serious illness or underlying medical condition; if you have any special medical problems, you should consult your physician to find out what is right for you.

The first nine chapters are organized around parts of the body; other chapters deal with such areas of wellness as stress management, getting a good night's sleep, and how to stay healthy while traveling. In the final chapter you will find information about choosing a doctor, diagnostic tests, medications, and other aspects of using the health-care system to stay well.

Skin, Hair, and Nails

Asked to name the largest organ of the human body, many people say the liver, but the correct answer is the skin. The skin (along with its glands), hair, and nails make up the body's integumentary system. The primary function of this system is to protect your body from outside elements, but it has many other functions as well. And like other bodily organs, it changes with the years. Some of these changes, such as wrinkles, we expect; others can be surprising or alarming.

Traditionally, skin has been thought of as just a passive envelope—a container for the more important parts of us. But it plays a more crucial role. The skin contains receptors for receiving the stimuli of touch, pain, pressure, and temperature, thus acting as the intermediary between the body and its external environment. It also is important in regulating body temperature, and helps prevent dehydration of the cells by deterring excessive loss of fluid.

The skin is also an essential part of the immune system. It prevents a number of harmful bacteria, viruses, and toxins from entering the body. For many years, scientists have known that the skin is laced with Langerhans cells, named for the medical student who discovered them in 1868. But not until 1978 did studies show that these cells have a major protective role. They actually "catch" microorganisms and other antigens and present them to the T-cells (a type of white blood cell), which then produce an appropriate immune response. Besides microorganisms, allergens of many kinds are also handled by the Langerhans cells. In fact, Langerhans cells may play a larger role. There is apparently some interchange between the lymphatic system and the skin and this interaction may prove to be a kind of staging ground for many immune responses—the field where the immune cells mount their strategies for dealing with all kinds of infections.

Thus, the intact human epidermis has an extremely able line of defense against harmful bacteria, fungi, viruses, and other would-be intruders. Unbroken skin is a tough terrain to penetrate, so an individual has almost no chance of catching a disease from a pay telephone, the handrails of a bus, a public toilet seat, or any of the objects people share daily. The one disease you might catch from an object is the common cold, which you can pick up by touching something that has been handled by a sick person. Even then you would have to infect yourself by touching your nose, eyes, or the inside of your mouth.

Skin survey

The changes listed below are benign and nothing to worry about—everybody can expect to have one or more of them. A few skin changes do call for medical attention, because they may be signs of cancer. These include moles that change their shape, size, or color (see below); a reddish patch that hurts or crusts over; a sore that won't heal; bleeding or ulceration. (Also see *cold sores* on page 360.)

Skin tags, or cutaneous tags. Small protrusions (less than half an inch) on a narrow stalk, usually flesh-colored or darker, and usually on the neck or upper body. Harmless, painless, and of unknown cause. No treatment is necessary. A doctor can remove a tag by freezing (cryotherapy) or burning (electrotherapy) if it is unsightly or subject to constant friction from clothing (like a shirt collar or bra strap).

Cherry spots, ruby spots, or cherry (or strawberry) angiomas. Bright red spots (flat or raised slightly), ranging from pinhead size up to a quarter inch in diameter. Usually on the trunk, arms, or legs. Formed by clumps of dilated capillaries. Harmless, painless, and of unknown cause. Can bleed heavily if punctured. No treatment is necessary. They can be removed by cryotherapy or electrotherapy, if you wish.

Liver spots, or age spots. Both terms are misnomers, since liver disorders don't cause these spots, which often appear around age forty, long before old age. Usually located on the back of your hands or on your face. May be yellow, tan, or brown in color and round, oval, or irregularly shaped. Flat, like freckles, and up to an inch in diameter, with a clearly defined border. Caused by exposure to sunlight, but not precancerous. Painless and harmless. No treatment is necessary. Bleaching creams won't remove them. (If liver spots change significantly in color, size, or shape, have a doctor check them.)

Senile purpura. Dark purple, irregularly shaped patches caused by small hemorrhages in sun-damaged connective tissue in exposed areas such as the face, back of the hands, and forearms. Painless and harmless. No treatment is required except for cosmetic reasons. These tend to fade within a few weeks.

Seborrheic keratoses. Wartlike, waxy, scaly growths, usually on the face, chest, shoulders, or back, seen chiefly in light-skinned people. Yellow, dark brown, or black. May start small and grow to more than an inch in diameter. Causes are unknown; seem to run in families. Painless, harmless, and not precancerous. Can be removed with cryotherapy or surgery.

Moles. Pigmented growths (flesh-colored, black or brown), usually small. Almost universal: adults typically have ten to forty. In most cases, harmless and painless. Some moles can become "dysplastic"—that is, they begin to grow abnormally and, if untreated, can develop into a serious form of skin cancer, malignant melanoma. These moles are asymmetrical and irregularly shaped and may contain different shades of brown, mixed with other colors. Any mole that grows or changes its shape and color requires medical attention. You should periodically check your skin for suspicious moles or growths. Remember to look on your back, the back of your legs, and other hard-to-see areas.

COMMON SKIN CONCERNS

Dry Skin

Though few people may think of it, dry skin is the most common cause of itching, particularly the allover itch or the itch that covers a wide area such as the back or legs. As you grow older, your skin produces less oil, which may aggravate the effects of winter weather. In winter, indoor heat and outdoor chill dry your skin. Frequent bathing, especially with soap, robs the skin of oils. Wool or synthetic fabrics next to the skin can make a person itch. So can perspiration or frequent swimming. If you have this kind of dry itchy skin, you suffer from xerotic or asteatotic eczema—eczema being the general name for skin inflammation. See if you can cure your itch as follows:

Hives

These red itchy welts, which may last for a few minutes or hours and may recur for weeks, have many causes. Allergic reactions to medication, food additives, specific foods, cosmetic ingredients, pollen, and animal dander may be involved. In rare cases, heat, cold, or sunlight may trigger hives. Emotional distress or underlying disease may also be factors.

Think of recent changes in your life: a new food, new medication, stress. See if it helps to avoid whatever you think caused the hives. If hives appear after you begin taking antibiotics, stop taking them and let your doctor know right away— especially if you also experience dizziness, wheezing, and/or breathlessness.

Cold compresses and calamine lotion can help relieve the itching. Over-the-counter antihistamines can also work, since histamine plays a role in producing hives.

•Take short baths or showers and use lukewarm water. Cut back to two or three a week. Sponge bathe the rest of the time.

•Discontinue deodorant soaps if you use them. Choose a milder soap and use as little of it as you can.

•If you take tub baths, add bath oil, cornstarch, or instant or colloidal oatmeal to the water.

•Pat yourself dry instead of rubbing.

•Apply a moisturizing oil or lotion, especially after a bath or shower. Avoid products that contain rubbing alcohol; don't use alcohol, which is drying, to combat itching.

•Make sure all clothing that touches your skin is well rinsed when washed. Try switching to a detergent that contains no perfume. Discontinue fabric softeners, bleaches, and other wash ingredients. (You may be able to return to your regular washing routine later.)

•Wear cotton instead of wool or synthetics. Permanent press and wrinkle-resistant fabrics may have formaldehyde or other irritating chemicals in their finish. Wash new clothing and towels before using them.

•Try not to scratch. You may irritate the skin further.

How moisturizers can help

Moisturizers work just on the skin's surface to relieve the flaking, itching, and tightness that characterizes dry skin. Despite the claims in ads, however, these creams and lotions can't penetrate and "nourish" the deeper layers of the skin, slow the aging process, or reduce wrinkling. Still, moisturizers can help relieve the symptoms of dry skin. There are two types of moisturizers:

Emollients (such as petroleum jelly, lanolin, and mineral oil). These work very

If you like expensive moisturizing creams, there's no harm in buying them. You may like the fragrance or the feel, or the design of the bottle. But what you're paying for is, in large part, the packaging and the advertising. An inexpensive cream with a few ingredients works in exactly the same way—and just as well—as an expensive one with ten to twenty ingredients.

Assessing an Itch

Hardly a day goes by that you don't get an itch. Itching (known medically as pruritus) is transmitted through the same nerve fibers that carry pain signals, and a persistent itch is certainly a first cousin of pain. Scratching usually alleviates the sensation, apparently by stimulating other nerves that slow down the itch messages traveling along the pain nerves—it's rather like drowning out an unpleasant noise with a louder one.

Sometimes just talking about the subject or even reading about it can make a person itch, and motional stress can also produce the sensation. The causes of some itches are obvious—insect bites, a sunburn, or poison ivy (which are covered on the following pages). Irritating as it is, such itching generally goes away by itself in a few days. Then there's the itch of athlete's foot, as well as "jock itch" in the groin or genital area (women, by the way, also occasionally get jock itch). These are generally brought on by fungus infections, and can often be cleared up by antifungal powders and

creams. Good hygiene and avoiding tight clothing or chafing underwear can also help.

Itching over a wide area may be caused by dry skin or, if a rash or irritation is present, by contact dermatitis (see page 294). Both these conditions are amenable to self care. However, *whether your itch is localized or generalized, you should go for medical help if self-treatment doesn't bring relief within a week or so.* Scaly silvery patches on your scalp, knees, elbows, and hands may be a sign of psoriasis, a skin disorder of unknown cause. You'll need a doctor's advice for treating it. Unexplained generalized itching can be a symptom of any number of serious disorders, including liver disease, diabetes, and some forms of lymphatic cancer.

So if you can't explain the itching and it won't quit, you should make sure it isn't a sign of underlying illness. Though it's probably only skin deep, there are a number of treatments your doctor can try, ranging from oral antihistamines to phototherapy.

much like your skin's natural oils; they form an oily barrier on the skin's surface that seals in moisture to some extent and thus blocks its evaporation.

Humectants (such as glycerin, sorbitol, lactic acid, and urea). These attract and hold water on your skin's surface.

Which moisturizer will work best for you? This depends on the moisturizer's ingredients and how chapped, dry, or sensitive your skin is. The simpler the moisturizer, the better. The more ingredients in a moisturizer—perfumes, colors, thickeners, emulsifiers—the greater the chance of a sensitivity reaction, especially if you have delicate skin. However, if you are prone to acne, overuse of any moisturizer may cause your skin to break out.

Contact Dermatitis

Contact dermatitis is a term used to describe skin irritation, itching, and inflammation caused by a substance that comes in direct contact with the skin—and which typically produces a rash or irritation.

Rashes or irritations are usually localized, which may help you discover what the cause is. For example, if your face is itchy and irritated, suspect a cosmetic. If your hands are cracked and itchy, suspect some chemical you handle (dish detergent, for example). This form of eczema, also known as allergic contact dermatitis, can be a reaction that takes years to develop, and sometimes you don't get it until several hours after you've come in contact with the allergen. Some people become allergic to nickel after having their ears pierced, and any form of nickel that touches the body produces intense itching and sometimes a rash).

Occasionally a previously tolerated medication turns into an allergen and causes itching. A less complicated form of contact dermatitis is caused by some irritant—art materials, antiperspirants, nail polish, or other cosmetic. You may experience anything from just itching to red swollen skin, blisters, and inflammation that mimic poison ivy. If you can identify the substance that's causing the itch and can discontinue using it, you may not need medical help.

Here are some home remedies that may ease itching from contact dermatitis:

•Try a cold compress and that old standby calamine lotion.

•Over-the-counter cortisone ointments and creams may help if the allergy or irritation is mild. As a rule, you should use creams or ointments only on dry rashes. If a lesion is oozing, use lotion or liquids.

•Be wary of "-caine" preparations, such as benzocaine. These deaden the itching, which may feel good momentarily, but they can cause secondary allergic reactions.

•As with any persistent itch, try not to scratch. This is especially important is you already have a rash or irritated skin.

Most cases of contact dermatitis are mild and hence never get reported. While true allergic reactions to cosmetics may be few, many people may be irritated by such products as deodorant soaps, bath salts, hair removers, hair straighteners, permanent-wave solutions, and hair dyes containing ammonia. Even if you don't think of yourself as having sensitive skin, be cautious about products that promise to kill bacteria or dissolve, curl, or straighten hair. They may leave you itching and burning, so follow instructions carefully if you do decide to use them.

Cosmetic Claims

If you've had allergic reactions, if your skin is very dry or oily, or if you've ever suffered from acne or other skin eruptions, you probably choose your cosmetics carefully. But you may be surprised at what the claims on the label actually mean:

Fragrance free, unscented. If you've recently switched to a new moisturizer and are wondering why your face itches, suspect the fragrance first. Of all ingredients, fragrances are the most likely to produce contact dermatitis. If you prefer to avoid fragrances for any reason, remember to check the ingredients- list of anything labeled "fragrance free." It can legally contain a small amount of fragrance to mask some unpleasant oily odor. Thousands of different fragrances are in use, and a single scent may contain hundreds of different substances, so it's nearly impossible to isolate the allergens, if any. Some fragrances are activated as irritants only when exposed to sunlight. Musk ambrette, a scent popular for after-shave lotions, is one such "photoallergen."

Hypoallergenic. Products with this label may be less likely to cause contact dermatitis, since "hypoallergenic" ("less allergenic")

should signal some effort on the manufacturer's part to eliminate the more common irritating ingredients—but there's no guarantee. The FDA has no list of allergens, nor any rules governing the use of this term on a label.

Allergy-tested, dermatologist-tested. Presumably the manufacturer, or possibly a real dermatologist, will have tested the product on animals or people, but there's no FDA regulation about the use of this term. Products without the label might also have been tested for potential irritants. (It is not in cosmetic manufacturers best interests for their products to be causing rashes.)

Natural. On cosmetics, as on foods, this term is meaningless. Nearly all cosmetics (and many other products, including medications) contain preservatives to ward off bacteria and fungi. "Natural" cosmetics, the customer might assume, would necessarily be preservative free. But this is often not the case. (A natural lotion with cucumber, milk, or other food products in it might need more preservatives, rather than less.) This may be a problem since, as is true with fragrances, some people are allergic to preservatives.

Caring for sensitive skin

If you tend to have allergic reactions to cosmetics, follow these tips:

•When you get cosmetics as gifts or decide to try a new line, use only one new product at a time. That way, if you have a bad reaction, you'll be able to nail the perpetrator at once.

•Don't skip the patch test whenever it's part of the instructions. If you're wary of any product, try your own patch test: put a dab of the new product on your forearm and cover it with a small bandage. Repeat daily for three or four days, and then wait another day or two. If you have no reaction, it's probably safe to use.

•If you do get a reaction and don't know what caused it, stop using all cosmetics. An over-the-counter hydrocortisone cream can help relieve itching or rash. Resume cosmetic use only after doing a series of patch tests, trying one product at a time until you find the culprit. If the irritation lasts more than ten days or is severe, see a physician.

•Remember that even a product you've used for years can suddenly turn into an irritant. The "new and improved" version of an old standby may contain an irritating surprise for your skin.

•Despite the price, expensive cosmetics are no more or less likely to cause irritation than others.

•As with any persistent itch, try not to scratch. This is especially important if you already have a rash or irritated skin. If you tend to scratch yourself while sleeping, cut your fingernails short—or try sleeping in cotton gloves.

Myth: Certain cosmetics can shrink your pores.

Fact: Although some products can cause a temporary reduction in pore size, within a short period of time your skin will return to its normal state.

Pore size is determined by heredity. People with oily skin have larger pores, and men tend to have larger pores than women. Acne can enlarge pores and squeezing pimples can permanently damage them. Since aging relaxes the skin, it tends to make pores bigger.

Astringents, fresheners, toners, bracers, and clarifiers are all designed to shrink or hide pores. The active ingredient in most of these is alcohol, which evaporates from the skin producing a cooling effect and thus a temporary tightening of the pores. Other ingredients with similar effects are witch hazel and salts.

Masks—soft ingredients that harden on the skin— are also designed to tighten pores. All of these products only work temporarily—the effects last about two hours.

Varicose Veins

Varicose veins occur when the tiny valves that regulate blood circulation in the legs malfunction. Doctors aren't sure why some people and not others are predisposed to this condition. Hereditary and, apparently, hormonal factors are at work: "varicosities" run in families, and of the more than 40 million Americans affected, women outnumber men four to one.

Causes of varicose veins

Prolonged standing or inactivity can cause varicose veins in people genetically inclined to develop them. Strain in the abdominal region—from repeated heavy lifting, pregnancy, or constipation—can also be a cause. Age is also an important factor. As the skin ages it becomes less elastic and therefore cannot support veins as firmly.

When you are standing, the heart pumps blood through the arteries to the legs with assistance from gravity. But muscle contractions are required to recirculate blood against gravity up through the veins—which lie just under the skin as well as deep in the legs—back to the heart. When the valves of the perforating veins do not work efficiently, blood accumulates, distending veins into a network of lumps that are visible just underneath the skin.

Preventing varicose veins

If you're prone to varicose veins, you may be able to head them off by avoiding prolonged sitting or standing in one position. Get up from your desk periodically and take a short walk. When standing, be sure to move around. Frequent walking or swimming can also help control a mild case of varicose veins. You can also try wearing elastic support stockings (with your doctor's consent). Don't wear tight shoes or garters or other constricting clothing.

Medical intervention

Varicose veins are usually more a cosmetic than a health problem. In severe cases, varicose veins may cause swollen ankles, itching calves, and leg pain. Sensitive and prominent veins can be unsightly and uncomfortable. Fortunately, doctors can remove them safely and permanently. One surgical method is called stripping, whereby distended veins are cut out or tied off. A second option, sclerosing, calls for the injection of a solution that hardens the affected veins and blocks the blood flow. The blocked veins form a kind of scar tissue and are eventually absorbed. In both instances, blood reroutes itself through veins that lie deeper in the skin.

Warts

Warts are caused by strains of human papilloma virus that can enter the skin through tiny breaks. Ordinary warts are slightly contagious; they spread most commonly from one location to another—for example, from finger to finger—on an infected person, rather than from person to person. (The exceptions are anal and genital warts, which are highly contagious and may contribute to the development

Varicose veins and exercise

In a leg with varicose veins, blood does not flow as efficiently toward the heart as in a healthy leg, so muscle contractions do not produce as great a drop in pressure. There is probably no danger of a vein bursting, but if you injure yourself you might experience excessive bleeding or bruising. If your veins are painful, you should probably avoid activity that requires you to tighten your abdominal muscles or strain (as in weight training), because this increases pressure in your legs. High-impact aerobics and running might also accentuate varicose veins. Indeed any intense exercise that increases blood flow, especially while you are standing, increases the pressure . However, walking and swimming may actually help you control a mild case of varicose veins. If you are currently following an exercise program and having no problems, there's no reason for you to change your routine.

of penile and cervical cancers. Warts on the larynx can also be dangerous. These three types always require medical attention.)

Warts never spread from one species to another: that old story about toads causing warts in people is just a myth. Warts are most common among children and young adults. Of the several million people who seek treatment for warts each year, about 70 percent are under forty.

Warts can occur anywhere on the body, but they look different depending on where they grow. On the face and tops of hands, they protrude as dry growths with a horny surface. On pressure areas such as the palms and soles, they grow inward. One of the most painful types is the plantar wart, a light-colored, flat growth on the sole of the foot, that may be spread through swimming pools or showers. Shower shoes can keep you from spreading or exposing yourself to such a wart.

Oddly enough, up to 80 percent of all warts (but not genital or anal warts) disappear by themselves, typically within two years, at least in children. This vanishing act has bred all kinds of legends and given credence to hundreds of home remedies. Huckleberry Finn recommended handling dead cats as a treatment for warts, and Tom Sawyer believed that spunk-water (stagnant water in an old tree stump) could cure warts, at least if you approached the stump backwards at midnight and recited the proper spell. Unfortunately, warts that have gone away (a process known as "spontaneous remission") can also return just as mysteriously.

Treating warts

If you think you have a wart, it's a good idea to see a doctor, since it might be another condtion. If it is a wart, the safest way to remove it is to have it done by a doctor. (There are various methods, including freezing, cauterization, and laser treatment.) Never cut a wart yourself, as there is a risk of bleeding, infection, and scarring. Drugstores sell salicylic acid products for the removal of warts, and if you decide to try one of these be sure to protect the surrounding skin, since it can get burned. Do not use these remedies on genital or anal warts. If you have any type of growth in the genital area, see your doctor right away.

Acne

Acne, bane of teenagers, also strikes adults. One study indicates that even in their fifties, 6 percent of men and 8 percent of women are affected by it.

What causes acne

Acne's causes at any age aren't completely understood. As in adolescence, acne flare-ups in adults are linked to various kinds of hormonal changes—for women, the hormonal fluctuations that accompany menstruation appear to be a factor. But contrary to conventional wisdom, you don't bring acne on yourself. It isn't a sign of poor health or the result of dietary indiscretions. Nor is it caused by masturbation or constipation.

Adult acne differs from the teenage variety. Teenagers are likely to get acne on the back, face, chest, and upper arms; in adults the outbreak is usually confined to the face. And in adult men acne is likely to be more serious. In both adult and adolescent acne the oil glands associated with the pores from which face, chest, and

The adhesive tape remedy

In an issue of **American Family Physician**, *Dr. Ruth Bolton mentioned adhesive tape as a cheap, noninvasive , and popular wart remedy. You wrap the area in several layers of waterproof tape and leave it for one week, then repeat the treatment. Sometimes the wart goes away. However, since ordinary warts frequently vanish by themselves without any treatment, it's hard to evaluate such remedies— if the wart does go away, you can never be sure why. If you have a persistent wart, the safest, surest way to remove it is to have it done by a doctor.*

back hairs emerge secrete too much sebum, the waxy lubricant that acts to retain moisture. Excess sebum clogs the pores and, if it remains beneath the skin, results in whiteheads. Blackheads occur if the plugs of sebum protrude above the skin. Angry red pimples appear if excess secretions invade and inflame surrounding tissue. The more extensive the inflammation, the more likely it will form abscesses and leave permanent scars and pits.

Adults can watch out for specific conditions that seem to aggravate acne: the use of oil-based cosmetics, for example, which block sebum from reaching the skin's surface naturally. The same goes for sweaty exercise in tight-fitting, nonabsorbent clothes or sweatbands, since sweating increases oil production. There is no scientific proof that chocolate, nuts, or colas can trigger flare-ups; but if they seem to for you, there's no harm in avoiding them. Flare-ups may also be related to emotional upset and too little rest—at least in some people.

Treatment and prevention

Acne can't be cured, but you can take steps to keep symptoms under control until they go away:

• Wash daily, but not too roughly or too often, with ordinary soap and water. Don't waste money on medicated cleansers (the medication just rinses away) or granular face "scrubs" (a washcloth does the same job). Facial saunas (actually facial steam baths) may aggravate acne.

• Use a drying lotion or cream. The most effective of these over-the-counter preparations contain benzoyl peroxide.

• Wear your hair off your face to keep your complexion free of scalp oils, and avoid greasy hair dressings.

• Use water-based makeup (or skip cosmetics entirely, if acne is severe). Don't overdo moisturizing.

• Avoid prolonged exposure to sunlight and ultraviolet lamps. These sometimes work to dry up acne, but can cause long-term skin damage, which can result in skin cancer, and thus are ill-advised.

• Don't pick at your face. Squeezing and picking increase inflammation and the risks of pitting and scarring. Ask your doctor if you can use a blackhead extractor (this device is available at most drugstores). If so, soften the area with hot wet compresses for about ten minutes first. Make sure your hands and the extractor are very clean.

• Severe outbreaks need the attention of a doctor, who can prescribe a wide variety of therapies, including lotions and ointments, antibiotics (taken orally or applied to the skin), and a drug called tretinoin, used in very resistant cases. (Tretinoin cannot be used by pregnant women, or those planning to become pregnant.)

Skin Cancer

Suntans are deceptive. People used to believe that a tan looked good and gave the impression of good health, but more and more people are getting the message that the sun causes skin cancer and premature aging of the skin. Exposing your unprotected body to anything but minimal amounts of direct sunlight is undeniably unhealthy, if not downright hazardous. The short-term effects of sunning yourself

Numerous studies have failed to show that even large amounts of chocolate trigger outbreaks of acne. In fact, there's little or no evidence that diet affects this skin disorder. A few people are allergic to chocolate and may develop a rash when they eat it—but that's not acne.

may be the pain and discomfort of a sunburn. In the long term the result is premature aging of the skin: the sun slowly but surely destroys the elastic fibers that keep the skin taut and young-looking, leaving it dry and wrinkled.

A far more serious danger from tanning is an increased risk of skin cancer, the most common of all cancers. The skin changes that result in cancer develop cumulatively and irreversibly in an individual over the years, and so may take decades to produce a malignancy. Men get skin cancer more frequently than women, and it usually shows up in older people, but no one is exempt. In fact, Americans are developing skin cancer at ever-younger ages because of the increasing amounts of time spent in the sun.

Exposure to the sun's ultraviolet radiation is know to promote three kinds of skin cancer *Basal cell carcinoma* is the most prevalent type, striking one out of every eight Americans, including people in their twenties and thirties, women as well as men, with 500,000 new cases reported annually in the United States alone. Fortunately, it is usually localized and curable when detected and treated early. *Squamous cell carcinoma* (100,000 cases annually) can also be cured if diagnosed early, but can otherwise spread and be fatal.

Melanoma, the least common of the three (32,000 cases annually), is also the most dangerous—though early treatment can result in a cure. Once rare, the incidence of melanoma has increased five- to sixfold worldwide over the past four decades. The lifetime risk is now about 1 in 105—and it may be 1 in 75 by the year 2000. Since 1973, the incidence has risen about 4 percent a year, even as the use of sunscreen has increased. And whereas melanoma was once a disease of the aging, now half of all those who develop it are between the ages of fifteen and fifty. Many scientists attribute some of this increase to the gradual destruction of the stratospheric ozone layer, which is allowing more ultraviolet radiation to reach the earth's surface.

Who's at risk

Surprisingly little is known about what causes melanoma. It is clear that the risk of the other types of skin cancer rises in proportion to the cumulative amount of time people have spent in the sun. But the sun's role in the development of melanoma is less clear. People who spend lots of time in the sun (such as farmers) do not have elevated rates of melanoma, though they do have higher rates of squamous and basal cell carcinoma. And melanoma sometimes turns up on parts of the body rarely exposed to the sun (such as buttocks and soles). Some researchers believe that intermittent sun exposure and severe, blistering sunburns, especially early in life, rather than simply years of sun exposure, cause melanoma. However, studies have been inconsistent about the role of sunburn.

People at highest risk for melanoma are the fair skinned—notably people with red or blonde hair, who freckle (especially on the upper back), and/or who have rough red patches on their skin (actinic keratoses) as a result of sunning. If, in addition, you have a family history of melanoma, or have had three or more blistering sunburns as a child or teenager, that also increases your risk.

Even if the only risk factor you have is fair skin, you still need to be cautious and protect yourself. One of the major steps you can take to prevent all forms of skin cancer is to reduce direct exposure to sunlight, use adequate sunscreens, and wear protective clothing. (See pages 301-304 for more specific guidelines.)

Sunscreens and melanoma

Some studies have found, ironically, that men who regularly use sunscreen have a higher risk of melanoma—perhaps because the sunscreens don't sufficiently block the particular ultraviolet rays that may be most important in the development of melanoma. Another possibility is that sunscreens allow people (especially fair-skinned ones) to stay in the sun longer before burning, and so give sunbathers a false sense of security.

Even if research confirms that sunscreens don't protect against melanoma, they do protect against other types of skin cancer, which are more common, as well as against sunburn and wrinkling. But the best safeguard of all is to limit your time in the sun.

Steps to early detection of skin cancer

Self-examination is the key to early detection. It isn't difficult—certainly no harder than the examination for breast cancer many women have learned to do. And it is vital; in the most successfully treated cases of malignant melanoma, for example, the patients themselves brought the melanoma to their doctors' attention early on. Pay special attention to areas that are habitually exposed to sunlight: your face, neck, and hands. Don't forget your scalp and the back of your ears. Use a mirror to check areas you can't easily see. Self-examination should be performed once a month. And don't forgo self-examination if you habitually stay out of the sun. While it's important to avoid excess sun exposure at any age, you cannot undo damage from past exposure, which is cumulative, starting in childhood. In fact, some experts believe that by age twenty the average American has already received 80 percent of the damaging ultraviolet rays that may lead to cancer in later years. In addition to self-examination, ask your doctor to include a total skin exam as part of your routine checkup. When examining your skin, be alert for the following signs; if you have any of them, see a physician at once.

Common signs of basal cell carcinoma

•A sore that doesn't heal. Have it checked if it hasn't healed after three weeks and it crusts, bleeds, or oozes.

•A persistent reddish patch. It may be painful, or crust and itch; or it may not bother you at all.

•A smooth bump indented in the middle. The borders will be rolled, and as it grows you may notice blood vessels on the surface.

•A shiny, waxy, scarlike spot. It may be yellow or white with irregular borders.

Common signs of malignant melanoma

•A mole that begins to enlarge, thicken, or change color. Some 70 percent of early-state lesions are identified because of recent enlargement, mottled color, irregular borders, or irregular surfaces.

Sunshine and Kids

The best time to defend against skin damage from the sun is during childhood, since the damage accumulates year after year and can't be undone. The following tips will help you protect your children:

•Cover up your children with long pants, a long-sleeved shirt, and a hat; especially if they have fair skin, blond or red hair, and light eyes.

•Keep infants and toddlers out of the sun as much as possible. Use a baby carriage with a hood or a stroller with a canopy or with an umbrella attachment.

•Try to schedule your children's outdoor activities in the early morning or later afternoon, since the sun's rays are most intense from 10 a.m. to 3 p.m.

•If your child is on medication, consult with your doctor or pharmacist to avoid possible adverse reactions to sunlight.

•Use a sunscreen with a SPF of 15 or higher. The regular use of a screen with SPF 15 during the first eighteen years of a child's life might reduce the lifetime risk of skin cancer by as much as 78 percent. For young children choose a milky lotion or cream, since this is less irritating than a clear solution, which may contain alcohol. Test the screen on the underside of the child's forearm to see if any irritation occurs. Apply the screen at least thirty minutes before the child goes into the sun to give it time to soak in, and reapply frequently; be careful around the child's eyes.

- A mole that suddenly begins to grow, or one that bleeds or ulcerates.
- A mole that has irregular rather than round borders.
- A mole with irregular pigmentation—some portions light colored, others almost black.

Treatment of skin cancer

When caught in time, basal cell carcinoma can often be removed by a doctor on an outpatient basis leaving only a minor scar. Once malignant melanoma is detected, the treatment is prompt surgical removal. If done in the early stages, the five-year survival rate from melanoma is 95 percent; the ten-year rate, 90 percent. If done during a later stage, when a tumor has begun to invade the surrounding tissues or other areas of the body, the survival rate drops sharply.

Sun Protection

A tan is damaging to your skin, whether you tan quickly or accumulate it slowly over a period of weeks. Though a suntan may protect you against sunburn, it does not protect you against accumulated radiation. All exposure to ultraviolet (UV) light is cumulative. Thus, the sun exposure you get at age ten can affect you adversely at age thirty-five.

Exposure to the sun thickens the skin while encouraging the production of melanin, a pigment that absorbs UV rays. This is the skin's defense against the sun. African Americans and other dark-skinned people probably don't need any sort of sunscreen because their high concentration of melanin protects them from UV rays. They seldom develop skin cancer and are less susceptible to sun-induced wrinkling. But in people who are not dark-skinned to begin with, repeated exposure to UV rays can result in the destruction of elastic fibers in the skin, which causes it to sag and wrinkle, and damages blood vessels. Even though people who tan easily appear to be less susceptible to skin cancer, they still need protection against UV rays.

Fortunately, protection is available in the form of a variety of over-the-counter sunscreen preparations. These oils, lotions, or creams contain compounds that minimize the damage inflicted on the skin by filtering out some or most of the sun's UV rays, which cause both suntan and sunburn. A sunscreen is a necessity, even if you're tan (unless you are naturally very dark-skinned).

Most sunscreens contain two or more active ingredients to protect against the two types of UV radiation (A and B) and most are water-resistant. Screens with sun protection factors (SPFs) higher than 15 are now far less likely to cause skin irritation. PABA (para-aminobenozoic acid), once the most common ingredient, often caused itching or rashes. It has mostly been replaced with PABA derivatives, such as padimate-O, which are less likely to irritate. Other common and effective sunscreen ingredients are cinnamates (such as octyl methoxycinnamate) and salicylates.

What an SPF means

Sunscreens are labeled with a Sun Protection Factor (SPF) number. This number tells you the relative length of time you can stay in the sun before you burn, compared to using no sunscreen. A product with an SPF of 8, for example, would allow

Protecting your lips

Your lips are one of the most sun-sensitive parts of your body. Here's a few tips geared specifically toward protecting them.

• Sun-blockers—such as zinc oxide—offer good protection for sensitive areas such as lips, but can be messy and unattractive.

• Lip sunscreens in stick form are most convenient to use, but—as they are waxy or greasy—they are generally short lasting. According to one study, the waxier or greasier a sunscreen feels on the lips, the greater the tendency to lick it off. A liquid or gel that is fully absorbed and cannot be felt on the lips will last longest.

• Colored lipstick offers partial protection against the sun for women; for full blockage, a sunscreen should be applied first. Ordinary lip lubricant such as petroleum jelly provides no protection.

Sunproof Clothing

Dressing properly for summer is a concern for people who are sensitive to the sun, have malignant or premalignant skin tumors, or are taking medication that is affected by sunlight. Yet even if you don't fall into one of these categories but plan to spend a day in the sun, you might consider the following factors affecting the amount of ultraviolet radiation that penetrates fabric:

Tightness of weave. This is the most important factor. Hold a garment up to a light bulb—if it allows lots of light through, it's loosely woven and probably inadequate to guard you against ultraviolet radiation.

Color and thickness of the material. Dyed fabric usually blocks more ultraviolet rays than undyed material. And the thicker the fabric, the better the protection.

In studying these criteria, researchers at Dryburn Hospital in Durham, England, found that tightly woven cottons are better protectors against the sun than nylon/polyester knits. Specifically, they showed that tightly woven blue denim, dark needlecords, and dark cotton prints are among the most protective options. They have a sun protection factor, or SPF, of more than 1,000. That means that if you wear such tightly woven cottons you can stay in the sun 1,000 times as long as you could with unprotected bare skin before you would burn. The researchers found that blue denim, for instance, allowed through only 0.1 percent of ultraviolet B rays (the kind that is most responsible for sunburn), compared to the 24 percent that penetrated a loosely knitted nylon jersey.

Be sun smart:
•Even if you are wearing a sunscreen, avoid long sun exposure.
•When you're outdoors, wear protective clothing and a hat with a wide brim. Sunglasses are also well worth the money (see page 335).
•When you're in sunlight for more than a few minutes, protect exposed skin by applying a waterproof sunscreen with a SPF of 15 or higher (see box opposite).

you to remain in the sun without burning eight times longer, on average, than if you didn't apply sunscreen. Thus if you're fair-skinned and would normally burn in ten minutes, a screen with SPF 8 would allow you eighty minutes before burning. Remember, these are only averages. The effectiveness of specific sunscreens varies from person to person—and also depends on how much you apply.

Studies have shown, however, that people tend to apply only about half the amount of sunscreen that the Food and Drug Administration (FDA) uses to determine SPF. Thus SPF 15 would drop, in effect, to about SPF 8. So if you're fair-skinned or will be outside for hours, either use a high-protection sunscreen (SPF 20 or more) or apply your sunscreen at frequent intervals.

What SPF doesn't tell you. Not all sunscreens with the same SPF offer the same protection, however. Although it is a fairly reliable indicator, the SPF pertains only to UVB rays—those mainly responsible for sunburn and skin cancer. Most of the active ingredients in chemical sunscreens effectively absorb UVB rays, but let through the longer-wavelength UVA rays, which researchers once thought would help you tan without harming the skin. Now it appears that UVA rays can damage the skin's connective tissue, leading to premature aging, as well as playing a role in causing skin cancer. There is, however, no rating system to indicate the degree of UVA protection, so two screens with the same SPF can offer very different protection against UVA rays.

Protection against UVA. The chemical compound avobenzone offers the fullest protection against UVA rays. There are two FDA-approved products that contain the compound—Photoplex and Shade UVAGUARD—and both are broad-spectrum screens that also protect against UVB. Both have an SPF of 15. Of the common ingredients in other sunscreens, benzophenones (such as oxybenzone) offer some protection against UVA rays, but less than Photoplex and Shade UVAGUARD. Benzophenones are used together with anti-UVB chemicals, such as padimate-O. Look for these names on the list of ingredients.

Physical blocks vs. chemical sunscreens

Even though chemical sunscreens with an SPF above 15 are sometimes referred to as sun blocks, they still allow some UV wavelengths to pass. The only true sun blocks are the opaque creams or pastes containing zinc oxide or titanium dioxide. Properly applied, they prevent any light from reaching the skin; thus they carry no SPF rating. They are good for the nose, lips, or other sensitive areas, but they can be messy to use and unattractive. Some sun blocks come in a variety of colors (versus the original white), which may appeal to some people, particularly children and teenagers. By contrast, chemical sunscreens are easier to apply and aren't very visible on the skin. Moreover, some high-SPF sunscreens now contain zinc oxide or titanium dioxide in highly pulverized form. These work just as well as sun blocks but are less messy and less opaque.

Do you need a waterproof screen?

If you spend a lot of time going in and out of the water, or if you are participating in activities outdoors that might cause you to perspire heavily, you may want to use a sunscreen that offers protection in the water. By law, products labeled "water-resistant" must protect at their SPF level even after you spend forty minutes in the water. "Waterproof" screens must do so even after eighty minutes in water. It's a good idea to use water-resistant or waterproof screens on children, since it may not be easy to reapply sunscreen to their skins after every swim.

Treating a sunburn

The best thing you can do for a sunburn is to soak the affected area for fifteen minutes in cold water (not ice water), or apply cold compresses—the same treatment that applies to all first-degree burns, which damage only the outermost layer of the skin. This provides some immediate relief from the pain, conducts heat from the skin, and lessens the swelling.

If you are sunburned all over your body, try an oatmeal bath. Scatter a cup of dry instant oatmeal in a tub of cool water and soak for awhile. The oatmeal soothes the

Don't assume that because your skin isn't red, it isn't getting burned. A sunburn becomes most evident six to twenty-four hours after sunning.

How to Select and Use a Sunscreen

•Choose a screen with SPF 15. If you're fair-skinned and will be staying outdoors for long hours, use one with an even higher SPF. Look for the seal of approval from the Skin Cancer Foundation which tests sunscreens with SPF 15 or higher for safety and effectiveness in blocking UVB.

•For greatest protection against both UVA and UVB, use Photoplex or Shade UVA-GUARD. Otherwise, look for a "broad spectrum" sunscreen which contains two or more ultraviolet-blocking ingredients. Many ingredient combinations work in concert to block a broader range of light waves and also wash off less easily.

•Apply the screen at least thirty to forty-five minutes before exposure to the sun. Studies show that this allows it to penetrate the skin for optimal effectiveness.

•Apply frequently and generously. A single application won't stay potent for long periods.

•Take into account the time of day and your location. UV rays are strongest between 10 a.m. and 3 p.m., so adjust your sunscreen strength and reapplication schedule accordingly. Intensity of the rays also increases the closer you are to the equator and the higher the altitude. If you're fair-skinned, you may need to wear protective clothing (see box, page 302), a hat, and a physical sun block on your nose and lips.

•If you're taking medication, ask your doctor or pharmacist about possible reactions to sunlight and interactions with sunscreens.

skin and reduces inflammation. (Cornstarch works equally well.) Greasy substances such as baby oil or after-sun creams seal in heat. Cooling lotions containing menthol or camphor may provide temporary relief by affecting the nerve endings and constricting superficial blood vessels in the skin, but they can be quite irritating and cause allergic reactions, especially in children.

If the burn is very painful, you may want to try a first-aid spray containing benzocaine, a topical anesthetic that also acts on the nerve endings in the skin. Using benzocaine, however, may sensitize the skin and lead to an allergic reaction upon subsequent applications of other medications in the "-caine" family. Do not use other "-caine" anesthetics for sunburn: they are readily absorbed into the bloodstream if the skin is broken and may cause immediate toxic or allergic reactions.

Aging Skin

Your skin changes as you grow older. With age, the skin gradually loses its elasticity and becomes thinner and dryer. Because of the effect of gravity, skin may begin to sag. When these developments affect facial skin, causing wrinkles and bags under the eyes, many people turn to moisturizers, skin compounds, and anti-aging formulas.

"Anti-aging" formulas: do they work?
Unfortunately, there is no such thing as youth in a bottle. Advertisements for skin care products may claim that they can prevent or reverse the effects of aging, but it has never been scientifically proven that they have any beneficial effect. While a moisturizer can help make the skin feel smooth, temporarily prevent moisture loss from the cells, and decrease the fine lines caused by dryness, no cream or lotion sold at the makeup counter—not even the ones that contain such exotic ingredients as grape seed or geranium oil, squalene (shark liver oil), collagen, and even human placental protein—can delay or reverse the effects of aging on the skin.

Retin-A. This vitamin A derivative (generic name, tretinoin) is a prescription drug approved by the FDA only to treat severe acne. Years ago, dermatologists began to notice that in some older patients the drug not only cleared up acne, but also smoothed out some wrinkles and reduced blemishes. Subsequent research found that Retin-A can reduce fine wrinkles, restore collagen formation, and produce rosier skin—to some extent. A small 1991 study concluded that the drug can help clear stretch marks; and a recent study found that it can help fade age spots. A manufacturer is now seeking approval from the FDA for tretinoin specifically as an anti-wrinkle drug, to be called Renova.

The drug's effect is usually subtle; it has little effect on deep or coarse facial wrinkles. The immediate effect of Retin-A is skin inflammation lasting two weeks to several months. In other words, for minor improvements, you may have a red, swollen, peeling face for a month or more. And you'll need to continue with the drug indefinitely to maintain any improvement (at a cost of more than $200 per year). No one knows what its long-term effects may be. Finally, since it isn't known how much Retin-A is absorbed through the skin, and high doses of vitamin A can cause birth defects, pregnant women—or those who may become pregnant—should not use the drug.

Collagen: not a miracle

Collagen, a type of protein, is the chief component of skin and connective tissue. Wherever it occurs it takes on the most efficient configuration, depending on its function. For example, in the tendons, which connect muscles to bones, collagen fibers arrange themselves in bundles to permit twisting and flexing, while in the skin the fibers are arranged in a flat crisscross pattern.

Some dermatologists promote collagen injections for minimizing scars and wrinkles. Performed carefully, the treatment is reasonably safe but quite expensive, and no one should expect long-lasting results. The injected collagen will be broken down by enzymes in about two years.

As an additive to cosmetics—which is one of its most common uses today—collagen is useless. Though it may come at a premium price, collagen cream is no better than any other kind. You cannot absorb the protein through your skin.

Minimizing Bags Under the Eyes

"Bags" under the eyes occur because fluid tends to accumulate there, where the skin is thinner than anywhere else on the body. With advancing age (and a little help from heredity) this puffiness may become more prominent or even permanent, since your skin gradually loses its elasticity and may begin to sag.

Other factors may be involved as well. In some people permanent bags may be due to a hereditary condition in which the fat that cushions the eyeball protrudes through weakened muscles. Certain medications, such as cortisone, and allergic reactions (to cosmetics, smoking, or air pollution, for instance) may aggravate matters. Generally, when your eyes are tired or irritated, accumulated fluids may make eyes puffy. Thyroid, kidney, or heart disease can all increase fluid retention, which may be particularly noticeable around the eyes. Not to be overlooked is the force of gravity: when you sleep or otherwise lie flat for a while, extra fluid may pool in the upper and lower lids.

Besides avoiding cosmetics that worsen the problem, there isn't much you can do about the puffiness. Sleeping with your head elevated on an extra pillow may be enough to allow gravity to drain the eye area. In severe cases the sagging tissue or excess fat under the eyes can be removed surgically. The operation is frequently performed on an outpatient basis.

Dark circles under the eyes also tend to be a family trait and to worsen with age. They seldom are a symptom of an underlying medical problem. What appears as a bluish-black tint is the blood passing through veins just below the surface of the skin. These "rings" may be darker when your eyes are tired, and during menstruation or pregnancy. If you wish, you can cover dark circles with special cosmetic concealers or regular makeup bases.

Retinol, retinyl palmitate, and other vitamin A derivatives. Because some doctors are reluctant to prescribe Retin-A for people who don't have acne, certain skin-care companies are promoting nonprescription skin creams containing vitamin A relatives as if these ingredients worked against wrinkles like Retin-A, but without the side effects. Despite the claims, the evidence that these other forms of vitamin A lessen wrinkles is far from conclusive. For instance, some animal studies have found that retinol (used in some Avon products) may improve the skin's connective tissue, which weakens with aging and sun exposure. But the amounts of retinol and other compounds actually used in these products may be too low to have any effect on the skin. And if the concentrations were increased, there would be a greater risk of side effects—and of toxicity if these vitamin A derivatives are absorbed through the skin.

Vitamins C and E. The theory behind using these two antioxidants on the skin is that if—and that's a big if—they penetrate the outer layer of skin and settle in the dermis, they may scavenge free radicals (created by ultraviolet rays) and retard skin damage. Unpublished preliminary research by scientists at Duke University Medical Center suggested that a high-concentration solution of vitamin C can be absorbed through the skin and seems to protect against sun damage in people. Other studies, mostly using animals, have had inconsistent results.

The research on the anti-aging properties of vitamin E has also had inconsistent results. The vitamin does have a legitimate use on the skin. Because it's an oil, it works as a moisturizer—that is, it keeps the skin's moisture from evaporating—whether it's used as a cosmetic ingredient or applied straight from the capsule. But, as such, it's no more effective than mineral oil, petroleum jelly, or other moisturizing ingredients. There have been reports of skin irritation caused by vitamin E as well as C.

Glycolic acid and other alpha-hydroxy acids (AHAs). Derived originally from fruit,

---

Is heavy sweating a dangerous sign?

If you are in good health, chronic heavy sweating is nothing to worry about.

Most sedentary people sweat anywhere from a negligible amount to two quarts a day, but heat and physical exertion can increase this output to as much as five to ten quarts. Age, race, sex, conditioning, and sensitivity to heat also affect the amount an individual sweats.

A few people suffer from hyperhidrosis (probably a genetic condition), perspiring so profusely that their clothing can become drenched in fifteen minutes. It is generally treated with topical antiperspirants. Sweat glands can also be removed, but because of subsequent scar formation such surgery is rarely recommended.

If you normally do not sweat much but suddenly start to do so, it may be due to fever and illness, or, in women, the onset of menopause.

Sweating can be dangerous if it leads to dehydration. Drink plenty of fluids—whether or not you are thirsty—before, during, and after exercise.

sugar, or milk, these "exfoliants" have been used for years by dermatologists in facial peels—sometimes with extreme irritation. They are supposed to make the skin smoother and slightly less wrinkled by making it shed or peel. Various over-the-counter creams and lotions now contain low levels of these acids (higher concentrations are available only by prescription). Many dermatologists believe that the concentrations of AHAs in such products are too low to have a significant effect on wrinkles.

Nayad and liposomes. These are found in many antiaging cosmetics. Nayad is a yeast derivative that's touted as a restorative for the skin's connective tissue. There's no published data to support these claims. Liposomes act as fatty envelopes that are supposed to help other ingredients penetrate the skin. Again, the manufacturers supply no data to support any of the claims—it's wishful thinking, at best.

The best defense against aging skin

If you can't live with your wrinkles, talk to a dermatologist about the pros and cons of Retin-A. Don't assume that these other creams and lotions will help. Rather than trying to remove wrinkles, prevent them. *The best preventive measure you can take is to stay out of the sun.* According to estimates from dermatologists, as much as 70 percent of skin damage comes from the sun.

This damage is cumulative, starting in youth. Thus much of what is considered an inevitable part of aging is preventable or modifiable. Avoid long periods in the sun; whenever you're in the sun, wear a potent sunscreen (some cosmetics contain sunscreen ingredients). Any moisturizer will help your skin appear smoother, though it won't get rid of wrinkles.

Soaps

Soap is simply a combination of fats and alkalis that lathers in water and cleanses dirt and oils from your skin. Manufacturers may add a wide range of ingredients to soaps—perfumes, deodorizers, lotions, extra fats, and even vitamins—and may claim that their soaps will moisturize, soften, or otherwise transform your skin. But the facts are:

•Any soap will get you clean.

•All soaps by their chemical nature may irritate the skin and remove natural oils. One way to soothe this irritation is to use a moisturizer after washing your hands or bathing.

•Deodorant soaps kill bacteria and cut down on body odor, but the antiseptics they contain may also cause dry skin or rashes as well as destroy helpful bacteria. This can increase the risk of skin infection, especially in the feet and under the arms. You are better off bathing frequently with some other kind of soap.

•Perfumed soap, though pleasant to use, may also irritate the skin. Regular perfume will last longer and smell better than the perfume in soap.

Personal soaps may cost anywhere from a few cents a bar to eight or nine dollars for a brand name in a beautiful package. The cleansing power, however, is the same, and the less expensive bar may actually contain fewer additives.

Your own preference is the best guide. If you like and can afford the soap you are presently using, stick with it, whether it is the generic bar from the supermarket or the eight-dollar kind with the heavenly perfume. Either one will get you clean. Neither will make you beautiful, successful, or moist.

Bar vs. liquid

Should you worry about contamination from a bar of soap? Studies of bacterial contamination, conducted during the 1980s, showed that bar soaps, even those containing germicides, swarmed with microorganisms after a week's use in a public washroom. But these studies didn't examine whether soap actually transmits germs to humans, let alone whether disease resulted, and a newer study suggests that a sloppy bar of soap may not be as threatening as it looks. When volunteers washed with contaminated soap bars (softened and then inoculated with two highly infectious strains of bacteria), researchers found that no detectable levels of the bacteria were actually transferred to the volunteers' hands. However, this study was small, the actual number of bacteria on sludgy soap may be higher than that used here, and only two strains of bacteria were measured.

Thus, the debate is far from over. Both the newer study and the old studies found that liquid soap dispensed from plastic containers remained uncontaminated. Liquid soap dispensers are certainly neater, and you may prefer them, as do most physicians. But recommendations to avoid bar soap on health grounds may be premature. It's important to remember that potentially harmful microorganisms exist on most surfaces, including money, doorknobs, and the hands you shake every day.

To prevent the spread of disease, you're obviously better off washing your hands often (and rinsing well)—even with the sloppy looking bar you may find in a washroom—than leaving them unwashed.

Antiperspirants and Deodorants

Almost 100 years ago the first commercial product to control body odor, Mum, was introduced on the market. Since then two kinds of preparations designed to minimize underarm sweating and odor have evolved—antiperspirants and deodorants. The first inhibit sweating; the second inhibit the bacteria that cause odor, or simply mask the smell. More recently, combination antiperspirant/deodorants—whether creams, roll-ons, sticks, or aerosols—have become prevalent on drugstore shelves.

Because antiperspirants affect the functioning of the body, the Food and Drug Administration (FDA) considers them drugs. Virtually all over-the-counter brands sold today contain an aluminum compound as their active ingredient. No antiperspirant can stop sweating completely. As for body odor, bathing is by far the best way to control and prevent it.

The effectiveness of specific antiperspirants varies from person to person. It also depends on a product's form—such as roll-on or spray—as much as on the brand, active ingredient, and/or formula. The reduction in sweating afforded by antiperspirants ranges from about 15 to 50 percent. Because they are applied directly to the skin and are rubbed in, sticks, roll-ons, and creams generally provide more protection than aerosols. Aerosols that spray on wet tend to be least effective.

Not only are aerosol antiperspirants less effective, they also have aroused safety

Deodorants and antiperspirants have been oversold. For many people, using their regular product two or three times a week, instead of daily, works just as well.

concerns. The problem is the fine mist hangs in the air near the mouth and nose when you spray an aerosol: some of it is inhaled. For this reason, many ingredients that are allowed in roll-ons and other forms aren't permitted in aerosols. Zirconium, for instance, was banned in aerosols by the FDA because it caused lung tumors in laboratory animals. Aluminum chlorohydrate is the only aluminum compound approved by the FDA for use in aerosols. In addition, aerosols can be irritating if accidently sprayed in the eyes. Despite these questions about safety and effectiveness, aerosols remain popular because they are quick and easy to use.

Unlike antiperspirants, deodorants control body odor without affecting sweating; the FDA considers them cosmetics. Unless you perspire very little, a combination antiperspirant/deodorant will be more effective.

The most common problems involving antiperspirants and deodorants are allergic reactions (caused, for example, by an aluminum compound, antibiotic, or perfume in a product) and skin irritation. There is no way to predict who will be allergic to what. Don't apply these preparations to broken (as immediately after shaving underarm hair) or sensitive skin, and switch to a brand with different ingredients if a rash or other irritation develops. Usually the rash will disappear as soon as you stop using the product.

SKIN FIRST AID

Burns

Superficial or first-degree burns—defined as a burn involving only the outer skin layer—can be the result of some minor household accident, such as grabbing the handle of a pan that's too hot or scalding yourself with hot water or steam. They are not dangerous, but can be extremely painful. The best way to treat a minor burn is not, as many people believe, butter; butter won't relieve pain and may cause infection if blisters form and then break. Cold (but not iced) water is by far the most effective first-aid treatment; it eases the pain as it cleanses. If you burn yourself, immerse the burn in cold water or hold it under cold running water for fifteen minutes. Continually applying fresh cold-water compresses will help if it's not practical to immerse the burned area. Afterwards, you can bandage it with sterile gauze pads held on by tape if you wish, but if blisters appear try not to burst them. Burn ointments are not necessary.

When to seek medical attention
A deep or extensive burn, especially one caused by hot liquids or contact with fire, electricity, or corrosive chemicals, requires immediate medical attention. Signs of a second degree burn are blistering, pain, and swelling. Sunburn that causes blisters, swelling, and oozing of fluid, is a second-degree burn and treatment by a doctor is advisable. Don't put anything on a second degree burn: creams or lotions may interfere with medical treatment the doctor will perform. Don't break blisters or peel damaged skin—you will only encourage infection.

Signs of a third-degree burn are lack of immediate pain (nerve endings have been destroyed), whiteness, and charring. Cover the area with sterile gauze, if possible, and get professional help.

Cuts and Scrapes

What is the best way to deal with the little cuts, abrasions, and scrapes of everyday life? Many remedies—from hydrogen peroxide to mercurochrome to antiseptic sprays and ointments—have enjoyed popularity over the years. The truth is, most small wounds don't need much doctoring.

Treatment

A simple two step process is the most effective method of treating a small wound. First, stop the bleeding—if there's any amount of it—by applying pressure with a clean cloth or tissue. If possible, elevate the wounded part above heart level to slow blood flow. (*Exception:* a puncture wound, from a nail or needle or similar long, sharp object should be encouraged to bleed as part of the cleansing process. See below for more information.)

Second, the main concern with any small wound is avoiding infection, and you can best accomplish this by cleaning the wound and keeping it clean. Cleanse a scrape or cut by swabbing gently with a clean wet cloth or holding the injured part under cold running water. Use a mild soap in the area, but try to keep it out of the wound per se. If there are dirt particles clinging to a scraped shin or elbow, remove them with tweezers (wash tweezers first and dip the tips in alcohol). If the wound is on the hand or finger and likely to get dirty, if the area needs protection from further injury, or if you'd just feel more comfortable not looking at the wound, a homemade or store-bought bandage is in order. This is really all you need to do for most wounds, which will heal in a week to ten days.

Unnecessary steps

Antiseptic solutions—rubbing alcohol, iodine, and hexylresorcinol—and hydrogen peroxide kill some microorganisms but they can also destroy skin cells. The FDA permits them to be sold for cleaning small wounds, and if you feel you have to use

---

When a Cut Needs Medical Attention

In any of the following situations, call your doctor, or go straight to the emergency room:

• If bleeding comes in spurts. This indicates that an artery may have been cut, and that you might not be able to stop the bleeding. Cover the wound with a large soft cloth, and if possible, elevate it above heart level. Press directly on the wound to help stop blood flow; apply an additional compress on top of the first, if necessary. Don't use a tourniquet, which can damage nerves.

• If a cut looks very deep, or if the edges of the wound gap open. A jagged cut, particularly from broken glass, is likely to need medical attention. If you need stitches, you should not wait more than six hours to get them.

• If a scrape is very large (for example, the whole length of your arm or leg) and there are bits of debris in it.

• If your face is cut. You may need plastic surgery to avoid scarring.

• If you think a wound has hidden dirt or debris in it.

• If you have a deep puncture wound, especially if it was made with a dirty object (a gardening tool for example), and if you haven't had a tetanus booster within the past five years. If more time has passed or you don't remember when you last had one, arrange to have a tetanus immunization as soon as possible. If any sign of infection (redness, pus, or fever) develops, get medical attention. You may need to soak the wound to keep the puncture open and encourage draining.

something, make it alcohol. Iodine can actually burn your skin under a tight bandage. Hydrogen peroxide can damage the outer layers of the skin and thus retard healing. Such solutions as mercurochrome and merthiolate (once medicine cabinet staples) contain mercury, which is highly toxic, and are not judged safe or effective by the FDA.

Antibiotic ointments—such as Bacitracin, Betadine, Neomycin, Neosporin, Aureomycin—may cause skin irritation and offer few benefits. Though the FDA allows first-aid antibiotic ointments to be sold over the counter, there's no evidence that they promote healing or can effectively treat an infection. Antibiotic ointments might be of some preventive value, however, if you have a cut finger and have to perform some task where its hard to keep your hands clean—or for scrapes and cuts on a child's hands and feet when the child is engaging in active outdoor play. Wash the wound first, and apply a small amount of ointment under a bandage, and repeat these steps if the wound gets dirty.

Overall, if a wound is small and is kept clean, the body's own immune system can adequately dispose of any bacteria that may be present. Be wary of any product that claims to "speed" or "promote" healing.

Holding the edges of a cut together will help minimize the chance of scarring. Try a "butterfly" strip, placing a regular adhesive strip over it, if desired.

Treating puncture wounds

A puncture wound caused by a nail or pin or other sharp object often doesn't bleed freely, so bacteria don't wash away and may be sealed in. If such a wound is not bleeding enough, press gently around the wound to encourage bleeding. Examine the wound and remove any foreign objects from it. Clean the wound with soap and water and cover it with a sterile dressing.

If the wound is deep or was made with a dirty object and you haven't had a tetanus shot within five years, contact your doctor about tetanus immunization. Go to an emergency room if you can't reach your doctor. If any sign of infection develops (severe swelling, redness, pus, or fever), get medical attention. You may need to soak the wound in warm water to keep the puncture open and encourage draining

A deep puncture wound on the hand may lead to an infection that is hard to combat; preventive antibiotic treatment may be advisable for such a wound. Any puncture wound of the head, chest, or abdomen requires immediate medical attention because of the possibility of internal injury. Numbness or tingling may indicate nerve damage, which requires medical attention.

Do you need a bandage?

For most small wounds, keeping it dry and exposed to air will make it heal faster. A scab helps protect the area from infection and shouldn't be removed until the wound has healed. However, some studies have shown for certain serious wounds covering *a large area,* moisture can aid healing and preventing scabbing can decrease the risk of scarring. New, flexible, transparent, waterproof bandages (called "occlusive" from "occluded," meaning to shut out) have thus been designed to retain moisture around the wound and protect it from bacteria and dirt. However, if a wound is draining, it can become infected unless the bandage is changed at intervals and the wound is cleaned. If you have a wound serious enough to need this kind of extensive treatment, you should probably be in a doctor's care.

If you do decide to use a bandage for a wound, how can you tell which type is best? Most people like to use ready-made bandage strips and keep a supply of them on hand. These come in a wide variety of shapes and styles for different small injuries. Old fashioned adhesive tape and sterile gauze are less convenient to use but are equally good for minor wounds, particularly for the occasional wound that a ready-made bandage won't cover. You should change any bandage when it becomes soiled or wet.

You can find the transparent, waterproof, occlusive bandages mentioned above in most drug stores; this new design has the advantage of not sticking to the wound itself. Though fairly expensive, they can be useful for some small wounds and abrasions such as a heel blister subject to chafing or a cut that needs protection from water. But don't use one on an infected wound.

As soon as you can comfortably do so, leave the bandage off. The warm, moist environment under a bandage is an excellent microclimate for breeding bacteria. A white, wrinkled appearance is a sign that the skin is too moist and has been covered by a bandage too long.

Animal Bites

If you are bitten by a dog, cat, other household pet, or by a wild animal, it's important to seek medical treatment immediately, since there is a risk of infection, rabies, and tetanus. Rabies in wild animals is common, especially along the Eastern Seaboard, but thanks to vaccination it is quite rare in domestic animals in this country and rarer still in humans. In 1993, however, an eleven-year-old girl died of rabies in New York State, the first person in the state to die of the disease since 1954. The disease is now so unusual that doctors were able to arrive at a diagnosis only after the child had died. Public health officials now think that she had contracted a form of bat rabies, but how transmission occurred may never be known.

Rabies and raccoons

Rabies is a viral disease transmitted by the saliva of infected animals. Any warm-blooded animal can carry it, but it's mostly found in raccoons, foxes, skunks and bats. (Being bitten by an infected animal is almost the only way humans are exposed to the disease, though airborne transmission might be possible in a heavily infested bat cave.) In humans, symptoms of rabies may include fever, pain, aggressive behavior, hallucinations, extreme weakness, and thirst. If left untreated until symptoms appear, rabies is fatal, but it can be caught and stopped if treatment is begun within ten days after exposure. A series of five injections—a version of the rabies vaccination discovered a century ago by Louis Pasteur—is very effective in combatting the virus. The treatment is expensive but less painful and less drawn out than it was years ago. Every year about 20,000 Americans get these shots. Serious side effects from the vaccine are virtually unheard of.

Raccoons, which thrive in great numbers as suburban scavengers, are now the chief source of rabies, and while rabid raccoons seldom attack people (one attack on a small child was reported in 1990), they do attack dogs and cats. Vaccination of pets, practiced since the 1940s, almost wiped out rabies in domestic animals. Then in the 1950s skunks and foxes became reservoirs of the disease in the wild, later to be outpaced by bats and then, in the 1970s, by raccoons, so that unvaccinated pets are now at greater risk of exposure. No human deaths have been attributed so far to raccoon rabies, but unvaccinated dogs and cats have died.

Though rabies has been prominent in the news lately, there's no reason to panic. Still, the following protective measures are important:

- •Be sure to vaccinate your cat or dog regularly. Ask for the shot that lasts three years. (Immature or very old animals need the yearly vaccine. Ask your veterinarian for advice.)
- •Don't let pets roam outdoors at night.
- •All wildlife, including raccoons, should be left alone or observed from a distance. In particular, don't try to make a pet of a raccoon, and warn children not to try to play with them or make friends with any wild animal. Keep garbage cans locked up to discourage animal scavengers. (Ferrets, including pet ferrets, are classified as wild animals and can carry rabies. They can, however, be vaccinated.)
- •Be wary of a raccoon or any other wild animal that appears tame or lethargic ("dumb" rabies) or else fearless or aggressive ("furious" rabies). Beware of any ordinarily nocturnal animal that is out in daylight. Such odd behavior might be a sign of rabies. Some rabid animals foam at the mouth.
- •If you're planning to travel in Asia, Africa, or Latin America, remember that dogs in developing nations are still a threat. Before leaving for a long stay in such a rural area, discuss pre-immunization against rabies with your doctor.

If you are bitten by any animal, *immediately wash the wound and any scratches thoroughly with lots of soap and water.* This can reduce your exposure to the virus, if it is present, and is the most valuable first step. *Then see a doctor without delay, or go to a hospital emergency room.* (You may not need to worry about rabies, but you may need a tetanus shot.) The doctor will decide whether to report the bite to your local health department. If it was a domestic animal that bit you, it may need to be confined and observed.

Health officials or the police can help locate the owner, if there is one, in order to find out whether the animal has been vaccinated. If it has been vaccinated within the last two years, you need not be fearful of rabies. But if bitten by a wild animal, you may need to begin treatment at once. Your doctor, in consultation with the health department, should advise you.

If you've been bitten by a poisonous snake, the most important task is to get to the nearest emergency room or other source of medical help at once. It's also important to try to immobilize the bitten body part and keep it below heart level. If possible, cleanse the wound with soap and water and cover it with sterile gauze or other clean dressing. (See page 584 for more detailed information.)

Insect Bites and Stings

Insect bites and stings are a common occurrence during the summer months (year round in warm climates). And while they are usually harmless—albeit, potentially painful—they can be dangerous for some people. Some insects also carry disease. Below are suggestions for warding off and treating the most common types of insect bites.

Bees, wasps, hornets, yellow jackets, and fire ants

These insects sting with venom that produces fierce burning, swelling, redness, and sometimes welts and itching in the areas around the sting. The best way to treat a sting is to wash it with soap and water. You may also obtain some relief by applying ice, calamine lotion, or a paste made by mixing baking soda or meat tenderizer and water.

If you've been stung by a bee, you'll have to remove the stinger as well (the bee is the only insect that leaves it behind). Don't pull at the stinger directly with tweezer or fingers, because it has a sack at the exposed end that can pump more venom into you if squeezed. Instead scrape the sack away cleanly with a sharp blade held against the skin, then remove the stinger.

Avoiding stinging insects. You can avoid being stung by taking a few preventive measures. Wear shoes and socks outdoors; when gardening, wear long-sleeved shirts, long pants, and gloves. Bees can mistake you for flowers, so avoid brightly colored clothes, floral prints, and sweetly scented perfumes, soaps, or lotions. Be cautious about eating outside, particularly sweet, drippy foods like ice cream or watermelon. If an insect is annoying you, don't swat it—either walk away or, if attacked by a swarm, lie down and cover your head.

Ticks

Ticks probably exceed all other pests in the variety of diseases they transmit to man and domestic animals. Tiny, wingless, louselike creatures, they range in color from brown to gray and from one sixteenth to one quarter inch in length. Many species are known to carry diseases such as Rocky Mountain spotted fever, Colorado tick fever, tularemia, babesiasis, and Lyme disease, to name a few. They occur in every part of the United States, though large numbers are concentrated in certain areas.

People usually pick up ticks from woodsy underbrush, tall grass, and the fur of free-ranging pets. The tick brushes against some part of the body and looks for a place to settle. It then bites the skin, embeds its head, and taps into a blood source, such as a small vein or capillary. As it feeds, the external part of its body swells to

---

Removing cactus spines

To remove very fine cactus spines from a child's skin:

First, use tweezers to remove as many spines as possible. Then apply a nontoxic household glue (definitely not Krazy Glue; use a glue like Elmer's Glue) to the skin with a cotton swab and top it with a single layer of gauze. Let the glue dry, then remove the gauze with the glue. The spines should come with it. It's much less upsetting for the child than extracting the spines individually, which can be difficult or impossible to do anyway. In a controlled study, this treatment worked better than any other method.

Obviously, the glue-and-gauze trick would work for grown-ups, too, and might even be worth a try with briars or multiple splinters.

Allergic Reactions to Insect Stings

For most people, the reaction to a sting is harmless, but about 3 percent of the population are so sensitive to the venom that even one sting can provoke their immune system to overreact drastically. This is known as anaphylactic shock (from the Greek *ana*, meaning "excessive," and *phylaxis*, meaning "protection"); it can include nausea, flushing, depressed blood pressure, irregular heartbeat, vomiting, and difficult breathing, and may lead to a coma and even death. In fact about fifty Americans die each year as a result of being stung by bees, wasps, or hornets. No other venomous animal, even snakes, kills that many. And this figure may be too low: experts suggest that an unknown number of deaths attributed to heart failure may actually be caused by stings.

Anyone who has experienced any symptoms of anaphylactic shock or any systemic reactions after being stung should know that reactions usually become increasingly severe with successive stings. Life-threatening reactions most often occur in people over thirty.

Fortunately, there are effective long-term and short-term treatments for those who are highly allergic. In the initial moments of a serious reaction, a dose of epinephrine (adrenalin) can arrest the attack. Your doctor can prescribe an emergency kit for you that includes a syringe and epinephrine, or an EpiPen, which comes with a spring-loaded mechanism that automatically triggers the injection of epinephrine when pressed against the skin. Take the kit with you whenever you go outdoors in bee season. If you get stung and must inject yourself, rub the site vigorously after the injection in order to increase the absorption rate.

Once a person is found to be allergic to bee stings, long-term treatment involves going to an allergist for regular shots of a serum made from insect venom. This may gradually desensitize the patient until a sting poses little serious harm. Recent studies indicate that this therapy can be discontinued after about five years without posing any future risk. (Followups were done for only about five years, not over a lifetime.)

as much as three times its original size. The bite is relatively painless; the real danger is the viruses or bacteria that the tick may harbor and that may infect you.

The best way to remove a tick. If you discover a tick attached to your skin, remove it immediately. The sooner it is removed, the less likely the chance of transfer of any infectious organisms. Don't try to detach it with your bare fingers; bacteria from a crushed tick may be able to penetrate even unbroken skin. Instead use a pair of fine-tipped tweezers. In fact, if you spend much time hiking or gardening in over-

Stings from Sea Creatures

Stingers include jellyfish, the Portuguese man-of-war, sea anemones, and some corals, all equipped with stinging cells called nematocysts. On contact with the skin, they discharge a small barb and a dose of toxin. You're more likely to encounter jellyfish and the Portuguese man-of-war while swimming; divers should watch out for coral and sea anemones. Sea urchins, which live on the sea bottom but may show up in shallow water, have poisonous spines that can puncture the skin even through thongs or sneakers.

Jellyfish. Only about one in ten species of these translucent, bell-shaped blobs produces severe reactions in humans. But if you do come into contact with a toxic jellyfish's trailing tentacles, you'll feel mild burning and stinging; long red weals that look like the marks of a whip will develop. If you have to pull the tentacles off, protect your hand with cloth or a glove to keep the stingers off your skin. To deactivate the stinging cells, wash with sea water, then apply rubbing alcohol, vinegar, or witch hazel. If possible, apply a papain-based meat tenderizer in paste form. This appears to break down the stinging cells (and the toxins in them) attached to your skin. A paste made of talcum, baking soda, or flour mixed with sea water may also help. When the paste is scraped off, the cells come with it. *Don't* rub the affected area or rinse with fresh water: this can discharge unactivated cells. If pain persists, a nonprescription topical anesthetic (such as one containing a "-caine" ingredient) can be applied.

The Portuguese man-of-war. Bright blue or purple and red, this is actually a colony of many individual jellyfish at two stages of development. The floating colonies are easy to spot, but not so their transparent tentacles, which can trail invisibly for as far as sixty feet. Contact with skin provokes red weals similar to jellyfish stings, but the burning and pain can be far more severe. Shortness of breath, nausea, stomach cramps, and shock may ensue. Treatment is similar to that for jellyfish stings (you can also try ammonia), but in some cases you may need to see a doctor.

Coral. On contact, some corals release toxins; fragments may break off and become embedded in your skin. Apply calamine lotion or rubbing alcohol, and if there is an abrasion, remove fragments with anything at hand: for instance, a towel, a handkerchief, tweezers, or a needle. Wash with soap and water.

Sea anemones. These flowerlike creatures live fixed to the sea floor; their waving tentacles equipped with stinging cells. If you step on one, follow the same measures as for jellyfish; do not rub the skin and do not rinse with fresh water.

Sea urchins. Also floor dwellers, sea urchins are protected with toxic spines; broken-off spines can cause secondary infections if not removed. A scrub with soap and water will get rid of some. Extract others with a sterilized needle or tweezers; a doctor may have to pull out the remainder. Hot compresses or immersion of the foot in hot water increases blood flow, which helps remove the toxins. Since the punctured foot may be numb, check the water temperature with your hand or uninjured foot.

If you're stung or stuck by any of these get out of the water as calmly as you can, and if possible identify the culprit so that you can choose appropriate first aid measures. If you didn't see what hit you, ask someone who knows the area. Check ahead of time on the hazards that may be lurking off the beaches where you plan to spend your vacation. Pack a small first aid kit with the following items: needles and tweezers, rubbing alcohol or calamine lotion, and meat tenderizer. Sea stings are rarely fatal, though when the reaction is severe, you should see a doctor as soon as possible.

grown areas, a pair of "tick tweezers" (available at many sporting goods stores) should be part of your first aid kit. To remove a tick, grip it as close to your skin as possible and gently pull it straight away from you until it releases its hold. Don't twist it as you pull, and don't squeeze its bloated body—that may actually inject bacteria into your skin. Afterwards, thoroughly wash your hands and the bite area with soap and water and apply antiseptic (such as rubbing alcohol). If you must touch the tick, cover your fingers with tissue; then wash your hands thoroughly.

Home remedies for tick removal—gasoline, petroleum jelly, kerosene, nail polish remover, or a hot match—have not been shown to be effective and may actually increase your chance of becoming infected from the tick. These methods may cause the tick to respond by secreting more of the infected organism.

Save the tick in a small container or jar labeled with the date, the body location of the bite, and where you think the tick came from. This way you can show it to your doctor if necessary.

Warding off ticks. The best treatment for tick bites, however, is prevention. Take the following precautions:

• Cover your body as much as possible. Wear long pants and a long-sleeved shirt with buttoned cuffs. Don't go barefoot. Tuck the shirt into your pants and your pants into your socks or shoes. Wear light-colored, tightly woven fabrics: it's easier to spot ticks on white or tan slacks than on dark ones, and the ticks may not be able to grab onto the tight weave of slippery materials such as nylon. A hat may help, too, since ticks like to settle on the scalp.

• In overgrown countryside, try to stay near the center of trails.

• Check yourself occasionally for ticks, especially when you're in underbrush or forests. Check your clothing, too; ticks often crawl around on clothing or even on the skin for a long time before they bite. Later do a thorough check of your entire body. Have someone look at your back and head if possible or use two mirrors. Shower and shampoo after your outing; this may help remove ticks that haven't yet begun to feed. Check your clothes too; wash them immediately to remove any ticks that may be hidden in creases. Inspect any gear you were carrying.

• Check pets after they've been outdoors. Remove ticks from them as you would from yourself.

• Inspect your children daily for ticks, perhaps before they go to bed. This is especially important during the summer, when they spend lots of time outdoors.

• One of the best ways to ward off ticks is to use an insect repellent containing DEET (see box on page 316). Also available are tick repellents that contain permethrin. The permethrin-based repellents are sprayed on clothing, not skin, and are effective for up to two weeks, even after laundering.

For information on how to keep your yard free of ticks and on Lyme disease, see pages 576-579.

Chigger mites

In April in the northern United States (year round in warmer climes), the newly hatched mite larvae climb the nearest plant and wait for a bird, snake, small animal, or human to brush by. The mite drops off the plant and attaches itself with a pair of jawlike claws. It doesn't burrow, like a tick, but clings for about three days before dropping off. During that time it feeds by secreting enzymes that liquefy skin cells. Chigger mites do not, as ticks do, feed off blood, nor do they spread dis-

Why a mosquito prefers one person over another is a complex question, since so many factors are involved. First of all, there are more than 150 species of mosquitoes in the United States, and not all are attracted to, or repelled by, the same things. Some don't even bite humans, preferring cold-blooded creatures such as snakes or turtles. Many body chemicals may attract or repel insects. And you may be more attractive to mosquitoes one day than another. Women, for instance, are more attractive to mosquitoes at various points in the menstrual cycle. Mosquitoes also seem to prefer body warmth and moisture, as well as certain parts of the body (such as the face and hands).

Are Insect Repellents Safe?

There is a relatively safe, effective insect repellent to drive off the bugs of summer. It's N,N-diethyltoluamide, mercifully known as DEET or deet, which will keep most chiggers, ticks, biting flies, mosquitoes, and other insects (except bees) at bay. Some popular brands of insect repellent have only a little of it; others are pure DEET.

The only trouble is that some of the chemical ultimately enters the bloodstream through the skin, traces of it showing up in urine. For most people this is of no concern. But a variety of allergic reactions to deet have been reported, as well as a few cases of toxic brain disease caused by the chemical, mainly in children. The higher the concentration of the chemical (some products are 100 percent DEET), the greater the risk.

Insect repellents containing the chemical compound Repellent-11 (also known as R-11 or 2,3,4,5-Bis (2 butylene) tetrahydro-2-furaldehyde) have been banned by the EPA because studies shows that it causes reproductive problems and tumors in lab animals that were fed it. Although you will no longer find repellents containing R-11 on store shelves, you may still have an old bottle or can of repellent in your home. Read the label carefully and don't use it if it contains R-11. Call the manufacturer to see if you can exchange it for a reformulated product or throw it away—but don't be casual about disposing it. Find out if your area has a household hazardous waste collection program. Otherwise tie several layers of newspaper around the repellent and dispose of it with other garbage.

If you want to use insect repellents, take the following precautions:

• Buy products with a lower concentration of DEET; these are safer, but have to be applied more frequently. Avoid brands that are totally DEET, since the risk of an adverse reaction is highest with them. (There is at least one repellent—called Skedaddle—designed specifically for children that contains only 10 percent DEET. It's effective for adults, too.)

• Don't use insect repellents on broken skin, such as cuts and scratches.

• Be very careful with infants and children, in whom the greatest number of serious reactions have been reported. Don't spray them (or anybody else) repeatedly over long periods, and don't use excessive amounts.

• When possible, use clothing as protection (long-sleeved shirts, socks, shoes, and loose-fitting trousers tucked into your shoes or socks). Applying repellent to clothing may also help.

• Don't reapply until necessary. Wait until flying bugs are circling close by.

If you—or a child in your care—develop a skin rash while using a repellent, discontinue its use. Severe reactions such as breathing difficulties or seizures are extremely rare. Should they occur, seek medical aid at once and be sure to tell the physician you were using a repellent; bring the can or bottle with you.

ease. But, these enzymes can provoke an allergic reaction resulting in two weeks or more of intense itching—which leads to the scratching that may result in serious bacterial infection.

If you're hiking through the underbrush, fend mites off by wearing a long-sleeved shirt secured at the wrist, waist, and throat; tuck your pants into your socks or boots. It also helps to apply insect repellent to exposed skin and to trouser and sleeve cuffs and shirt fronts. If a mite does attach—they look like a tiny red fleck—a needle, small knife, or even your fingernail will remove it.

Starch baths and calamine lotion help relieve itching. Lindane and crotamiton (a prescription drug) kill mites; crotamiton also alleviates itching. For more serious attacks, your doctor may prescribe an oral antihistamine or topical steroid cream to control the itching. If you do develop a secondary infection due to scratching, an antibiotic may be needed.

Poison Ivy and Poison Oak

You may remember the old saying "Leaves of three, let it be." It's a reminder that poison ivy and its cousin poison oak consistently have three leaves. But beyond that these plants can vary tremendously—which is why many people don't recognize them and end up in misery each year. They can grow as woody vines or shrubs. The leaves can be dull or glossy, from one to five inches long, and have edges that are saw-toothed, lobed, or smooth. Though usually green, in autumn they can turn yellow or pink; in spring they often bear small green or white flowers that mature into berries in late summer.

The plants, which belong to the aptly named genus *Toxicodendron,* are widely distributed. The only states that have no toxicodendrons are Nevada, Hawaii, and Alaska. Poison ivy grows throughout the rest of the United States except California, which is where one type of poison oak is concentrated. Another form of poison oak grows in the southeastern states. In damp areas like swamps or bogs, you may encounter poison sumac, a small tree or shrub related to poison ivy that has seven to eight leaflets on each stem.

People who think they're immune to these plants are usually inviting trouble. Often people aren't affected after their first or second exposure. But four out of five become sensitive after several exposures to urushiol (uh-ROO-she-all)—the chemical in the oil secreted by these plants—which causes itching and burning along with a red, blistery rash. Usually the rash begins a few hours after exposure, but it may not appear for several days. And you need not touch the plant itself. Urushiol is extremely hardy—it doesn't evaporate or lose its power. You can pick it up from an old tool you used in the garden a year before, or from an old shoe you wore in the woods and that got contaminated. Stored leaves can retain their potency for five years. In addition, dogs and cats that have brushed against the leaves carry the irritating oils on their fur, and may transfer it to you.

Prevention and treatment

Here are pointers for avoiding poison ivy—and for taking care of the rash if you get it:

•Be observant when gardening or out in the woods. Remember that poison plants may cling to the ground, or grow up the trunks of trees, or along fences. They may look like shrubs or bushes or small trees or vines. Leaves may be dull or glossy, with saw-toothed or smooth edges, but always grow in triple clusters. In autumn the leaves may turn pinkish. In summer poison ivy has white berries.

•If you're in an area where these plants grow, wear gloves and other clothing that protects your extremities. Lightweight fabrics aren't much good, as urushiol can penetrate them. Avoid touching your face or other bare areas.

•If you think you may have brushed up against poison ivy or oak, remove your clothing carefully, wearing gloves, and wash everything (separately from other clothes) in strong detergent. Wipe off shoes.

•Wash your dog or cat (carefully, wearing gloves) if you think the animal has walked through poison ivy.

•If you think you've gotten the sap on your skin, wash with soap and lots of water within fifteen minutes. This can help ward off a reaction.

•If you break out, try not to scratch, because scratching may lead to infection.

Nonprescription hydrocortisone

Hydrocortisone has long been known to be useful for treating certain skin conditions, especially insect bites and rashes or itches resulting from hypersensitivity to plants, cosmetics, and the like.

Recently, it became available in a 1 percent formulation—twice the strength of the old 0.5 percent kind. While the 1 percent ointment is more likely to relieve itching and promote healing in some cases, it can also make matters worse if applied to the wrong skin disorder. Hydrocortisone generally should not be used by itself on any eruption caused by fungi, viruses, or bacteria (for example, athlete's foot, ringworm, cold sores, or infected areas). If you're sure what your problem is—say, an allergy to a new soap, or a mosquito bite—then try the new ointment. But if you aren't sure, or if hydrocortisone hasn't helped within seventy-two hours, see a doctor. And avoid using it over long periods if your skin eruption is extensive.

But contrary to myth, it won't cause the rash to spread. The water inside the blisters does not contain urushiol. Thus, poison ivy can't spread from one person to another. You can't transmit it to a child, for example, by hugging him when you've a rash on your arms. (If you still have urushiol on your skin, however, you could in theory spread it by touching someone.)

•Try home remedies—cold compresses, cool baths, calamine lotion or cream, baking soda. Over-the-counter cortisone cream may also help. If the rash is very extensive or extremely painful, a doctor may prescribe stronger cortisone treatments or antihistamines. Either way, you'll probably be rid of all traces of the problem in less than three weeks.

•Don't believe anyone who tells you that eating a poison ivy leaf will "desensitize" you. It may make you very sick.

•Ridding your yard of poison oak and ivy is easier said than done. You can try chemical herbicides, but you risk killing other plants. You can still get a rash by picking up the dead plants, so wear heavy protective clothing when pulling them up; then bury the plants. But if possible, let the plants be and don't go near them.

Frostbite

Frostbite can be insidious—if you've been out in the cold a while and your extremities already feel cold and numb, you may not notice that it has set in. Frostbite comes in three categories, from mild to serious: frostnip, superficial frostbite, and deep frostbite.

While the treatment for each type of frostbite varies, two guidelines are applicable to all three types: never massage or rub frostbitten areas (with or without snow), and do not apply any ointments.

Frostnip. The first hint of this stage of frostbite is numbness, followed by a whitening of the tissue—a change that can take place very quickly. Frostnip usually affects the nose, ears, hands, or feet. If possible, get out of the cold. The best treatment is direct application of warmth—blow on the areas, or get someone else to do so; if your nose is frostnipped, apply your warm hands. If it's your hands that are freezing, put them in your warm armpits. Your skin will probably burn and tingle as it warms, but there should be no lasting injury.

Superficial frostbite. This type of frostbite requires medical attention, but there are some steps you should take first. The area will appear very white and waxy and will feel hard on the surface, yet will have its normal resilience in the lower layers. (When checking, press very gently). Get out of the cold, and warm the areas, preferably by immersion in warm water (100 to 105°F—a temperature that should feel comfortably warm, but not hot to undamaged skin). Keep adding warm water as necessary, but take care that it doesn't get too hot. Avoid dry heat or uncontrolled heat sources such as campfires. Don't try to walk on frostbitten feet, and avoid the temptation to rub frostbitten hands or fingers. The warming process may be painful. On the way to the emergency room or doctor, keep the area warm.

Deep frostbite. In this stage, the tissues may be blotchy or blue and will be very hard, without any underlying resilience. Don't try to administer first aid or thaw the tissue. Wrap the frozen area in a blanket or other soft material to prevent bruising, and keep it elevated on the way to the hospital.

Hair is found all over the body, except on the palms of your hands and soles of your feet. A strand of hair is composed of two parts: the shaft—the part of the hair that we see—consists of dead cells; the follicle, which lies just under the skin, is composed of the root and connective tissue. Cells proliferate in the follicle and manufacture a protein called keratin. As more and more cells are produced, the other cells move up and out of the follicle and die, thus creating the shaft of the hair. As long as the follicle remains intact, new hair will be produced. Hair stops growing when the follicle is damaged.

Protecting your hair from the elements

A strand of hair is not as simple as it looks, and its very structure makes it vulnerable to such elements as the sun's ultraviolet rays, the chlorine in pools, beauty-shop chemicals, and detergent shampoos. The cells in the hair shaft's thin outer layer (the cuticle) overlap like scales to protect the shaft's inner mass of fiber (the cortex). Normally this shaft is covered with a protective lubricant, sebum. Sun, salt, and chlorinated water draw moisture from the hair shaft, strip away the sebum, and can damage the cuticle. If the cuticles' scales crack or warp, the roughened hair surface loses its natural sheen, and the unprotected fiber of the cortex frays or "splits," resulting in frizzy, dry hair.

Even worse, pool water can leave blond or gray hair green-tinted. This occurs when copper compounds found in algicides or leached from water pipes bond to the hair and penetrate the cortex, thus acting as a pigment. (People with dark and unbleached hair don't face this problem because the hair shafts' dark pigment, melanin, disguises the green.) In the past, if your hair turned green, all you could do was wait until the hair grew out. But several new gels or shampoos that may help remove discoloration have come on the market.

One way to keep your hair, dark or light, in good health despite exposure to the elements, is to use a hair conditioner. Some of the claims made for conditioners may be commercial hype, but they really do work on a temporary basis by coating the hair with a lubricant, natural or synthetic, that temporarily replaces stripped-away sebum. Other conditioner ingredients bond to the hair, helping to smooth down the cuticle (thereby restoring sheen); still others reduce the static charges that result in flyaway hair. Conditioners (which are mildly acidic) also help balance the pH of shampoos (which are usually mildly alkaline).

Keeping hair healthy

•If you swim or spend a lot of time outdoors, go easy on coloring, permanent waving, hot combs, heated rollers, and blow-dryers.

•Wear a hat in the sun.

•Wear a rubber bathing cap, but don't expect it to keep your hair completely dry. Before you put the cap on, comb conditioner into your hair.

•After your swim, rinse out salt or chlorine with tap water and, if it is available, use shampoo.

•Dry your hair by wrapping it in a towel. Blot and squeeze, don't rub or pull, and don't brush wet hair. Use a wide-toothed comb instead.

Myth: Your hair reveals the state of your health.

Fact: While it is true that hair produced during illness is likely to be of poor quality, hair is not generally an indicator of health. (The exception is that some types of heavy metal exposure can be diagnosed by carefully executed hair analysis.) Companies that promote "hair analysis"—claiming that they can judge the state of your health, evaluate your overall nutritional status, or screen for disease—are perpetrating a fraud. While mineral content of the hair can be readily quantified, factors such as age, sex, race, season, hair length, and color, and even the action of shampoo vary results so much that it is practically impossible to form a standard that would indicate health or illness.

Dandruff

Mild dandruff isn't so much a medical problem as a cosmetic concern. Your whole body continually sheds outer layers of dead skin. Usually the process isn't noticeable, but when the scalp sheds skin, flakes can get trapped in the hair and collect with dirt and oil. The result may be unsightly, but it's generally not a cause for alarm; dandruff doesn't signal hair loss, for instance.

There's no way to prevent dandruff from forming, but frequent shampooing can help keep it under control. An ordinary shampoo may work if used often enough—usually every two to four days. Dandruff shampoos may control it for a few days longer, usually by helping to slough off the scales. Look for these effective anti-dandruff ingredients: zinc pyrithione, sulfusalicylic compounds, selenium sulfide, or coal tar. (While there is some concern that hair dyes containing coal tar—see page 323—may be carcinogenic, dandruff shampoos have much smaller concentrations of coal tar, and are considered safe and effective by the Food and Drug Administration [FDA] and dermatologists.) Use special care with products that contain any of these ingredients—they can hurt your eyes. And since continually using any shampoo may leave a residue build-up, alternate it with another dandruff shampoo, or regular shampoo.

Consult a doctor if more extreme symptoms develop. Severe flaking, crusting, itching, and redness may be signs of medically treatable problems.

Hair Loss

Hair loss afflicts millions—and not just men, though their hair loss is often the most noticeable. Most women, too, experience some degree of hair loss as they grow older. In our culture, and many others, thinning or vanishing hair is bad news. For one thing, hair is usually an obvious give-away of a person's age—and beautiful, thick hair is the symbol of sex appeal and youth in everything from Renaissance verse to television commercials. Throughout life, people are identified by their hair-type: straight-haired, curly-headed, blonde, brunette, redhead—and later, perhaps, "silver-haired," or "bald," and the transition is hard for some people.

Hair is not living tissue like the skin but is composed of a protein called keratin, which is also the building block of fingernails and toenails. Each hair grows from a root enclosed by a follicle, a small pocket in the skin, which is nourished by blood vessels. Hair grows according to a genetic program (hormones are also involved), about half an inch a month; each hair grows for two to six years, then rests. Part of your hair is growing and part is resting at any given moment. After the rest stop, the hair falls out, and it's normal to lose from 50 to 100 hairs a day (not many out of 100,000 in the average youthful head). The shape and size of each scalp hair determines its appearance, and this varies not only from hair to hair but from one person to another and by genetic type. Very thick, round hairs (as in a typical Chinese head of hair) have a geometry that makes them lie flat and straight. Africans and those of African descent tend to have flattened hair shafts, with a resulting tendency toward tight curls. Blondes have more hair—thinner, more elliptical hair shafts compared with the flat or round kind—than other people. Blonde and brown hair, of course, may be straight or curly.

When a hair falls out, a new one presumably grows in, but the catch comes when it doesn't—when more falls out than grows back in.

Why hair may fail to replace itself

Many things can cause sudden, dramatic hair loss. In women, contributing factors can be the hormonal changes of pregnancy and its aftermath, as well as oral contraceptives (taking them, or ceasing to take them—and this problem is less common with the newer pills). In both men and women, severe emotional stress, fad diets if pursued to the point of malnutrition, thyroid disorders, anemia, and various drugs and medications, particularly chemotherapy for cancer, can cause hair loss. So may large doses of vitamin A. The scientific term for hair loss is "alopecia," and thus hair loss caused by constantly wearing tight-fitting wigs or hats is called "friction alopecia." "Traction alopecia" is hair loss caused by pulling hair too tight in ponytails or braids, so that it falls out. In most cases, hair begins to grow again once the underlying problem is corrected, or corrects itself.

More serious is "alopecia areata," which causes loss of hair in patches and is thought to be an autoimmune disorder. It can proceed to complete hair loss, and affects about 2.5 million people in the United States. This condition can sometimes be treated successfully, and anyone who suffers from it should see a dermatologist. Occasionally it simply goes away by itself and new hair grows in.

Any sudden hair loss, of course, is reason to consult a physician.

Androgenetic alopecia: thinning hair

By far the most common form of hair loss is determined by our genes and hormones: it is androgenetic alopecia, usually called male and female pattern baldness. About 35 million American men have male pattern baldness, the receding hairline that eventually turns into a bald pate (sometimes with very fine thin hairs replacing the original growth). By age fifty half of all men of European origin will experience this kind of hair loss, which can begin as early as age twenty. Some other genetic groups—Asians, some Africans and African Americans, and Native Americans—seldom or never get bald in this manner. Though the exact process that shuts down the hair follicles has yet to be explained, the male hormone testosterone plays a role.

Female pattern baldness usually begins about age thirty, becomes noticeable around age forty, and may be even more noticeable after menopause. The pattern of female hair loss is usually an overall-all thinning—two hairs where five used to be—rather than a bald area on top of the head—though women may have a receding hairline, too. It's thought that about 20 million American women have such hair loss. As in males, hair follicles simply shut down, with hormones playing some role in the process.

It's impossible, at present, to prevent this kind of hair loss, though good hair care practices may at least slow down hair loss and keep the hair you've got in good condition. It used to be impossible, too, to replace lost hair, and mostly it still is. But a new drug as well as surgical techniques offer some hope for a few people—at great expense, to be sure, and with sometimes less than satisfactory effects. Certain cosmetic remedies work to some extent, especially if hair loss is not extensive. And at least cosmetic remedies are inexpensive and less risky than drugs or surgery.

How to handle thinning hair

Always handle your hair gently, particularly if it is thinning. Avoid crash diets. Don't over-brush your hair: grandmother's hundred strokes a day wasn't great advice, particularly if your hair is thinning. Avoid hairbrushes and combs that pull your hair. Exposure to sunshine and swimming-pool chemicals should be minimized—wear a hat in the sun and a cap in the pool.

Use a mild shampoo, and avoid rough rubdowns with a towel. If possible, dry your hair naturally. Blow-dryers, hot rollers, and curling irons can damage hair roots, as well as hair shafts. Perming is all right, though (like dying) it does dry out your hair. But avoid anything (such as tightly fastened rollers or teasing and back-combing) that tends to pull the hair out at the roots.

Minoxidil—does it work?

This prescription drug, marketed as Rogaine by the Upjohn company, which developed it, is approved by the FDA for stimulating hair growth. It is the topical form of minoxidil, a potent oral medication for high blood pressure. When minoxidil was being tested, it was found serendipitously to promote new hair growth, sometimes in places where hair was unwanted. Next it was shown to stimulate hair growth when applied to the skin as a solution. Nobody knows how and why Rogaine works—when it does work. It is far from being a miracle. It was first tested on men. In clinical trials, only 39 percent of the men using it experienced moderate hair growth (a thin fluff), and only 8 percent did better than moderate. The majority—61 percent—had little or no hair growth. Younger men did much better than older ones. Some men did report a slowing of hair loss around the temples and the hairline. However, Rogaine stimulates new hair growth only on the top of the head. According to Upjohn, a man who still has some hair in the balding area is more likely to respond than the slick-headed. If you're entirely bald, Rogaine probably won't help.

Rogaine is now being prescribed for women. In one clinical trial, according to Upjohn, about half the women had some new hair growth, but only 12 or 13 percent experienced moderate growth.

In some people, Rogaine may produce itching and skin irritation; its long-term side effects remain unknown. But its two most dramatic drawbacks are these: it costs about $600 a year to use the stuff, and it's a lifetime proposition: if it does make your hair grow, you have to keep using it indefinitely. Otherwise the new hair falls out.

Hair implants

Hair implantation is a form of cosmetic surgery in which patches of skin with healthy hair follicles are transplanted into balding or bald areas. Usually, patches are taken from the back of the scalp and moved to the top of the head. The transplanted hairs always fall out, but new ones grow in a few weeks. Another method is called scalp reduction—i.e. the bald patch is partly excised and the areas of the scalp that still have hair are pulled closer together. Obviously, surgery works best to correct male pattern baldness rather than the overall thinning of hair that most women experience.

Hair transplants are better than they used to be, for doctors can now use micrografts, instead of transplanting larger patches of hair, and can place them in small incisions, "feathering" the hairline so that it looks like natural hair. There is also less risk of scarring using this technique. But it is still a long, laborious, and expensive procedure requiring a series of office visits, sometimes at long intervals. Transplantation is not covered by most medical insurance, and the cost can easily run to $10,000.

Unsatisfactory results are no longer as likely as they once were, but they are a real risk—a "doll's hair" look, scarring, and patches of thin transplanted hair over scalp sections that continue to grow bald, or loss of hair that leaves the scars from transplantation visible.

If you decide to go this route, choose your surgeon with care, and beware of seductive advertising brochures showing "after" photos of men with thick, wavy hair. Ask to see some real people whom the doctor has treated. The best way, actu-

---

Hair-loss remedies that won't work

No product sold over the counter in drugstores or health food stores or by mail will make your hair grow, including high doses of vitamin A, which actually promote hair loss. None of the following are worth trying:

- *Wheat germ oil.*
- *Lanolin.*
- *Special diets (unless you are severely malnourished from a crash diet or an eating disorder).*
- *Protein and amino acid supplements.*
- *Vitamin supplements, taken orally or applied to the scalp.*
- *So-called vasodilators, products to rub into the scalp that supposedly increase the blood supply*
- *Massage, special combs, or electrical stimulation.*
- *Suturing a hairpiece to your scalp. This surgical technique, advertised as a "lifetime answer to baldness," hasn't been banned by the FDA, but it entrails such risks as chronic infections, scarring, blood poisoning, and even brain abscesses. It's also quite uncomfortable.*

ally, to find a surgeon is through a referral from a satisfied customer, but even then you should be sure the doctor's credentials check out. Check with the Department of Plastic Surgery at your nearest university medical school.

Cosmetic remedies you can try

Resort to camouflage. Especially for women, a short haircut and such hair cosmetics as sprays, gels, and mousses can hide thinning. Hair dyes can minimize the visual and psychological effects of hair loss. Permanent dyes, of course, can dry out the hair shaft if they are used over long periods, but they won't injure the root or promote additional hair loss. Whether using a dye at home or going to a salon, don't skip the patch test for possible allergic reactions. At home, follow package directions carefully.

Or try out a wig or hair piece. One cosmetic trick that may work for women: buy a powdered eye shadow the color of your hair and apply it lightly to your scalp in the thin spots. It's harmless and may make thinning hair less noticeable.

Hair weaving?

Also called "hair intensification," or "hair integration" means adding to thin hair by weaving or braiding wefts of human hair or synthetic fibers into existing hair. Apart from the expense (anywhere from $50 to $2,500), this poses two problems: first, it may be difficult to keep your hair and scalp clean. And second, it stresses existing hair and may cause it to fall out. The American Hair Loss Council advises that only people with plenty of healthy hair should consider hair weaving. And even they should plan to keep the "intensified" hair for only a few weeks.

Hair Dyes

About one third of American women and an unknown percentage of men use hair dyes, most of which contain coal-tar dyes. Because they work better, last longer, and look more natural, coal-tar dyes have almost entirely replaced plant derivative dyes (such as henna) and metallic dyes (the kind you apply every day for gradual darkening). In spite of their superior cosmetic qualities, the use of coal-tar dyes can cause severe skin allergies in some people. Moreover, in 1978 two chemicals found in coal-tar dyes—known as 4-MMPD and 4-MMPDS—were shown to cause cancer in animals.

Curiously enough, though, the FDA has no power to ban hair dyes. According to the Food and Drug Act of 1938, coal-tar dyes have a special status among cosmetics, and the FDA cannot take them off the market. The FDA does require that packages warn about possible skin irritation. In 1978 the FDA proposed that a cancer warning be posted on hair dye packages. Rather than comply, many companies "voluntarily" removed 4-MMPD and 4-MMPDS from their products. This sounded reassuring to the public, but in fact these dyes were simply replaced with similar ones whose carcinogenic qualities had never been tested.

Most of the studies evaluating hair dye safety have involved feeding large quantities of dye to laboratory animals. According to cosmetic manufacturers, this is a far cry from putting a small amount on your scalp every four weeks or so. Yet the scalp is a highly sensitive area, and hair dyes do penetrate the skin. Some human

Myth: Worry can turn hair white.

Fact: *Nothing turns hair white but the gradual decrease of pigmentation that occurs with age. Shock or stress does not affect hair color. Graying, whether it comes with the normal process of aging or prematurely, has a genetic basis. If you are Caucasian, you'll begin graying on average at about age thirty-four; average black begins graying at forty-four.*

Whenever it happens, hair turns gray or white when pigment ceases to be produced in the hair root, and new hairs grow in that are gray or white. Overnight graying rarely if ever occurs. In any case, it has never been documented.

It is impossible that pigmented hair could simply shed its color without benefit of a bleach. There is, however, a rare type of scalp disorder, known as **alopecia areata,** *which causes hair to shed rapidly. This might leave remaining unpigmented hairs looking all the whiter—hence the "overnight" myth.*

studies have revealed no increase in the risk of breast or bladder cancer, while others do show increased risk.

But one recent study of half a million women, published in the *Journal of the National Cancer Institute,* reported that even using hair dyes for twenty years does not increase the risk of breast, stomach, brain, lung, or other cancers. Indeed, those women who dyed their hair had a lower risk for urinary tract cancers than women who never used dyes. The one possible worry was among women who had used black hair dyes for twenty years or more—who accounted for only 0.6 percent of all hair-dye users. Black dyes did appear to increase their risk for non-Hodgkin's lymphoma and multiple myeloma—relatively rare forms of cancer. If you have used black dyes for many years, this could mean you have increased your risk, but not that you are likely to get either of these cancers. If hair has anything to do with them, it is only one of many factors.

Based on this study, women—and men—who use hair dyes (except permanent black ones) need not worry that they're increasing their cancer risk. Still, the National Cancer Institute advises people to check hair dye labels and avoid any with the following ingredients, which have been shown to cause cancer when fed to laboratory animals: 2,4-diaminoanisole sulfate, also known as 4-MMPD and 4-MMPDS (no longer used); 4-amino-2 nitrophenol, also known as 2-nitro-p-phenylenediamine; direct black 38; direct blue 6; lead acetate.

Safety guidelines

If you do dye your hair, follow these suggestions:

•Women who are or might be pregnant should avoid dyes entirely, since some may pose a risk to the fetus.

•Dye your hair as infrequently as possible, and don't leave the dye on your head longer than the instructions tell you.

•Try frosting or streaking instead of methods that call for applying dye to the entire scalp.

•Wash your hair and scalp thoroughly after dyeing.

•Avoid using dyes regularly over a period of many years.

•Check the label of henna and metallic dyes. Henna can only dye hair bright red; a product that does anything else may have coal-tar supplements. Metallic dyes often contain lead acetate.

N A I L   C A R E

Fingernails are simply another form of skin, a hardened protein called keratin that has a high sulphur content. Contrary to popular belief, the calcium content of nails is very low. Fair-skinned people appear to have pinkish nails; others may have brown or black ones, according to the skin color underneath. Healthy-looking fingernails are more often than not a sign of good health. But changes in color and appearance are not necessarily a sign of illness. Although a careful physician will always look at the nails, diagnosing or predicting any generalized ailment would be impossible on the basis of nails alone.

Among the nail problems that cause anxiety from time to time are:

Brittleness. Like dry skin, this is likely to worsen in winter. Frequent immersion in water—particularly if chlorine, soap, or detergent is added—makes nails break. Wearing rubber gloves will help if dishwashing is causing the brittleness. So will wearing warm gloves outdoors in the winter.

White spots. As a rule these result from minor injury. White spots seldom indicate any vitamin or mineral deficiency; they will vanish as the nail grows.

Ridges. Longitudinal ridges are not unusual; they may be genetic, and they do become more prominent as you age. If you have transverse furrows (known as "Beau's lines") that begin at the base of the nail, one thing to suspect is excessively rigorous manicuring. Pressure with a manicure tool can cause pits or bumps in the nail; so can biting your fingers. Furrows may appear after such illnesses as measles, pneumonia, or other severe infections, but they are not symptoms of infection.

Discoloration. Cigarettes, hair dyes, and even the tints that sometimes leak out of nail polish can discolor your nails. An injury may also be the culprit.

Separation of nail from nail bed. This condition, along with alterations in the nail texture, may be a sign of psoriasis, a disorder of the skin, often mild and often confined only to fingernails. Like brittleness, it may be caused by, or aggravated by, exposure to water, detergents, soaps, and even nail hardeners. An allergic reaction to nail polish is also a possible cause.

Reversal of the normal nail curvature (spoon nail). This may indicate iron deficiency, especially in older children.

With the exception of spoon nail, none of these problems is likely to be significant. Nevertheless, your nails are one of many indicators of health. Any dramatic changes in their texture, shape, color, or growth rate may be a signal to seek medical advice.

Are nail products safe?

Under most circumstances nail enamels, hardeners, and polish removers won't do you any harm. Nevertheless, you should read the labels, as with any product, and be aware of the problems nail products can sometimes cause.

First, polish remover is very drying to nails and cuticles, so use it sparingly and as infrequently as possible. Don't remove nail enamel every day. Make repairs by reapplying enamel.

Second, nail plates (the visible nails) are very porous and dry quickly. Enamels waterproof the nail plates, so when the skin under them gets wet, it stays moist longer and thus is subject to infection, especially if you accidentally injure the nail bed. If you notice signs of infection (pain, redness, pus), see a doctor.

Third, some nail product ingredients can produce allergic reactions. One such component is called toluene-sulfonamide formaldehyde resin. This can cause rashes on the fingers or around the eyes, since buffing or filing nail enamel—or even blowing on it as it dries—can cause small particles to enter the air. For a hypo-allergenic enamel, look for one without formaldehyde resins. "Hardeners" are particularly likely to contain them.

Caution on artificial nails

What are the long term effects of artificial nails? Sculptured nails are more likely to damage nails than other products. They are formed by mixing a powder and liquid containing acrylics and peroxide; this mixture is applied to the nail plates and, after it dries, filed and shaped like a real nail. Methyl methacrylate, which can

Nail growth

•Rate of nail growth varies from person to person and from finger to finger. The nail of the middle finger grows fastest, the thumbnail and little-fingernail lag behind.

•Right- or left-handedness affects nail growth—nails grow faster on the hand you use most. For unknown reasons nails grow faster in the premenstrual phase in women. Male nails grow slightly faster than female, perhaps because the nail plate is bigger. Hormones may also play a role.

•The nails of well-nourished people grow faster than those of the undernourished, but no specific food, mineral, or vitamin accelerates nail growth—not even that old standby gelatin.

•It takes 5½ to 6 months for a nail to grow from cuticle to tip, so your nails are a mini-biography. A ridge caused by an injury near the cuticle line in May will still be visible in October.

cause skin inflammation and splitting of the nail plate, was once a common ingredient of the sculpting powder, until the FDA enjoined American manufacturers from using it. However, you've really no way of knowing what's in the mix the manicurist may apply, since manufacturers seldom specify what's in wholesale nail products and, in any case, some salons may use imported products containing methyl methacrylate.

A potential hazard for manicurists is repeatedly breathing the vapor from such solvents as toluene, found in a wide range of nail products. This chemical may cause damage to the bone marrow and liver, as well as irritation to the throat and lungs. Cyanoacrylates (found in Krazy Glue, for instance), another nail-sculpting ingredient, can also produce irritation and splitting, and particles may enter the air during filing.

Stick-on nails—preformed plastic nails glued to the nail bed—are not so bad, as long as cyanoacrylates are not in the glue. However, wearing artificial nails for long periods can damage the natural nails because the artificial nails form an airtight cover. Thus stick-on nails should be removed at least once a year to give the real nails a breather.

Eye Care

Your eye is an intricate structure that efficiently performs myriad tasks: it receives and transmits thousands of visual messages per minute, automatically adjusts its lens to changing light conditions, focuses incoming light, and produces its own fluids for lubrication and cleansing and fighting off infection. Healthy eyes perceive the world both centrally and peripherally—and simultaneously. Your central vision enables you to read this page, while your peripheral vision lets you see the person entering a door to your right, without turning your head. Moreover, though each eye sees separately, both eyes together produce "binocular" vision—that is, the brain perceives a single image, thus giving you three-dimensional depth perception and a coherent picture of your surroundings.

Nevertheless, for most of us this miraculous system has its flaws: 54 percent of us wear corrective lenses, and few people (especially as they age) have what's called 20/20 vision in both eyes. That's an arbitrary measure of perfect vision—meaning that your eye can read what a normal eye can read at a distance of twenty feet in daylight. You might have perfect vision in your right eye but 20/50 vision in the left—that is, using the left eye only, you have to stand at twenty feet to read what a normal eye can read at fifty feet. (The larger the second number, the worse the vision.) Problems related to refractive errors (that is, faults in focusing light) fall into three categories: astigmatism (distorted or partially blurry vision), myopia (nearsightedness), and hyperopia (farsightedness), including presbyopia (the farsightedness that accompanies aging). All these problems can be corrected or at least helped with proper lenses.

An eye-care checklist

1. Wear goggles or safety glasses when working with power tools or dangerous chemicals that might splash, and when playing racquetball and other high-risk sports. More than a million Americans injure their eyes every year playing sports, at work, and in other activities. Be wary of flying objects—twigs coming out of a lawn mower, even a cork exploding from a bottle of sparkling wine (cover the cork with a towel and point it away from your face; ease it out, rather than popping it).

2. Avoid tanning booths and sunlamps, which can cause irreversible damage to your eyes or even blindness. If you insist on getting an artificial tan, wear opaque goggles. Shutting your eyes is not enough.

3. Don't share eye cosmetics; buy them in small amounts and replace them every four to six months (that's how long the preservatives last). "Tester" products that other people have used in a store may be contaminated, so try them on the back of your hand, not around your eyes.

4. Wear sunglasses with ultraviolet-coated lenses outdoors on sunny days, even in winter. Studies suggest that lifelong exposure to ultraviolet rays promotes cataracts.Wearing a hat in the sunshine protects your eyes, too.

5. Consider wearing protective glasses or goggles (any type of plastic lens will do) on windy, snowy days. Cold wind and weather dry your eyes, and dryness paradoxically makes them "cry"—uncomfortable for anybody and a real problem for contact lens wearers.

6. Avoid working in bad light. While it's a myth that reading in bad light will ruin your vision, you'll be less prone to headaches in adequate glare-free lighting—and you'll work more efficiently and pleasurably.

7. Stick with daily-care lenses if you wear contacts. Sleeping with contact lenses can lead to infections.

8. Avoid habitual use of over-the-counter eye drops as a remedy for redness (see box on page 332). They do whiten the eyes by constricting blood vessels, but too frequent use can actually irritate the eye, making it redder, and can cause allergic reactions. Use other eye drops only as directed by a doctor.

When do you need an eye checkup?

Schedules for eye checkups vary according to your age and other factors. The U.S. Preventive Services Task Force recommends the following:

All children should have their eyes examined at age three or four, before starting school. Another vision check at age thirteen may be a good idea, since this is when refractive problems may develop.

For most adults, it's not necessary to have eye exams on a regular basis. Obviously, any eye problem or change in vision requires a visit to an ophthalmologist or optometrist.

People at risk for glaucoma should be screened for the disease as frequently as their eye-care professional recommends: high-risk groups include those sixty-five and older, African Americans, the severely nearsighted, diabetics, and those with a family history of glaucoma.

Eye-care specialists

Over the course of a lifetime, most people will need the services of the following types of vision specialists:

Ophthalmologists are certified doctors of medicine—with several years of residency training beyond medical school—who specialize in medical and surgical care of the eye. As such, they have the greatest range of expertise among eye-care specialists. In addition to testing vision and prescribing corrective lenses, ophthalmologists diagnose and treat all sorts of eye disorders, from minor infections to conditions like glaucoma that can lead to blindness.

Optometrists diagnose refractive errors and prescribe lenses, screen for glaucoma, and identify other disorders. They are not medical doctors, but they have completed a three-year university science program plus a four-year program at a school of optometry. In some states, optometrists can also diagnose and treat specified eye diseases—but if a disorder outside their expertise is apparent, an optometrist would refer you to an ophthalmologist.

Opticians do not test vision nor prescribe treatment for any sort of eye problem; rather, they are practitioners who fit and sell corrective lenses as prescribed by an ophthalmologist or optometrist.

The most common eye problem

Most people are never troubled by anything other than faulty focusing—so-called refractive defects, which occur because light entering the eye isn't precisely focused on the retina, the "film" inside the back of the eye. In most cases the problem is either nearsightedness—in which near objects are more clearly focused and distant objects are fuzzy—or farsightedness, in which close-up vision is blurred. Another common refractive defect is astigmatism, a distortion caused by an uneven cornea or lens. Presbyopia, a fourth common condition, is caused by an impaired ability to change focus as a result of weakened eye muscles and rigidity in the lens. This problem gradually develops with age, such that most people need help in correcting their vision by their mid-forties, even if only for reading (see page 332).

Fortunately, all of these focusing problems can generally be easily remedied with corrective lenses, which are now worn by about half of the population, either in the form of eyeglasses or contact lenses. You should consult with your eye specialist as to which corrective measures are best for you.

Other common eye problems are covered in the chart on the next page.

Eye Problems, Minor and Major

Condition	Comments	Treatment
Dry eyes	Discomfort usually due to insufficient tear production, though certain eyelid abnormalities or surface infections may also be responsible. Overflowing tears, ironically, are often a symptom, produced in response to underlying dryness. Postmenopausal women often susceptible. May also be a side effect of certain drugs (diuretics, antidepressants) or associated with arthritis.	Extreme dryness can damage eyes, so professional diagnosis is a good precaution even in mild cases. "Artificial tears" (nonprescription eye drops) are often completely effective, though some may be allergic to the preservatives in them. Avoiding hair dryers, smoky, overheated, or very dry rooms may also help. Glasses can cut down evaporation in the wind.
Blepharitis	Scaly, red eyelids, inflamed around the margins. May be accompanied by dandruff.	Wash twice daily with warm salt water, a solution of baking soda, or soap and water. If it does not clear up, consult a doctor, who may prescribe an ointment.
Foreign bodies	Such debris as eyelashes and specks of grit usually require no medical attention, unless embedded in the eye.	Don't rub your eye; pull the upper lid over the lower and roll your eye. If that fails to remove the debris, flush the eye with plain water. Blowing your nose may help. If discomfort persists or becomes acute, or if you think something is embedded in your eye, go to a physician or the emergency room. Never try to remove a foreign body that appears lodged in the cornea (the covering over the iris) or that has penetrated the eye.
Sty	A pimple on the eyelid caused by an infection in the eyelash follicle or the oil gland. Red, painful inflammation like a small boil.	Apply warm compresses three or four times a day. Don't burst, squeeze, rub. Avoid rubbing eyes, which spreads infection. Should subside in a week or so without medical attention. If sties occur frequently, see a doctor.
Conjunctivitis (pinkeye)	Infection or inflammation of the thin membrane or conjunctiva that covers eyeball and inner eyelid. Highly contagious if caused by bacteria or viruses, not catching if produced by allergies or irritants.	Usually clears up in a week. To avoid spreading an infection to your other eye, or to other people, avoid touching or rubbing the eye. Wash away discharge with tissue; separate your washcloths and towels from family wash. Don't use contact lenses or eye makeup, which can spread infection to the other eye. Consult a doctor if discharge is severe, redness get noticeably worse, eye is very painful, or vision is persistently blurred. Antibiotic eye drops should clear up most bacterial infections.
Glaucoma	Most common form called chronic open-angle glaucoma: fluid pressure within the eye gradually rises, and in time damages optic nerve, narrowing field of vision and eventually leading to blindness. Symptomless in early stages. Not contagious; always affects both eyes. (See page 339 for more information and recommendations on testing for glaucoma.)	Early diagnosis and treatment essential. Medications to reduce eye pressure come in pill or eye-drop form; these drugs are effective in preserving vision and must be taken for life. Laser and conventional surgical techniques useful in some cases. Regular checkups necessary: glaucoma may worsen or improve with no symptoms, and medication may need to be adjusted.
Cataracts	Not a growth, but a gradual clouding and hardening of the lens of the eye (located behind the pupil). Most commonly associated with aging, though can be caused by injury or diabetes. Painless, but eventually causes hazy or blurred vision, or sensitivity to light, or the impression of having a film over the eyes (see page 338).	Surgical removal of the lens; replacement with intraocular lenses (implanted in the eye), with contact lenses, or with eyeglasses. Surgery usually performed on outpatient basis. Treatment is safe and 90 percent effective at improving vision.
Detached retina	A tear in or dislocation of the eye's back layer of light-sensitive cells and nerve endings. May be caused by a severe blow but more commonly by a shrinking of the vitreous inside the eyeball, which may occur with aging. Severe nearsightedness also a risk factor. Complete loss of vision may result. Symptoms: dramatic onset of floaters and flashers (see page 334), or sudden wavy, watery quality in vision, or loss of central vision. Diabetes is a risk factor.	Essential to seek treatment immediately. Go to nearest emergency room. Many treatments now available, including laser or surgical repair, which can successfully correct early retinal detachments in 90 percent of cases.

Contact Lenses: Options New and Old

About 24 million Americans now wear contact lenses. Two out of three of them are women, and six out of seven under age forty-five. For most wearers, contacts are both comfortable and safe, and can be superior to glasses in correcting vision problems. Not everyone can wear them, however, and they won't correct all vision problems. But they are a boon to all who dislike the look of glasses and the hindrance they can pose in sports and exercise. Choosing contact lenses used to be easy: there were hard lenses (now rarely used) and soft lenses. Today there are many more and better options, including more for people with special needs, such as those with astigmatism, those who have had cataract surgery, or those who need bifocals. The chart on the next page sketches the pros and cons of various kinds of lenses.

A note about extended-wear lenses

During the past five years, extended-wear contact lenses have been the one of the fastest growing segments of the contacts market. Some extended-wear lenses are disposable. Extended-wear sounds great: you wear the lenses day and night for up to a week and then clean and disinfect them. If they're also disposable, you never touch them except when you first put them in and then throw them out. But several studies have shown that overnight use of lenses increases the risk of infection or ulceration of the cornea (the eyeball's transparent covering). One 1994 study, in the *Archives of Ophthalmology*, found that people who wear lenses overnight have an eight times greater risk of corneal ulcers than other lens wearers. The risk of infection appears to increase with each consecutive day you wear the lenses without removing and cleaning/disinfecting them. Thus a few years back, the FDA advised that lenses not be worn for more than seven consecutive days and nights. But even one night may be too much, so it's safest to remove the lenses each night. If you're considering extended-wear lenses, discuss the risks with an eye-care specialist.

Where to go

The key to getting the right contacts is using a skilled eye-care professional—this is even more important than with eyeglasses. No one type or brand of lens is right for everyone. The lenses must suit your vision, your eyes, and your lifestyle. Only optometrists and ophthalmologists prescribe lenses. They, as well as opticians, may also fit and sell them (regulations and practices vary from state to state). Chains of discount optical stores offer huge stocks and low prices. Lenses can also be bought mail-order, sometimes directly from the manufacturer. Be leery of stores or companies that advertise cut rates. The lenses they offer may be of older design, bought by the store at bargain rates. In some cases, discount stores may offer no follow-up care at all beyond a booklet and a kit of solutions.

The way to judge a practitioner is not by price but by the time he devotes to prescribing and fitting lenses and particularly to follow-up care. A first consultation and fitting should take at least an hour, and the practitioner should give you precise instructions for inserting and removing the lenses, as well as a demonstration of proper lens care. Follow-up visits are a necessary part of professional care.

Remember, the lenses themselves cost very little. What you pay for—and should insist on—is continuing professional supervision and advice.

Contact trouble spots

The following conditions, situations, and products may make wearing lenses temporarily impractical:

- Very low humidity—from dry heat, air conditioning, or extremely dry weather—can make lenses uncomfortable. So can airplane cabins, wind, blow-dryers.
- Cold pills and diuretics decrease the amount of tears, causing discomfort.
- Watery eyes from colds or allergies can make lenses uncomfortable.
- In some women, pregnancy, menstruation, or birth control pills. can cause dry eyes.
- Tobacco smoke and other types of air-borne irritants can be a problem.
- Apply eye makeup carefully after inserting lenses, and don't use cosmetics that are likely to run into the eye. Avoid putting makeup on the inside edge of the eyelid.
- Avoid aerosol sprays.while wearing lenses.
- If you experience minor eye fatigue, especially toward the end of the day, change to regular glasses. It never hurts to give your eyes a rest.

A Guide to Contact Lenses

Type	Comment	Advantages	Disadvantages
Rigid gas-permeable (RGP) lenses	Have largely replaced standard hard lenses. Made of semi-flexible plastic that allows oxygen through. Cost $200-$300.	Generally give better vision than soft lenses. Can correct some refractive problems, such as astigmatism, that most soft contacts can't. More flexible, comfortable, and easier to get used to than standard hard lenses. Easiest to care for. Durable, usually lasting several years, so least expensive. Least likely to cause infections.	Require consistent wear to maintain adaptation. Less comfortable than soft lenses at first; may require a week to adapt. Can occasionally be dislodged from eyes, which limits their value for sports.
Daily-wear soft lenses	By far the most common type. Made of flexible plastic that allows oxygen through. Water content varies. Cost $150-$275.	More comfortable and easier to get used to than RGP. Fit well because larger. Hard to dislodge, so good for sports.	Vision may not be as sharp as with RGP. Can't correct all vision problems. Require careful, daily cleaning/disinfecting. Less durable than RGP; may tear when handled. Usually need to be replaced at least once a year.
Extended-wear lenses	Available in RGP or soft. Cost $225-$375.	Can be worn for up to seven days without removal or cleaning. Very thin, so may be more comfortable and easier to get used to.	Increased risk of infection, so frequent cleaning/disinfecting is recommended. Soft lenses are fragile. Can't correct all vision problems. Usually need to be replaced at least once a year. May require more office visits.
Disposable lenses	Soft lenses worn for up to fourteen days, if removed at night. Cost $300-$600 per year. One-day disposables now available.	Less chance of deposit build-up.	Increased risk of infection if worn overnight. Expensive, especially if discarded daily. Can't correct all vision problems. Vision may not be as sharp as with RGP. May tear.
Planned replacement lenses	Soft lenses that are replaced biweekly, monthly, or quarterly. Cost $300-$600 per year.	Need less care. Available in most prescriptions.	Can't correct all vision problems. Vision may not be as sharp as with RGP.
Bifocal lenses	Soft or rigid. Various options, including monovision (one lens for distance, one for near), simultaneous vision, or segmented vision. Cost $375-$500.	Better choices than in the past. Monovision is simplest solution.	May be hard to adjust to and may compromise vision. As with bifocal glasses, not everyone can adapt to these. Depends on individual needs and motivation. Requires expert fitting.
Toric lenses	Correct a variety of astigmatisms. Soft (sometimes disposable) or rigid. Cost $275-500.	Improved choices for people with severe astigmatism. Stable on the eyes when blinking.	Difficult to fit and expensive.

Lens care

Caring for most types of lenses is a daily job that demands a commitment of time and money. Many different kinds of lens solutions and several systems of lens care are available. Some products may contain preservatives (to keep them sterile) and other potentially irritating ingredients. What works for one person may produce an allergic reaction in another. Not all brands of solution are interchangeable, so don't experiment without professional advice.

Rigid lenses need daily rinsing and cleaning, and the lens case must be cleaned and refilled each night. Daily- and extended-wear lenses may require as many as five products, including special cleaners and "wetting" eye drops for lubricating lenses every so often. And all soft lenses must be disinfected by storing them in special disinfecting solutions or in electrically heated disinfecting units. Again, professional advice is always necessary.

Reading Glasses and Bifocals: New Options

Most people over forty-five begin to need glasses to read small print, even those who still have excellent distance vision. This perfectly normal condition, called presbyopia (meaning "old eyes"), occurs when the lens of the eye becomes less flexible and thus less able to change shape and focus on close objects, especially in dim light or when a person is tired.

All that's needed to correct presbyopia is a set of reading glasses. These can cost $100 or more if prescribed by a specialist; yet over-the-counter glasses, which cost around twenty dollars or less, may be just as effective. These glasses must meet the requirements of the American National Standards Institute (ANSI) and of the Food and Drug Administration (FDA), including impact resistance tests.

There's an important caution, however: over-the-counter reading glasses won't correct nearsightedness, astigmatism, or other refractive defects, and buying a pair of them is no substitute for an eye exam. Many people, especially those over sixty-five, should see an eyecare specialist at regular intervals for a glaucoma test and an examination. If your vision is changing rapidly, consult an optometrist or ophthalmologist to make sure that magnifying glasses are all you need.

When you pick out nonprescription reading glasses, be sure you have the time to try on several pairs and read the test cards provided. You might also carry along a book or newspaper for testing. Glasses will usually be marked with a number ranging from 1.00 to 4.00, indicating the magnifying power. (Low magnification would be 1.25 or 1.50, high would be 3.00 and above.) Start at the low end and work your way up, holding the card at a comfortable reading distance.

Progressive lenses. Someone who has no other refractive problems needs only a

Myth: Eyeglasses that are too strong can make your vision worse.

Fact: Eyeglasses can't worsen your vision or damage your eyes. If you think your reading glasses are too strong or if you have difficulty with a new prescription, you should certainly see your ophthalmologist or optometrist. It makes no sense to wear glasses that seem too strong or otherwise unsatisfactory—they're uncomfortable and can interfere with your daily life, and might cause you to have an accident. But they won't actually hurt your eyes. Going without your glasses doesn't hurt them either (unless you have a special eye problem for which glasses are part of the treatment).

Over-the-Counter Eye Drops

Most are safe, but they are rarely necessary. Normal eyes do not need "cleansing," "soothing," or "refreshing" solutions. Your tears, which contain antibacterial agents, are the most effective eye cleansers of all. Though they may be soothing, over-the-counter drops can mask symptoms of serious eye infection and diseases. If there's irritation or redness for more than a day or two, seek professional advice. In no case should you continue using eye drops for more than a day or two.

Nonprescription eye drops come in three types: artificial tears to soothe dry eyes (such as Aqua Tears, Tears Plus, Muro Tears); decongestants, which whiten the eyeball (Visine, Murine Plus); and eyewashes, which "irrigate" the eye.

Artificial tears can temporarily soothe eyes, but are needed only by people with serious eye problems. Most contain preservatives that can cause allergic reactions. People with dry eyes should humidify their houses and avoid dry environments—two steps that can reduce the need for artificial tears.

Decongestants, too, can provide temporary relief to eyes irritated by air pollution, chlorinated pool water, or fatigue. But they can have an irritating effect all their own. Don't use them more than three times a day.

As for eyewashes, they may feel refreshing, but they have no medicinal effect and are no more effective than cold tap water. Many over-the-counter eyewashes contain boric acid, which is a very mild antibacterial and wouldn't help at all if you had an eye infection.

Any liquid you put in your eyes should be sterile, and should therefore be bought in a drug store. There's one exception: emergencies. If you get dirt or a toxic chemical in your eye, there won't be time to find a sterile solution—just wash your eye with plenty of tap water.

If you wear contact lenses, use only drops recommended by your eye-care specialist.

pair of reading glasses. But depending on their existing vision problems, people who already wear corrective lenses will eventually need bifocals or even trifocals—glasses with two or three kinds of vision correction, as the names imply. Until recently, these visual fields were necessarily divided by a "break" in the lens. With the progressive lens type of bifocal, the lens is manufactured to provide a gradual change in correction from top to bottom. "Erase the line between youth and middle age" is the slogan that's appeared in ads and on billboards for one brand of progressives. And indeed some people who need only reading glasses sometimes opt for progressives in order not to have a pair of reading glasses perched halfway down their noses.

Progressive lenses are less common in the United States than in Europe, where more people use them than regular bifocals. The lenses are also expensive—roughly three times what half-glasses usually cost at the optometrist or optician, and about twice as expensive as conventional bifocal lenses. As an article in *Optometric Economics* pointed out, "for dispensers, the extra cost of progressive addition lenses… means bigger margins."

Progressive lenses have some of the same disadvantages as regular bifocals or trifocals—they are usually hard to get used to, and you may trip and fall if you forget that the bottom half of your glasses is for close work, not for making your way downstairs. (Simple reading glasses are less of a nuisance, since people tend to take them off when not reading, the chief hazard being mislaying them.) In addition, progressives have a smaller near-field for reading, because the focus changes gradually. As with bifocals, some people simply can't adapt to progressives, which tend to have greater peripheral distortion than other lenses, and thus can be a problem for people doing a lot of close work. Nevertheless, some people adjust to them and really like them. If you want progressives, you would be wise to compare before you buy, and to discuss the matter with your eye-care professional. They're harder to prescribe and fit than regular bifocals, so you'll need somebody who is experienced in fitting the newer type of lens. You may have to return for instruction more than once.

Bifocal contacts: practical for some. If you wear contact lenses for another vision problem and now need help for close work, another option is bifocal contact lenses, rather than a pair of reading glasses to be worn with your contacts. In a small study of middle-aged contact lens wearers at the University of California at Berkeley, two out of three preferred bifocal contacts over the lens/glasses combination. But these lenses won't work for everybody. They do reduce vision somewhat, as well as the ability to do close work. And the participants in the study were highly motivated—that is, they had volunteered to take part because they were eager to be rid of reading glasses.

Better bifocal contacts are being introduced on the market. Another option some people have been experimenting with is called monovision—wearing a near-vision contact lens in one eye and a distance-vision one in the other, so that you see with one eye at a time. Surprisingly, some people find it works well. If you want to investigate bifocal contacts or monovision, discuss your needs thoroughly beforehand with a professional experienced in fitting them.

Eyes and eye makeup: recommendations

Eyeliner, shadow, and mascara usually pose no danger to the user. Well-packaged eye makeup is almost always clean and virtually uncontaminated (it contains preservatives to keep it that way). Still, some women get eye infections from eye makeup. It's all a matter of care. Follow the suggestions below and opposite to keep your eyes safe.

•Wash your hands before applying makeup to your eyes. Your fingers can carry bacteria.

•Keep applicators and containers clean. Wipe dust off your makeup area and containers with a damp cloth.

•Take care not to scratch your eye with an applicator.

•Buy mascara in small amounts. If it or any eye product is more than a few months old, throw it out. Because women tend to keep mascara around for months or years, it is the most commonly contaminated eye makeup (the effectiveness of its preservatives declines in just three or four months).

Radial Keratotomy: Surgery for Nearsightedness

Radial keratotomy (RK) is an operation that aims to correct nearsightedness, also known as myopia. It's thought that around 11 million Americans are myopic—an abundance of potential customers. Advertisements for RK promise a new life without contact lenses or eyeglasses. But we suggest holding on to your prescriptions at least long enough to consider the risks along with the benefits.

The shape of the eyeball and cornea is one factor that determines how the eye focuses light. If the cornea is too convex, the result may be nearsightedness. In RK, which requires extreme precision, small cuts are made in the cornea to flatten it, so that the point of focus on the retina is corrected. This outpatient procedure, done under topical anesthetic, came into wide use in this country in the 1980s. The fee ranges from about $1,500 to $2,000 for each eye. It's advisable to have one eye done at a time to see what the results are, though many doctors do both at once. It's possible to correct just one eye and leave the other nearsighted, for reading. This is called monovision (you see at a distance with the corrected eye) and will delay the need, eventually, for reading glasses.

The operation should be done only after young adulthood because myopia may continue to worsen into the early twenties. According to Dr. Penny Asbell, a spokesperson for the American Academy of Ophthalmology, "Very few patients will have perfect vision [after RK]. You have to have realistic expectations." Results are predictable: about 75 to 95 percent will end up with 20/40 vision, not perfect but good enough to pass a driving test.

Keep the following points in mind:

•A government study, called PERK (Prospective Evaluation of RK) has followed 435 people who had the surgery in 1982-83. Five years later, as reported in 1990, 36 percent of the 323 people who had surgery on both eyes still needed glasses. Overcorrection was a problem for a few people—they became farsighted. But recent studies report a lower incidence of overcorrection. Then, too, the surgical technique has been improved since the PERK patients had RK. Correction appears to be better now, at least initially.

•But it's still not known what the long-term results of RK will be. That is, no one knows what the repaired eyes will be like in fifteen, twenty, or thirty years.

•The best candidates for the operation are those with mild to moderate, stable myopia. Those with severe myopia should not undergo RK.

•The operation weakens the eye and may make it more vulnerable to injury.

•It may be more difficult to treat cataracts in people who have undergone RK.

•RK is usually not reimbursed by health insurance (check with your insurance company). Make sure follow-up visits are included in the fee, as well as further surgery if your eyes prove to be undercorrected.

•With or without RD, you will no doubt need reading glasses eventually.

On the horizon

Something slightly better than RK may be waiting down the line—a procedure using an excimer (or cold laser) that can flatten the cornea without cutting it. Approved for use in many other countries, this treatment, as of early 1995, was being done on an experimental basis here, pending FDA decision for general use. It will probably cost about as much as RK. While it's less traumatic to eye tissue, it

Floaters

Floaters—those spots or lines that drift across your eyeball from time to time—are generally nothing to worry about. Called "entoptic phenomena," they are sloughed off retinal cells "floating" in the vitreous—the jellylike substance that fills much of your eyeball. Floaters tend to appear when you tilt your head or suddenly glance up or down, causing cellular debris to cross the center of the retina.

But, in rare instances, floaters can be a danger sign. Flashing lights, a sudden onset of floaters, or a rapid increase in them (especially if they are confined to one eye or appear in large clumps), blurry vision, or partial shading of your visual field may indicate that your retina has—or is about to—come loose. If you have such symptoms, call an eye doctor or go to the emergency room at once. Don't wait until the next morning, as a detached retina, when untreated, can lead to blindness.

takes longer for its effects to become noticeable. Postoperative pain is said to be worse, and patients may have to wear glasses for a few weeks after the procedure. Again, it's not magic, but like RK it can often produce good results.

Begin by consulting an ophthalmologist at a major eye clinic who does not perform RK. If you decide to go ahead, get a referral to an experienced surgeon skilled in RK.

Sunglasses

Sunglasses are no mere fashion statement: good ones provide safe, comfortable vision. Indeed, everybody who is outdoors in the sun needs sunglasses, and not just in the summer. *Any sunglasses are better than no sunglasses.* But some models offer more protection than others.

If you think that the best sunglasses are the darkest ones, you may be looking for trouble. Unless they have a coating to absorb ultraviolet (UV) light and blue light, dark lenses still allow damaging radiation to enter the eyes. While most sunglasses provide comfort in the sun—that is, they block high-intensity visible light and reduce glare sufficiently—many don't provide adequate UV protection. Exposure to UV rays over the years can damage the lens, potentially leading to cataracts, and has been implicated in damage to the cornea and retina. Of the million cataracts removed each year in the United States, it's estimated that up to 100,000 may be sun-related and thus preventable. That's why eye specialists now recommend that everyone wear UV-absorbing sunglasses whenever they are in the sun—not just during the summer or at the beach.

Even fewer sunglasses block blue light, which recent research suggests may be a potential danger to the eyes over the long term. So if you're looking for maximum protection, the best sunglasses are those that block most or all blue light along with all UV rays. How do you find such glasses? While you usually get what you pay for, a high-price, high-tech model is no guarantee of protection. Here are factors to consider when buying sunglasses:

Do they block as much UV rays as possible? The tint in sunglasses blocks some visible light, but not UV rays. Clear glass or plastic will absorb a certain amount of UV rays. But special chemicals need to be added to the lens when the glasses are made to do the best blocking job. (You can have your clear lenses treated so they also will block virtually 100 percent of UV rays.) Labeling for UV and visible light blockage is voluntary, and there are no government standards. If possible, buy glasses that meet the standards of the American National Standard Institute (ANSI). Look for the following ANSI labels: *General Purpose*—medium to dark tinted lenses for use in any outdoor activity. *Special Purpose*—for very bright environments, such as skiing, tropical beaches, and mountain climbing. *Cosmetic*—lightly tinted lenses for use in shopping and other around-town uses. Glasses without a label may be fine, but it's hard to be sure.

Do they block enough visible light? Excess light can damage the retina. Lenses should block 75 to 90 percent of visible light, thus transmitting only 10 to 25 percent of it. Some brands bear labels stating this "transmission factor." If this information isn't stated on the label, try on the glasses and look in the mirror—if they're dark enough, you won't be able to see your eyes. However, avoid glasses that are too dark, as they could cut your vision too much and contribute to falls or other mishaps. Ask the clerk if you may step outside for a moment to test the glasses in bright light.

Do they block blue light? Beyond UV rays on the spectrum is violet/blue light (400 to 510 nanometers), which may play a role in degeneration of the macula (the area of the retina with greatest acuity) over a long period of time. There is controversy about the danger of blue light. Some scientists think that lifetime exposure may damage the retina and contribute to blindness; others think that these fears are exaggerated. Blue light is of most concern if you:

• Spend much of your time outdoors, especially where the sun is most intense—at high altitudes or where sunlight is reflected off water, sand, or snow.

• Are fair-skinned and blue-eyed.

• Have had cataract surgery, which removes the eye's UV-absorbing lens. Be especially careful if you've had a lens implanted that has no UV protection.

• Have a personal or family history of macular degeneration.

• Are regularly taking medication, such as tetracycline, that increases your sensitivity to UV rays.

Lenses that absorb blue light are tinted yellow, brown, or amber. Generally, these also provide comfort from glare, particularly for older people. However, since lenses that block all blue light distort some colors, you may prefer a partial block. The amount of protection a particular brand offers may be indicated on the label; otherwise, you should consult your eye-care professional.

Size. Make sure that the lenses are large enough to protect against light coming in from the sides, top, and bottom of the frames. Wraparound sunglasses can be

---

Special Needs, Special Lenses

If you do a lot of driving, are an avid cyclist or fisherman, or spend long hours at certain other outdoor activities or sports, the following types of lenses offer special characteristics that may best suit you.

Polarized lenses. These are usually made by sandwiching a polarizing filter between pieces of tinted plastic or glass to block glare reflected at certain angles from water, wet or sunlit roads, a car hood, or any other horizontal surface. They are good for fishermen, boating enthusiasts, and drivers; however, polarized lenses may bring out distracting patterns in some windshields. Unless specially treated, polarized lenses provide little protection against ultraviolet rays and blue light.

Mirrored lenses. The thin metallic coating (over a tinted lens) on mirrored lenses acts as an extra buffer against strong light and offers excellent protection against overall glare. This makes them useful for water and snow sports. Some mirrored lenses block more than 90 percent of all visible light, but not necessarily 100 percent of UV rays. The mirrored coating scratches easily.

Photochromic lenses. Made of light-sensitive glass (rarely plastic) that adjusts to light conditions, photochromic lenses are good for cyclists, golfers, and other people who are in constantly changing light. They don't work well in a car, however, since the interior isn't that bright and the windshield blocks much of the UV radiation that stimulates them. If you're considering sun-sensitive lenses, make sure they get dark enough when you go outside, and remember they may take several minutes to adjust to light conditions. How dark they become largely depends on their thickness and the temperature. Photochromic treatment is not by itself effective against all UV rays and blue light.

Gradient lenses. Many drivers and pilots prefer single-gradient lenses (darker at top than at bottom), which allow them to see the dashboard or instrument panel easily. Because of the glare reflecting off the snow or water, skiers and fishermen often prefer double-gradient lenses, which are darker at the top and bottom than in the middle. Gradient lenses can be polarized, photochromic, or mirrored.

particularly effective. Small, round glasses may be fashionable, but they don't provide as much protection.

Fit. Sunglasses shouldn't slip down your nose. A study from the University of Massachusetts Medical Center has shown that when glasses slipped even just one quarter inch from the forehead about 20 percent more UV rays entered the eyes.

Color. Gray, followed by green, lenses have traditionally been considered best because they distort colors least. Brown and amber lenses are now gaining favor for certain sports or activities; not only can they help block blue light, they may also enhance contrasts in haze or fog. Fashion tints such as purple can greatly distort colors, particularly traffic lights. Check color accuracy by looking outdoors.

Glass or plastic. There are pluses and minuses for each type. If you toss your glasses around, glass may be better because it resists scratching, but thick glass lenses can be heavy. Plastic is lightweight and doesn't fog up much, but it scratches, and scratch-resistant coatings are easy to smudge. Both materials need to be specially treated for adequate protection against UV rays. Lenses made from polycarbonate (a special plastic) are often used by cyclists since they have improved impact resistance.

No distortion. Distorting lenses won't harm your eyes, but they may give you a headache. You can test sunglasses for distortion in the store. When shopping for nonprescription sunglasses, hold them at arm's length and look at a straight line in the distance. Slowly move the lenses across that line; if the line sways or bends, the lenses are imperfect. Look through the periphery as well as the center of the lenses. (This test will not work for most prescription lenses, some of which cause a straight line to waver or curve.)

How to choose. Your best bet, particularly if you have special needs, is to talk to an eye-care professional, who will have technical data from manufacturers. However, you can buy protective sunglasses at other retail outlets, provided you ask the right questions about the amount of visible light, UV rays, and blue light absorbed by various brands. Don't go just by how the glasses look on you.

Eyestrain and Computers

Of the millions of people who spend their workdays in front of video display terminals (VDTs), many suffer from eyestrain (visual fatigue, headache, eye irritation, and similar symptoms). But are these problems peculiar to working at a computer? Some studies show that such complaints were judged no worse than those caused by any close work and were not unique to video display terminals. However, clinical findings at the School of Optometry at the University of California at Berkeley suggest that working regularly at a video display terminal may cause a premature loss in the eye's ability to focus. This evidence was preliminary and the conclusions were based on people who had come to the clinic with eye problems—not on a controlled study. Still, of 153 patients who averaged six hours a day at a video display terminal for four or more years, more than half had difficulty changing focus. Presbyopia, or loss of ability to focus with advancing age, accounted for half of these problems. The other patients, though, were in their twenties and thirties and should have had good focusing mechanisms. Eyeglasses corrected the problem.

The conclusion is: if you work at a computer screen, you should have your eyes checked annually. (And when you do, tell your eye-care professional that you work at a screen.) Also:

•If you already have corrective lenses, you may need a special prescription for work at a terminal. Regular reading glasses, designed to focus at about eighteen inches, may not be right for terminal work if the screen is farther away.

•Bifocals may not be well suited for video display terminal work because the near-vision part of the lens is designed for looking down. Even trifocals may not help, since the field of vision in the medium-distance range will be too narrow to take in the whole screen. If you wear glasses and use a video display terminal, you'll probably find that single-vision lenses are best for this distance.

There are other ways as well to cut down on VDT eyestrain:

•Choose nonreflective glass screens, and eliminate reflected glare from windows or light fixtures. Overly bright light can be worse than inadequate lighting.

•Keep the reference document as close to the screen as possible and at the same level, so that you needn't change reading focus as you work. Light it at the same intensity as the screen.

•Keep your screen ten to fifteen degrees below the straight-ahead eye position.

•Take regular breaks—fifteen minutes every hour or two—to perform other work. Frequently look away from the screen to rest your eyes momentarily.

Cataracts

Until recently, cataracts were thought to be an inevitable part of growing older. Now, however, there's hope that with good health habits you may be able to postpone or, in some cases, prevent them. The lens of your eye, which focuses light on the retina at the back of the eyeball, is normally colorless and clear. With age, however, the lens may grow cloudy and opaque, impairing your vision—a condition called a cataract. Although cataract surgery, in which the lens is removed, is almost always successful, cataracts are still a major cause of treatable blindness worldwide. In the United States. over a million cataract operations are performed each year, accounting for about 12 percent of the entire Medicare budget.

It's long been suspected that smoking increases your risk of cataracts, and that the risk rises with the number of cigarettes smoked. In 1992, the *Journal of the American Medical Association* published two studies (one involving 17,000 male physicians, the other 69,000 female nurses), both of which showed a strong association between cigarette smoking and cataracts, with the heaviest smokers running the greatest risk. In an accompanying editorial, Dr. Sheila West of the Johns Hopkins Hospital in Baltimore estimated that at least 20 percent of all cataracts could be attributed to smoking. No one knows exactly how smoking damages the lens, but smokers are about twice as likely to develop cataracts as nonsmokers.

Lifelong exposure to ultraviolet light also promotes cataracts, which are most common in regions where the duration and intensity of sunlight are greatest. You can protect yourself by wearing ultraviolet-protective sunglasses. A hat with a brim is a good idea, too, especially when the sun is brightest.

Finally, what you eat may affect your risk of cataracts. In cataract formation, it's suspected, the lens of the eye is damaged by free radicals. These are highly reactive oxygen molecules created by ultraviolet light, cigarette smoke, and other environmental factors, as well as by the normal process of oxidation in the cells themselves. The body combats the destructive action of free radicals with the so-called antioxidants. Among the most essential of these chemical "good guys" are three nutrients—vitamins C and E and beta carotene (the plant form of vitamin A). Eye fluids are rich in vitamin C, presumably a protective factor. There's some evidence that vitamin-rich diets may forestall or prevent cataracts. Nurses in the new study who had taken vitamin C supplements for ten years had a lower risk of cataracts. A high intake of spinach seemed most consistently associated with a lower risk.

The causes of cataracts are not completely understood. There's no guarantee that not smoking, eating a diet high in vitamins C and E and beta carotene, and protecting your eyes from ultraviolet light will keep you cataract-free as you grow older, but these measures may help. And they have obvious auxiliary benefits, including a lower risk of some cancers and heart disease.

Glaucoma

Glaucoma, a disease of the eyes marked by increased pressure within the eyeball that can ultimately damage the optic nerve, currently affects about two million Americans. It cannot be prevented, but it can be treated and sometimes cured by surgery or laser treatment. If it is caught early, it need not result in blindness.

Open-angle glaucoma, the most common type, has nearly no symptoms in its early stages; its earliest sign is a painless increase in eyeball pressure, which can only be measured by an eye-care specialist. Side or peripheral vision may be affected, but only gradually. Those at high risk for developing glaucoma are:
• anyone with a family history of the disease;
• African Americans;
• the severely nearsighted;
• diabetics;
• anyone over age sixty-five (up to 3 percent of whom may have the disease);
• anyone taking certain blood-pressure medications or cortisone.

Accurate screening for glaucoma is best done by ophthalmologists or optometrists, who can perform a specialized type of measurement of the pressure within the eye called tonometry; dilate the pupil for a complete look inside the eye; and carry out measurements to detect subtle losses of peripheral vision. Studies have shown that a combination of screening procedures is more likely to uncover early glaucoma than the simple hand-held tonometer used by many primary care physicians. According to the American Academy of Ophthalmology, a complete ocular examination should be done at least once between age thirty-five and forty-five and repeated every five years after age fifty. Those who fall into any of the risk groups should begin routine testing at an early age.

While open-angle glaucoma at first has no symptoms, there is a rarer type that manifests itself by a sudden blurring of vision, a halo effect around objects, redness of the eye, and possibly nausea and vomiting. Anyone with these symptoms should immediately seek medical help, since glaucoma of this type can quickly damage the optic nerve.

Ear, Nose, and Throat

Disorders of the ear, nose, and throat—such as hay fever, the common cold, hoarseness, and hearing loss—are troublesome afflictions that affect nearly everyone at one time or another. While not life threatening, such problems can cause considerable distress and discomfort. Fortunately, there is much that you can do yourself to prevent or alleviate them.

Colds

Though people don't die of colds and seldom develop serious complications from them, the discomfort can be debilitating. A cold is by definition temporary and self-limiting. The symptoms vary but usually include a runny nose, sneezing, a sore or scratchy throat, hoarseness, coughing, and general malaise, as well as occasional low-grade fever (more often found in children than adults), and muscle aches and pains. Inflamed membranes in the nose and throat may cause discomfort day and night, making normal life (including sleep) difficult.

What causes colds

Researchers know more than they used to about how colds are transmitted and about the viruses that cause them. At least 200 different cold viruses exist, the most common being the rhinoviruses ("nose viruses"), which are estimated to cause 30 percent of all colds. Rhinoviruses tend to infect people in late summer and early autumn. Other types of viruses, not so well understood, are more likely to cause winter and early spring colds.

A sure way to "catch" a cold virus to which you are not already immune is to get a dose of it directly in the upper nose, where the temperature and humidity are ideal for its growth. In laboratory experiments, putting rhinovirus in the noses of volunteers almost always gives them a cold, no matter what their state of physical or emotional resistance or whether they are cold and wet or warm and dry. Three possibilities exist for getting cold viruses into your nasal passages: they may travel through the air (from the sneezing or coughing of others); they may be transmitted through direct contact (shaking hands with a cold sufferer, for example, and then touching your eyes or nose); or they may spread via a telephone, toy, or cup used by a cold sufferer. One study has found that airborne transmission is common in adults, whereas children tend to transmit secretions directly.

But, in fact, unless the virus gains access to the upper nose, the body has many lines of defense against it. Simply putting a cold virus near the nose usually has no effect, because it cannot penetrate the skin. The mucous membranes of the mouth are usually an effective barrier, so that kissing is not an efficient way to spread a cold. Simply being in the same room with a cold sufferer won't do it. Workers in the same office usually don't share colds. They may have colds at the same time, but they are due to different viruses. Family members, though, do tend to share their colds. The three factors that primarily influence transmission are the amount of time spent around the cold sufferer, the volume of his secretions, and the amount of virus in them.

Who is most susceptible?

No one knows what makes a person prone to colds in general or to any particular cold. Although newborns are thought to be immune to 20 percent of rhinoviruses (they get the antibodies from their mothers), they quickly lose their immunity. Small children are the most susceptible to colds, and can have six or eight a year. People who spend a lot of time with children, such as teachers, also tend to have numerous colds. Most people believe that being overtired or under emotional stress can "bring on" a cold. Others blame industrial pollution. There's no proof one way or another. There is evidence, though, that smokers are more likely to catch colds and to have longer-lasting symptoms than nonsmokers. Tobacco smoke paralyzes the hairlike projections that line the nose and throat. Thus, these cilia are less efficient at moving mucus out.

Because of the great variety of viruses, it is unlikely at present that one vaccine could be effective against all colds. To track down every virus type and make a "magic bullet" for each would be a horrendous and probably futile task. (Through genetic technology, it may one day be possible to identify a common genetic component in all cold viruses so that one vaccine would cover all of them.)

Yet in one sense, every cold is your last—from that particular virus for a period of time. One compensation for growing older is that you develop immunity to a progressively larger number of viruses and thus catch fewer colds. By age sixty, most people have one cold per year, if any.

The weather factor

Colds do occur seasonally—peak periods in the United States are September, October, and early spring—and it is hard to keep from blaming them on the weather. Puzzlingly enough, researchers have never been able to connect cold viruses with the weather. (One theory says that people catch colds in September because the schools open then, and the most susceptible population—that is, children—begins transmitting viruses.) Getting chilled or undergoing rapid weather changes cannot cause you to catch cold. At least in the laboratory, low temperatures do not seem to increase susceptibility. In one study reported in the *New England Journal of Medicine*, one group of volunteers in a 40° temperature was exposed to cold viruses, while another group received its viruses in an environment warmed to 86°. Both groups caught colds at about the same rate.

Some people believe winter is a prime time for colds because indoor heat removes humidity from the air, which dries out your nasal passages and makes you more susceptible. But while dry air may make you feel more uncomfortable if you already have a cold, there is no evidence that it increases your susceptibility.

The best way to avoid colds

The most effective way to keep a cold from spreading is hand washing. If you have a cold, remember that it spreads via your fingers, so wash them often in soap and warm water. If you are around people with colds, wash your hands often and try to avoid putting your fingers to your nose and eyes. Try not to share objects with cold

Inhaling heated vapor (medicated or not) with devices that shoot steam up the nose (like the Viralizer) has no effect on the course of colds or flu, or on the germs that cause them. And studies have found that such devices do not relieve cold symptoms.

Cold and Flu Products: Do They Help?

Decongestants. Available in pill form, nose drops, or inhalers, decongestants constrict blood vessels in the lining of the nose, open nasal passages temporarily, and may dry up mucus. They can also have a rebound effect—an increase in swelling and more congestion than ever if overused. In some people they can increase heart rate, induce insomnia, and elevate blood pressure.

Pain relievers. Aspirin, acetaminophen, and naproxen sodium (Aleve) can relieve fever and muscle aches. Ibuprofen relieves muscle aches but not fever. Children under sixteen should not take aspirin, which may cause Reye's Syndrome. Pregnant women, especially in the last trimester, should avoid aspirin and ibuprofen. Alcoholics or people with liver or kidney disease should avoid acetaminophen. In treating a sore throat, avoid aspirin-containing chewing gum and aspirin gargles. Aspirin applied directly to the mucous membranes won't reduce pain and can act as an irritant.

Antihistamines. These drugs are effective against hay fever but may make cold congestion worse; they can dry up secretions, but may also make mucus too thick, and thus difficult to expel by coughing up. They can also induce drowsiness.

Cough syrups. Coughing serves a useful purpose by clearing secretions from your throat. Thus cough suppressants should not be used for wet productive coughs, unless the cough prevents you from sleeping. Try hot drinks, steam, or hard candies instead. For a dry, nonproductive cough, suppressants may help you get a good night's sleep. Cough medicines that are expectorants can help to loosen mucus.

Combination cold medicines. Both children and adults should avoid those drugs that combine a variety of ingredients for "fast" relief of a whole range of symptoms. The active ingredients may work against each other, and none is likely to do much good.

Comparing pain relievers

In an Australian study published in the Journal of Infectious Diseases, *sixty healthy volunteers were exposed to a cold virus and then given aspirin, acetaminophen (such as Tylenol), ibuprofen (such as Advil or Nuprin), or a look-alike placebo for a week. Both aspirin and acetaminophen increased nasal congestion, while ibuprofen and the placebo did not. None of the drugs affected the multiplication of the virus significantly, though subjects taking aspirin or acetaminophen tended to have longer periods of viral multiplication. Whichever pain reliever you choose, stick with one type at a time. If you wish, you can also take a decongestant to temporarily relieve nasal congestion.*

sufferers—their telephones, pencils, typewriters and other tools, drinking glasses, towels, or bars of soap. Paper towels and paper cups are worthwhile investments during cold season. See that used tissues are disposed of promptly and properly. They should be discarded in a plastic-lined receptacle or paper bag, or in any manner that makes rehandling them unnecessary.

Though megadoses of vitamin C have been highly touted as a means of "heading off" a cold, no clinical trial has ever shown vitamin C to be more than marginally useful; there's really no reason to think that it will prevent or cure a cold or noticeably relieve symptoms. Megadoses of vitamin C—defined as more than ten times the Recommended Dietary Allowance (RDA) of 60 milligrams—may cause side effects, including nausea, abdominal cramps, and diarrhea. Chewable vitamin C tablets can erode tooth enamel.

Managing a cold: what helps, what doesn't

There is little or nothing that a doctor can do for the common cold. Antibiotics, including penicillin, cannot cure or alleviate a cold, nor is it wise to take antibiotics in an attempt to prevent later bacterial infection. *Take antibiotics only when your doctor prescribes them—and certainly don't take them on your own for a cold or flu.*

Most colds last a week or less, but two-week colds are not unheard of (see box on page 343 for determining if your condition is more than a cold). Your symptoms, however uncomfortable, are a sign that your body's defenses are working against the virus. Keep the following pointers in mind for your general well-being:

•Don't automatically "take something" for a cold or insist on giving medicine or vitamins to a child. Many over-the-counter cold medications made for adults contain ingredients that are harmful when taken by children.

•A salt or sugar-water gargle (one quarter teaspoon of salt or one table-spoon of Karo syrup added to eight ounces of water) can be helpful in relieving sore throat symptoms.

•Saline nose drops (also one quarter teaspoon of salt to eight ounces of water) may clear your nasal passages.

•"Drink plenty of fluids" is time-honored advice, but there is no evidence that increasing fluid intake will do anything but increase the need to urinate. Drink as many fluids as you want—they ease a dry throat—but you don't need to force yourself or anyone else.

•Hot drinks, on the other hand, are definitely comforting. In one study, chicken soup (as compared with cold water and hot water) was shown to increase the flow of nasal secretions. The taste and aroma was thought to be part of the therapy, as well as inhalation of the vapor. Some other hot soup might do as well, depending on your preferences and the availability of the soup. Tea with honey is not bad, either.

•Hot alcoholic beverages or a shot of brandy may sound tempting, but alcohol dilates blood vessels and may produce more nasal congestion. Overindulgence, obviously, may bring on stomach upset and headache. Pregnant women are advised never to drink.

•Bed rest will not cure a cold or even alleviate symptoms, but if you feel exhausted or your symptoms are distractingly painful, rest at home—either in bed or just around the house.

•If a child has a cold, going to school will do him no harm. But for the protection of other children, a child in the first stages who has a severe runny nose should probably stay at home. The most infectious period generally begins about a day before symptoms appear and lasts only another day or two

•Increased humidity in the air you breathe can sometimes make you feel better, at least temporarily. Hot-water vaporizers offer some advantages but can cause burns and scalding. Use a cold-mist vaporizer or humidifier if you wish. There is no value in adding medications to the water. Remember that humidifiers can harbor molds, which may cause allergic reactions. Clean the tank daily, rinsing with a mild solution of chlorine bleach and refilling with fresh water.

•There's no harm in exercising if you feel up to it, but you should never force yourself if you feel too tired or unfit, or if you have a fever. A break of two or three days in your exercise program won't be a significant setback.

•A red and sore nose and lips, caused by mucous secretions and aggravated by nose blowing, can often be relieved with petroleum jelly or skin lotion.

It's not possible to "sweat" a cold out of your system. Therefore, steam rooms and saunas are of no help. Still, steam rooms, because of their increased humidity, may help you feel better temporarily.

Is It More Than a Cold?

There's nothing a doctor can do for a cold. Some symptoms, however, should tip you off that what seems to be a cold may be something more serious requiring professional care:

•Oral temperature above 103°.

•Severe pain in the chest, head, stomach, or ears.

•Enlarged neck glands.

•In a child, shortness of breath or wheezing (particularly difficult breathing), marked irritability or lethargy.

•Sore throat combined with oral temperature that remains above 101° for twenty-four hours.

•Oral temperature that remains above 100° for three days.

•A fever, sore throat, or severe runny nose that persists for more than a week.

Hay Fever

Hay fever is a misnomer: it's not usually caused by hay and does not produce a fever. What it does produce is persistent sneezing, swollen nasal passages, acute discomfort, and usually a clear discharge. The proper name is allergic rhinitis, and it's thought that 32 million people in the United States and Canada are affected by it. According to the American Academy of Allergy and Immunology (AAAI), Americans lose 3.5 million workdays annually because of this condition. Ragweed, grass, and tree pollens are the worst culprits, along with mold spores. Flower pollens are too heavy to be airborne (bees carry them), so they are seldom a cause of hay fever. Grass and tree pollens become airborne in spring—the first allergy season each year. But ragweed gets going in the late summer and early fall (except on the West Coast, where it is less common), followed by an upsurge of molds and fungi that live in decomposing leaves. Many molds are present year round, indoors and out. Some allergies are set off by animal dander (actually, a protein in the animal's saliva, which is transferred to the fur during grooming and then dries and sheds with the dander), feathers, cosmetics, cigarette smoke, and dust mites, as well as other indoor pollutants. Dust mites peak in warm, humid weather.

The first step in controlling, maybe preventing, hay fever is to find out what you are allergic to. Maybe you know already, from years of experience, that it's grass pollen in early spring, or ragweed in the fall. If you don't know, you should see a physician or allergy specialist, who may be able to determine what sets you off. If your problem is feathers, animal dander, or a cosmetic, you'll probably be able to avoid it entirely.

If you're allergic to molds, raking leaves can cause itchy eyes, nasal congestion, and difficult breathing. The risk of allergic reaction is less if you rake freshly fallen leaves, since it takes a day or two for leaves to decompose and for molds and mildew to develop.

More accurate pollen counts

If it's pollen that bothers you, you'll be interested to hear that the AAAI now sponsors a nationwide network that collects and broadcasts more accurate pollen counts. Various collecting stations all over the country do pollen and mold counts up to three days a week, which are then faxed to AAAI, which in turn faxes them to radio stations and newspapers. The counts are given either numerically or described as "absent," "low," "moderate," "high," and "very high." According to the AAAI, there's no accurate way to forecast pollen counts. But if you hear that pollen counts have risen, you can at least carry medication when you leave the house, or postpone outdoor activity until things clear up.

What to take if symptoms get bad

If you can't eliminate the cause of your discomfort, over-the-counter antihistamines may help control symptoms. (A decongestant may also bring temporary relief.) The drawback is that most antihistamines cause drowsiness. Three effective prescription antihistamines are less likely to have this side effect: Seldane (generic name, terfenadine), Hismanal (astemizole), and Claritan (loratidine). In addition, two cortisone-based inhalants, beclomethasone and flunisolide have proved effective against inflammation, and some doctors prescribe them. Cromolyn sodium, an anti-asthma drug, can be prescribed as a nasal spray or eye drops. It actually prevents the outbreak of symptoms.

You should talk to your physician about these treatments. If your symptoms are severe, an allergy specialist may also recommend allergy shots. These desensitize you to specific allergens and eventually allow your body to tolerate them. Many people find the shots really do reduce symptoms. And it's not always necessary to repeat them annually. Avoid over-the-counter nose-drops and sprays, which may provide temporary relief, but over the long haul cause the nasal passages to swell more than ever. This is known as the rebound effect.

How to sidestep allergens

•When pollen counts are high, people with severe allergies should stay indoors if possible, especially between 5 a.m. and 10 a.m., when pollens are most prevalent. You may be surprised to learn that a dog or cat that goes in and out of the house can carry pollen indoors. Use an air conditioner, if you have one, in the car as well as your home. But be sure you keep the filters clean, or you may end up blowing allergens around.

•The few controlled studies on air-purifying machines have found that they have little, if any, effect on allergens. Very small air cleaners cannot remove dust and pollen. Electrostatic precipitators, which electrically charge airborne particles and use polarized metal plates to pull them out of the air, can pollute indoor air with ozone, aggravating allergy symptoms. The best type of filter is the HEPA (high-efficiency particulate arresting)—effective but expensive.

•Don't smoke, and avoid smoky environments. Insect sprays, fresh paint, and other households chemicals can also be irritating.

•If you're allergic to dust and dust mites, remove some or all carpets and soft furnishings. Keep floors and furniture dust-free. Get rid of feather pillows; use synthetic materials instead. Enclose your mattress in a plastic casing. Wash clothing frequently.

•If you're allergic to your pet, the best remedy is to find another home for it. Or at least try to keep it out of your bedroom.

•If molds and fungi set you off, get somebody else to do the yard clean-up in the fall.

Hoarseness

It has long been known that high noise levels can cause hearing loss over time. But the noisy modern world may have an effect on your speaking voice, too. As the noise around you increases, you tend to shout over it and thus alter the quality of your voice. In addition, more people these days work in jobs requiring heavy telephone use. Trying to sound authoritative, people sometimes unconsciously pitch their voices lower than is really comfortable.

Your vocal cords react just like any other tissue strained by overuse: they resist. Typical symptoms are hoarseness, dry cough, and increasing difficulty in producing normal sound. Continued irritation can result in small benign growths—known as vocal nodes or polyps—on your vocal cords.

Protecting your voice

How can you head off these problems or minimize the damage and get your natural voice back? One way is to follow some of the rules professional entertainers follow to protect their voices:

- Avoid talking over background noise. Wait until the hubbub subsides.
- When using the telephone, speak softly. If you have to be on the telephone for long periods, a phone rest or a headset may lessen the strain on muscles in your face, throat, and neck, thus relieving some vocal cord tension. Try to rest your voice between telephone calls.
- Be aware of voice pitch. Don't pitch your voice unnaturally high or low.
- If you are hoarse or your voice is squeaky, rest your vocal cords. This means that for two or three days you should speak only when absolutely necessary and in a soft, breathy voice. Don't whisper. That puts more pressure on your vocal cords than speaking softly.
- Keep your vocal cords well lubricated. Increase your fluid intake. Increase the humidity in your surroundings. Avoid alcohol and cigarettes. A glycerine throat lozenge may be helpful, but avoid cold pills containing decongestants or antihistamines, which may dry your throat.

If hoarseness, voice change, or discomfort lasts more than two weeks (and you don't have a cold or allergy), check with your doctor. When all other measures fail, surgical treatment for polyps may be an option. Many chronic voice problems can be solved with the help of a speech-language therapist. Such therapists are usually certified by the American Speech-Language-Hearing Association and licensed by the state; your throat specialist should be able to refer you to one.

Nosebleeds

Unless you've had a blow to the nose, a nosebleed usually starts and stops spontaneously. The dry air of wintertime can be a major factor. So can the low humidity of an airplane cabin. The septum (nose partition) is the most common site of bleeding. When the fragile membranes in the forward part of the nose dry out, they crack easily, and it doesn't take much to damage blood vessels that lie just beneath their surface. These thin membranes offer very little supporting tissue, especially as they grow more delicate with age. Inflammation from a cold, an allergy, or sinusitis can also weaken the tissue. Picking your nose can also make it bleed.

Thus blowing your nose hard can set off a nosebleed; so can picking or hard rubbing—and, of course, a bump or blow. If you have a history of nosebleeds, it may help to use a home humidifier. Avoid repeated rubbing or picking.

The following measures usually stop a nosebleed quickly:
- Sit up so that gravity will lower pressure in the veins. To keep blood from running back into the throat, tilt your head forward a little.
- Pinch the fleshy part of the nose (between the bridge and the nostril) with your thumb and index finger for five to ten minutes, breathing through your mouth. Applying ice probably won't help, since it's really pressure, not temperature, that stops the bleeding.
- After the bleeding stops, don't blow your nose too hard or too often. Sneeze through an open mouth, and avoid strenuous sports for a few days.

Apply a little petroleum jelly with your fingertip or a small cotton swab just inside the nostrils several times a day for a week to keep membranes moist. If your nose bleeds on plane trips, try using petroleum jelly before you depart.

In people past middle age, nosebleeds sometimes start farther back in the nose,

The right way to blow your nose

Despite popular belief, it's not possible to rupture the eardrum by blowing your nose too hard. The sensations you may feel in your ears while blowing are due to vibrations resulting from pressure changes. But you can give yourself a bloody nose if you blow hard enough, by breaking blood vessels in your nose. And if you're suffering from an upper respiratory infection and have heavy nasal discharge, forcefully blowing your nose may send bacteria from the nose to your ears and so contribute to an ear infection. The best advice is still to blow gently.

beyond the fleshy area. And a blow to the nose can also result in bleeding farther back in the nose (posterior bleeding). This type of nosebleed is harder to stop; it can cause significant blood loss and require medical help if it doesn't cease within a few minutes.

A nosebleed doesn't herald a stroke, nor does it necessarily signal hypertension, as some people believe. Of course, those with hypertension who take aspirin or other blood-thinning drugs may have more frequent episodes of nosebleed. If the bleeding doesn't cease with simple remedies, you should see a doctor.

Swimmer's Ear

Just as you needn't be an athlete to get athlete's foot, you needn't be a swimmer to get swimmer's ear, also known as "jungle ear"—though you don't have to be in a jungle to get it either. *Otis externa* is the medical name of this painful, itchy condition, which is a bacterial (sometimes fungal) infection brought on when water containing infectious agents gets trapped in the outer ear canal. Swimming is the most common cause of this problem, but some people may get water in their ears from showering or washing their hair. The longer the water remains in the ear, the likelier it is that any microorganisms will breed.

To prevent swimmer's ear, take these simple precautions:
• After swimming, shake your head to remove water trapped in your ears.
• Gently dry the external ear with a corner of a towel. Don't insert cotton swabs or anything else into the canal to dry or clean your ears. This could cause injury, remove protective earwax, and encourage infection.
• If you are prone to ear infection, use antiseptic eardrops—particularly if you've been swimming in a lake. You can buy these without a prescription at any drugstore. Or make them yourself: mix equal parts of white vinegar and rubbing alcohol, and put one or two drops of this solution in each ear with a medicine dropper. This solution restores the natural acid balance of the ear canal and helps dry it out, as well as killing bacteria. If alcohol irritates your skin, use vinegar diluted with water. If, despite all efforts, your ear begins to itch, use the drops three times daily.

If the ear swells and becomes painful and the triangular piece of cartilage in front of the ear opening becomes sore to the touch, or if you have a discharge from the ear canal, you need medical care. Antibiotic drops and irrigation of the ear canal are effective treatments. People who are prone to itchy ears or ear infections may need to have a doctor check their ears and remove excess wax before swimming season starts. If you have ever had a perforated eardrum or have ever had ear surgery, get medical advice before using eardrops and before swimming.

Hearing Loss

The ear is a remarkable piece of sound-receiving equipment, designed to last for decades without repair or replacement parts. With age, this receiver inevitably grows less acute; hearing loss makes social communication a chore for half of all men and a third of all women over sixty-five. But some of this hearing loss is preventable and much of it is modifiable.

Excessive noise: a common cause of hearing loss

Few people realize that excessive noise can accelerate age-related hearing loss. Currently, the Department of Labor sets some limits for allowable exposure to noise in the workplace, or at least requires that workers be given protective devices, but no government agency protects us from the din of the casual environment or from the recreational noise we inflict on ourselves.

A decibel is a physical measurement used to express the relative intensity of sound; a whisper produces 20 decibels (dB), an ordinary conversation, 60. The decibel scale is logarithmic—each rise of 10 dB represents a tenfold increase in physical energy; a rise of 20 dB, a hundredfold increase. However the perception of sound does not follow the same logarithmic scale. For example, at a moderate sound level, an increase of 10 dB may be perceived as only a doubling of volume. Sounds become annoying around 70 dB (a vacuum cleaner), and potentially damaging at 85 or 90 dB (a motorcycle close by). Electronically boosted Mozart isn't any easier on the ears than rock music. Headphones mercifully shield innocent bystanders, but they can damage the user's hearing over the long haul. Millions of people now use headphones—while working, while exercising, or on long plane flights—and even a cheap set can put out more than 110 dB. (The Environmental Protection Agency has proposed that industrial workers be exposed to no more than 85 dB for eight hours and recommends that exposure time be cut in half for every 3 dB over this amount. Thus enduring 106 dB for three minutes is the equivalent of eight hours at the recommended maximum level.) Studies have suggested that people tend to listen at high volume, but it's hard to specify at what point hearing loss begins, for the decibel level interacts with the length of exposure. Decreasing one but increasing the other keeps the risk more or less constant. The longer you're subjected to the noise, the harder it is on your ears.

Reducing noise

There are many common sense ways of avoiding hearing loss:

- When wearing headphones, never use the music to drown out other noise. If

The Right Way to Clean Your Ears

Some people use cotton swabs or even bobby pins to clean wax from their ear canal (the tube leading to the eardrum). Such objects can push wax up against the eardrum and temporarily impair hearing. They can also irritate the delicate skin of the canal or, far worse, perforate the drum.

Wax build-up isn't a problem for most people. It serves to protect the eardrum against dust and other irritants, as well as potential sources of infection such as fungi and bacteria. In the normal course of events, ear wax gradually dries up in small particles and migrates to the outer ear, where it falls out of the ear or is washed off. All you need to do is wash your outer ear regularly. It's also okay to use your well-washed little finger to wipe off wax near the outer part of the canal.

If wax does accumulate, take the following steps. Using an eyedropper, put a drop or two of warm (not hot) mineral or vegetable oil in each ear twice a day. Then, using a bulb syringe, flush with warm water, holding your head upright and then turning it sideway to allow the water to drain. (If you have a perforated eardrum, however, never put any liquid in your ear.)

Over-the-counter earwax softeners are harmless, but no better than mineral oil. Don't use hydrogen peroxide or any product that causes fizzing in your ear, since they cause pressure to build up and might injure your eardrum.

If your ear remains blocked because of impacted wax, consult your doctor.

you want to use headphones while your companion watches the ball game on television, perhaps you should move to another room rather than compete with the television noise. If you're in a bus that is making a deafening racket, lay your headphones aside. If you can't hear any sounds around you, you've got the volume too high.

•If background noise in any setting drowns out a normal conversational voice, you should try to escape or reduce the noise as soon as you can. If you have to shout to be heard, something is wrong.

•If you must be exposed to high noise levels while you are working or commuting, give your ears a break during leisure time. Don't go to the noisiest restaurant or nightclub in town.

•If you have to be in noisy environments frequently, carry a pair of earplugs and use them. They won't keep you from hearing a concert, for example; they'll just keep the decibels from damaging your ears.

Combating hearing loss

Even with precautions, however, age-related hearing loss is still a problem for many people. Most hearing problems can be alleviated by a hearing aid, yet only about one-third of those who need hearing aids actually have them.

It isn't easy to admit to hearing impairment; it's too often taken as an embarrassing sign of "old age." But the truth is that most people suffer some degree of hearing loss after age fifty. This age-related degeneration of the inner ear—called presbycusis, from the Greek meaning "old hearing"—results in lowered sensitivity to high frequencies (you don't catch those high notes or the doorbell the way you used to) and a loss in the ability to discriminate among speech sounds (people seem to mumble). Or you may be aware of a persistent low hiss or ringing in the ears.

Any one of these symptoms should send you to your doctor for advice. Don't go first to a hearing-aid dealer. If your doctor recommends a hearing aid, you'll need his written prescription, and you should take your hearing test results along so that the dealer can match the hearing aid to your particular problem.

Medicare will pay for an evaluation of your hearing loss if requested by a physician, but not for the aid itself. It pays to shop around. Look for a dealer who'll give disinterested advice and reliable after-sales service. Most dealers also offer a thirty-day free trial of any aid you select. All hearing aids consist of a microphone, amplifier, speaker, volume control, and battery. Most people want a model worn behind or in the ear, or fitted to a pair of glasses. Some people may be able to wear an aid that fits entirely inside the ear or even in the ear canal. (These smaller devices tend to distort sound and are useful only for mild hearing loss, but new technology offers marked improvements.) People with severe hearing loss may still need the type worn in a shirt pocket with a wire connection to an ear receiver. Many newer types of assisted hearing devices are being developed, one of which should be able to help you even if your hearing loss is marked. Don't assume, however, that only the most expensive model will do. Get one that seems to meet your needs, and ask your doctor to check it.

Tips for coping

If you know someone with hearing loss (with or without a hearing aid) there are many ways to make life easier for him. Indeed, a little thoughtfulness in this domain can counteract the tendency among some elderly people to withdraw from normal conversational give-and-take into depressed isolation.

When you talk to someone with a hearing problem:

•Speak a little louder, more distinctly, and in short, simple sentences. Don't shout; shouting distorts.

•Don't overarticulate. Just be sure to face your listener squarely.

•Make sure your mouth isn't obstructed by food, chewing gum, a cigarette, or your hands.

•Make an extra effort to bring hearing-impaired persons into the conversation.

If you have difficulty hearing:

•Don't be shy. Ask people to repeat or slow down if you don't understand.

•Cut out background noise. Turn off the radio or TV during conversation.

•In noisy places, station yourself near sound-absorbent surfaces (curtains, books, or upholstered seating) and stay clear of echoing expanses of plaster and glass.

•Above all, don't ignore even mild hearing loss. Delay in dealing with it can only intensify it, sometimes irreversibly. And it could be a sign of another medical problem that needs attention. Let your physician decide.

Tinnitus

Most of us hear faint ringing sounds occasionally when there's no external noise. Usually such sounds last a few minutes or, at most, several hours. But if ringing or other noises in your head are persistent, you have tinnitus. Though the term is from a Latin word meaning "to ring like a bell," people with tinnitus may actually hear many sounds, from buzzing, tinkling, and humming to popping and clanging.

Researchers estimate that about 36 million Americans have occasional or constant tinnitus. About 10 million have such severe symptoms that they have sought medical help. The rest experience a low level of noise—usually in both ears but sometimes in just one—which can still be a nuisance, interfering with work, social life, and sleep. The onset of tinnitus doesn't signify that you will become seriously or permanently deaf, but tinnitus is often associated with some hearing loss—though it does not cause it. About 80 percent of Americans who have some hearing loss also experience tinnitus.

Tinnitus has been described by one expert as someone "listening to old age sneaking up on him," since the great majority of tinnitus sufferers are middle-aged or older. It usually comes on slowly, with intermittent episodes that may become chronic as you age. But some young people also experience tinnitus.

Causes of tinnitus

While it's true that the sounds of tinnitus are all "in your head," they are nevertheless real. The physiological or neurological cause of such subjective sounds isn't always known, but they are a symptom of something that has gone awry in the auditory system. For example, infections of the middle ear or a perforated eardrum can provoke tinnitus, as can a build-up of wax or dirt in the outer ear. One of the most common causes is exposure to loud noises such as gunshots, jet engines, jackhammers, chain saws, rock music, or industrial machinery. Tinnitus has also been linked to tumors of certain cranial nerves, head injuries, and excessive use of alcohol and aspirin.

There is a less common form of tinnitus—"objective" tinnitus—in which the sounds you hear can also be heard by your doctor listening with a stethoscope. Usually these sounds are produced by either movement of the jaw (the temporomandibular joint) or the flow of blood in major blood vessels of the head and neck.

Medical treatment

There is no standard drug or medical procedure to relieve tinnitus. If you hear persistent ringing or other noises, you should see an otologist (ear specialist) or an otolaryngologist (ear, nose, and throat specialist). He can determine if it is due primarily to an ear condition or to other medical conditions. For instance, if the underlying cause is otosclerosis (a fusing of minute bones in the ear), surgery may help relieve tinnitus. If a middle-ear infection is involved, it may be treated with antibiotics. When conductive hearing loss, such as that caused by wax in the ear canal, is involved, treatment is almost always successful. However, when the cause is unknown—which is generally the case—the chances of medically correcting tinnitus are quite small.

Nonmedical treatment

There are nonmedical ways of relieving tinnitus that have proven effective. Perhaps the most promising method is to drown out the sounds of tinnitus with less bothersome sounds. For the many tinnitus sufferers with hearing loss, the ambient sounds picked up by a hearing aid can reduce or even eliminate tinnitus of medium or low pitch. A newer device that has been quite successful is the tinnitus masker, which is worn like a hearing aid and emits a steady, monotonous noise like wind in trees or the hum of an electric fan—a sound that quickly becomes familiar and can be easily ignored. One benefit of such a device is psychological: one of the most disturbing aspects of tinnitus is your lack of control over the noise, and a masker gives you back that sense of control. Masking devices must be approved by the Food and Drug Administration (FDA) because of the potential risk they pose if too loud. They are sometimes combined with hearing aids.

One expert estimates that almost 60 percent of patients with severe tinnitus can be helped by using a hearing aid, masking device, or combination device.

Self-help

Alcohol, caffeine, nicotine, and aspirin can all make tinnitus worse, so reducing your intake of them can help alleviate the condition. One of the only preventive steps you can take is to avoid loud noise; use ear plugs when necessary.

Since stressful situations often seem to aggravate tinnitus—and tinnitus in turn is stressful—almost any type of relaxation technique may help you cope. Some tinnitus sufferers have reported that biofeedback helped them temporarily. Claims have also been made for hypnosis and acupuncture.

Another way to deal with tinnitus is to join a self-help group, which can offer support as well as information about new techniques and treatments.

Dental Care

There is more to good dental hygiene than simply brushing your teeth every day. If you pay only superficial attention to your teeth and gums—or ignore them altogether—you risk developing a dental disorder that can require expensive and time-consuming treatment, or worse, can result in the loss of one or more teeth. Fortunately, dentistry has made enormous strides in the past few decades. Fluoridated drinking water and fluoridated toothpastes, along with dental sealants, have made cavities and fillings almost a thing of the past, while improved preventive care and therapy for periodontal disease may eventually do the same for toothlessness. Through root canal therapy and restorative dentistry, severely decayed teeth can be saved, and even lost teeth can sometimes be successfully replaced with dental implants.

Furthermore, the role that we can all play in our own dental health has become clearer. Most tooth decay and subsequent tooth loss is preventable with proper oral hygiene (along with regular visits to the dentist). This section covers the right way to take care of your teeth at home and addresses other topics of dental care that may require professional intervention.

Basic Self-Care

The aim of dental self-care is to prevent the buildup of *plaque*—a gummy film made up of saliva and bacteria that adheres to your teeth, especially along your gum line. Plaque control is the best way to avoid tooth decay and periodontal disease as well as bad breath. Not only does plaque lead to cavities, it also eventually combines with certain minerals in saliva to form *tartar* (also called calculus). These deposits, above and below the gums, lead to periodontal disease—called *gingivitis* in its earlier reversible stage (the chief symptom of periodontal disease are bleeding, swollen and receding gums, bad breath, and, ultimately, loose teeth. Destruction of the underlying bone and loss of teeth occur in advanced stages. Obviously, it's worth taking every possible step to prevent all this.

Steps for clean, healthy teeth and gums

Here are the essentials of good oral hygiene:

How much. Your first line of defense is brushing thoroughly at least twice a day, and flossing once a day. *Total time: five minutes a day minimum* for the brushing and flossing, in order to thoroughly clean all tooth surfaces, especially those between the teeth.

The right way to brush. Use a brush with soft bristles (hard bristles can damage the gums), and hold it at an angle pointed toward the junction of teeth and gums. For your upper teeth, point your toothbrush up at a 45-degree angle to the gum line; for the bottom teeth, point the brush down. That will help clean out plaque that may lurk at the gum line. Remember that the goal is not so much to polish flat

Dental Anxiety

An estimated 35 million Americans suffer from some degree of anxiety over visiting the dentist, and another 12 million can be classified as true phobics. Fortunately, dentists are becoming more and more aware of the problem and have developed many ways to help patients relax—everything from fish tanks in the waiting room to video games to be played while in the dental chair. According to the American Dental Association, most dental squeamishness can be traced to an unpleasant childhood experience. Making a child comfortable with dental treatment from the outset can do much to eliminate anxiety in adulthood. The following tips will show you how to make your child's dental visits more pleasant.

•Don't put off a child's first dental visit until a painful condition has occurred. This will only teach the child to associate the dentist with pain. Your child's primary teeth are important, so have them examined as early as your dentist and pediatrician recommend.

•Emphasize to your child that the dentist is a friendly doctor. Never threaten a child with a visit to the dentist as punishment.

•Avoid passing on any fears about dental treatment you may have to your child. Studies have shown that parents and other family members often provide negative reinforcement about dentists. Dental treatment is not as painful as it used to be. In fact, thanks to widespread fluoridation and new developments such as dental sealants, many kids today have no cavities at all. And when dental work is necessary, modern equipment and techniques minimize the discomfort.

•Many dentists will postpone treatment until the second visit so that the child can become familiar with the surroundings. Ask the dentist to explain to your child what is being done and why it is necessary, and to use the "tell, show, do" technique—where the dentist demonstrates the procedure first—with your child during any treatment.

•To help your child relax, play a cassette tape of a favorite story at the dentist's office.

According to a recent national poll, everybody knows that brushing is very important for maintaining healthy teeth, and almost everybody agrees that flossing and regular dental checkups are equally important. But knowing isn't always doing. Only half of us see a dentist twice a year, and 29 percent don't even go once a year. While 80 percent say that flossing is important, only 36 percent actually do floss daily.

surfaces as to clean between the teeth and in the spaces where teeth meet gums. Use enough pressure so that you feel the bristles against your gums, but don't press so hard that you do damage, particularly if you have periodontal disease. You can use a circular brushing motion or an up-and-down one. A back-and-forth scrub is not recommended. Brush the outside and inside of your teeth, using short, gentle strokes, then brush the biting surfaces. Brush the gum line as well as the teeth. Brush all chewing surfaces carefully; hold the brush vertically to reach the inside surfaces of the front teeth.

The right way to floss. Though flossing is as important as brushing for healthy teeth and gums, surveys show that most Americans don't do it. Waxed floss is designed to glide easily between tightly aligned teeth, but most studies have found no difference between it and the unwaxed variety in terms of plaque-removing efficiency. Some brands of waxed floss use "natural" components: beeswax, aromatic oils, spices. These added substances provide no advantage over plain floss, other than possibly providing you with incentive to adhere more faithfully to a daily flossing routine.

Follow these tips for quick, safe, effective flossing:

•Break off about a foot and a half of floss. Wind most of it around the middle finger of one hand and then wind the other end around the same finger of the other hand. Unwind from the full "spool" as you work.

•Hold the floss taut between thumb and forefinger, with about an inch of floss between them.

•Don't snap the floss into your gums. Use a gentle sawing motion. Remember, you're after plaque on the side of the tooth.

•When you reach the gum line, curve the floss into a C-shape and slide it very carefully between tooth and gum until you feel resistance. Pull the floss down against the side of one tooth, then reinsert and repeat for the adjacent tooth.

•Don't forget the far side of your rearmost teeth.

•If you are just starting to floss, your gums may bleed for the first few days. As the plaque is removed, your gums will heal and bleeding should stop. If it doesn't, see your dentist.

Limit the amounts of sweets you consume. Or at least try to brush as soon as possible after eating them. This is particularly important for older people, whose roots may be exposed.

See your dentist twice a year for an evaluation, and thorough cleaning and removal of accumulated tartar. Go more often if you have a problem that needs more frequent attention.

Last but not least. Don't rely on the "magic" in any dental product to protect your teeth. You'll find many gadgets and high-tech appliances on the market. These aids can be a help, particularly if used as recommended by a dentist to help combat periodontal disease. But there's no magic in dental hygiene—the most effective plaque fighter and tartar controller is you.

Choosing toothbrushes and and toothpaste

Toothbrushes. Look for soft nylon bristles with rounded or tapered ends rather than stiff natural bristles, which are much more likely to fray, damage gums, and become contaminated with food particles. Flexible, water-repellent nylon bristles are also smaller in diameter and able to remove plaque between teeth and around gums more efficiently. When you buy a new brush (every three or four months, or sooner if the bristles begin to mat), choose a compact head that can be maneuvered to any part of the mouth, particularly if your jaw is small. The shape of the handle doesn't really matter in most cases—use a bent or straight one, as you prefer.

Electric toothbrushes. These are not necessarily more effective. They may, however, save you time and may be useful for people with certain physical handicaps.

One special type of electric toothbrush is Interplak, which has ten soft bristle tufts that rotate at high speed, continually reversing direction. The bristles can get between teeth and reach most, if not all, tooth surfaces. Rotodent and Braun are other electric models that are specially designed to provide thorough cleaning. Some dentists and periodontists recommend these, especially for heavy plaque formers. It may be possible to get the same cleaning from a manual toothbrush, but it might take more time and more work. These toothbrushes aren't cheap, but they cost far less than dental visits for gum problems that result from chronic plaque buildup. Some dental insurance policies will pay for the devices.

Toothpastes. Though it's theoretically possible to get your teeth clean without toothpaste, it's still better to use toothpaste. Any toothpaste, or even baking soda, acts as an abrasive and cleans tooth surfaces. Thorough flossing and brushing with any toothpaste will remove plaque. The plaque-removing ability of one toothpaste is no greater than any other; a toothpaste's pleasant taste and clean aftertaste, however, can be an incentive to brush.

The benefit of fluoride. Fluoride really does reduce tooth decay—a fact established long ago in studies of children's teeth. And according to research published in the *Journal of the American Dental Association*, fluoridated toothpaste also reduces cavities in adults. Though older people tend to get fewer cavities than kids, gums

Myth: Young children don't need to floss.

Fact: *According to the American Dental Association, parents should floss their children's teeth from age one and a half until the children are eight years old, when they will probably be able to do it themselves. Children should be supervised, however, so that they do not injure their gums.*

recede with age, exposing the softer root surfaces to decay. You don't outgrow your need for toothpastes containing fluoride—even if the drinking water in your community is fluoridated. Fluoride toothpastes most commonly contain sodium fluoride or sodium monofluorophosphate. Both are effective. Any fluoride toothpaste with the American Dental Association (ADA) seal will do the job.

"Tartar-control." Toothpastes containing zinc chloride or pyrophosphates decrease tartar buildup on the tooth's exposed surface, according to several studies. One study suggested that a toothpaste with pyrophosphate, used twice a day, decreased tartar buildup on tooth surfaces by 36 percent over a three-month period, and by 46 percent over six months, compared with a regular fluoride paste. Even if a "tartar control" toothpaste bears the ADA seal on its label, this is only a partial endorsement stating that while such toothpastes may reduce the formation of tartar above the gum line, they have not as yet been shown to affect tartar formation below the gum line. Thus manufacturers cannot claim that these toothpastes have any therapeutic effect on periodontal disease. They are not a substitute for dental care and regular professional cleanings. Furthermore, any agent that cleans away plaque will reduce new tartar, whether it's marked "tartar control" or not. *Indeed, dental floss is still the best plaque remover and "tartar-control" agent.*

Another potential antiplaque weapon is sanguinaria or bloodroot (an herb with antibacterial properties), which is the active ingredient in some rinses. So far, there's no conclusive evidence that products with sanguinaria are any more effective than regular toothpastes.

Desensitizing toothpastes. Dental hypersensitivity is not a disease but a symptom—of a root exposed by receding gums, or possibly of a fractured tooth or a cavity. If a tooth or teeth become sensitive to heat and cold, you should check with your dentist. But if you have chronic hypersensitivity with no underlying cause, you may need a special desensitizing toothpaste containing potassium nitrate, sodium citrate, or strontium chloride, for instance. Four or five brands are available with the ADA seal. To get fluoride protection when you're using a desensitizing toothpaste, look for a brand with added fluoride and use a fluoride rinse.

Dental rinses

Brushing thoroughly twice daily with a fluoride toothpaste and flossing once a day will be adequate dental hygiene for most people. But if you want added protection against decay, you can use a fluoride rinse after brushing. The ADA recommends a fluoride rinse for everyone (except children under six). Rinsing once a week seems to be effective for children. The benefits for adults, however, haven't been as well studied. Rinses contain either stannous or sodium fluoride—both effective in preventing decay.

Keep in mind, though, that a fluoride rinse is only extra insurance. No rinse or mouthwash can take the place of brushing with a fluoride toothpaste and daily flossing of your teeth.

If you are taking good care of your teeth, you don't need an antiplaque mouthwash any more than you need a "tartar-control" toothpaste. Studies have shown that antiplaque rinses do decrease plaque to some extent. But brushing and flossing do a better job.

A prescription rinse. Peridex, a prescription rinse that bears the ADA seal, is usually prescribed for those with symptoms of gum disease. It contains chlorhexidine,

Baking soda is no better or worse than any other toothpaste, except that it lacks fluoride, which helps prevent cavities and is important for adults as well as children. However, there are baking soda tooth powders and pastes on the market that do contain fluoride, and these would be as good a choice as any other toothpaste. Baking soda by itself is a good cleaning agent; if you prefer to use it plain (thus skipping the other ingredients, which are harmless but not essential for dental health), you might use a fluoride mouthwash in addition.

an antibacterial agent that sticks to the teeth and provides a longer antiplaque action than most other ingredients, which lose their effect after you spit out the rinse. Peridex is particularly useful for people with trench mouth or other infections; for those who have just had gum surgery; and for handicapped people who can't adequately clean their teeth. However, some patients may develop unpleasant side effects—discolored teeth and fillings, along with a brown film on the tongue. Professional cleaning can correct these.

Accessory aids

Nothing can replace brushing and flossing, but there are a few new implements that make flossing easier and more effective, plus other devices that take up where toothbrushes leave off. These are particularly useful if you have crowns, bridges, other orthodontic elements, or any hard-to-reach tooth surfaces.

Filament floss. Marketed under the trade name Super Floss, this improved floss has been given the seal of acceptance by the ADA. Each length has three parts: a stiff threader section, a fatter central section of nylon-mesh filaments, and a final section of regular floss. The threader gets under bridgework and other orthodontic work so that you can pull the filament "brush" after it. You gently move this section back and forth to get rid of debris and plaque. Then using the third section, you finish with a regular flossing.

Shred-proof floss. For most people, finding a floss that doesn't shred or break is no problem. But for people with tight contacts between their teeth, there are two relatively new brands—Glide and Precision—that are made of a teflon-like material that doesn't shred: it slips easily between very tight teeth and won't tear on sharp edges. It does cost more, though.

Floss handle. This useful plastic device looks like a miniature coping saw and is a good utensil for people who lack the dexterity needed for normal flossing. You simply thread your floss through its two ends. Ready-threaded, throwaway, miniature versions are also available.

Floss threaders. These small plastic loops help you thread regular floss through the space between connected crowns and under bridges. First you pass the threader between your teeth, put the floss through the loop, then pull the floss through.

Interdental brushes. These look like tiny bottle brushes, and they're excellent for cleaning between widely spaced teeth, between teeth and bridges or crowns, and areas where the gum has formed a pocket because of some degree of gum disease. Studies show them to be more efficient than floss for removing plaque between widely spaced teeth. You either throw them away when they become matted, or fit replacement brushes to toothbrush-shaped handles. They come in a variety of sizes, so you can shop around for the one right for your teeth.

Rubber tips. You can buy toothbrushes with pointed soft rubber tips affixed to the ends of their handles. Or look for replaceable tips fitted to the end of a handle; some devices have a rubber tip at one end and an interdental brush at the other. The tips are useful for routine plaque removal, for gently stimulating the gums, and for removing debris trapped in orthodontic bands, around the margin of a crown, or around bridgework. Note, however, that studies show that in most cases regular use of an interdental brush or floss can accomplish these jobs equally well.

Toothpicks. These old reliables have been upgraded from the round, hard, splintery picks that are a standby in some restaurants, to flatter, round-tipped versions

---

Mouthwash and bad breath

Chronic halitosis, or bad breath, is most often caused by periodontal disease (infection of the gums). It can also stem from a multitude of sources ranging from something as simple as food particles lodged between the teeth or a dry mouth to more serious conditions like respiratory or gastrointestinal disorders. Other contributing factors include smoking, alcoholic drinks, and such foods as garlic and onions. Mints and mouthwashes will temporarily quell bad breath. But they cannot cure the underlying problem. Avoid strong-smelling foods, and if you smoke, stop. Floss daily, and brush after each meal (or if you can't, at least rinse out your mouth).

If you practice good dental hygiene (brushing and flossing daily) and still have chronic bad breath, consult your dentist to make sure that periodontal disease is not the reason. And if it's not, see a physician to eliminate the possibility of lung or gastric disorders.

that soften in contact with saliva, massage gums, and remove trapped debris. Sold in matchbook-style packs, they're a useful adjunct to a brush and floss in getting rid of plaque. Special toothpick holders are also available that help to better manipulate a toothpick.

Whatever dental aids you adopt, remember never to force anything between your teeth or into bridgework or other dental work. This can damage gums.

Special Concerns

Cleaning crowns and bridges

If you have had to replace a tooth, or teeth, with a crown or a bridge, you may have assumed that since the new "tooth" is artificial, you need not be so particular about dental hygiene. After all, a crown or a bridge can't get cavities. But in fact, you need to work even harder at keeping these artificially restored teeth clean than people who still have their natural teeth. Though a crown covers most of a tooth (usually one that has undergone root canal or has had extensive decay), what remains of the original tooth is still subject to decay. And a crown or bridge (an artificial tooth attached to two abutting teeth) can attract and hold plaque, thus increasing your risk of periodontal disease, which could lead to bone loss and destruction of the bridge support.

A study published in *Annals of Dentistry* showed that periodontal disease and bone loss were significantly higher around crowns and bridges. Another study, reported in the *Journal of Prosthetic Dentistry,* indicated that crowns that meet the gum line were associated with inflammation of the gums.

Why would crowns and bridges promote gum problems? First, the materials in the restored tooth may irritate the gums, increasing their vulnerability. Second, the comparatively rough surface of the crown encourages bacteria to stick to it. And finally, bacteria can penetrate the space between the crown and the tooth, even if the fit is tight. Theoretically the fit should be perfect—and indeed your dentist should check regularly to make sure your crowns do fit correctly and that the cement has not deteriorated—but perfection in restorative dentistry is impossible to achieve. According to Dr. Dennis Tarnow at New York University, even a properly fitted crown can promote inflammation, and an improper fit can increase the incidence of periodontal disease.

If you have crowns or bridges, here's what you can do:

•Thoroughly floss at least once daily and brush at least twice.

•In addition, brush at the gum line with a soft brush. You can use your toothbrush or a small end-tufted brush designed for the purpose, available at most drugstores. Aim the bristles at a 45-degree angle to the gum line. Brush gently so as not to hurt your gums.

•Try wetting the brush with an antiplaque mouthwash and brushing the gum line before you apply toothpaste. Ask your dentist to recommend a mouthwash.

•If you have extra space between your teeth, the best tool is an interdental brush—a tiny brush tip at the end of a handle, which is also excellent for cleaning between artificial and natural teeth.

•Use the rubber tip, or stimulator, that comes on some toothbrushes to clean the gum around the crown. Or try interdental sticks, which look like toothpicks.

Mercury in dental fillings

According to the American Dental Association, "for the vast majority of dental patients, mercury-containing amalgams present no health hazard." There's no evidence to support the claim that the mercury used as a hardener in silver dental amalgams can leach into your bloodstream in significant amounts and thus, supposedly, cause a variety of conditions, ranging from insomnia to multiple sclerosis. Nor is it dangerous to breathe the vapor when fillings are being ground down in a dental procedure.

Researchers conducting tests on 1,100 people with amalgams found levels of mercury in their urine of less than 20 micrograms per liter; according to the American Conference of Governmental Industrial Hygienists, there's no need to be concerned unless levels exceed 150 micrograms.

• For cleaning fixed bridges, you'll need a floss threader to get the floss between the bottom of the bridge and your gums, as well as perhaps special brushes.

• Ask your dentist about a dental irrigation device (such as Waterpik). Several models bear the American Dental Association's seal of acceptance. They can help remove trapped food debris.

Semiannual dental visits are particularly important for people with restored teeth. Next time you go, discuss the tools and techniques of preventive home care with the dentist or hygienist.

Avoiding gum problems. Several studies have indicated that patients with restored teeth had no significant problems with them, so long as they were given (and followed) good instruction in dental care and had their teeth cleaned regularly by a dentist. If you are undergoing restorative dentistry, ask your dentist for suggestions and instructions for special care. Anything that exerts undue pressure on a crown or bridge, such as nail-biting and tooth grinding, can displace a restored tooth. Be sure your dentist checks for fit and stability at your regular visits.

Dental sealants

Sealants are a plasticlike coating applied to the biting surface of the teeth to create a barrier against food particles and bacteria. When applied to children's teeth, they can prevent up to 80 percent of all cavities. Some dentists are prejudiced against sealants because the earliest sealants, which appeared in the mid-1970s, produced a fragile and easily dislodged coating. But today's sealants are far more advanced.

Why are sealants helpful? Fluoride and brushing are effective against cavities on the smooth surfaces of the teeth, but they have little effect in preventing cavities on the biting surfaces—and that's where 80 percent of the cavities in children under fifteen occur. Dental sealants that are brushed on the pits and fissures of the teeth form a tight protective seal against decay. Durable and invisible once applied, the sealant is most effective on the permanent molars and premolars—teeth with what dentists call "pits and fissures," which are least likely to be protected against decay by fluoride and are hard to keep clean. Other teeth may also be sealed, depending on their susceptibility to decay. In combination with fluoride, sealants virtually guarantee a cavity-free mouth.

The teeth to be sealed must first be cleaned and the enamel lightly etched with acid to improve the bonding of the plastic to the surface. Then liquid sealant is applied to the chewing surfaces with a brush. The material is then exposed to high-intensity light to harden it. The procedure is painless. It costs less to seal a tooth than to fill a single cavity.

The American Dental Association and the U.S. government recommend sealants for all children. Dentists sometimes also apply sealant to the teeth of very young children and young adults, but usually only if they're highly prone to tooth decay. The coating may last up to seven years and is easily replaced if it wears down. Sealants have been well studied for efficacy and safety. If your children or grandchildren don't have them, this may be a good time to ask why not.

Sensitive teeth

At some time or another you may suddenly find that heat, cold, certain foods, or brushing and flossing bring on a temporary but acute toothache. The first step is to see your dentist and make sure there is no underlying problem that needs treat-

---

Is chewing gum an aid to dental hygiene?

It can be. Gum-chewing stimulates copious secretions of saliva, and saliva helps neutralize tooth-decaying acids in dental plaque. The chewing action also helps squeeze the saliva into the spaces between the teeth.

Frequent chewing, however, can inflict harmful stress on jawbone and gum tissue. Since most chewers favor one side of the mouth over the other, the favored side is over-developed, which can lead to jaw pain. Constant chewing can also erode biting surfaces, crack fillings, and loosen inlays, allowing the possibility of recurrent decay.

For dental health, the key to chewing is moderation: chew on a piece of sugarless gum within five minutes of finishing a meal, and chew for fifteen to twenty minutes, no more.

ment—a cavity, nocturnal tooth grinding, a dying root, or a fractured tooth. You may simply have what's called dentin hypersensitivity, a common problem. Exactly what's going on inside the sensitive tooth is uncertain, but one theory is that it's the movement of fluids deep inside the tooth that stimulates the nerves. Whatever the mechanism may be, wear and tear on the teeth—for example, overzealous brushing or constant grinding, which causes enamel to thin—is usually responsible. Acidic foods, such as citrus fruits and juices or wine, may cause sensitive teeth to ache. Fortunately, dental hypersensitivity can be treated and cured.

You may need instruction in gentler brushing techniques. You'll probably be advised to try a desensitizing toothpaste such as Sensodyne or Denquel. (Be sure to buy a brand with the seal of the American Dental Association.) These contain compounds, such as strontium chloride and potassium nitrate, that can reduce the painful nerve response, though it often takes a month or so of regular use for this to occur. Meantime, you may want to avoid foods that seem to aggravate the condition—such as hot coffee, ice cream, wine, or grapefruit juice.

If the toothpaste doesn't help, fluoride treatments, though expensive, can reduce sensitivity. Sealants and resins, applied to sensitive areas, may also be useful. If nothing else works, root canal therapy may eliminate the problem.

Wisdom teeth

At one time apparently the jaw had room for three sets of molars. But today the third molars, or wisdom teeth—*dens sapientiae*—often cause trouble. Sometimes they are badly positioned and crowd the second molars. Sometimes they fail to grow through the gums, a condition called impaction. A partially exposed wisdom tooth may decay because of overlying gum tissue that makes it hard to clean. Impacted wisdom teeth can also cause pain and swelling.

No wonder that removal of wisdom teeth is one of the most common forms of dental surgery today. It is often prescribed even for young patients before the roots of their wisdom teeth have fully formed. But if you have a wisdom tooth (impacted or not) that doesn't cause you trouble, don't assume you should have it removed.

One school of dentistry says any wisdom teeth should be extracted to ward off future problems. But there is no evidence that a dormant wisdom tooth will necessarily harm the alignment of your teeth. A consensus report from the National Institute of Dental Research counsels general caution instead. Remove wisdom teeth only when there is clear evidence of trouble: infection, pain, a cyst, non-reparable cavities, or a threat to the second molars. (If you engage in contact sports, you should consider extraction, since there is some evidence that an impacted wisdom tooth seriously increases the risk of jaw fractures during such sports as football or boxing.)

If your dentist recommends extraction and you have any doubts, you should seek a second opinion.

Canker sores and cold sores

These very common sores are often confused because they both usually occur in the mouth area. They're also similar in that there's little you can do about them but let them run their course, like a cold. But there are crucial differences—in appearance, causes, and specific locations.

Canker sores, those small craterlike lesions that can occur on or under the tongue

Novocain is the best and most common local anesthetic for dental work. It's safe, effective, and has almost no side effects. Laughing gas (nitrous oxide) also has a good safety record, but it can cause nausea and vomiting. Laughing gas should be reserved for people with high levels of anxiety about having dental work performed. For long complicated procedures, laughing gas may not be adequate; the advice and perhaps presence of a trained anesthesiologist is important.

or inside the cheeks, have not been proved to have a viral origin, nor are they contagious or a sign of disease. Painful and irritating as they are, they usually go away in about a week, with or without treatment. That's the good news. The bad news is that doctors aren't sure what causes them, and there is no known remedy.

Canker sores have bothered humanity since ancient times. Hippocrates coined the medical term for them—*aphthous stomatitis*—in the fourth century B.C. Canker sores seem to be brought on by stress in some people; stress can also be a side effect. Heredity may play a role, and some women find that the sores recur with menstrual periods. Some people believe that food allergies can cause an outbreak. There's no proof, but it certainly won't hurt to follow your hunches.

Another suspect is trauma—the kind that comes from biting your tongue or the inside of your cheek, or from using a hard-bristled toothbrush. If you unconsciously bite the inside of your cheek, try to kick the habit. Any mouth injury can get infected. If you are prone to canker sores, stay away from anything that can hurt the lining of the mouth, such as hard-bristled toothbrushes and bones in meats. If canker sores become very painful, ask a pharmacist to recommend an over-the-counter anesthetic drug or protective gel to reduce pain and inflammation. And if the lesions don't heal fully within two weeks, see your doctor.

Cold sores (or fever blisters) are tiny blisters that occur most frequently on the lips and adjacent skin, though occasionally on gums or the nose, and often appear in clusters. Unsightly and sometimes painful, they are usually caused by a virus called herpes simplex 1, which is different from the virus that causes genital herpes. The infection is contagious, but most people have already contracted the virus in childhood or early adulthood (though often with no symptoms), so it is unlikely that an adult would "catch" the virus by, say, kissing someone with a cold sore.

The sores usually go away in a week or two, but they tend to recur, often in the same spot. The virus lies dormant in the body until triggered by factors such as a cold, fever, fatigue, sunlight, or emotional stress. An over-the-counter anesthetic ointment can help relieve pain. A prescription antiviral ointment may suppress the virus if applied early. Other products (such as the amino acid lysine) have been suggested for treating cold sores, but there's no conclusive evidence that they work.

Teeth grinding

Teeth grinding during sleep, known as bruxism (from the Greek *brychein*, meaning "to gnash the teeth"), can indeed cause facial soreness and pain, headaches, and fractured or abraded teeth, as well as the jawbone pain known as TMJ (temporomandibular joint syndrome). Up to 20 percent of the population may grind their teeth at night, but are seldom aware of it.

Occasionally, a malocclusion—that is, teeth that don't fit together properly or are improperly positioned—may cause bruxism. In such cases, corrective dentistry (selective grinding or braces) may solve the problem. Conversely, tooth grinding can cause a malocclusion.

Emotional upsets, anxiety, and occupational stress may also play a role. Psychotherapy, counseling, or relaxation therapies are sometimes recommended.

Dentists often supply plastic or rubber tooth-guards, known as splints, which protect the teeth during sleep. One small study found that hard splints were effective in reducing bruxism in eight of the ten patients; soft splints did not work as well. Thus a hard splint is worth trying.

Dental X-rays should not be done routinely, but only to diagnose specific conditions. The radiation exposure is small, but there's no point in getting X-rays you don't need. Your dentist or hygienist should cover you with a leaded apron during the procedure. Pregnant women should postpone X-rays if possible.

TMD

This form of jaw trouble was, until recently, called temporomandibular joint (TMJ) syndrome, but was recently rechristened temporomandibular disorders (TMD). The new name, it was hoped, would more accurately reflect the complexity of the disorder. Either way, the term refers to a grinding or clicking sound, plus pain or discomfort, when you open your mouth—a feeling that your jaw has come unhinged. In most people this is not serious, but it can persist painfully. For unknown reasons, 90 percent of TMD sufferers are women. Jaw muscles become sore, chewing is difficult, and pain spreads to the facial and neck muscles and persists around the clock. Headaches, toothaches, and earaches may also be part of the syndrome. Most people with these symptoms consult a physician or dentist—both may be needed for a diagnosis. Not all jaw and facial pain is caused by TMD, so other conditions have to be ruled out.

Causes: there can be many. What causes TMD has been a matter of dispute—emotional stress is often cited—but there is probably no single cause. The bones, ligaments, and muscles of the jaw hinge are a complicated mechanism, and many factors can adversely affect the joint, particularly in combination:

• Teeth clenching and grinding (bruxism) can cause muscle spasm, or be caused by it—and muscle spasm, in turn, produces still more spasm. Many experts think this (and the emotional stress that sometimes leads to teeth clenching and grinding) is at the root of most cases of TMD.

• Malocclusion (teeth that don't fit together properly) can throw the jaw out of line.

• Internal derangement of the jaw or other orthopedic problems of the joint (such as arthritis, degeneration of the bone, injury, or developmental disorders) can play a role.

• Bad posture, particularly thrusting the chin forward, can strain the neck muscles and those of the jaw. Beware also of gripping a phone between your shoulder and cheek during a long conversation, or of carrying a heavy shoulder bag for long periods on the same shoulder. Strained neck and shoulder muscles can affect the muscles in your jaw.

• A blow to the jaw can result in TMD, as can whiplash.

• Chewing gum or too many chewy foods (bagels, beef, candies, or dried fruits) can promote or aggravate TMD.

Treatments: varied but complicated. The first line of treatment is simple self-care. Going on a soft diet for a few days (and giving up gum chewing, if you chew gum) can help. Aspirin, ibuprofen, or acetaminophen can reduce pain and muscle spasm. Cold or hot compresses to the jaw may help. Experiment to see which is best for you, or apply ice and then moist heat to the jaw. Rest your jaw as much as you can. Squelch cavernous yawns (hold your chin in place with your fingers). Correct any poor postural or other habit that may be contributing to your problem. Try gentle exercises to relax neck muscles: roll your head in circles, or stretch your chin toward each shoulder in turn and hold for a few seconds. You may need the help of a physical therapist or other practitioner with experience in body mechanics.

In addition, your dentist may be able to correct your bite simply by grinding a few tooth surfaces. Bite plates or splints, fitted over the biting surface of your teeth, can also help stabilize the bite and eliminate nocturnal tooth grinding. Muscle relaxants may be prescribed if over-the-counter painkillers don't break the

Dentist-to-patient: is there an AIDS risk?

According to the American Dental Association, the risk of HIV transmission between dentist and patient is extremely low—and certainly no reason for you to skip dental visits or feel anxious. The Centers for Disease Control and Prevention (CDC) have identified five dental patients "believed to have been infected" with HIV during visits to the same Florida dentist—these are the only cases out of the millions of dental procedures that are performed each year. (How this happened may never be known.)

To prevent the spread of any disease, dentists and their hygienists and assistants are strongly advised to wear masks and new latex gloves with each patients, and to follow correct procedures for disinfecting reusable equipment and disposing of disposables. These precautions should protect both provider and patient. Anyone who is HIV positive should, of course, let the dentist know before beginning treatment.

pain/spasm cycle. If you believe that emotional problems are contributing to your TMD, try to pinpoint the source of stress or unhappiness and do what you can to alleviate it. Some kind of psychological counseling may be worthwhile. For nearly everybody, measures such as these will cure or control TMD.

Surgery can make matters worse. In severe and persistent cases, however, surgery is sometimes advised. Be cautious about agreeing to any kind of irreversible treatment. One type of TMD surgery, reported in the *Wall Street Journal* in 1993, had tragic results. About 25,000 people with TMD underwent a procedure—touted as "state of the art"—in which a Teflon-laminated implant was inserted into the jaw joint. Manufactured by Vitek, a Houston company, these implants were to serve as a kind of shock absorber, but not only did they fail to alleviate TMD symptoms in most cases, they also often damaged the bone and left some people permanently disfigured and disabled. In 1990, after several complaints had been lodged and the company had withdrawn the devices, the FDA took action against the company, and it went out of business. In 1993 a Texas court, in response to an FDA suit, ordered a batch of similar implants from another manufacturer destroyed.

Surgical techniques exist for extreme cases, but consider surgery only as a last resort. As with any surgery, get a second opinion.

Saving a knocked-out tooth

If you or a child of yours knocks out a tooth, the last thing you should do is throw it away. Pick it up, replace it in the socket if possible, call your dentist, and get to his office as soon as you can. Research shows that you have a 50 percent chance of a successful replantation if you get to the dentist within thirty minutes. Accomplishing this may not sound difficult, but don't underestimate the trauma of the situation: blood and confusion may delay you. Try to remain calm and rational—saving a tooth is definitely worth the effort. And even if more than thirty minutes elapse, take the tooth to the dentist anyway and let him decide what to do.

Follow this step-by-step post-accident procedure:

• After finding the tooth, rinse the it gently in tepid tap water, holding it by the crown (nonroot) surface. Don't scrub the tooth—this could injure the surface root tissue needed for successful replantation.

• Call the dentist to inform him of your imminent visit. Unless he tells you not to, gently insert the tooth in the socket. To seat the tooth properly, bite down firmly on a clean handkerchief or piece of cloth for at least five minutes; keep biting down with moderate pressure until you get to the dentist's office.

• If reinsertion at the scene of the accident isn't possible, place the tooth, bathed in saliva, under your tongue or inside your cheek until you get to the dentist's office. If a child is so young that he may swallow the tooth, transport it in a plastic cup or bag filled with milk or tap water and a pinch of salt.

Dental implants

Thanks to the fluoridation of water and improved dental treatment, most people under thirty-five today have had remarkably little tooth decay and, in the future, are likely to have less periodontal disease than their parents and grandparents. In contrast, many older Americans have lost some or all of their teeth. For them, there's an alternative to removable dentures, fixed bridges, and missing teeth—dental implants, which has become one of the hottest areas in dentistry.

What is a cracked tooth and how should you treat it?

It is a fracture in the tooth enamel caused by wear and tear, aging, grinding your teeth (bruxism), chewing ice, gum, nuts, or hard candies, or biting down hard on a bone, pit, or other hard object. It may be hard for a dentist to diagnose a cracked tooth because the crack may not be visible, even on an X-ray. The first symptom is usually pain in the tooth when you bite down hard or discomfort when inhaling cold air through the mouth.

A crack can get larger and deeper with further wear and may cause serious injury to the tooth or promote infection. In some cases, grinding down the chewing surface of the tooth may relieve pressure on the bite and keep the crack from opening when you chew. However, a crack won't heal, and you'll probably need some kind of restorative dentistry, such as a crown.

Unlike conventional crowns and bridges, which rely on remaining teeth for support, a dental implant consists of an artificial tooth or bridge attached to the underlying jawbone. First an anchor (usually made of titanium) is surgically embedded in or placed on top of the bone. Most often this procedure is done under local anesthetic on an outpatient basis. You then have to wait for up to six months for the bone to grow around the anchor and hold it firmly in place; meanwhile you may wear a temporary denture. Sometimes the post that will hold the replacement tooth is already attached to the anchor when it is implanted; other implants require additional surgery to attach the post to the anchor later on. After the gums have healed, the artificial tooth, bridge, or denture, is finally attached.

Implants can replace one or more teeth, provide support for a partial denture, or be used to attach a full denture. The implanted tooth can't be removed by the wearer, who treats it like a natural tooth and can expect it to last a decade or more. Dental implants are likely to be more comfortable, convenient, and stable than dentures. But for many people who can manage well enough with conventional crowns, bridges, and dentures, the following potential hitches of implants may well outweigh the advantages:

•Not everyone is a candidate. You need to have healthy gums and adequate bone in your jaw to support the implant. You must also be in good general health: any condition, such as diabetes, that would make healing difficult would rule out an implant.

•The procedure takes many months, can be painful, and is expensive. Expect to pay anywhere from $500 up to $2,500 per implant, depending on how much work is needed. Dental insurance rarely covers implants.

•As with any surgery, there's the risk of temporary adverse effects, such as swelling and residual pain. There's also a small risk of more serious complications, such as nerve or sinus injury.

•If new bone does not grow around the anchor, the implant may be unstable and/or lead to an infection. Occasionally implants put additional stress on the bones in the jaw, which can lead to bone deterioration and the loosening of the implant. In general, however, new techniques and materials have improved the long-term reliability of implants. Implants tend to be less successful in the upper jaw, because the bone there is less dense than in the lower jaw.

•Once you have an implant, meticulous oral hygiene (brushing, flossing, and regular dental visits) is essential. The seal between the implant and the gums is never as complete as it is with a real tooth, so there's always a risk of infection.

•It's essential to find a practitioner experienced in this specialty. Start by consulting your own dentist. Oral surgeons, periodontists, prosthodontists (specialists in tooth replacement), and even some general dentists perform implantations, sometimes working in teams. Ask about the practitioner's training, and how many implantations he has performed.

Digestive Disorders

The digestive system is divided into a number of sections: the mouth, the esophagus, the stomach, the small and large intestines, and the rectum. The digestive organs and glands—the liver, gall bladder, and pancreas—are also part of this system. It is the main job of the digestive system to take in food; to break it down so the nutrients can be absorbed by the body; and to eliminate waste.

Disorders of the digestive system afflict nearly everyone at one time or another. This section covers the most common digestive disorders—many of which are preventable or are treatable at home.

Constipation

Constipation, defined as failure to have a bowel movement after three days or more, can usually be alleviated or prevented altogether by drinking plenty of fluids, exercising regularly, and eating a diet that features high-fiber foods—grains (including unprocessed wheat bran), fruits, vegetables, and legumes. Fiber provides bulk in the intestine and absorbs water, thus making bowel movements easier. As your grandmother may have told you, prunes are particularly effective in preventing constipation, as are raisins and figs. Besides drinking an adequate amount of fluids and forming good dietary and exercise habits, you should allow yourself time for bowel movements. Medical authorities advise that you never ignore the urge to defecate, even when it may not be convenient to interrupt your routine. If you follow these guidelines, constipation should not be a problem for you.

Laxatives are not the answer

In spite of what the laxative advertisements say, the human intestine does not have to function according to an exact schedule. It is okay for a person to have a bowel movement once a day, twice a day, every other day, or perhaps only three times a week, according to most doctors and the National Institutes of Health. What is normal for one person may not be normal for another.

Worry about "irregularity" leads many people to rely unnecessarily on laxatives or enemas. Recently a Food and Drug Administration Advisory Review Panel on laxatives and similar products expressed the view that Americans are too concerned about the health implications of bowel movements. We spend more than 400 million dollars annually on laxatives—a mostly useless expenditure that fails to promote normal bowel movements or accomplish any health objective. While a mild laxative may occasionally be appropriate if your eating or exercise habits have been altered by travel or some other circumstance, relying on laxatives can actually cause irritable bowel syndrome or other problems that will *intensify* constipation. A laxative is a drug and should not have a permanent place in your medicine cabinet.

Constipation that lasts longer than a week is a signal to consult a doctor, for it can occasionally be a symptom of some underlying disorder.

Diarrhea

Simple diarrhea is common and has many causes: among them, bacterial or viral infection or eating contaminated food or drinking water. In addition, specific types of diarrhea can occur after taking antibiotics and with excessive use of certain over-the-counter antacids. People who are lactose-intolerant—that is, they have trouble digesting milk products—may also suffer from diarrhea if they eat dairy products.

Diarrhea occurs when too much water is passed along with the stool during a bowel movement. Normally, fluids in the digestive tract are mostly reabsorbed through the intestinal walls, so that fecal matter solidifies as it travels through the digestive tract. If something interferes with the effectiveness of that process, you'll pass excess fluid as you defecate.

Fortunately, simple diarrhea is usually self-limiting—it gets better without treatment in a day or two. However, diarrhea can be serious, particular for children and the elderly, because of the risk of dehydration. And, at any age, diarrhea requires prompt medical attention if it lasts more than forty-eight hours or is accompanied by any of these symptoms: severe abdominal cramping, blood in your stool, or lightheadedness or dizziness (indicating dehydration). You should consult a physician if you get frequent bouts of diarrhea or if you have alternate bouts of diarrhea and constipation since this may be a sign of a potentially serious underlying disorder.

Prevention

Food poisoning is the most easily prevented cause of diarrhea. It's simply a matter of taking precautions when preparing, cooking, and storing food. (For information on how to prevent food poisoning, see page 380.) People who are lactose intolerant should avoid the dairy products that seem to trigger symptoms or drink milk treated with lactase. Avoid taking megadoses of vitamin C; too much vitamin C can cause diarrhea.

Treatment

First and foremost, drink water, fruit juices, or clear broth to help restore fluid balance. In addition, avoid alcohol, caffeine, milk and dairy products, and any products containing the sweeteners sorbitol, xylitol, and mannitol, most commonly found in sugarless gums, vitamins, and diet foods. If you suspect a drug you are taking could be the cause, stop using it—unless it is a prescription drug. In that case, consult your doctor.

Some over-the-counter medications to alleviate diarrhea can be useful in certain cases. Products containing loperamide (brand name Imodium), diphenoxylate hydrochloride, or bismuth subsalicylate can be helpful for run-of-the-mill diarrhea Products containing attapulgite, or kaolin (kaopectate), pectin, and atropinelike substances are generally *not* effective. If you suspect food poisoning, however, you are probably better off letting it run its course; you want to get the harmful bacteria out of your system. But in that case, consult your doctor just to be sure.

(Traveler's diarrhea is a separate issue and is discussed on page 485.)

Flatulence

Although most belching is due to swallowing air, most gas passed from the rectum is produced in the bowel. There's no need to fret about passing gas occasionally—everyone does it. Though on occasion it can be an acute social embarrassment, it's not a symptom of bowel cancer or other serious disease.

The offending gases, including hydrogen, methane, and carbon dioxide, are produced when bacteria that are normally present in the large intestine cause incompletely digested carbohydrates to ferment. The only real way to cut down on flatulence is to cut down on foods that contain these indigestible carbohydrate residues—particularly legumes like beans and lentils. Intestinal gas is also common in people who can't digest the lactose in milk and some dairy products (see page 370). If you are bothered by excess flatulence, simply cut down on, or avoid, the foods that intensify the problem for you.

How to reduce gas

•Soak beans before cooking to remove some of the carbohydrates that cause gas. You must discard the soaking water and then boil the beans in fresh water.

•Chew food thoroughly. If you gulp it, you swallow harder-to-digest lumps that remain longer in the intestine, where their residue may ferment.

•Avoid constipation, which slows down the passage of food through the gastrointestinal tract, thereby stepping up fermentation. Eat high-fiber foods and drink plenty of fluids.

•If you have problems digesting lactose, avoid regular milk. Stick to cheese, yogurt, and special lactase-treated milk.

•Don't expect relief from over-the-counter remedies. Antifoaming agents (such as simethicone), found in some "antacid-antigas" preparations, merely change large gas bubbles into smaller ones—hardly a remedy for flatulence. Bulk-forming laxatives can actually promote the kind of fermented residues that cause the problem in the first place. As for products containing "activated charcoal," there's little or no evidence that they can actually absorb gas in humans, as claimed. They can, however, interfere with the absorption of some medicines.

Heartburn

The most common cause of heartburn is "gastroesophageal reflux"—the backup of stomach contents into the lower esophagus, where gastric acids produce a burning sensation and discomfort. This can occur when there's too much pressure in your stomach—or sometimes a loosening of the muscle band (sphincter) separating the esophagus from the stomach—during the digestive process.

Occasional heartburn is no cause for concern. Repeated reflux can, however, lead to injury of the esophageal lining. If you frequently have heartburn, the following steps can help prevent or alleviate it:

•Don't overeat.

•Avoid tight clothing, especially waist-pinching belts.

•Try to avoid constipation by increasing your fluid and fiber intake. This will

---

Myth: Carbonated beverages relieve nausea.

Fact: Fluids—especially carbonated ones—are hard to keep down on a queasy stomach. What often works best for nausea is eating a cracker (or other dry food) and lying down for a while.

Drinking cola or ginger ale may be a good way to restart the eating cycle and to replenish any fluids lost through vomiting. But these beverages must be at room temperature and flat, and you should drink them in small sips. Carbonation bloats an already upset stomach and may actually cause more vomiting.

Apple and grape juices at room temperature are also good choices. Avoid citrus juices, however, since their acidity can further irritate the lining of the esophagus, and they often contain hard-to-digest pulpy solids.

Antacids: How to Spell Relief

Over-the-counter antacids are so popular because most are effective, fast-working, and easy to use—neutralizing stomach acid and inhibiting the action of pepsin, a potentially irritating digestive enzyme.

All antacids are safe when used occasionally by healthy people. But no over-the-counter medication is without its risks. Daily use of antacids can mask a serious problem, such as a peptic ulcer. In extreme cases, the "heartburn" may actually be an incipient heart attack. Taken regularly without a doctor's supervision, antacids may cause bowel irregularities (constipation or diarrhea), aggravate kidney disorders, and cause other disorders. And prolonged use can actually cause an increase in the production of stomach acid if you suddenly stop taking the antacids—this is called acid rebound.

Here are nine tips for effective antacid use:

•Try to eliminate the cause of frequent heartburn or upset stomach (excess fatty food, alcohol, stress) instead of making antacid use a part of your daily life.

•Use antacids only occasionally for indigestion or heartburn. If symptoms persist despite antacid use, see your doctor.

•Liquid types generally neutralize acid more effectively than tablets. Chew tablets thoroughly to help them dissolve quickly in the stomach—and drink some water after swallowing them.

•If one brand doesn't work well, try another. Some formulations are more potent than others.

•Antacids may interfere with the absorption of many drugs (such as antibiotics, digitalis, and anticoagulants). If you take prescription medication, consult your pharmacist or doctor before using antacids.

•If you are on a salt-restricted diet, avoid sodium bicarbonate antacids, which contain whopping doses of sodium.

•Seek medical help immediately if your "heartburn" is severe and accompanied by chest pain, nausea, vomiting, weakness, breathlessness, fainting, and/or sweating. It may be a heart attack.

•Pregnant women and people with ulcers or kidney problems should consult a physician before using any antacid.

•If you are using antacids only to increase your calcium consumption, take doses yielding no more than 1,000 to 1,500 milligrams of calcium a day—and avoid aluminum-based antacids, which can actually deplete calcium.

Comparing antacid types

Sodium bicarbonate (such as Alka-Seltzer, Bromo Seltzer, Brioschi, and Rolaids). Ordinary baking soda, usually in effervescent form. For short-term use only: frequent use may interfere with kidney or heart function, promote urinary tract infection, and disrupt the body's acid balance. High sodium content—for instance, two Alka-Seltzer tablets have 550 milligrams. Brands containing aspirin can upset stomach and aggravate ulcers.

Calcium carbonate (such as Tums, Alka-2, Titralac, and Amitone). Good source of calcium—500 to 800 milligrams per tablet. Limit dosage according to instructions. May cause constipation.

Aluminum compounds (such as Amphojel and Alternagel). Less potent and slower acting than other types. Some types may promote calcium (or phosphorus) depletion, and are not recommended for those with high calcium needs, such as postmenopausal women. People with kidney problems should check with a doctor before using. May cause constipation.

Magnesium compounds (such as Philip's Milk of Magnesia). May cause diarrhea.

Aluminum-magnesium compounds (such as Maalox, Di-Gel, Mylanta, Riopan, and Gaviscon). May have the same side effects as either aluminum or magnesium compounds in some people, but generally less likely to cause constipation or diarrhea. Some brands add simethicone, which is supposed to reduce gas (or at least reduce the size of gas bubbles), but which has never been proven to provide relief.

Generic antacids are also available.

Don't take an antacid that contains aluminum if you are taking any prescription drug—first consult your doctor or other health-care provider. The FDA now requires the labels on such antacids to warn about possible drug interactions, notably reduced absorption of prescription drugs.

help prevent straining during bowel movements, which can increase abdominal pressure and encourage heartburn.

•Don't eat just before retiring, or lie down for a nap right after a meal. It helps to stay upright for at least several hours after eating.

•Put the force of gravity to work—don't sleep flat. Try elevating the head of your bed by at least six inches or more. (Wood blocks or a couple of fat phone books under the bed frame legs should do the trick.) This may be the single most important mechanical alteration that heartburn sufferers can make.

- Limit your fat intake, since fat slows the emptying of the stomach.
- If you're prone to heartburn or have eaten a heavy meal, avoid chocolate, alcohol, peppermint, and spearmint. Highly flavored after-dinner liqueurs, often thought of as aids to digestion, may make you feel worse. Caffeine may be an irritant, as may tomatoes and citrus fruits and juices.
- Birth control pills, antihistamines (often found in over-the-counter cold remedies), valium, and other drugs can promote heartburn. If you are taking any type of drug regularly, ask your doctor if it might be the cause of your heartburn.
- Don't smoke. Nicotine adversely affects the tone of your esophageal sphincter and thus can contribute directly to heartburn.
- If discomfort continues or recurs frequently, see your doctor.

Your stomach growling is the sound of your digestive juices mixing with gas as they move through the digestive tract. You are more likely to hear this noise when you're hungry because you tend to salivate more then and swallow more air.

Ulcers: A New Treatment

An ulcer is a craterlike sore in the stomach or intestinal lining—called a gastric ulcer when in the stomach, a duodenal ulcer when in the first portion of the small intestine. (A peptic ulcer, another familiar term, is one that occurs in any part of the digestive tract exposed to gastric acid and the enzyme pepsin.) Ulcers are usually painful, and they can lead to complications such as severe bleeding. What causes them? Many factors may contribute. Most recently it's been discovered that a common bacterium, *Helicobacter pylori,* is present in the stomach or duodenum of almost all people with ulcers. People who often take large doses of aspirin, ibuprofen, or other nonsteroidal anti-inflammatory drugs (NSAIDs) are at risk for ulcers, because these drugs may damage the stomach lining, and then digestive acid makes the lesion worse and interferes with healing.

Cigarette smoking is another factor that seems to promote ulcers, though it's not clear how. Smoking definitely slows down the ulcers' healing. Food has also been blamed—coffee, tea, cola beverages, and spicy foods, as well as alcohol use. But no food has ever been shown to promote ulcers. A bland diet with lots of milk and cream was once the routine treatment for ulcers, but now that's known to be counterproductive. Milk actually stimulates the production of stomach acid. Emotional stress, chronic anxiety, and even an "ulcer-prone personality" have all been blamed, too. But calm, happy people, as well as tense, unhappy ones, get ulcers. There is no "ulcer personality." Nevertheless, a recent study at the Centers for Disease Control and Prevention in Atlanta (published in *Archives of Internal Medicine*) did suggest that people who perceive their lives as stressful may be somewhat more likely to get ulcers.

The discovery that *Helicobacter pylori* may play a role in ulcer formation is good news, because antibiotics kill this organism and thus may offer a cure in some circumstances. How these bacteria are transmitted is unknown. A recent study at the Veterans Affairs Medical Center in Houston showed that antibiotic treatment could be helpful against ulcers. The 109 patients in the study, all suffering from an ulcer recurrence, were known to have the bacterial infection. One group underwent a two-week course of antibiotics, along with the standard ulcer drug ranitidine (brand name Zantac) that decreases the production of stomach acid. Another group took only ranitidine. Only 1 percent of those who had undergone the antibiotic therapy had a recurrence of ulcers in the year they were followed. But half the patients taking only ranitidine had a relapse within twelve weeks, and nearly all had a relapse within a year.

Still, antibiotics aren't a magic bullet. Doctors have been reluctant to treat all ulcers with antibiotics, and more research is clearly needed. Some people can take one of the standard ulcer drugs and never have a recurrence. Furthermore, *Helicobacter pylori* is not a factor in all ulcers. NSAID-induced ulcers, for instance, would not necessarily respond to antibiotics.Nor should you take antibiotics just because you have gastric symptoms, unless you're sure you have an ulcer. But if you do have recurrent ulcers, you should discuss antibiotics with your doctor. And before any ulcer is treated with antibiotics, it's important to establish that *H. pylori* is present (via biopsy or blood tests).

The best plan, as always, is to try to avoid ulcers, and not to experience a recurrence if you've ever had them. These measures can help:

•If you must take aspirin or other NSAIDs regularly, take the smallest possible dose and always take it with food. Enteric-coated aspirin is a good idea, but check with your doctor before changing.

•Quit smoking, if you smoke.

•Though no food is known to cause ulcers, it won't hurt to avoid foods that seem to give you indigestion or cause pain.

•If you drink alcohol, drink moderately and never on an empty stomach.

Irritable Bowel Syndrome

The symptoms typically include cramping (often on the left side of the abdomen, but it may mimic heartburn or backache), bloating, and an urgent need to move your bowels. The stool may be loose and watery, and you may notice white mucus in it. Eating may make you feel worse, and defecation or passing gas brings relief. You have no fever or bleeding, and you can't think of anything you've eaten or done to have brought this on. Mysteriously, the diarrhea may give way to constipation, but you may still have abdominal pain and a lot of gas. The condition may correct itself and then return when you least expect or want it—for example, before an important occasion about which you already feel tense.

This is irritable bowel syndrome, also known as spastic colon, mucus colitis, or nervous bowel. It's a common abdominal complaint, probably the most common reason for visits to gastroenterologists. It usually develops in late adolescence or early adulthood, and affects twice as many women as men. It does not lead to cancer, does not require surgery, is not caused by any known physical abnormality, and is not the same thing as inflammatory bowel disease—a much more serious disorder that may produce ulceration of the intestinal wall. But it's still a chronic disorder and is more difficult to cope with than the occasional bout of diarrhea or nervous stomach most of us experience from time to time.

Diagnosis and treatment

No one is sure exactly what causes irritable bowel syndrome—some doctors attribute it to emotional stress, or food allergies, or an as-yet-undetermined physiological disorder. If you frequently suffer from the symptoms of irritable bowel

Myth: The colon requires cleansing.

Fact: *Fears of "auto-intoxication" of the colon lead some people to fasting (to "purify" the body), periodic "cleansing" of the intestines (with laxatives), and most extreme, colonic irrigation. The last involves inserting a tube through the rectum and far into the large bowel, and then pumping in pints of warm water, which may contain such additives as soap suds, herbs, coffee grounds, or other allegedly therapeutic substances. Some of the risks are severe cramps, rupture of the colon, injury to the lining of the colon walls, infection from micro-organisms in improperly cleansed equipment, disturbance in body fluid balance, and dependence on colonic irrigation for elimination.*

Colonic irrigation won't cure headaches, skin problems, or any disease. Some theories of the origins of colon cancer suggest that regular bowel movements are important in preventing cancer—but that doesn't call for colonic irrigation (just a high-fiber diet).

syndrome, you should make an appointment with your doctor, who can rule out more serious disorders such as gallstones, bowel diseases such as colon cancer, and ulcers. The inability to digest lactose (milk sugar), caused by an enzyme deficiency, can also produce the same symptoms (see below).

Your doctor may quiz you about your diet and advise against certain foods. However, when it comes to treatment, irritable bowel syndrome is poorly understood, and existing therapies are not known to have lasting success. Once the diagnosis has been made, there are a number of treatments that may help, such as antispasmodics to control diarrhea, tranquilizers for temporary relief of anxiety, and bulk laxatives (high in fiber) or stool softeners to relieve constipation, if necessary. If symptoms persist, your doctor may also suggest some form of psychotherapy.

Once you know the diagnosis, it helps to remember that what you've got won't turn into something worse. It's chronic but not progressive. Though no food or category of foods is a known or even suspected culprit, there's no harm in watching your diet, and if certain foods seem to set off symptoms, try avoiding them. A high-fiber diet (fruits, vegetables, and whole grains, taken with plenty of fluids) is known to promote normal bowel function.

Emotional stress and anxiety are certainly associated with irritable bowel syndrome, but don't let anyone tell you it's all mental—or that your emotional makeup is the cause. If anything, the reverse is true—chronic bowel problems cause a lot of stress, and frequent bouts of irritable bowel syndrome can seriously interfere with the normal conduct of your life. Some studies have shown that patients who didn't improve with medical treatment and who also had psychological problems such as depression could benefit from psychiatric treatment.

However, according to Dr. William Whitehead of the Johns Hopkins University School of Medicine, while emotional upset can make intestinal symptoms worse, there's no evidence that irritable bowel is itself a psychiatric disorder. Rather he believes that depression may be a result of having the disease—or at least that anxious and depressed people are more likely than others with the syndrome to see a doctor, because they tend to worry more about their symptoms. Thus "brief psychotherapy focussing on better ways of coping with current problems…may be superior to medical management alone."

Lactose Intolerance

Many people cannot digest more than a small amount of milk because of its lactose (milk sugar). The inability to digest milk occurs because the enzyme *lactase,* which breaks down the milk's *lactose* in the intestines, is produced in increasingly smaller quantities in most people after infancy. Virtually all human infants depend on milk for survival and digest the nutrients in it, including lactose. However, early in childhood, most people start producing less lactase. In these people, who are termed lactose intolerants or lactose maldigesters, drinking milk may produce such symptoms as gas, stomach cramps, and diarrhea. Lactose intolerance can also develop later in life because of digestive disorders. (A few people, including infants, may be allergic to the protein in milk, but that's not lactose intolerance.)

According to a recent study, only about 30 percent of all peoples, chiefly those who have depended historically on herding and dairy products, retain their ability to digest lactose throughout adulthood. These include northern Europeans, some Mediterranean peoples, and their descendants in the Americas, as well as such African peoples as the Masai. Asians are mostly lactose intolerants, as are West Africans and their descendants in the Americas. So are 80 percent of Native Americans, half of all Hispanics, and even about a fifth of Caucasians.

Not all lactose intolerants have to give up regular milk, however. There are degrees of tolerance and intolerance for milk. Although the ability (or loss of ability) to digest lactose is an inherited trait, drinking habits also depend on custom and preference. For people who are truly lactose intolerant, there are many lactose-reduced products and treatments available. But they are an added expense and a bother to use if you don't really need them. Keep these facts in mind:

•Bloating, flatulence, and stomach cramps aren't always caused by lactose intolerance; it's not a condition that comes on suddenly. You can do a simple test for lactose intolerance at home. Drink two glasses of milk on an empty stomach and see if symptoms occur during the next three to four hours. If so, repeat the test using lactase-treated milk. If you now have no symptoms, you probably have a lactose intolerance. But if you have chronic gastrointestinal discomfort, you should see a doctor.

•Studies have shown that many true lactose maldigesters (classified as such by lab tests) can consume moderate amounts of milk and dairy products without symptoms, particularly if the milk is part of a meal. Whole milk causes fewer problems than skim, because its fat slows the rate of stomach emptying.

•Fermented milk products such as yogurt with active cultures, are usually easier to digest than milk. Most yogurt is low in lactose anyway, and the bacteria in it help break down what milk sugar there is. But as much as 30 percent to 70 percent of the lactose originally in the milk may remain in the yogurt, for lower lactose, look for yogurt made with bulgaricus cultures—or just experiment until you find a brand that agrees with you. Cheese should be no problem, since most lactose is removed along with the whey when the cheese is made.

•Acidophilus milk or buttermilk may not be any better for people sensitive to lactose; the degree of fermentation is variable, and so lactose content also varies.

•If you are lactose-intolerant, drink lactose-reduced milk, which is available in most markets. This type of milk contains about 70 percent less lactose and tastes sweeter than regular milk. You can also buy lactase tablets or liquid in drugstores or grocery stores and add them to the milk yourself; five drops per quart can break down over 70 percent of the milk sugar in about twenty-four hours (for greater reduction, let the treated milk stand for forty-eight to seventy-two hours). If you add drops to commercially treated milk, you can eliminate nearly all the lactose.

•You can also swallow lactase tablets or capsules just before you consume a milk product, but that's usually less effective than adding drops to the milk itself.

Diverticulosis

Diverticulosis, is a condition, not a disease. It occurs when tiny pouches (diverticula) form in the wall of the colon. These are small, self-contained hernias that appear to be related to aging, not diet or lifestyle. People under thirty-five seldom have them, but one in ten Americans over forty does, and about one in every two by age sixty. The colon wall thickens as we age, and the pressure inside increases, causing small protrusions. This condition has no symptoms and is not usually serious. However, in a small number of people diverticulosis can turn into diverticulitis, an inflammation of the colon that may have dangerous side effects. Caused by blockage of the diverticula and a subsequent overgrowth of bacteria, diverticulitis may cause severe pain and requires prompt medical treatment.

The best way to head off diverticulitis is to avoid constipation and straining during bowel movements. Don't take laxatives, however, which can irritate the large bowel. Keep your dietary fiber at the recommended level of thirty to forty-five grams daily, or even higher if constipation remains a problem. Eat fruits, vegetables, and whole grains. Wheat bran, which you can add to casseroles and baked goods, is especially helpful. These are good practices for the health of your digestive tract, whether you have diverticulosis or not.

Myth: Decaffeinated coffee is safe for people with digestive problems.

Fact: *Decaffeinated coffee stimulates the flow of stomach acid almost as much as regular coffee. Though caffeine is a mild stimulant of stomach acid and digestive juices, the principal components in coffee that provoke this flow (with consequent irritation of stomach ulcers) are apparently introduced during the roasting process whether the beans have been decaffeinated or not. Increased acid flow can also exacerbate heartburn, so people with ulcers or chronic heartburn should avoid regular coffee and decaf. Other coffee substitutes include caffeine-free herbal teas and grain-based beverages such as Postum, Pero, and Cafix. These unfortunately, may also stimulate stomach acid.*

Hemorrhoids

If there's any comfort in having hemorrhoids it's that they are so common. The tissue of the anus is a cushion of blood vessels, connective tissue, and muscle. A hemorrhoid is not a growth but an inflammation and enlargement of the natural tissue, caused by excess pressure in the abdominal and/or anal area. Thus pregnant women often get hemorrhoids, which may disappear after the birth. Genetics and obesity may also play some role. The most common cause is constipation and straining at stool. Sitting a lot may make existing hemorrhoids more painful.

The first symptom of hemorrhoids is usually rectal bleeding or bright red blood in the stool—a mild symptom that by itself does not indicate that any drastic treatment, such as surgery, is in order. If you notice blood, however, you should not just assume you have hemorrhoids, but get a doctor's evaluation. Unfortunately, in a very small number of cases, bleeding may be the first sign of gastrointestinal disease, including cancer. Hemorrhoids may exist outside or inside the rectum; it's the latter location that causes the most pain.

Preventing hemorrhoids
Though hemorrhoids may not be avoidable in all cases, prevention is always the best policy. Here's how:

•To avoid constipation, eat a high-fiber diet—fruits, whole grains, and vegetables—and increase your fluid intake. This will increase fecal bulk and thus prevent straining at stool. Avoid large amounts of meat and highly refined foods.

•If you are chronically constipated and nothing seems to help, get a doctor's advice, rather than self-prescribing laxatives.

•Careful personal hygiene can also cut down skin irritation. Be sure to keep the area very clean. But anything that abrades or irritates the skin should be avoided—even too-zealous cleansing.

•If you have hemorrhoids or know you're prone to them, don't use rough toilet paper, but clean gently with wet paper or premoistened wipes.

•Avoid lifting heavy objects.

If you already have hemorrhoids

Try frequent warm sitz baths and bed rest if the hemorrhoids are painful. Avoid sitting long hours. If your job is sedentary, stand up now and then and take a short walk. If you're sitting through a long performance, take advantage of intermissions and walk around. Exercise seems to help, too. Some people find that certain foods, such as nuts, coffee, or alcohol, aggravate hemorrhoids. You can try eliminating foods that seem to be making matters worse.

Many people rely on over-the-counter remedies, and last year the FDA made major changes in its rules for these products. Some ointments, suppositories, and foams will be taken off the market because they had never been proven effective. No over-the-counter preparation will be permitted to claim to relieve internal pain (there are no nerve endings inside the rectum); all must be labeled for external use only. Claims must be limited, since these products can offer only temporary relief of symptoms. Products that claim to shrink tissue must carry certain cautions (people with heart disease and diabetes should not use them, for example), and they must also advise sufferers to seek medical help if the condition worsens or fails to improve. In addition, a number of ingredients were banned (lanolin alcohol, turpentine oil, and camphor) as potential irritants or because they were ineffective. In fact, the most useful ingredients in these products are likely to be zinc oxide or petroleum jelly—both of which cost less if bought on their own.

Surgery: the last resort

If home remedies don't bring relief, your doctor can prescribe suppositories, injections, and other therapies. Surgery is the most invasive treatment, and you should consider it only if your primary physician advises it. It's always wise to seek a second opinion before having surgery. Don't let your first stop be a surgeon's office or a clinic that advertises quick-fix laser treatment ("In and out the same day"). Some people may need surgery, but there's no such thing as surgery that's pain-free and complication-free.

Anal Itching

Anal itching—known medically as *pruritus ani*—is generally regarded by physicians as a simple problem that home remedies can alleviate. Very rarely, persistent anal or rectal itching may be a sign of serious infection, so if it does not respond to simple treatments or the passage of time, see a doctor. Pinworms, rare in families without small children, are one possible cause that requires a doctor's advice.

Common causes

The majority of cases are caused by skin irritation from fecal soilage. In older people or in anybody with a touch of diarrhea, seepage of fecal matter may occur. As people grow older, anal skin becomes more irregular and harder to clean; people with hemorrhoids (which may trap small fecal particles) are more prone to itching. At any age haste may contribute to bad hygiene. One doctor blames pruritus ani on dispensers that give out toilet tissue one sheet at a time. Too much hygiene, such as rubbing energetically with dry toilet paper, can injure the skin, too. Another precipitating factor may be constipation.

Once the itch starts, many factors can exacerbate it. Such as walking, sitting—particularly prolonged sitting on a plastic seat—and such activities as bike riding. Hot weather and sweating, tight clothes that compress the buttocks, and nonabsorbent nylon panty hose and underpants may make matters worse. Some experts think stress may be a factor in anal itch.

Home remedies

Don't scratch; it only causes further irritation and invites infection. Meticulous, gentle cleaning provides relief. A bidet would be a convenience, but a shower is just as efficient. Wash the area gently with soap and water, taking care to rinse thoroughly, and don't wipe with dry tissue. Pat yourself dry with cotton. When away from home, carry a few premoistened, individually packaged wipes—the kind you'd use for a baby. If leakage is your problem, wear a small cotton pad against the anal opening and change it frequently. Wear under garments with cotton crotches, and generally avoid tight clothing. Go easy on cycling activities until you feel better. Corticoid lotions or creams can be effective if used for a short time. Avoid the "-caine" creams sold for topical relief, since they can often further inflame sensitive skin.

Anal Fissure

An anal fissure is an elongated ulcer—or crack—in the skin lining the anal canal. Fissures usually result from constipation and the passage of hard stool, stool that is inadequately emptied, or in association with hemorrhoids. Subsequent bowel movements can irritate the fissure and cause spasms of the sphincter muscle—which can be extremely painful—and sometimes bleeding.

Prevention and treatment

The best way to prevent anal fissures is to avoid constipation by eating a diet high in fiber along with drinking plenty of fluids.

If you experience pain during bowel movements, or notice any bleeding, don't simply assume it is an anal fissure. See your doctor to rule out potentially more serious conditions. If your doctor diagnoses anal fissure, avoiding constipation can help make them less likely to cause pain. Warm sitz baths can help ease the pain of spasms. Your doctor may prescribe stool softeners. Cleaning the anal area after each bowel movement is also important: use moistened cotton (and soap if necessary), then pat dry with dry cotton. A fissure will usually heal within two to three weeks.

Food Poisoning

It is estimated that 33 to 50 million Americans get sick each year from foodborne bacteria, yeasts, molds, or viruses. Every home, and every person, is host to a variety of bacteria that can cause serious illness if they get into food and multiply. You can get mild food poisoning without realizing it. When people come down with a "bug" accompanied by symptoms such as headache and stomach distress, it's often dismissed as "stomach flu" or "twenty-four-hour virus"—but it may be food poisoning. Food poisoning is more than just a stomach ache; some types of bacteria and viruses can cause severe illness which can be fatal in the elderly, in children, in diabetics, in alcoholics, and in individuals whose immune systems are depressed, such as cancer patients. Anyone with prolonged symptoms should see a doctor.

Food poisoning is primarily caused by a number of different bacteria and some viruses, with bacteria being responsible for the majority of cases. Just about every type of food—unless it has been sterilized—has bacteria in or on it, but most of them are harmless. In addition, bacteria can be introduced into foods from external sources. For example, some types of bacteria are always present on the skin; others are found around sores, pimples, or infected wounds. Soil and dust are also homes to bacteria. Household pets, insects, individuals with poor sanitary habits (such as not washing their hands after going to the bathroom) and those who are ill and handle food can all transmit bacteria, as well as viruses, into food.

Still the mere presence of bacteria or viruses in food isn't enough to make you sick. They cause problems only when the food is improperly handled and prepared. Heat inactivates most viruses, and bacteria are relatively harmless unless they are allowed to multiply. Bacteria begin to multiply quickly in food left at room temperature and thrive on food that is kept warm on a stove. Moist foods, such as stuffing or cooked rice, are especially susceptible to bacterial growth. Refrigeration retards the growth of bacteria, and cooking at high temperature kills most of them. But if food has been left out long enough, some types of bacteria can form a toxin that will survive heat or freezing.

The most common type of food poisoning

The bacterium salmonella is by far the most frequent cause of foodborne illness and it is rapidly becoming even more prevalent. In the 1970s, poisoning by salmonella, called salmonellosis, accounted for about 740,000 reported cases of food poisoning each year; researchers now project that estimates could be upward of four million cases annually. The number of cases may actually be higher, since many individuals

Steam tables and chafing dishes are often not hot enough to prevent dangerous bacteria from growing. Hot food has to be kept at a temperature of about 140 to 165°F to prevent food poisoning, so beware of food that has been kept warm for more than two hours.

Microwaving Microbes

While microwave ovens cook foods quickly and tend to destroy fewer vitamins than conventional cooking methods, they also may heat foods unevenly and leave some parts undercooked. This leaves open the possibility that bacteria may survive cooking. To be sure that your microwaved food doesn't cause food poisoning, follow these guidelines:

•To be sure that foods cook evenly, rotate all foods at various intervals during cooking.

•Check the internal temperature of meat and poultry to be sure that they are cooked all the way through.

•Wrap plastic made to be used in microwave ovens around the dish, or cover it with glass or ceramic. The trapped steam will help decrease evaporation and will heat the surface. Prick a hole in the plastic wrap to vent steam. The plastic wrap shouldn't touch the food.

•Allow microwaved food to stand covered after cooking. Heat concentrated on the inside will radiate outward through the food, cooking the exterior and equalizing the temperature throughout. Food will taste better this way, too, since it will be consistently hot.

•Thaw meats before cooking in a microwave oven; most models have defrost settings for this purpose. Ice crystals in frozen foods are not heated well by microwaves and can leave cold spots.

•If you're used to conventional cooking, remember that the more food you're microwaving, the longer it will take. For example, four baked potatoes will take much longer than two.

Types of Food Poisoning

Disease/Organism	Sources of Infection	When Symptoms Begin	Symptoms
Campylobacteriosis (*Campylobacter jejuni*)	Food can become contaminated during processing of meat and poultry. Sources of infection include raw or undercooked beef and poultry and raw milk. Can also be present in untreated water and in shellfish.	2 to 5 days	Fever, diarrhea, abdominal cramps, and bloody stool
Botulism (*Clostridium botulinum*)	Improperly processed, low acid canned goods (usually home canned products), such as green beans; foods contaminated by soil and then left in an oxygen-free environment, such as potatoes coated with oil or butter, at room temperature.	8 to 36 hours	Nervous system affected: double vision, problems swallowing, trouble breathing. Can be fatal.
Perfringens food poisoning (*Clostridium perfringins*)	Grows rapidly in large portions of food that are cooling slowly or at room temperature. Can grown in any dish made with meat or poultry as well.	8 to 24 hours	Abdominal pain and diarrhea. Sometimes nausea and vomiting. Symptoms are usually mild, but can be more severe in the ill and the elderly.
Salmonellosis (*Salmonella*)	Raw or undercooked beef and poultry, or foods contaminated by coming into contact with them. Raw or undercooked eggs or products made with them. Food handlers with poor hygiene.	12 to 48 hours	Nausea, vomiting, abdominal cramps, fever. Can be fatal in infants, the elderly, and individuals with depressed immune systems.
Shigellosis (*Shigella*)	Food can become infected by a food handler with poor hygiene and can cause illness if the food is not cooked properly. Multiplies when food is kept at room temperature for long periods.	1 to 7 days	Abdominal cramps and pain, nausea, vomiting, diarrhea, bloody stool, fever. Can be serious in infants, the elderly, and those with depressed immune systems.
Staphylococcal food poisoning (*Staphylococcus*)	Food that has been coughed or sneezed on or otherwise handled in an unsanitary manner. Staph is present on the skin, around pimples and boils, and thus can be introduced into foods by a food handler with a skin infection. It is particularly common in foods that require a lot of handling, such as tuna or potato salad. Multiplies rapidly at room temperature.	1 to 8 hours	Nausea, vomiting, abdominal cramps, diarrhea.
Cholera (*Vibrio cholera*)	Fish and shellfish from waters infected with sewage.	1 to 3 days	Diarrhea and abdominal pain. Can be mild or severe. Cholera can be fatal.
Parahaemolyticus food poisoning (*Vibrio parahaemolyticus*)	Fish and shellfish. Proliferates in warm weather.	15 to 24 hours	Abdominal pain, diarrhea, nausea, fever, headaches, chills, bloody stool.
Gastroenteritis (*Enteroviruses, rotaviruses, parvoviruses, and norwalk*)	Viruses present in human intestine. Can be passed on by food handlers with poor hygiene. Also in shellfish from waters contaminated with sewage.	12 to 48 hours	Vomiting, nausea, diarrhea.
Infectious hepatitis (*Hepatitis A*)	Can be passed on by a food handler who has the disease. Also in shellfish from contaminated waters.	15 to 50 days	Fatigue, jaundice, nausea. Can cause liver damage. Can be fatal.

and even doctors mistake salmonellosis for intestinal flu. The increase in salmonellosis has been attributed principally to high-speed mechanical methods of slaughtering and eviscerating animals, especially poultry. According to a variety of estimates, at least half of all raw chicken marketed is contaminated by salmonella and/or campylobacter. Of course, any animal may harbor salmonella—no cow or chicken is completely free of bacteria. Mechanical evisceration and other processing methods simply increase the bacteria count. But no matter how an animal is killed and dressed—even if by hand on your own farm—it must be handled carefully, kept refrigerated or frozen, and never eaten raw. If you follow the guidelines for handling foods on page 380), you should have no problem.

foods on page 380)

If the Power Fails

Power outages are common and, if they last long enough, can cause havoc in the freezer and refrigerator. According to guidelines from the U.S. Department of Agriculture, first of all, do not open appliance doors. A well-stocked freezer provides its own insulation and should stay at a safe temperature for up to two days without power; a half-full freezer may last up to twenty-four hours.

If dry ice is available for the freezer, you can bring it home in a cardboard box or picnic cooler. Don't touch dry ice—it will instantly freeze your skin. Handle it with gloves or tongs in a well-ventilated area, and avoid inhaling the fumes. Don't lean into a freezer in which dry ice has been stored; there is no oxygen left to breathe. Twenty-five pounds should keep a full freezer (ten cubic feet) safe for three or four days, and a half-full freezer for two or three days. Dry ice will stick to plastic wrap, so put it on an empty shelf, or insulate packages of food with pieces of cardboard.

A nonfunctioning refrigerator will hold food safely for up to six hours in a cool room. You can add block ice to the main compartment and dry ice to the freezing compartment. (Do not put dry ice in the main compartment: it might freeze the contents.)

FROZEN FOODS

Frozen food	Thawed but cold (under 40°)	Thawed and held above 40° for up to two hours
Meat, poultry	refreeze	cook and serve, or cook and refreeze
Casseroles, stews	cook and serve	cook and serve
Dishes made with cream, milk, eggs	cook and serve	discard
Hard cheese, butter, margarine	refreeze	refreeze or refrigerate
Vegetables	refreeze (may lose quality)	cook and serve
Juices	refreeze (may lose quality)	refreeze

If frozen food is thawed and held for over two hours, treat it like refrigerated food—see below.

REFRIGERATED FOODS

Discard after eight hours above forty degrees:	milk, cream, soft cheese, mayonnaise, raw meat or poultry, lunch meat, hot dogs
Discard after one day:	fruit juice
Discard after five to seven days:	fresh eggs
Keep as long as they look and smell okay:	fresh fruits and vegetables, hard cheese, butter, margarine, open containers of mustard, pickles, jelly, etc.

Take special precautions with vacuum-packed prepared foods. These sous-vide foods, as they are called, are fresh, raw ingredients that are packaged in a plastic pouch from which all the air has been removed. Because these foods are in an oxygen-poor environment they carry a risk of botulism if they are not kept cold during shipping and storage.

Safe to Eat?

Most of the time, if a food looks suspicious, you should go with your instincts and throw it away—but not always. Some foods may look as if they are spoiled or moldy, but are actually safe to eat:

Hard cheeses, such as Cheddar, that have turned partly moldy are safe if you cut off the mold and a generous slice of the cheese underneath. (Mold on blue cheeses such as Roquefort, Stilton, and Gorgonzola are harmless.)

Mayonnaise is thought to be a common cause of food poisoning, but it is actually a preservative to some degree—the vinegar and/or lemon juice in it make it sufficiently acidic to inhibit bacterial growth.

Oil that has clouded is not spoiled. Any oil will cloud at cold temperatures and clear when warmed.

Cooked ham has an iridescent film that is harmless. Ham has a high fat and water content; these ooze out and reflect light like oil on a puddle.

Chocolate with white spots is caused by separation of cocoa fat.

Raw eggs, too, can be a source of salmonella. But in these cases, poor handling may not be the cause. Researchers suggest that the bacteria come from inside the hen, rather than by the usual route of cracked or dirty eggshells. While raw or soft-cooked eggs—or foods made with them such as eggnog or Caesar salad—are potentially risky, commercial products made with eggs, such as mayonnaise, are safe because the eggs have been pasteurized.

There have also been periodic reports that the rise in salmonellosis is due to the practice of feeding antibiotics to cattle, pigs, and poultry to enhance their growth—a practice that has allowed antibiotic-resistant strains of salmonella to flourish. However, the evidence implicating animal antibiotics as a cause of illness in humans is far from conclusive. And in any case, the routine use of antibiotics is much less widespread than it was during the 1980s. Indeed, except for treating sick animals, it has almost been eliminated from the beef industry.

Common symptoms

Contaminated food can look, smell, and taste perfectly fine. The only way you know you've eaten it is when you experience the symptoms (of course, if a food looks off, throw it away). Never test to see if leftovers—or any food—have spoiled by tasting them. Even a small taste of contaminated food could contain enough bacteria or toxin to make you sick. The most common symptom of food poisoning is diarrhea. Other symptoms include abdominal pain, nausea, vomiting (sometimes severe), and sometimes fever. The onset of symptoms can occur anywhere from one hour to seven days after eating contaminating food, depending on the infectious agent. (Hepatitis A, however, has a longer incubating period.)

Botulism—rare but dangerous

Botulism is caused by potent toxins produced by the spore-forming bacterium *Clostridium botulinum*, which is common in soil. Any food that is contaminated by soil and is subsequently carelessly washed or mishandled may be a source of botulism. However, this microbe produces poisons only at temperatures above 38°F and under certain conditions—notably an almost complete lack of oxygen—and therefore is quite rare, especially in this country.

Canned foods are a potential source of botulism. Modern commercial canning methods have gone far toward eliminating botulism from canned foods, but outbreaks still occur as a result of home canning. Though contamination usually causes cans to swell, the absence of swelling does not guarantee safety. Other possible warning signs of botulism in canned foods are gas bubbles, discoloration, and milky liquids that normally should be clear.

While botulism is generally associated with canned foods, studies have found evidence of new trends. In one case, for example, onions sauteed in butter carried the toxin and in another, potato salad was the culprit. The salad had been made from leftover baked potatoes, which had sat unrefrigerated overnight and had been wrapped tightly in aluminum foil, thus creating the airless environment the spores require. With the onions, the butter coating deprived them of oxygen, and in addition the dish had been left at room temperature for several hours.

Even if the spores are present, however, toxin won't be produced unless food is left at room temperature for *at least* twelve to twenty-four hours *and* under relatively airless conditions—for example, a tight wrap or a coating of fat. The spores can be destroyed only by moist heat at 248°F under pressure (in a pressure cooker, for instance) for thirty minutes, but the toxin will be inactivated if the food is brought to the boiling point (212°F) for ten minutes. Thus if the onions or potatoes had been thoroughly reheated, they would not have made anybody sick.

Safety for Mail-Order Food

Americans send about one billion dollars worth of mail-order food each year, especially as holiday gifts. Many of these foods—from baked turkeys and hams to smoked fish and cheesecakes—are highly perishable. Large shippers use sophisticated packaging systems to keep food from spoiling, but sometimes goods arrive in an unsafe condition. People who receive food in questionable shape may simply throw it away, not wanting to complain about a gift (anyway, it didn't cost them anything). Worse yet, they may take a chance and eat the spoiled food and get sick. By thinking ahead you can avoid many of the problems that may arise with mail-order food.

When ordering a gift
•Set a workable delivery date for any perishable food you're sending. Find out how long the mailing should take and make sure someone will be home on or around that date to receive it. If people are out of town, the food may end up sitting and spoiling at the Post Office or parcel-delivery office.
•Unless there's no other option, don't send perishable food to a friend's office, where it may be left unrefrigerated for many additional hours.
•Make sure the package will be labeled "perishable" on the outside. It will stand a better chance of being handled properly.

When receiving a gift
•If it was frozen when shipped, then raw, cooked, or smoked meat, poultry, and fish should arrive frozen or at least hard in the middle. If the food has never been frozen, it should be firm and cold—at or below 40°F. The same is true for canned or processed foods (including most vacuum-packed foods) that are labeled "keep refrigerated." Some smoked fish, if it has been highly salted, doesn't need to be refrigerated.
•Baked hams (except dry-cured hams) should arrive cold. Many canned hams must be kept cold even when unopened because they are only pasteurized and not sterile; their labels say "keep refrigerated."
•Cheese should have no mold—unless, like Roquefort and other ripened cheeses, it is supposed to. If mold has grown, cut it off along with a thick slice underneath.
•Cheesecake should arrive fully frozen.
If you have a question about food you receive, or think you deserve a replacement delivery or refund, call the mail-order company. Most reputable firms have customer-service telephone numbers and offer money-back guarantees.
Remember, it's the company's responsibility to deliver food in good condition, but it's your responsibility to make sure someone is there to receive it.

When is it safe to eat food from a dented can?

As a general rule, if the seal of the dented can isn't broken—that is, if the contents aren't exposed to air—the food is safe to eat. However, the following signs should tell you when not to buy a damaged can:

The can is leaky*. A stained label, a dented seam, or rust should make you suspicious.*

Its ends bulge*. This is a possible sign of botulism.*

Odor. *If the food has an off odor, or spurts out of the can when you open it, don't eat it.*

The symptoms of botulism poisoning do not involve the digestive tract, as with most food poisoning, but the nervous system: sudden marked weakness, difficulty in breathing, swallowing, or speaking, and double or blurred vision. Seek medical aid at once if such symptoms occur, and try to bring any of the offending food that may be left. Botulism need not be fatal if diagnosed early.

Preventing food poisoning

There are a number of simple steps you can take to prevent food contamination and reduce your risk of getting sick from tainted food:

- Keep your refrigerator below 40°F and the freezer below zero.
- Always refrigerate raw meat or poultry immediately. Don't keep it refrigerated for more than two or three days.
- Wash your hands thoroughly before you handle food. The proper way is to use soap and warm water for at least twenty seconds, working the soap into the hands, including the fingernail area and between the fingers.
- Use a fresh dish towel every time you cook.
- Keep pets away from food preparation areas.
- Defrost frozen foods only in the refrigerator, in the microwave, or under cold running water. Use a microwave only if you plan to cook the food right away or re-refrigerate it until cooking time.
- After preparing raw meat or poultry, wash the utensils, counter, cutting board, and your hands—anything that touched it—thoroughly in hot soapy water before making a salad or handling vegetables.
- Marinate meats and poultry only under refrigeration. And don't put cooked meat back into an uncooked marinade or serve the used marinade as a sauce unless you heat it to a rolling boil for several minutes.
- Cook rare beef to at least 145°F (pink, not red). Pork and chicken should, of course, be thoroughly cooked—not pink at all.
- Don't serve barbecued meat on the same plate you used for the raw meat and don't use the cooking utensils for serving.
- When eating out, pass up the steak tartare and any other uncooked meat.
- Hold foods at room temperature no longer than an hour before or after cooking. Don't leave normally refrigerated foods sitting out. Given the right conditions, the bacterial content in some foods can double in twenty minutes.
- Promptly refrigerate leftovers, particularly anything with a coating (bread or fat) or a tight wrapping. Divide large amounts of leftovers—such as sauces, soups, stews, and casseroles—into smaller containers so that they cool faster.
- Store all starchy stuffing (rice, bread) separately from the poultry in which it was cooked.
- If you can fruits and vegetables at home, ask your county health department for guidelines about safe procedures to protect against botulism.

Sexuality and Reproduction

Topics concerning sexuality and reproduction are discussed more openly than ever before. And yet, despite—or because of—changing attitudes and scientific advances in this area, many people are confused or misinformed about choices that can directly affect their health, particularly with regard to birth control and sexually transmitted diseases. This section includes essential information on these two topics and other concerns that can be self-managed. (You should consult your doctor for any type of sexual dysfunction; likewise, you should see your doctor or gynecologist if you become pregnant and for any problem related to pregnancy.)

Birth Control

The ideal contraceptive is 100 percent safe, 100 percent effective, convenient, and yet doesn't interfere with the sex act or hamper the potential to reproduce. To date, no birth control method meets those conditions. At the same time, the variety of contraceptives is greater than ever and there are additional variables to consider when choosing among them. Condoms, for example, are widely promoted because they also reduce the chance of contracting sexually transmitted diseases—or STDs—such as gonorrhea and chlamydial infection as well as HIV (the virus that causes AIDS) and herpes. And oral contraceptives, which pose some risks for certain women, particularly those who smoke, are now known to protect against some types of cancer and other disorders. (Methods such as coitus interruptus and periodic abstinence—known as "natural family planning" and based on monitoring of ovulation patterns and abstaining from sex at times of fertility—are not covered in this chapter because of their high failure rate.)

More than half of all American women between the ages of fifteen and forty-four use some form of contraception. Unfortunately, American women have more unplanned pregnancies and more abortions than women in most industrialized nations, according to a study by the Alan Guttmacher Institute in New York, a nonprofit organization that studies population issues. Moreover, the most common method of preventing unwanted pregnancies in the United States, especially after age thirty, is not contraception but sterilization, which is largely irreversible.

Our national reluctance about using contraceptives stems partly from the belief that all available methods pose medical risks, an apprehension based on the early problems associated with birth-control pills and an awareness of the pelvic infections caused by the Dalkon shield (an intrauterine device, or IUD, that was withdrawn from the market). There are additional reasons: in many other industrialized countries women have easier access to advice about contraceptives. Also, Americans have fewer methods of contraception to choose from than do women abroad. (Most western European countries market IUDs and birth-control pills not available in the United States.) Since not every type of contraceptive is appropriate for every woman, nor for every stage of her reproductive life, the more choices available, the

Comparing Contraceptives

Type and Estimated Effectiveness	Advantages	Disadvantages	Comments
Male condom (rubber, prophylactic, sheath) 85-90%	Latex condom protects against STDs, including HIV and herpes. May often protection against cervical cancer.	Must be applied immediately before intercourse. Rare cases of allergy to rubber. May break, may blunt sensation.	More effective when the woman uses a spermicide. Non-prescription.
Female condom (with spermicide) 74%	Some effectiveness against STDs, including HIV. Offers women a choice if partner refuses to use male condom. (However, no clinical studies. Not known to be as effective as male condom.)	Must be handled carefully and used correctly to avoid breakage.	New one must be used for each act of intercourse. Nonprescription.
Vaginal spermicide (used alone) 70-80%	Available over the counter as jellies, foams, creams, and suppositories. Active agent usually nonoxynol-9.	Messiness. Must be applied no more than 1 hour before intercourse. May cause rash.	Best results occur when used with a barrier method (condom or diaphragm). Nonprescription.
Diaphragm (with spermicide) 82-94%	No side effects. Can be inserted up to two hours before—rather than during—intercourse. May protect against pelvic infections and human papilloma virus, but not HIV.	Increased risk of urinary tract infection. Rare cases of allergy to rubber.	Must be used with spermicide. Prescription.
Cervical cap (with spermicide) 82-90%	Less fragile than diaphragm; can be left in place for up to 48 hours; spermicide needn't be replaced for subsequent intercourse.	Can be hard to insert or remove; may cause unpleasant odor. Test must be done before fitting of cap.	Approved only for women with a normal Pap smear prior to use and after 3 months of use. Prescription.
Birth-control pill (oral contraceptive) 99% (combination) 97% (mini)	Most effective reversible contraceptive. Results in lighter, more regular periods. Protects against cancer of the ovaries and uterine lining. Decreases risk of pelvic inflammatory disease, fibrocystic breast disease, and benign ovarian cysts. Does not affect future fertility.	Minor side effects similar to early pregnancy (nausea, breast tenderness, fluid retention) during first 3 months of use. Major complications (blood clots, hypertension) may occur in smokers and those over 35. Must be taken on a regular daily schedule. No STD protection.	Combination types contain both synthetic estrogen and progesterone (female hormones). Mini-pill contains only progesterone and may produce irregular bleeding. Prescription cost: $20 to $30 monthly.
Implant (Norplant) 99%	Effective for 5 years with no further effort. Can be removed anytime. Does not affect future fertility.	Menstrual cycle irregularity. In some women, weight gain, headaches. Removal of the device may be uncomfortable. No STD protection	Hormones, progestin only. Released from 6 silicone rubber tubes implanted under the skin. Prescription cost: about $500 for implant, $100 for removal.
Injection (Depo-Provera) 99%	Good choice for women who have trouble remembering OCs and who don't like Norplant.	Menstrual cycle irregularity. In some women, weight gain, headaches. No STD protection.	Progesterone given by injection once every 3 months. Prescription cost: about $50 per injection.
Intrauterine device (IUD) 95%	Once inserted, usually stays in place. Two types available in the United States: Progestasert (which requires annual replacement) and ParaGard (effective for up to 8 years).	May cause cramping, Increased risk of pelvic inflammatory disease. If pregnancy occurs, increased risk that it may be ectopic (tubal).	Should be used by women who are over 25, have had a child, and have no history of pelvic inflammatory disease or tubal pregnancy. Prescription.

more likely she is to find one she is comfortable enough with to use regularly—the only way birth control devices can be effective.

Recently, a woman's choice of contraceptives has significantly widened. Two long-term and very effective hormonal methods have been introduced: Norplant and Depo-Provera. Norplant consists of six tiny capsules that a doctor inserts under the skin of a woman's upper arm, using a local anesthetic; the capsules release a constant low flow of a hormone that prevents ovulation. Norplant provides protection for five years. Depo-Provera is an injection lasting about three months. The Food and Drug Administration (FDA) has also approved a condom for women that may prove even more effective than the male condom against certain STDs—though its effectiveness for disease prevention and contraception has not been as rigorously tested. However, at least it offers some protection for women whose partners refuse to use the male condom. And unlike the male condom, which can only be applied to the erect penis, the female condom can be inserted in advance. Besides this, improvements have been made in many methods during the past decade; moreover, users have come to realize that some contraceptives have advantages in addition to preventing unwanted pregnancies. At the same time, with the incidence of STDs on the rise, preventing conception is not the only concern. Condoms must also be used to prevent infection as well.

Aside from abstinence, there are four basic types of contraception for women:

Barrier methods. Used during intercourse, and applied just in advance of it, these methods—which include condoms, the diaphragm, and the cervical cap—prevent sperm from reaching the egg. (Another barrier method, the sponge, is no longer marketed.) They should be used in combination with spermicides, which can also be used alone (although spermicides alone provide only limited protection).

Hormonal contraception. This involves modifying sex hormones to imitate the natural suppression of fertility that occurs during pregnancy and breast-feeding. Birth-control pills (OCs, or oral contraceptives) contain estrogen and a form of progesterone and prevent ovulation. Others (the "mini-Pill") contain progesterone only and cause the cervical mucous to thicken so that the sperm cannot reach the egg. Progestin or other forms of progesterone can be delivered via implant (Norplant) or long-lasting injection (Depo-Provera).

Intrauterine devices (IUDs). These small plastic devices are inserted into the uterus; how they prevent conception is not well understood. They may alter the uterine environment or inhibit the transport of sperm. Of the two now on the market in the United States, ParaGard is covered with copper, which gives it its contraceptive properties, and the other (Progestasert) delivers progestin.

Surgical sterilization. For women this means tubal ligation, which involves sealing the fallopian tubes to prevent transport of the egg.

For further details on availability, advantages, and disadvantages of each method, see the chart on page 382.

Women, who are more often responsible for choosing and using a contraceptive, have wider choices than men. So far, the only definitely reversible contraceptive for men is the condom. The other option, aside from abstinence, is permanent sterilization, or vasectomy, which entails tying off the vas deferens, thus preventing the transport of sperm to the penis). Vasectomy is now available at comparatively low cost and offers the advantages of efficacy, safety, and convenience. Its only drawback is its significant degree of irreversibility.

Norplant caution

Since Norplant became available in 1991, about one million American women have had the contraceptive capsules implanted (and more than 25,000 physicians and nurses have been trained to do the implants).

Norplant appears to have side effects similar to those of the Pill, such as prolonged bleeding or spotting between periods. But it can also have other potential adverse effects, ranging from heart attack to strokes, and is not recommended for smokers or hypertensives, or women with liver disease or blood clotting disorders.

Some users have also complained of lengthy and painful procedures when the capsules are removed—which usually takes fifteen to twenty minutes when the capsules are correctly implanted. if you opt to use Norplant, it's important to find an experienced practitioner to perform the implant.

Oral contraceptives: benefits and risks

Oral contraceptives for women are easier to use and more reliable than any other method of birth control. Yet surveys show that Americans tend to overestimate the risks of the Pill and underestimate its benefits. The following information should help you put the Pill into perspective—though, naturally, new research on the Pill will probably continue to raise issues about its use. As a basic safeguard, you should always consult your physician before you decide to start—or stop—taking an oral contraceptive.

Oral contraceptives contain compounds chemically related (but not identical) to both estrogen and progesterone, the two major female hormones that define a woman's reproductive cycle. Estrogen and progesterone, if taken orally, go from the digestive tract into the liver, which breaks them down. Synthetic hormones used in oral contraceptives travel intact through the liver into the main circulatory system, where they effectively shut down the reproductive cycle. Because of the presence of these hormones in the blood, the hypothalamus—a gland in the brain—doesn't stimulate the production of FSH and LH (sex hormones involved in ovarian function). Ovulation ceases and pregnancy cannot occur. Even if ovulation should occur (and some experts think it may), implantation of the ovum is impossible because the uterus is unprepared.

In the 1960s and 1970s, oral contraceptives contained up to three times as much estrogen and ten times as much progesterone as the pill of the 1980s. The "low-dose" Pill has been proven as effective and is much less likely to cause side effects or increase long-term risk of disease. Properly used, low-dose oral contraceptives are almost 100 percent effective.

The cancer risk. Though estrogen alone may promote cancer, today's oral contraceptives contain progesterone as well, and the combination is known to be protective against cancers of the cervix and uterine lining (endometrium). An additional advantage is that women who take oral contraceptives are more likely to have annual pelvic examinations and Pap smears—a proven method of detecting reproductive cancers at a more curable stage.

So far, the evidence on oral contraceptives as a promoter of breast cancer is unclear or unconvincing; some studies show oral contraceptives not to be linked to breast cancer, others suggest they might be. A further difficulty in gathering accurate evidence is the relatively recent advent of the low-dose Pill. Since breast cancer develops slowly, and its causes are unknown, scientists have to survey many women over many years to answer the question. Thus there's been time to study women using the old, high-dosage Pill (with inconclusive results, as noted), but not those on low-dose oral contraceptives. Studies of low-dose oral contraceptives, it's thought, will fail to demonstrate any link with breast cancer. But some women with particular risk factors should proceed with caution (see next page).

Heart disease and stroke. In the 1960s the Pill was shown to have another potentially hazardous side effect—an increased likelihood of heart attacks and blood clots. While a woman is using high-dose oral contraceptives, her risk of coronary artery disease is 4.7 times higher. But this is far less serious than it sounds, because for women in their twenties the risk of heart disease is extremely small: less than 1 in 500,000. A fivefold increase in that age group brings the odds to 1 in 100,000. Even this small risk has been reduced by low-dose oral contraceptives, so that increased risk of heart disease among users of the Pill has been shown to be negligble.

Antibiotics and oral contraceptives

A few antibiotics can interact with some oral contraceptives (OCs) to cause breakthrough menstrual bleeding and, possibly, to reduce the effectiveness of OCs in preventing pregnancy. Though reports of such side effects have been few, it's long been known that ampicillin and tetracycline, for example, as well as some tranquilizers, can reduce the effectiveness of OCs. What's known about interactions is based on experience with OCs containing estrogen. Women taking the newer progestin-only pills may not need to worry.

Nevertheless, if you are on the Pill, you should always discuss this with a doctor who's prescribing antibiotics or any other drug for you. Don't hesitate to bring up the matter yourself if the doctor doesn't. (A qualified pharmacist can be a good source of information.) It might make sense for you to switch contraceptive methods if you must take antibiotics or other medications.

Moreover, a recent major study indicates that women who have stopped taking the Pill, even if they took it for a decade or more, are at no more risk for heart disease or stroke than women who never took the Pill at all. This reassuring news is based on an eight-year follow-up of the subjects of the Harvard Nurses' Health Study, conducted on a group of nearly 120,000 nurses aged thirty to fifty-five when the follow-up began. About 7,000 were taking the Pill at the time; about 50,000 had taken it in the past.

Previously, researchers focused on women who were currently taking the pill. This was the first major study to examine the residual cardiac effects on long-term pill users, many of whom took the original "big pill" of the 1960s.

Who should avoid using oral contraceptives? Smokers, diabetics, and women with high blood cholesterol levels or high blood pressure (since all these factors increase the risk of coronary artery disease) and women who have had cancer of the reproductive system or breast cancer should avoid oral contraceptives. Women who have a family history of breast cancer, who have had surgery for benign breast disease, or have other risk factors for breast cancer should consider using other methods. In addition, women are generally advised not to use oral contraceptives throughout their reproductive lives, as such complications as blood clots are more likely to occur after thirty-five. At this age, switching to another method is advised.

Male condoms: how effective?

More than a decade into the AIDS crisis, Americans are still debating about condoms. One of the most common arguments made by those afraid of "pushing" condoms is that condoms are not foolproof in preventing pregnancy or sexually transmitted diseases such as AIDS. This "all-or-none approach" was discussed by two scientists from the Centers for Disease Control and Prevention in the *New England Journal of Medicine:* "Nothing in medicine, or in life for that matter, always works….We agree that abstinence and mutually faithful sexual relationships with uninfected persons are the only guaranteed methods of preventing the sexual transmission of HIV [the virus that causes AIDS]. This does not mean, however, that we should withhold information about ways of reducing risk from those who do not find this approach feasible. Moreover, the absolutist line of reasoning does not take into account that condoms may be effective more than 90 percent of the time and that even delaying the transmission of HIV is beneficial, both to individuals and in changing the dynamics of the epidemic as a whole." In fact, condoms offer the only known effective protection against HIV transmission.

Another essential point is often overlooked: *most of the time, condom ineffectiveness is due to human failure, not product defects.* Thus education about condoms is the surest way to make them more reliable. Women, as well as men, should know the basics of condom use. Studies have found that many people are still making the most basic kinds of errors when using condoms—for example, choosing the wrong type of lubricant, or not holding onto the rim of the condom when withdrawing from intercourse. And many aren't using condoms at all.

Three potential problems can undermine condom effectiveness: breakage, leakage, and improper use. Breakage rates depend on the type and duration of sexual activity. Lack of lubrication (or use of an oil-based lubricant) also increases the chance that a condom will break. A 1989 survey by Consumer Reports estimated that about one latex condom in 140 breaks. As for leakage, standard water tests

Whatever your age, use a condom every time you have intercourse if there is any risk of sexually transmitted disease. No other contraceptive, however foolproof as a birth control device, offers any protection against STDs. Even if you or your partner has been sterilized, so that pregnancy is not a concern, you still need to use a condom to protect yourself against STDs.

have revealed that the major brands' leakage rates meet the Food and Drug Administration's requirements of fewer than four failures per 1,000 condoms.

While in theory condoms should be 100 percent effective, in reality they aren't. As a contraceptive, they are about 90 percent effective. That's substantial, but hardly surefire, protection. Failure rates vary not only from brand to brand, but also from batch to batch—as well as according to the users' age, education, and the amount of experience they've had with condoms. But you can take steps to enhance condom effectiveness. Researchers estimate that when condoms are used properly, failure rates can be as low as 1 to 2 percent.

Improving your odds

Use a new condom for every act of intercourse. Inconsistent use offers little protection. Also follow these guidelines:

Buy latex. About 1 percent of condoms are made from "lambskin" (actually lamb gut), which is more porous than latex; though such condoms block sperm, some viruses, including HIV, can get through them. Thus manufacturers aren't allowed to claim that these protect against STDs. People allergic to latex can try wearing a lambskin condom under a latex one.

Buy fresh. When stored in the proverbial cool, dark, dry place, condoms can last three to five years. Latex deteriorates faster when exposed to light, temperatures over 100° F, humidity, and air pollution. Glove compartments and hip pockets do not provide ideal storage conditions. Buy from a busy, reputable store, where the stock is likely to be fresh. Remove the condom from its sealed wrapper only when you're ready to use it. If it looks dried-out or discolored, discard it.

Use a water-based lubricant or prelubricated condoms. Adequate lubrication helps lessen the chance of breakage. Use only a water-based lubricant, such as K-Y jelly. Oil-based products, including petroleum jelly, mineral oil, cold cream, vegetable oil, and hand lotion, should never be used; they can cause latex to deteriorate in as little as one minute and thus break. The label should say that the lubricant is safe for use on latex. "Water-soluble" isn't necessarily water-based. Researchers have found that even college graduates familiar with precautions against oil-based lubricants are often fooled by products such as Vaseline Intensive Care or Johnson's Baby Oil that wash off with water but are nonetheless oil-based.

Buy nonoxynol-9. This spermicide has been shown to kill HIV in lab studies. But recent studies have raised questions about the spermicide's efficacy in actually preventing HIV transmission. Still, nonoxynol-9 is known to help prevent the spread of most other STDs and probably of HIV as well, so if you use prelubricated condoms, look for ones that contain the compound. In addition, since prelubricated condoms contain only small amounts of nonoxynol-9, a woman should probably also use a vaginal spermicide containing nonoxynol-9 for added protection.

Buy a good design. A well-designed condom has a reservoir tip, a bubble or nipple that provides a place for semen to collect. If your condom doesn't have this feature, don't pull it on so tightly that it's snug; leave a quarter- to half-inch space at the tip. The condom should be long enough so that a surplus of rubber at the open end forms a rolled rim or seal at the base of the penis. Avoid novelty condoms unless the label says they offer protection against STDs.

Wear it right

•Handle a condom carefully. Fingernails and rings can damage it. Don't unroll it until you are ready to put it on; once unrolled, it is more difficult to put on. Use a different condom if the one you have feels brittle or gummy. Don't wait until the last minute to put it on—it could be too late.

•Place the condom against the head of the erect penis. If you aren't circumcised, pull back the foreskin first. Squeeze out the air from the reservoir end or the space you've left at the tip. Unroll the condom to the base of the penis.

•Immediately after ejaculation, before the penis gets flaccid, hold the condom's rim to the base of the penis while you withdraw so the condom doesn't leak or slip off. A study at Emory University found that half of all condom failures were due to condoms slipping off during withdrawal.

A condom for women

Until recently, a woman has had no way, except abstinence, to protect herself against sexually transmitted diseases. Making certain that her partner uses a latex condom has been the only means of having safe—or at least "safer"—sex. The catch, from the woman's point of view, is that the man must not only agree to use the condom, but must use it properly. If he refuses to use one, her only recourse is to refuse intercourse. In any case, while condoms do offer reasonable protection against syphilis, gonorrhea, chlamydia, and HIV (the virus that causes AIDS), they may not protect either partner from genital warts or herpes.

In 1994, however, a new form of protection came on the market after being approved by the FDA—the female condom or vaginal pouch. Packaged in a small envelope, it's a seven-inch-long, loosely fitting pouch or bag made of thin polyurethane. At its closed end is a flexible ring, which is inserted like a diaphragm ring and covers the cervix. At the open end of the pouch is another flexible ring, which rests against the vulva and holds the condom in place outside the vagina. The condom comes with a cream lubricant and can be used with a spermicide as well. It has several advantages over the male condom:

- It's the woman who chooses to use it.

- She can insert it before intercourse (an advantage over the male condom, which must be put on the erect penis and thus requires a disruption of lovemaking).

- When correctly used, the part of the condom outside the vagina covers the area around the vagina as well as the base of the penis during intercourse—and thus offers better potential protection against genital warts or herpes.

- The pouch is made of polyurethane, which has been shown in lab tests to offer better protection against the passage of viruses than latex. Thus it may be more effective against HIV. Yet it is thin and pliant and does not block sensation. It can also be safely used by people who have an allergy to latex.

But it has some disadvantages as well. Though the manufacturer says the pouch is as effective a contraceptive as other barrier methods, additional studies remain to be done about its effectiveness. Thus if you decide to use it, it may make sense also to use a more reliable contraceptive, such as the Pill. Moreover, both partners must take care that the device does not slip inside the vagina and that the penis is inserted in the pouch, not outside it. The polyurethane is tough, and tearing is not likely—but as with the male latex condom, not impossible. In that event, intercourse must stop.

The pouch is sold in drugstores; no medical consultation is necessary. The manufacturer advises changing it for each act of intercourse. Unlike a diaphragm, it can be safely removed when intercourse is over. For any woman not in a long-term monogamous relationship—and not sure of her partner's sexual past—the new condom might well prove to be a lifesaver.

A recent government ruling requires that oral contraceptives, Norplant, Depo-Provera, IUDs, and lambskin condoms be labeled, stating that they prevent conception but do not protect against STDs. Labels on lambskin condoms must also state that users should add a latex condom as a means of protecting against STDs.

Vasectomy: benefits and risks

Vasectomy (the severing of the tube through which sperm travel from the testicles to the penis) is probably the safest and most effective means of contraception—its success rate is more than 99 percent. In recent years, about 500,000 men have been getting vasectomies annually, and today more than 15 percent of all American men over forty have had a vasectomy. At the same time, several widely reported studies suggested that vasectomy may increase the risk of prostate cancer, the most common malignancy among men. Two large Harvard studies, published in 1993 in the *Journal of the American Medical Association (JAMA)*, found that men who had a vasectomy had a higher risk of developing prostate cancer than other men; specifically, men who had a vasectomy at least twenty years earlier had an 80 percent increased risk. Many men are undoubtedly worried—enough so perhaps to avoid vasectomy or, if they've already had one, to consider having the operation reversed.

There are several good reasons why a fear of prostate cancer based on these studies should *not* cause you to avoid vasectomy—and certainly should not lead you to seek to reverse it. Though the association between vasectomy and prostate cancer in the two Harvard studies was statistically significant, it was relatively weak and may still have been due to chance. Earlier studies of prostate cancer risk and vasectomy have had inconsistent results: at least three found a link, and three did not. A review of six previous studies on vasectomy and prostate cancer risk by researchers at the National Institute of Child Health and Human Development found that all of the studies were biased in a number of respects or failed to meet other scientific standards of inquiry. For example, men who undergo vasectomies may, for various reasons, receive more medical care than men who haven't, and therefore vasectomized men are more likely to have prostate cancer detected—even though their rate of cancer may be no higher than that in the general population.

In addition, a panel of experts convened by the World Health Organization in 1991 concluded that the link between vasectomy and prostate cancer was "unlikely." Another expert panel convened in 1993 by the National Institutes of Health concluded that any link may be due to bias in research or to chance—and that health-care providers "should continue to offer vasectomy and perform the procedure." There is also no plausible biological explanation for a vasectomy–cancer link. One theory is that the operation may increase the level of male hormones, which are known to stimulate the growth of prostate cancer. But while a few studies have shown a slight hormonal change, most studies have found no change at all.

Finally, risk factors for prostate cancer, other than aging and a family history of the disease, have not been firmly identified. While the researchers adjusted their data for some possible risk factors (such as diet and smoking), there's no way of knowing whether other, still-unidentified risk factors for this cancer were equally distributed in the studies between men who had opted for vasectomy and those who had not. These "confounding factors" are a problem in population studies.

Bottom line

No method of contraception is completely risk-free—usually women are the ones who face the risks. Vasectomy still appears to be one of the safest means of contraception.Other studies are underway and more are planned, so the picture may become clearer in the next few years. Meanwhile, if you were planning to get a vasectomy, don't rule it out because of these studies. In one of them, men who had a vasectomy actually had a *lower* overall death rate than men without vasectomies.

If you have had a vasectomy, don't consider having it reversed in the hope that you will thereby lower your risk of prostate cancer: there is absolutely no evidence that it will. The American Cancer Society and other experts recommend that all men who are between the ages of fifty and seventy have an annual prostate exam. To be on the safe side, men who have had a vasectomy should be doubly certain to be screened.

Vasectomy facts

Along with fears about a possible risk of prostate cancer, men may also be scared off of getting a vasectomy because they believe the operation is painful, complicated, or that it will reduce sexual pleasure and prowess.

In fact, vasectomy is fairly simple and straightforward—the procedure takes about twenty minutes in a doctor's office, and the cost for it averages about $600 (which some insurers will cover). Furthermore, it has no effect on sexual desire, achieving an erection, or experiencing orgasm.

Reversing a vasectomy is not nearly so simple, however. It usually requires general anesthesia and can cost upwards of $10,000; insurers generally don't cover it. Moreover, its success rate is well under 50 percent. Therefore, men should only undertake a vasectomy if they are certain they won't want children in the future.

Sexually Transmitted Diseases

Sexually transmitted diseases, or STDs, are among the most prevalent kinds of infections in the United States, with millions of new cases reported every year. In recent years, AIDS has received far more attention than any other STD. Yet researchers have identified more than twenty sexually transmitted diseases, and the most common ones—listed in the chart on page 390—affect an estimated one out of four Americans. Some of these have risen dramatically: the incidence of syphilis, for example, which is highly curable with penicillin, began increasing in the 1980s after years of declining (though it began declining again in the 1990s). Anywhere from 500,000 to one million Americans are thought to become infected with herpes each year. And medical consultations for genital warts in the United States increased from 169,000 in 1966 to more than two million in 1988.

All of these diseases, including AIDS (see page 392), are so-called because they are transmitted by sexual contact, usually sexual intercourse. Syphilis, like AIDS, can also be spread by infected blood. And the herpes virus, if mouth sores exist, can be transmitted by kissing. But sexually transmitted diseases are not transmitted by toilet seats, towels, dishes, or other objects; by ordinary contact such as shaking hands, sharing meals, or using the same telephone; or by mosquitoes or other insects. Organisms that cause sexually transmitted diseases usually die within minutes outside the body.

If you have been in a mutually monogamous sexual relationship, sexually transmitted diseases are very likely not something you need to worry about. But anyone who has had multiple sexual partners, or has a relationship with someone who has multiple partners, may be at risk. *All of the diseases covered here are preventable.* Most are also treatable. Syphilis, gonorrhea, and chlamydia can be cured with antibiotics. Genital herpes, genital warts, and AIDS cannot be cured, but they can be treated or managed. However, no sexually transmitted disease can be accurately diagnosed and treated without professional help. *There are no home remedies, so see a doctor or other health-care professional if you get infected.*

Preventing sexually transmitted diseases

Apart from abstinence, the most reliable preventive is long-term monogamy with a monogamous partner. If you're healthy and have a long-term monogamous relationship with a healthy partner, you're at no risk. But if you have not had a long-standing monogamous relationship, always take the following protective measures:

Use latex condoms and a spermicide containing nonoxynol-9. These provide protection—though not infallible—against infection (see page 386). Jellies, foams, creams, and condoms containing nonoxynol-9 are recommended, since this chemical appears to kill many microorganism and *may* help prevent transmission of the virus that causes AIDS. Remember that nonbarrier forms of birth control (oral contraceptives, IUDs) offer no protection against sexually transmitted diseases. While a diaphragm and cervical cap protect against pregnancy, they are *not* reliable against infection. Use a condom and spermicide in addition. Note: condoms may not offer adequate protection against genital warts.

Know who your partner is. It's risky to have sexual intercourse with someone you have just met, or someone you won't be able to locate later.

A Guide to STDs

Disease	Symptoms and Course	Complications	Treatment
Syphilis. Bacterial infection. Treatable and curable, though damage in later stages is not reversible. Historians argue whether it originated in the Americas or Europe and Asia; records of the disease go back to the time of Columbus's voyage. After declining in this century in the United States, the number of cases began rising in the 1980s. If untreated, it is chronic and ultimately fatal.	Up to twelve weeks after infection, a painless sore (chancre) appears on genitals, mouth, or elsewhere. Lymph nodes may enlarge. Chancre more obvious in men; if vaginal, rarely noticed; heals without scarring. About 6 weeks later, fever, rash, and flu-like symptoms may occur, then disappear and later reappear. Symptoms may vanish but the infection will not.	Years later, brain and spinal chord damage, blindness, insanity, and death may result. Can cause miscarriage and birth defects; can be contracted by fetus in utero.	Even if no symptoms are present, diagnosis can be made by a blood test, but results may be negative for up to twelve weeks after exposure. Antibiotics, taken as prescribed, are a dependable and relatively inexpensive cure.
Gonorrhea. Bacterial infection. May not have immediately detectable symptoms. Known since ancient times. Chronic and progressive. If untreated, can result in physical disability and infertility. Spreads by direct contact with infected mucous membranes in genitals, mouth, and throat. Estimated one to two million new cases each year.	Symptoms (if any) noticeable within two to ten days of infection: painful urination, vaginal or penile discharge, sore throat (if contracted through oral sex), rectal pain or discharge (if contracted through anal sex). Possibly heavy menstrual bleeding or bleeding between periods.	If untreated, may cause arthritis, skin sores, and heart or brain infection. Common cause of pelvic inflammatory disease (PID), which may damage Fallopian tubes, leading to ectopic pregnancy (potentially fatal to the mother). Can cause permanent sterility in both women and men. Infants infected during birth may become blind.	Diagnosed by a smear or culture. Antibiotics, taken as prescribed, are a reliable cure; some strains resistant to standard antibiotics can be treated by newer drugs.
Herpes. Caused by two types of herpes virus: type 1 commonly produces cold sores around mouth; type 2 produces genital outbreaks. But both viruses can infect either area, causing roughly the same symptoms. Chronic but not progressive or fatal. No cure. Transmitted by direct contact with an active sore or virus-containing genital secretions. Virus establishes itself permanently in nervous system, staying dormant for months or years. Can spread silently, since some people may shed viruses while asymptomatic. An estimated 30 million people are infected.	Within ten days after infection, flu-like symptoms—muscle aches, swollen glands, fever, and sometimes shooting pains in legs or abdomen; followed by painful blisters and sores, usually on genitals or mouth. Symptoms subside without treatment, but sores recur at unpredictable intervals in 90 percent of cases. First outbreak is usually most severe, but in some cases may be so mild as to go unnoticed.	Infants may acquire herpes during birth, resulting in central nervous system damage or death. Caesarean delivery may be necessary for infected mothers. Frequent recurrences can result in depression. But in many cases, herpes becomes less severe with time.	Diagnosis confirmed by a scraping or culture. Does not respond to antibiotics. Acyclovir, a relatively new, expensive drug (ointment or capsule) is not a cure but can ease symptoms and may reduce length of attack. If taken continually, this drug usually prevents recurrences. For an outbreak, warm compresses, sitz baths, and aspirin may relieve discomfort. Herpes support groups may be helpful in combatting depression and other emotional problems that sometimes result from the disease.
Chlamydia. A bacterial infection. Thought to be the most common curable sexually transmitted disease in America today (estimated four million cases annually). Chronic if untreated. Like other sexually transmitted diseases, spreads by contact with infected mucous membranes. Can occur simultaneously with gonorrhea.	Similar to gonorrhea: within twenty-one days painful urination, vaginal or penile discharge, abdominal pain, possibly urethral itching. Symptoms may be very mild (possibly going unnoticed) and can go away without treatment, only to produce later complications. High percentage of women have no symptoms.	In women, leading cause of pelvic inflammatory disease (PID), which may result in ectopic pregnancy or sterility. In men, can lead to diseases of the urinary tract and sterility. Babies born to infected mothers are subject to eye infection and pneumonia.	Diagnosed by lab test. Antibiotic treatment, taken as prescribed, is a reliable cure.
Genital warts. Caused by human papilloma virus (HPV). Warts appear on, in, and around the genitals, or in the mouth and throat. Highly contagious, spread by intimate bodily contact. HPV is a recent discovery as a cause of cancer in humans.	Within eight months of infection, local irritation and itching, followed by soft, flat, irregularly surfaced wartlike growths that may increase in size. May cause no symptoms. If inside vagina or cervix, usually detectable only by physician.	Strongly associated with cancer (cervical and possibly penile). Infants born to mothers with human papilloma virus may develop warts.	Immediate treatment is essential. Can be removed chemically or surgically. Virus remains latent: warts often recur. Infected women should have annual Pap smear. Drugstore remedies for other kinds of warts are useless and may be harmful.

A Vaccine for Hepatitis B

A liver infection that can vary greatly in severity, hepatitis B is spread by direct blood contact, sexual intercourse, contaminated needles, and blood transfusions—much like HIV, the AIDS virus. The hepatitis B virus may also pass through cuts or scrapes in the skin or can be transmitted via saliva on a shared toothbrush. About 300,000 new cases are diagnosed each year.

Most infected people develop no symptoms, or else just flu-like symptoms and jaundice that clear up by themselves. But about 6 to 10 percent of infected adults, and up to 50 percent of children, become chronic carriers who face potentially fatal complications, notably cirrhosis and liver cancer. (In contrast hepatitis A is spread primarily through contaminated water and food and is not chronic; hepatitis C, much less common, is transmitted mainly by transfusions. Thanks to screening tests used by blood banks, the risk of getting either the B or C virus through transfusions has dropped greatly.)

There is no cure for hepatitis B, but there is an effective vaccine with minimal side effects. Unfortunately, parents and physicians have been slow to accept the idea of immunization—perhaps because of the high cost, and an unwillingness to believe that the disease is a real danger to people not designated as "high risk." The high-risk groups include:

- Intravenous drug users.
- Health care workers.
- Anyone living with an infected person
- Sexually active gay men.
- Heterosexuals with multiple partners
- Recipients of certain blood products.
- Children of immigrants from regions where hepatitis is common, such as Southeast Asia.
- International travelers who plan to spend six months or more in areas where infection rates are high.
- Infants born to infected women (all pregnant women should be tested). Vaccination will prevent about 90 percent of these infants from becoming chronic carriers

While efforts to vaccinate health care workers and gay men have shown positive results, the incidence rate has continued to climb among other groups. One problem is that 30 to 40 percent of those who come down with hepatitis B have no known risk factors.

The U.S. Public Health Service, the American Academy of Pediatrics, and other physician groups have advocated that all infants be immunized routinely against hepatitis B. Like some other immunizations, hepatitis B requires three injections and confers long-term immunity. The cost is about sixty dollars for the three shots—though the cost would decline if the vaccine were more widely used.

If you have children in your care or are expecting a baby, it's worth asking your doctor about the vaccine. If you fall into any of the risk groups listed here, you should also take steps to protect your health. (Travelers can call the the Centers for Disease Control and Prevention in Atlanta for information about vaccinations before going abroad.)

Be observant. Don't have sexual contact with anyone who has genital or anal sores, a visible rash, a discharge, or any other sign of venereal disease. But being observant is not a substitute for knowing your partner.

Be informed. Recognize the symptoms of STDs and seek medical treatment at once if you notice them in yourself. A lesion, blister, sore, discharge, or rash in the genital or anal area should be a signal to seek medical help. If you're at risk for STDs, persistent unexplained flu-like symptoms and abdominal pain are other signals to see your doctor.

Be responsible. If you think you may have been exposed to a sexually transmitted disease, don't have sex again until you've seen a doctor and been diagnosed and, if necessary, treated. If you are infected, inform your partner or partners and advise them to seek medical help. Remember, no STD confers immunity: you can be reinfected with the same disease. Refrain from all sexual activity (even if you have no symptoms) until your doctor tells you you're cured—and until your partner has sought treatment and been given the same assurance. (See the chart on the previous page for advice about herpes and genital warts, which are not curable.)

Remember that syphilis and hepatitis B, like HIV (the virus that causes AIDS), can be transmitted by contaminated needles. Make sure such instruments used in tattooing, acupuncture, even ear piercing are sterile (or, better yet, disposable). And, of course, intravenous drug users should never share needles.

Inform others. If you have adolescent children, make sure they understand what sexually transmitted diseases are and how they can be transmitted and prevented. If they are not sexually active now, don't assume they'll remain inactive. Sex education classes in school can help, but don't rely on them exclusively. There's no substitute for parent–child discussions about sexuality.

It bears repeating that STDS are transmitted by sexual contact, primarily, and by contaminated needles (with regard to hepatitis B, syphilis, and HIV). Two possible exceptions: a person with fever blisters (caused by the herpes virus) can spread the disease by kissing alone, and a carrier of hepatitis B can spread the virus by everyday contact.

AIDS

Acquired Immune Deficiency Syndrome—AIDS—is the clinical name of a disease recognized as a worldwide epidemic. It is also one of the most dangerous health problems of modern times. AIDS is caused by a bloodborne virus that attacks and eventually destroys the body's immune system. It is a sexually transmitted disease, and although the virus is most likely to pass from one person to another during anal intercourse, it can also be transmitted during vaginal intercourse and possibly—though so far not definitively—during oral sex. AIDS can also be spread via contaminated hypodermic needles and syringes, and—if donated blood is contaminated—blood transfusions. In addition, an infected mother can pass the virus to her child in utero or during delivery.

In Africa and Asia, AIDS is primarily a heterosexual disease. In the United States it has been confined primarily to certain well-defined risk groups—male homosexuals, intravenous drug users, and hemophiliacs (because they need frequent transfusions). AIDS can be transmitted between heterosexuals by vaginal intercourse, but the rate of infection by this route seems to be low—although it increases with frequency of intercourse and especially with multiple partners.

Once AIDS develops it is fatal. So far there is no cure, and no vaccine to prevent the disease. New vaccines are in various phases of testing, but making a successful vaccine has proven to be a far more difficult effort than researchers had imagined.

What we know so far

Not all the news about AIDS is bleak. In 1983, only three years after the disease was first fully described, scientists discovered its cause. The virus, known originally as HTLV III and now simply as HIV (Human Immunodeficiency Virus), is an infectious agent known as a retrovirus, which has the ability to take over certain cells and interrupt their normal genetic functioning. While none of this may sound particularly hopeful, what is amazing is how much scientists already know about the virus. None of the deadly infectious diseases of modern times has so quickly met scientific understanding. The AIDS virus can already be cultured in a laboratory; scientists have devised reliable tests to detect its presence in blood samples.

Secondly, we know that the disease is hard to catch. The virus is not transmitted through air or water. Nor does it travel easily from person to person, as other infections may. Until a vaccine can be developed, halting the spread of AIDS must depend solely on educating those at risk—all sexually active people, particularly those who have not lived in strict, long-term monogamy. Though education may not be the ultimate weapon, it is an effective and powerful means of controlling the spread of the disease.

Indeed, thanks to education efforts, the rate of new HIV infection in the gay community in the United States has declined. And thanks to several new drugs and improved ways of managing HIV infection, there is hope of slowing the course of the disease, improving the quality of life for people with AIDS, and enabling them to live longer.

Yet by all accounts, the worst is yet to come. Although the rate of infection in the United States is no longer accelerating, both the number of new infections with HIV and the number of full-blown cases of AIDS are expected to continue rising sharply at least into the mid-1990s. As of 1994, at least one million Americans were infected with HIV; more than 175,000 Americans have already died of AIDS. By the turn of the century, there will be at least 80,000 children orphaned by AIDS in the United States, many of whom will themselves be infected.

Most alarming, the worldwide epidemic is spinning out of control. Since the epidemic took hold in the early 1980s, about 16 million adults and one million children have been infected with HIV, according to the World Health Organization, and more than two million cases of AIDS have been reported—though the actual number of AIDS cases is very likely much higher. If AIDS advances at its present rate, the organization estimates that 30 to 40 million people will be infected with HIV by the year 2000. Other estimates put the number of cases at over 100 million.

These predictions need not come true, since some of those people are not yet infected, and education could save many of their lives. In addition, new therapies such as the drug AZT and other AIDS antiviral drugs could positively affect the survival rate. Unfortunately, though, misconceptions about AIDS continue to persist, despite the wide coverage of the disease in the mass media. What follows are some of the leading myths about AIDS and the facts established at present.

Myth: AIDS can be transmitted by casual contact with an infected person—a handshake, a cough, or sharing bathrooms, toilets, and bathing facilities.

Fact: The AIDS virus has never been transmitted via food and drink, and cannot penetrate intact human skin. It can only be spread by sexual intercourse or the exchange of blood or blood products with an infected person, or by an infected mother to her unborn child. There is no known risk of non-sexual infection in daily life. In numerous studies of families caring for AIDS patients here and abroad, not one case of AIDS occurred in a family member who was not the sexual partner of the victim or the newborn child of an infected woman.

The Highest Risks

It's not who you are, *but what you do and with whom you do it,* that puts you at risk for contracting AIDS. The following are known to be high-risk practices:

- Sharing drug needles or syringes.
- Anal sex (with or without a condom) with someone who might carry HIV antibodies. The virus is passed easily during anal sex.
- Unprotected vaginal or oral sex (without a condom) with someone who might carry HIV antibodies. Obviously, the more times you have unprotected sex, the greater your risk. Sex with prostitutes is particularly risky.

In addition, some recipients of blood transfusions between the fall of 1978 (when HIV first appeared in the United States) and May 1985 (when blood donor screening became routine) may have been at risk for infection, particularly if they received the blood in San Francisco or New York City or if they had multiple transfusions. Hemophiliacs, who also receive donated blood products, may also have been at risk during those years. Since 1985 the risk of infection from transfusions has been minimized thanks to rigorous screening of donated blood (see box on page 396).

AIDS Terms

AIDS-related complex (ARC): milder clinical symptoms (such as fever, weight loss, diarrhea, and swollen glands) caused by the AIDS virus. About 25 percent of people with AIDS-related complex will develop full blown AIDS within three years. Also, a substantial number of people have died from ARC without developing AIDS.

ELISA (enzyme-linked immunoabsorbent assay): a simple test for detecting the antibodies that form in the blood in response to an invasion by the AIDS virus. If antibodies are present, the patient is "AIDS positive." The results of ELISA need to be confirmed by the Western blot assay.

Opportunistic infections: once AIDS destroys the body's immune system, certain otherwise controllable infections, such as a specific type of pneumonia, may gain a foothold and eventually cause death.

High-risk sex: any unprotected sexual contact with a person who might be carrying the AIDS virus.

MYTH: AIDS is a disease of male homosexuals and intravenous drug addicts. Other people have nothing to worry about.

FACT: Of the nearly 412,000 reported cases of AIDS in the United States as of mid-1994, the vast majority were homosexual or bisexual men or intravenous drug users; the rest were hemophiliacs and others who had received contaminated blood, or heterosexual sex partners of infected persons. Of the more than 5,000 children under age thirteen diagnosed with AIDS, most were born to AIDS-infected parents, and the rest had hemophilia. *But while the two main risk groups remain for the moment well defined, anybody who has unprotected sex can get AIDS.*

In the United States, male homosexuals still run the highest risk of contracting the disease sexually—a relatively small percentage of newly diagnosed AIDS cases in the United States can be traced to heterosexual transmission. When it is transmitted heterosexually, women appear to be at greater risk than men: the virus is far less likely to pass from woman to man during conventional intercourse than from man to woman. More than 100,000 American women have been infected, and the numbers are rising sharply, especially among poor African Americans and Latinas.

The frequency of sexual contact appears to be more important than the form. Though a single contact can spread AIDS, people who have multiple sexual partners are in considerably more danger than those with fewer partners. Prostitutes, both male and female, are more likely to be infected by AIDS and to transmit it, since in addition to frequent exposure, many use intravenous drugs.

In Africa and Asia, AIDS has been spread primarily by heterosexual transmission: according to a report from the Harvard-based Global AIDS Policy Coalition, 70 percent of HIV cases worldwide are heterosexual. In one study in Africa, 340 heterosexual subjects were tested for HIV antibodies, a sign of infection; all of the subjects had reported frequent sexual contact with prostitutes among whom HIV infection was known to be rampant. Of these men, 11.2 percent (thirty-eight men) tested positive for the antibodies, all of them infected through vaginal intercourse. Significantly, among this group, nearly two out of three had a previous history of genital ulcers, compared with just under one out of five of the 302 who tested negative. This suggests venereal diseases, such as herpes, that cause genital ulceration may predispose to HIV infection. Indeed, a higher rate of AIDS transmission in people with genital ulcers has been confirmed by studies in the United States.

MYTH: AIDS could spread rapidly through the general population.

FACT: Based on a number of studies, the estimated risk of becoming infected with the AIDS virus from a single sexual encounter can be as low as 1 in 5 million. This assumes your sexual partner is not in any known risk group for AIDS (but whose infection status is unknown). If a condom is used, the odds rise to 1 in 50 million—far greater than winning a lottery or being struck by lightning.

At the other end of the spectrum, one sexual encounter with a person infected with HIV poses a risk of infection of 1 in 5,000 if you use a condom, and 1 in 500 if you don't. This margin diminishes sharply as the number of sexual encounters rises: 500 sexual encounters with an infected person would pose a 9 percent risk of infection if condoms are used, and a 66 percent risk without condoms. Therefore, in their efforts to contain the spread of AIDS, health experts emphasize the need to limit the number of sexual partners and to choose them carefully. Unless you and your sex partner are both sure you are not infected, you need to take precautions: use condoms and a spermicide, and avoid high-risk practices such as anal intercourse. Couples who have not been monogamous for at least ten years may wish to consider testing (see page 398).

MYTH: The AIDS virus is something new— probably a product of the lax sexual mores of modern times.

FACT: Our knowledge of the AIDS virus is new, but retroviruses are a part of the natural world and are no more likely to manifest divine wrath than any other infectious agent. As early as 1910 an American scientist isolated and studied a retrovirus that causes cancer in chickens. Dr. Robert C. Gallo, head of the team that discovered the first human retrovirus (the agent responsible for a form of leukemia), theorizes that it may have originated in Africa centuries ago and have been spread around the globe by the slave trade and other commercial ventures in the period after the discovery of America. Nor are sexually transmitted diseases anything new; they have been carried around the world for centuries. Syphilis, once regarded as retribution for sinful habits, can now be completely cured with adequate penicillin. AIDS too may one day be curable with proper treatment.

MYTH: Children with AIDS should be barred from schools to protect other children.

FACT: So far as is known, no case of AIDS has ever been transmitted from one child to another at school. Some parents fear that a bite from an AIDS-infected child might transmit the virus. But the virus only rarely appears in saliva, and even then not in sufficient quantities to cause infection. The Centers for Disease Control in Atlanta has stated that "casual person-to-person contact as would occur among school children appears to pose no risk." Similarly, the non-infected siblings of an infected child will not acquire the virus from him.

MYTH: AIDS can be spread by mosquitoes and bedbugs.

FACT: No case of AIDS has ever been traced to insect bites, and there is every reason to think such transmittal is impossible. AIDS viruses are scarce even in infected blood, and the amount of blood on a mosquito's proboscis is minuscule.

Myth: AIDS is a disease of young people.

Fact: In the United States, adults over fifty account for about 10 percent of all cases. AIDS-related symptoms are less likely to be diagnosed among these older people because doctors may assume that they are not at risk for the disease.

Facts About Blood Transfusions

About four million Americans a year receive transfusions, most of them using donor blood. How likely are they to contract AIDS? It is true that before blood screening was possible, a small number of people receiving donated blood did contract AIDS. But although the risk that makes the headlines is AIDS, and people tend to worry about it most, the chances of acquiring some form of hepatitis from a transfusion have always been greater than the chance of infection by HIV. In any case, today you are running very little risk of any type of infection from a transfusion, according to the Department of Transmissible Diseases of the American Red Cross.

There is no such thing, of course, as an absolutely safe blood supply, but there have been major innovations such as new tests for infectious organisms, as well as improvements in the sensitivity of these and other tests. Donated blood is now subjected to seven different tests for diseases, including syphilis, two kinds of hepatitis, and HIV. Paid blood donations have been outlawed in some states, and the practice has generally been discontinued (except for plasma, which is treated to eliminate viruses). Volunteer donors are carefully screened. Nevertheless, doctors are still trying to keep transfusions to a minimum.

Why, since screening is mandatory for donated blood, does some contaminated blood slip through? Because there is a period—the so-called antibody-negative window—when an infected donor can transmit the HIV virus but hasn't yet developed enough antibodies to be picked up by standard screening tests. A second problem arises from the possibility that the virus may hide in immune-system cells in a small number of people and thus not be detectable.

Recent studies by the Red Cross put the chances of transfusion-related HIV infection at only one case per 225,000 units of blood; but a study of 12,000 heart patients in Baltimore and Houston (as reported in the Annals of Internal Medicine) found the risk to be higher—about one in 60,000 units. The difference, though, is that the Red Cross studies were much larger and included data from low-risk areas of the country. (Risk varies according to infection rates in your part of the country—it's lower outside big cities.) Dr. Kenrad Nelson, who headed the study of heart patients, pointed out that the risk of getting AIDS from a transfusion was "very small and decreasing."

The risk from not getting a transfusion when you need one greatly outweighs the small risk of an infection. Also, if you know you'll need a transfusion, there are alternatives to traditional blood banks (see page 494).

Furthermore, if insect bites could spread AIDS, the whole population would now be randomly infected—children and the elderly, the celibate and the promiscuous—since mosquitoes don't confine their attentions to groups with any particular profiles and practices.

MYTH: In hospitals that treat people with AIDS, staff and other patients alike are in danger of getting the disease.

FACT: For the same reasons that AIDS is not transmitted in a family setting, it is unlikely to be spread in a hospital. AIDS patients are mainly admitted to hospitals because they are suffering from "opportunistic" infections that are life-threatening. As with other infected patients, the hospital staff uses special isolation procedures for blood and tissue samples, as well as for hospital equipment.

Accidental self-puncture with an AIDS-infected needle is a possible danger for health care workers. However, in a survey of 2,500 health care workers who had been carefully tested for AIDS, about 750 of them had experienced accidental spills of bodily fluids of AIDS patients or had been stuck accidentally by contaminated needles; of these, only three workers—all of them stuck by needles—had developed AIDS antibodies.

**MYTH: Everyone who tests "AIDS positive"
currently has the disease.**

FACT: Testing positive (after a confirmatory test) simply means that a person has been exposed to the HIV virus and has developed antibodies to it. No one knows what percentage of antibody-positive people will develop the disease. And because the disease can be so slow to develop, it will be years before scientists have the answer to this question.

**MYTH: Sexual abstinence is the only sure way
to protect yourself against AIDS.**

FACT: If you have had a lifetime sexual partner, and both of you have been monogamous, you are not at risk for AIDS. Any person who has multiple partners, or has a sexual relationship with someone who has multiple partners, may be at risk. Fortunately, condoms provide a nearly foolproof AIDS preventive: the AIDS virus cannot penetrate an intact condom. Unless you are certain that you and your sexual partner have not been exposed to AIDS, the use of condoms must be habitual for any intimate sexual encounter.

Who needs an AIDS test?

Dread of AIDS is universal, and many Americans (with or without good reason) now wonder whether they or someone in their families or among their friends has been infected with the AIDS virus. How can they find out? Should everybody be tested? Or only those in high-risk groups? Or nobody?

The test is fairly simple. A blood sample from the arm is analyzed in a laboratory. What the test detects is not the presence of the AIDS virus—the human immunodeficiency virus, or HIV—but of antibodies that the immune system produces after the virus enters the bloodstream. The first stage of the testing is known as ELISA (enzyme-linked immunoabsorbent assay). Should it prove positive, it is followed by a confirmatory test known as the Western blot assay.

The accuracy of the combined tests is high. In a high-risk population, virtually all people who test positive will truly be infected, but among people at low risk the false positives will outnumber the true positives. Thus for every infected person correctly identified in a low-risk population, an estimated ten noncarriers will test positive. Such testing of low-risk groups creates more problems than it solves. False negatives may occur, too. Indeed, it has been recently discovered that in rare instances carriers of the virus may not start to produce antibodies for years.

Testing positive: benefits and drawbacks

Many people have resisted testing, in large part because all they could do if they tested positive was wait helplessly for symptoms to occur. However, evidence has been accumulating that the antiviral drug zidovudine (commonly known as AZT) and several other similar drugs may delay the progression to AIDS in symptomless individuals infected with the HIV virus. Furthermore, researchers have found that a lower dose of the drug works as well as a high dose, and that neither dose produced significant side effects. (In contrast, many people who don't start taking AZT until they have AIDS symptoms suffer serious side effects, notably anemia.)

The improved prospects that may be afforded by early treatment with AZT (as well as drugs to reduce the risk of the type of pneumonia that eventually strikes most AIDS patients) *offers people who think they may have been infected the best reason yet to be tested for HIV.*

People in high-risk groups would also seem to have much to gain from being tested. One situation is fairly clear: anyone who is at high risk and is contemplating parenthood should certainly consider being tested. The chances of an infected mother transmitting the AIDS virus to a fetus or a newborn run from one in three to one in two; and infected babies almost always develop the disease and die. Besides, pregnancy may accelerate the disease in an infected but still healthy woman. No one infected with HIV should become pregnant or father a child, and thus a test can be of crucial importance.

Why not mandatory screening?

Mandatory programs would very likely drive infected people underground and delay their seeking medical care. Since AIDS is not a disease spread like tuberculosis or measles, quarantine is not likely to be helpful, either. Depriving AIDS-infected people of jobs, medical attention, medical insurance, access to public facilities or to education would not protect the healthy.

Keeping people in lifelong quarantine—even if no civil rights issues were involved—would also divert tax money that could better be spent on scientific research.

It is true those who test positive will often need extensive counseling; some have become chronically depressed or even suicidal. Thus people should undergo testing only where adequate counseling is available. And there are social and financial risks in getting a positive result. According to a report in the *Journal of the American Medical Association,* in a small Midwestern town, one young man tested positive, only to learn that his doctor had notified the local health department, which did not keep the information confidential. The man was then fired from his job, and the loss of his job meant loss of health insurance.

However, in addition to the possible benefits offered by AZT and other drugs that have come on the market, there are two good reasons to be tested. First, if you know you are infected you can avoid passing the virus to others. This means either abstention from sex or limiting sexual activity to safer practices. Second, you can inform your sexual partner or partners and encourage them to protect others. These two reasons should be motivation enough for people at high risk to be tested. Also, a doctor can monitor you, administer drugs, and perhaps offer preventive treatment for some opportunistic diseases.

But a person willing to abstain from sex or practice safer sex in order to protect others can do so without having the AIDS test. Indeed, anyone not in a long-term and strictly monogamous relationship should practice safer sex. For some people, it may be easier psychologically to alter behavior without taking the test. Others may want to know. Some people may refuse to change their practices even if they know they carry HIV, although this is morally (and perhaps legally) unjustifiable.

Negative test—potential risks

If the test result is negative, everyone involved will be relieved, but there are pitfalls here, too. A person who does not wait at least twelve weeks after his last possible exposure to the virus may test negative but develop antibodies later. So to be absolutely certain, some people who test negative feel obliged to repeat the test. A negative test can be damaging, too, if it leads to a sense of invulnerability: the fallacy "I've taken risks and didn't get it, so this proves I'll be okay" could be deadly. Whether the test result is negative or positive, the practical result has to be the same: safer sexual practices.

That's why the so-called "AIDS-free singles' clubs" that have sprung up around the country are so dangerous. To join you have to test negative for AIDS and then promise to refrain from sex with nonmembers. But people who are infected could test negative if they take the test too soon. And testing negative does not guarantee that a person is safe forever.

Getting an AIDS test

If you decide in favor of testing, try to ensure confidentiality, and make certain that counseling will be available. If you live in New York City, Washington, D.C., or San Francisco, you can be tested at a clinic where anonymity is the rule: you will be required to fabricate a name or use a number. In a number of states, you have to give your correct name and show identification, though confidentiality requirements are specified. In others, positive tests are usually reported to the health department. And in a few, contact tracing is mandatory. That is, you will be asked for the names of your past sexual partners, who will then be notified if your test is positive.

To find out where to be tested and to discuss other issues, you can start by calling your doctor, your local or state health department, an AIDS hotline, or the American Social Health Association hotline, which can give you the number of your state's AIDS coordinator. In big cities, you can locate so-called alternate test sites (which provide free or low-cost testing) through your local health department. Do not have your insurance company billed for the test, whatever the result may be. Insurance companies "bank" such information, and you may, in effect, be blacklisted for future life or health insurance. If you are at low risk and test positive, have the test repeated at another lab.

Menstruation

For most women, menstruation creates no medical problems: even the most uncomfortable symptoms are not permanent, nor do they usually indicate any serious underlying condition. Yet this stage of life, as is true of menopause (see page 402) can create physical and emotional problems, and few women escape some form of discomfort or anxiety—in part because patterns of menstruation are as unique as each individual. Here are the problems you are most likely to encounter and the remedies that are most effective.

Dysmenorrhea

The Greek-derived word dysmenorrhea, meaning painful menstrual flow, is a term for what most women call "cramps." Besides pain in the lower abdomen or back, women may also experience nausea, diarrhea, vomiting, and jumpiness. When it occurs, menstrual pain always comes at the beginning of a period and may last up to three days. It chiefly affects women twenty-five and under; for reasons not well understood, dysmenorrhea tends to vanish as women grow older, especially after the birth of a child.

Although it can cause emotional distress, dysmenorrhea is not psychological in origin. The discomfort comes from uterine spasms, which temporarily deprive the muscle of oxygen. These spasms are triggered by prostaglandins, hormonelike substances that the body sometimes releases in excess. The high level of progesterone characteristic of ovulation is what triggers the prostaglandins. Thus cramps are a fairly sure sign that ovulation has taken place.

Remedies. For centuries women have relied on home cures for cramps—hot drinks, massage, stretching exercises, keeping warm. No specific exercise for relieving dysmenorrhea exists, and there is no scientific evidence that any of the old tried-and-true remedies really work. Yet personal experience cannot be discounted; different things work (or don't work) for different people.

Effective, inexpensive medications that suppress prostaglandins are available without prescription. They include aspirin and ibuprofen, the same drugs that are useful for headaches. If you usually have cramps, you may want to begin taking such an anti-prostaglandin the day before you expect a period and to continue for a day or two. (For more information on these pain relievers, see page 519).

Oral contraceptives are another highly effective treatment for cramps, since they prevent ovulation and hence high levels of progesterone and prostaglandin production. They are available only by prescription and must be taken on a regular basis, not just when symptoms appear. Smokers and women over thirty-five have to consider other risks in taking oral contraceptives (see page 384). Nevertheless, when cramps are truly incapacitating, oral contraceptives may be a practical option.

Premenstrual syndrome

Most women can tell when a period is about to start: tension, increased irritability, and breast soreness are common symptoms, as are a small weight gain, headaches, a craving for certain foods, and fatigue. For many women, the tension evaporates in a burst of energy and feeling of well-being just before a period starts. Others find premenstrual symptoms minor nuisances that vanish after a few days. But for some women, the problems remain and may intensify over a two-week period.

Thus from ovulation until the start of a period, some women's emotional tension and physical symptoms may severely disrupt their personal and professional lives. Premenstrual syndrome (PMS) has received a great deal of attention in recent

---

New Advice for 70 Million Women

The U.S. Public Health Service has advised that all women capable of becoming pregnant—about 70 million Americans—consume 0.4 milligrams of folacin daily, from food or supplements, in order to ward off birth defects. Folacin (also called folic acid or folate) is one of the B vitamins, and it is now recognized as a potent factor in preventing neural tube defects—including spina bifida (a crippling defect in which the spinal cord is improperly encased in bone) and anencephaly (which prevents part of the brain from developing).

Studies in the United States and elsewhere offer strong evidence that folacin combats these defects. Government experts think that the number of neural tube defects—which now number about 2,500 a year—could be cut in half. Other research has shown that folacin may also be a significant factor in protecting women against cervical cancer.

Since neural tube defects, when they do occur, happen in the first two weeks of pregnancy—long before most women know conception has taken place—women shouldn't wait until they become pregnant to begin consuming high levels of folacin. In fact, they need to start building folacin stores at least twenty-eight days before becoming pregnant.

Folacin is plentifully supplied by leafy green vegetables, broccoli, dried beans, whole grains, citrus fruit and juices, peanuts, and wheat germ. If your diet is rich in these foods, you should be getting enough folacin; most other foods contain modest amounts of folacin. If you aren't sure your intake is sufficient, consider taking a supplement. But remember that, as with many other nutrients, excess amounts of folacin offer no advantage—and consuming more than 0.8 milligrams is not advised. (High folacin intakes may make it impossible to diagnose vitamin B_{12} deficiency, which can lead to anemia and damage the nervous system.

Important note: A woman who has already given birth to a child with neural tube defects should consult her doctor about folacin supplementation before planning another pregnancy.

Having Babies at Any Age

One of the big news items of the last decade was that increasing numbers of women were postponing childbearing until their thirties, sometimes until their forties. And what was instantly dubbed "retirement pregnancies" made headlines worldwide: a fifty-nine-year-old British woman gave birth to twins, and an Italian woman in her sixties was reported to be pregnant. These, of course, were in vitro fertilizations; that is, a fertilized ovum or embryo had been implanted in these women, a technique previously used to treat infertility chiefly in premenopausal women. Does this mean postmenopausal pregnancies will become commonplace? Perhaps. But the procedure is very expensive and not always successful. "How old is too old?" is a highly controversial issue, since it's only applied to women.

The birth rate among older women is on the rise. In 1991, about 10,000 first babies were born to American women aged forty to forty-four. By the year 2000, it's estimated that one baby in twelve will be born to a woman thirty-five or older.

Some studies have shown that as women grow older, they run a greater risk of miscarriage, premature birth, birth defects, having a low-birth-weight baby, and of having complications. Yet other research suggests that the risks of delaying pregnancy until late in the reproductive years (after thirty-five) are not related to age at all but to pre-existing disorders such as high blood pressure or diabetes that may worsen with age. A 1987 study in the *American Journal of Epidemiology,* however, was solidly reassuring, finding no evidence of increased risk of low birth weight or of premature delivery in women having their first pregnancy after age thirty compared with younger women. Complications did increase, but with good management, both mother and baby were healthy.

Still, recent studies continue to show that women older than thirty-five are at higher risk for miscarriage and birth defects, as well as for Caesarean delivery—although the latter may reflect physician/patient anxiety rather than an absolute need for Caesareans. In addition, fertility in women declines with the years. None of this means, however, that it's inadvisable to have a baby when you're over thirty-five or even in your forties. A woman attempting a first pregnancy at thirty-five or older should take the following precautions:

- If pregnancy does not occur readily, seek professional advice early. If either partner needs treatment for infertility, the sooner it is begun the better.
- All women should avoid cigarette smoking and caffeine and alcohol consumption just before and during pregnancy; these increase risk of miscarriage and other complications.
- All women who may become pregnant should increase their intake of folicin, a B vitamin that is known to prevent certain birth defects (see previous page).
- Women over thirty-five should consider amniocentesis to determine whether there are genetic abnormalities in the fetus. Genetic counseling for couples is a good idea.
- Try to embark on pregnancy before the age of forty, since fertility declines quickly after that, and the chances of genetic abnormalities in the fetus increase. Nevertheless, women in their early forties can still conceive and bear healthy babies.

years: courts in France and England have accepted it as a mitigating factor in criminal cases, and some people even cite it as evidence that women ought not to hold high political office. Yet doctors have never agreed on what it is, what causes it, how many women suffer from it, or how to treat it. One difficulty in diagnosing PMS is that some of the more disturbing emotional symptoms (irritability, depression, binge eating, and wide emotional swings) may in some cases not be tied to the menstrual cycle at all.

Remedies. Treatment with diuretics and the same anti-prostaglandin drugs that are known to relieve dysmenorrhea have helped some women but not others. Women may also find it helpful to keep a daily diary of their cycles, noting what the symptoms are and exactly when they occur and disappear. If these symptoms do not fall within the two weeks preceding a period, they are probably not connected with menstruation. Women who tend to have swelling in the hands, ankles, and abdomen can predict this by means of their diary.

Myth: Douching is part of good feminine hygiene.

Fact: *Vaginal tissue is self-cleaning. Douching is not necessary after a menstrual period or after intercourse, and—another myth—postcoital douching should never be relied on as a contraceptive. Indeed, if you use a spermicidal foam, a douche can wash it away. Some vaginal discharge is normal, and odors, if any, probably originate from the external genitals; both can be taken care of with soap and water. If an unusual odor, a discharge, itching, or other discomfort leads you to suspect an infection, you should see your doctor.*

At least one major study has linked douching to ectopic (tubal) pregnancy, a potentially life-threatening condition. Moreover, some douches contain chemicals that may seriously endanger the health of a fetus if absorbed. Thus, pregnant or potentially pregnant women should not douche.

Since salt intensifies the tendency to retain water, you can head off this symptom by going on a reduced-sodium diet. Increasing water intake will help as well, since water is a diuretic.

As with dysmenorrhea, no specific exercise will relieve PMS. Nevertheless, in at least one study, a small group of women with PMS had fewer symptoms after they began a weekly running program. They averaged only forty-one miles per menstrual cycle (about $1\frac{1}{2}$ miles a day), but the subjects reported improvement in a wide range of problems from breast soreness to irritability. As investigators pointed out, the therapy had beneficial effects, although more research is needed to prove why.

Menopause

Menopause signals the end of a woman's fertility, but not necessarily the end of her sexuality. Indeed, some women, freed of worries about birth control, pregnancy, and the bother of having a monthly period, report that their sex lives are better than ever. And not all women need or want hormone therapy at menopause. But every woman needs to know about it to make her own decision.

More than 40 million American women are over fifty now—that's greater than one third of the female population—and their numbers will increase dramatically during the next decade. Yet menopause, the issue that affects every one of them, is poorly understood even by scientists and, until lately, was seldom discussed.

What is menopause?

It's a gradual biological process (except as a result of surgery), culminating in the cessation of ovulation and menstruation. In a three- to five-year period, known as the perimenopause, preceding a woman's final menstrual period, her ovaries begin to produce less and less estrogen and progesterone, the two major female hormones. (Two other hormones, known as follicle-stimulating hormone and luteinizing hormone, which are produced by the hypothalamus and regulated by the pituitary gland, act with estrogen and progesterone to orchestrate ovulation, menstruation, and, if fertilization occurs, pregnancy.) During the perimenopause, menstrual periods may become irregular, unusually light, or unusually heavy. Ovulation (the monthly release of an egg) declines and stops.

This culminates in the cessation of menstruation, usually about age fifty. Estrogen production does not completely stop: the ovaries still produce a little, as do fat cells and the adrenal glands. Menopause is complete when a woman has been without a period for a year. Women who have hysterectomies (the surgical removal of the uterus) also experience an abrupt cessation of menstruation, but their ovaries continue to produce hormones and the actual menopause will occur naturally later. However, if their ovaries have also been removed, they experience an abrupt menopause, sometimes with more severe symptoms than a natural one, and earlier onset of at least some aspects of menopause—bone loss, for example.

Estrogen and progesterone play many roles in a woman's body, affecting many tissues including the breasts, skin, vagina, bones, blood vessels, and digestive system, in addition to the reproductive process and organs. When production of these important hormones declines, many changes are to be expected, both short- and

When does menopause occur?

About half of all women stop menstruating by age forty-eight; by age fifty-two, 85 percent will have reached menopause. There's no evidence that median age at menopause has increased for American women, though age at menarche (onset of menstruation) has declined. Women who have never had children also tend to reach menopause earlier. If a woman ceases to menstruate before age forty, it's not considered true menopause, but "premature ovarian failure," though the results are the same. Ethnicity, marital status, genetics, and geography don't seem to influence menopause. Smokers, however, experience menopause, on average, two years earlier than nonsmokers, though no one understands why.

long-term. It's important to remember, though, that some women have none of these symptoms, some have mild and largely tolerable symptoms, and some find them so severe as to require medical advice.

Symptoms of menopause

Hot flashes, or hot flushes. About 60 percent of American women experience these sudden feelings of intense heat, accompanied by sweating and a flushed face, and followed by a clammy feeling. Sometimes an "aura" precedes the flash—you know you're going to have one. Heart rate increases, your body temperature fluctuates. All this is caused by a shortage of estrogen, which is somehow involved in regulating body temperature, but the hot flash is as yet poorly understood. By day, the hot flash can be embarrassing and disconcerting, and can result in sweat-soaked clothing. By night, hot flashes or "night sweats" disrupt sleep. A woman may awaken several times in sweat-soaked sheets and feel exhausted the next day.

If hot flashes are disrupting your life, you should certainly see a doctor. Hormone replacement therapy, or HRT (see page 404), can put a stop to hot flashes and night sweats. The following self-care measures may also prove helpful.

• Dress in layers, with a porous fabric like cotton next to your skin. Avoid woolens. If a flash starts, take off your top layer. Try drinking a glass of cold water or juice if a flash is starting. At night, keep a thermos of cold water handy.

• Sleep on cotton sheets, and keep your bedroom cool.

• Avoid alcoholic beverages, highly spiced foods, or anything else that seems to provoke hot flashes.

• When you have a hot flash in public, try to remain calm and retain your sense of humor. You are probably less conspicuous than you think. Men, too, can get hot and begin sweating in social or workplace situations and will have to take their jackets off.

• Remember, this won't last forever. Hot flashes are worse right at the early part of menopause. They usually subside and then go away entirely within three to five years.

Mood swings, irritability. It's a myth that the menopausal woman is raging, depressed, and unpredictable—though for many years doctors have believed that menopause caused depression and even psychosis. Recent studies, however, have shown that a majority of women greet the cessation of menstruation with relief. Their children may be grown or nearly grown, and midlife for many women is a time to refocus their energies and begin anew. For women who are in good health, menopause is rarely a major crisis.

Some women do feel angry and depressed, of course, and do experience mood swings. Those suffering from night sweats and other troublesome symptoms may be irritable from lack of sleep. At midlife, too, women may be coping with professional and marital problems, may be dealing with adolescents, and may be assuming responsibility for the care of grandchildren or older relatives. All this might contribute to depression, but the influence of hormone deficiencies on emotions is a matter of debate. Studies suggest that women with young children are more likely to be depressed than menopausal women.

According to a review of findings in a recent government report to the U.S. Congress on menopause from the Office of Technology Assessment (OTA), "understanding of the relationships among aging, the menopause, and behavioral change

Take precautions

Though rare, pregnancy can occur during perimenopause, when a woman still occasionally ovulates. Women should continue using some form of contraception until menopause is complete (one year after the final period). They should remember, too, that if they have new sexual partners, menopause is no protection against STDs. Older women as well as men are just as susceptible to STDs as the young.

is incomplete. Many studies have relied on small samples of self-selected women seeking treatment for symptoms. As a result, the actual prevalence of minor psychological symptoms directly related to lowered levels of ovarian estrogen remains speculative at best."

Vaginal dryness. As women grow older, vaginal walls become thinner and more vulnerable to injury. Another common consequence of menopause is a decline in vaginal lubrication, which may lead to pain during sexual intercourse. This, not the decline in estrogen, is probably the chief reason for reduced sexual desire in menopause. Vaginal dryness can be corrected with HRT, or (if that is the only menopausal symptom), with vaginal creams containing estrogen, or with plain water-soluble lubricants. When intercourse becomes pleasurable again, women will resume sexual activity. Many women, relieved to be freed from birth control and worries about pregnancy, report an increase in sexual pleasure in their fifties. However, more research needs to be done on female sexuality after menopause.

The two most important long-term consequences of menopause are the thinning of bone mass known as osteoporosis, and the increased risk of heart disease. The risk for both can be reduced with HRT (see below), as well as by other preventive measures (see pages 18 and 428).

Alternative treatments for menopausal symptoms

Medical science knows little or nothing about nondrug or dietary remedies for hot flashes, vaginal dryness, and other menopausal symptoms. Because tofu contains a form of plant estrogen, it's often vigorously promoted to women as a cure for hot flashes. Vitamins (particularly vitamin E) and minerals, garlic, herbal remedies (chamomile, hops, catnip, and passion flower), and special diets and exercise programs also have their advocates.

There's nothing to back up these products besides the claims of their promoters. Ginseng, for instance, like tofu, is a source of plant estrogen and is a popular menopausal remedy. (It comes in capsules, teas, powders, and syrups.) Yet no studies have ever been done to test ginseng against menopausal symptoms. And since herbs and herbal remedies are not regulated by the Food and Drug Administration (FDA), it's hard to be sure whether a given product contains a lot of ginseng or none at all. So even if ginseng were helpful, there may not be enough of it in the ginseng tea you buy to have any beneficial effects.

There's no harm in trying home remedies. Though not known to counter menopausal symptoms, vitamins from foods and from supplements—such as vitamin C, vitamin E, and beta carotene (the plant form of vitamin A)—may be beneficial for other reasons. Tofu may or may not have medicinal properties, but it's good food. A healthy diet is advantageous for a woman at any time of life. Being sedentary is not good for anybody, and while there's no proof that exercise can prevent hot flashes, there's plenty of proof that regular aerobic exercise (such as brisk walking) will increase a woman's sense of well-being, help her control her weight, and delay or prevent bone loss and coronary artery disease.

Hormone replacement therapy

Estrogen and progesterone play a role not only in ovulation, menstruation, and pregnancy but in many other tissues and functions of a woman's body: bone-building, blood cholesterol levels, the breasts, skin, and hair. It's been known for many years that estrogen replacement therapy (ERT, meaning estrogen without any progesterone added) after menopause can help keep bones strong as well as alleviate other menopausal symptoms such as hot flashes. Recently, too, it's been shown to lower the risk of heart disease.

But some concerns cannot be brushed aside. Over the years, ERT has been shown to increase the risk of cancers of the endometrium (uterine lining). ERT may also increase the risk of breast cancer, though perhaps only when therapy is long-term (ten years or more). Another suspected risk of unopposed estrogen is gallbladder disease and gallstone formation.

For these reasons, ERT has been largely superseded by hormone replacement therapy, or HRT, consisting of low-dose estrogen and progestin (a synthetic form of progesterone). HRT is just as effective against hot flashes and other post-menopausal symptoms and is less likely to cause endometrial cancer (the added progesterone has been shown to reduce the risk of uterine or endometrial cancer). Women who have had hysterectomies, however, still take ERT, since they are not at risk for endometrial cancer.

The problem is that the long-term effects of HRT are not as well understood as those of ERT. Some evidence is accumulating, but no one yet knows how HRT will affect the risk of breast cancer. Nor has it been shown that HRT protects against heart disease as effectively as ERT.

Benefits vs. disadvantages of HRT

While it may have many benefits, HRT does have its downside. It may cause monthly bleeding or spotting, and some women experience other menstrual symptoms along with the bleeding (breast tenderness, bloating, irritability). For a woman enjoying the freedom of life without menstruation, this can be discouraging. According to the report to Congress from the OTA, studies of women who take HRT indicated that they gave high priority to the short-term impact of HRT, such as reducing hot flashes, but were less concerned with reducing long-term risks such as heart disease and osteoporosis. That is, their choices suggest that they value immediate quality of life over quantity of life, or long-term concerns. Yet it is certainly worth thinking ahead to the diseases that affect many women in later years—osteoporosis and heart disease.

Only you, *in consultation with your physician,* can decide whether HRT is for you. Menopause is not a medical condition automatically requiring drugs. Some women do very well without HRT. Nevertheless, all women should be informed about the following aspect of HRT:

•HRT can alleviate hot flashes, moodiness, and night sweats, as well as sleep disturbances caused by lack of estrogen. It will also help relieve vaginal dryness. Women who have been experiencing painful intercourse because of lack of vaginal lubrication may find that their sex lives improve. There's no evidence, though, that any kind of hormone therapy will alleviate depression or contribute to a sense of well-being. Nor can it keep a woman looking young for life.

•HRT can unquestionably slow bone loss and prevent fractures just as well as ERT. However, even ERT will not prevent bone loss forever. A study of women age sixty-eight to ninety-six who were taking ERT, published in the *New England Journal of Medicine,* showed that while estrogen had beneficial effects on bones right after menopause, it had little impact on women older than seventy-five, who have the highest risk of fracture. Still, if you are at risk for osteoporosis, HRT is definitely worth considering as you approach menopause.

•Estrogen appears to protect premenopausal women from coronary artery disease (CAD) and heart attack, but no one is sure how it works. What is known is that when estrogen production declines at menopause, a woman's blood cholesterol may rise. However, this is by no means uniform or universal, and other factors are also clearly at work.

ERT does have a positive effect on blood cholesterol, and some experts think it may also lower blood pressure. A widely publicized 1993 study from the *New England Journal of Medicine* found that low-dose estrogen raises high-density lipoprotein, or HDL—the good element of cholesterol, and lowers low-density lipoprotein, or LDL—the bad element; thus protecting against arterial disease. Estrogen therapy, therefore, might be appropriate for postmenopausal women with elevated cholesterol levels.

There is good evidence that estrogen taken orally after menopause reduces the risk of cardiovascular disease by 40 to 50 percent. And a large study from the National Heart, Lung, and Blood Institute found that estrogen therapy reduces the risk of stroke. (Oral contraceptives containing a form of estrogen actually increase heart attack risk very slightly, but this is significant only for smokers or women who already have some form of cardiovascular disease.)

Many studies have explored these issues. A large-scale ten-year study (also from the *New England Journal of Medicine*) of almost 50,000 nurses who had taken estrogen since the onset of menopause showed that they had reduced their risk of heart disease by half. Their risk for stroke was not affected. Some experts hailed the study, declaring that the benefits of taking estrogen had now been conclusively shown to outweigh the risks. But not everybody is convinced. There could be confounding factors: women who take estrogen tend to be health-conscious women with access to medical care, and they are at lower risk for heart disease anyway.

HRT, although safer in other respects, may not have the same protective effect against heart disease that estrogen alone appears to have. Progestin may diminish the good effects of estrogen on blood cholesterol. The only way to find out is by clinical study—and while some work is underway, much remains to be done.

Sex and Aging

We live in a culture that until quite recently has disapproved of sexuality in people past their reproductive years, viewed it as distasteful, or preferred to think it nonexistent. And yet experts in the field indicate that, in the absence of disease, sexual expression may endure throughout life. At Duke University ongoing research into sexual activity among the aging found that 80 percent of men in their late sixties continue to be interested in sex. At the age of seventy-eight or older, one in four men continues to be sexually active.

Researchers have found that women, too, retain their sexual abilities and interests throughout life. Decreased sexual activity in older women quite often arises from the lack of a partner rather than a lack of interest. While the *intensity* of sexual interest may generally decline with age, individuals may continue to be sexually active at age sixty, seventy, and beyond.

Myth: If you're over sixty-five, you only need a mammogram every few years.

Fact: All experts say that an annual mammogram for women over fifty saves lives. And the older you are, the higher your risk. Yet older women, according to the National Cancer Institute, are less likely to follow the guidelines than younger ones. The latest data show that fewer than 40 percent of women over fifty get both an annual mammogram and a breast exam. See page 501 for recommendations and guidelines on getting a mammogram.

Whether sexual expression is heterosexual or homosexual, a person with a happy sex life in youth and middle age is more likely to maintain it in old age. This does not mean, however, that sexuality cannot be developed later in life. The physiological and biological changes of midlife may change the nature and possibly the frequency of sexual activity. Some of these changes may be decidedly for the better: a postmenopausal woman no longer has to worry about contraceptives, menstrual periods, and the possibility of pregnancy. After children leave home, couples may have more privacy and more time for sex. In middle age and after, people can be interested in the quality rather than the quantity of sex. Nevertheless, sexual capabilities do alter with time, and remaining sexually satisfied is largely a matter of knowing what changes to expect as you age, and how to adjust.

What to expect as you get older

Postmenopausal women may find intercourse painful at times due to a decrease in vaginal lubrication. The vaginal wall thins and may be less elastic. As discussed on page 404, a lubricating jelly or cream—or hormones prescribed by your doctor—may be helpful in correcting diminished vaginal lubrication.

Older men may find that they feel less sexual urgency, that erections are sometimes delayed or partial, and that the moment of ejaculation is less well defined. This is neither a reflection of decreased sexuality, nor a symptom of impending impotence. Rather, it is the result of physiological changes: your body secretes less testosterone (the hormone that regulates sexual performance and desire) and conducts nerve impulses more slowly. In addition, the arteries in the penis are less able to maintain the blood pressure necessary for a full erection.

These changes needn't be alarming; indeed, they can be turned to advantage since they can allow a man to prolong foreplay, sustain intercourse longer, and delay orgasm until the moment when both partners will be most satisfied. Many people find that more leisurely lovemaking is a bonus. A woman of any age requires on average thirteen minutes of arousal and direct stimulation before climaxing, but only three minutes may elapse between arousal and orgasm in a young man. Aging lengthens this time between your sexual arousal and climax, bringing it closer to your partner's timetable.

Problems that are sexual

Nearly everyone experiences a diminished sexual response from time to time, due to such routine difficulties as fatigue, stress, or acute illness. For some people, however, this becomes a chronic problem.

Impotence. Whether occasional or frequent, impotence—the inability to achieve and maintain an erection—is not the inevitable result of aging, but the reported rate of impotence does increase with age. More than ten million American men are chronically impotent. By the age of fifty-five, 18 percent of men report the problem; by age sixty-five, that figure increases to 30 percent; and by the age of seventy-five, 55 percent of men report suffering from impotence.

Up until just a decade ago, more than 90 percent of all cases of impotence were blamed simply on emotional causes. During the past ten years, however, doctors have come to believe that at least half, and perhaps as many as three quarters, of all cases have a physiological basis as well. Medical problems such as diabetes, Parkinson's disease, liver or kidney disease, and lower back problems have been linked to

Counteracting impotence

• Avoid drinking too much alcohol. Impotence among men in their late forties and early fifties is associated more often with excessive alcohol consumption than with any other single factor.

• Maintain an active and regular sex life. In one study of men over sixty, those who engaged in more frequent sex had significantly greater blood levels of testosterone.

• Not every sexual experience has to end with orgasm. Thinking that you must achieve a climax can make you anxious, which can result in impotence. Instead, you and your partner can agree to focus on caressing and kissing rather than having an orgasm. This may relieve performance anxiety.

• Though zinc supplements have been reputed to cure impotence, there is no evidence to support this claim. While a zinc deficiency can cause a drop in testosterone levels, this doesn't mean that taking zinc will boost testosterone above normal levels.

impotence. Other causes are medications, including prescription drugs (especially those for hypertension) and some antihistamines and decongestants, which may cause temporary impotence; and lifestyle habits such as excessive alcohol consumption, drug abuse, and smoking. When a medication or habit is the cause, the remedy is fairly straightforward. Most cases of impotence, however, have a psychological component—anxiety, depression, or marital problems are common causes—and about 80 percent of these cases can be overcome with psychotherapy.

When a man who experiences impotence awakes at night or in the morning with a full, firm erection, the cause of the impotence is most likely psychological. But for any case of chronic impotence, a doctor should first be consulted to rule out any physiological causes. If the doctor suspects a physiological cause, he can perform tests to see if blood flow into the penis is adequate and check whether spinal cord problems might be involved. Nearly all forms of impotence can be at least partially corrected by various methods ranging from a special vacuum device that draws blood into the penis to surgically implanted prosthetic devices. And as research on impotence continues, treatments that are equally or even more effective, and less intrusive, may become available.

Sexual dysfunction in women. Frigidity is the label used for a wide range of sexual dysfunctions in women. The term misleadingly implies coldness, and has been inappropriately used to describe women who become sexually excited but are unable to achieve orgasm through intercourse alone. This "failure" is in fact the norm: surveys indicate that an estimated 70 percent of women fall into this category; most women need direct stimulation of the clitoris to have an orgasm. True frigidity, a lifelong inability to become excited, may be the result of sexual repression, anxiety, or guilt, and can often be treated by psychotherapy. As with male impotence, however, frigidity may have organic causes that can be medically treated.

Maintaining sexual satisfaction

None of the changes that you go through as you age need limit your sexuality. However, as people grow older they may find it wise to emphasize other aspects of sexuality (kissing, affectionate behavior, new positions) and to remember that coital performance is not the inevitable, or the only, expression of sexual love. Another point to bear in mind: according to William Masters of the Masters & Johnson Institute in St. Louis, continuing sexual activity as you get older helps to slow sexual changes that are physiological. Indeed, the best predictor of a satisfying sex life in later years is a satisfying sex life in the middle years. Even if you are currently without a sexual partner, experts say that if you stay physically active in general, and take other steps to keep in good health, you should be able to resume a rewarding sex life in the future.

How to find sexual counseling

Since many sexual problems have a psychological basis, psychotherapy is often suggested to help solve them. If you are having sexual problems, turn to your doctor first, since he will be in the best position to assess your physical condition. If counseling is in order, a referral from your doctor is probably the best way to find a properly certified sex therapist, although some family practitioners may have training in sexual therapy.

Muscles and Joints

Nearly everyone has experienced stresses and strains to those parts of the body responsible for movement: the bones and muscles; major joints like the knee and ankle; and the tendons and ligaments—the soft connective tissues that transmit movement among muscles and joints. Though sometimes referred to as sports injuries, these mishaps can occur not only during sports and exercise, but during such everyday activities as brisk walking, climbing stairs, housework, or gardening. The injuries range in severity from minor bouts of muscle soreness to tears or sprains that may take weeks to heal. Fortunately, the likelihood of injury can be reduced through conditioning exercises and by observing certain precautions.

In the following pages you will find an overview of activity-related problems: the steps you can take to protect specific body parts; what to do if you sustain a muscle or joint injury; and how exercise can help you cope with two problems related to aging—arthritis and osteoporosis. This section doesn't discuss the injuries that physicians refer to as "direct trauma," such as broken bones and severe cuts and bruises, which usually require first aid and, often, a doctor's care. Most of the injuries covered here can often be managed without professional help.

Preventing Aches and Pains

From runner's ankle and biker's knee to tennis elbow and swimmer's shoulder, there is hardly a sport or exercise that doesn't have some type of aggravating problem associated with it. Despite the proliferation of names, most injuries associated with exercise or sports activities fall into a few broad categories. An understanding of these basic types may help you avoid injury, minimize the damage when you are hurt, and speed your recovery. Don't let concern about injuries keep you from exercising, though. A number of studies show that the benefits of exercise far exceed the risk of injury.

Muscle soreness

When you exercise, you intentionally use certain muscles to increase their strength and endurance. As your body adapts to these efforts (depending on their intensity), you are likely to experience minor aches, twinges, and soreness. For example, one type of discomfort, called ischemic pain, occurs when muscle tissue doesn't have enough oxygen to continue working. This is the ache you feel when you attempt to perform more sit-ups or lift more weight than you are accustomed to, and it disappears when you stop exerting yourself or when you reduce the intensity of the workout, such as by slowing down or using lighter weights.

After any unaccustomed, strenuous exercise, you may experience a painful stiffness called *delayed-onset muscle soreness* (or DOMS, as it is sometimes referred to by physiologists). This type of discomfort occurs most often to weekend athletes who exercise only occasionally or among frequent exercisers who suddenly increase the intensity of their workouts. Typically, it sets in a day or two after a game or workout and can last a week or more.

Physiologists believe that this soreness may be a symptom of microscopic injury to muscle tissue, but there is no evidence that it leads to long-term damage. Often the injury appears to be brought on by activity that has an "eccentric component"—that is, one requiring your muscles to produce a force while lengthening. Ordinarily, muscles shorten when they contract, as when you lift a weight; this is called a concentric contraction. In contrast, when muscles lengthen, as when you lower a weight, the action is called eccentric. Running downhill, when your legs must extend in stride, and, at the same time, resist gravity, is another example. Most exercise—running, brisk walking, aerobic dance, calisthenics—has an eccentric component to it, during which some muscles are elongating and at the same time producing enough force to slow down a movement.

Prevention. Unfortunately, there is no proven way to prevent delayed-onset muscle soreness. Some people believe that stretching after exercise can help prevent it, but studies have failed to confirm it. (Still you should not forego stretching since it has other benefits.)

What does work to minimize muscle soreness from unusually hard activity, according to research, is to do some mild training beforehand. If you plan a hiking trip, do some exercise with an eccentric component—for example, walk down long flights of stairs every day during the preceding week or two.

Relief. Once your muscles are stiff and sore, resting for five to seven days can ease the discomfort. However, "active" rest may be better: according to recent research, relief from DOMS may be best achieved by repeating the activity that caused the soreness at a much lighter intensity.

If you become very uncomfortable and you want to take a pain reliever, don't use aspirin or ibuprofen. New evidence suggests that aspirin and ibuprofen (for instance, Advil or Motrin), block the production of prostaglandins, which help stimulate muscle repair. Acetaminophen (Tylenol), which has no anti-prostaglandin effect, is probably your best choice for relief. Applying ice can help; so can massage.

Muscle cramps

Though they are harmless and do not involve injury, few things are as painful as common muscle cramps. Cramps, also called spasms, can occur in any muscle at any time, but they most often occur in the calf or foot, and usually while you are lying in bed or playing sports or exercising. Cramps remain something of a mystery, and it's seldom possible to pinpoint why they occur. Still, some general facts about cramps can help prevent or alleviate them.

Nighttime calf cramps usually strike in bed at night as a result of contracting the calf muscles by suddenly pointing your toes or by lying with the feet in that position. (Swimmers, who kick with their toes sharply pointed, can suffer calf spasms similar to nocturnal leg cramps.) If you exercised strenuously earlier in the day, your muscles may tighten while you sleep and thus cramp. Similarly, if you're not used to them, wearing high heels may cause cramps. In general, as you age you may find that you experience leg cramps more frequently. Certain medications, notably diuretics, may also promote cramps.

Athletes' cramps occur during exercise for a number of reasons. The imbalance of

---

Can liniments help?

Liniments and balms are popular, convenient methods for producing a feeling of heat or cold in muscles. But their effect is only superficial—the active ingredients stimulate sensory nerve endings in the skin just enough to produce sensations of heat or cold that may temporarily mask the pain of sore muscles. The massaging action can increase blood flow and help relax muscles. But since the heating action isn't real, it does little or nothing to promote healing. Never put a liniment over a wound or cover it with a heating pad or elastic bandage. Severe burning or blistering can result.

minerals called electrolytes (potassium and sodium) in the blood, which often results from excess sweating and dehydration may cause muscles to cramp. Another common cause is overexertion or muscle fatigue, marked by excessive tightening of the muscles and/or a buildup of lactic acid in them. Poor conditioning may also contribute to cramps.

Prevention. If you seem predisposed to nocturnal calf cramps, don't point your toes while stretching, and try not to sleep with your toes pointed. Sleep on your side, and don't tuck in your blankets and sheets too tightly, since these can bend down your toes.

Stretching your calf muscles can also help (see page 414), as can drinking plenty of water before and during exercise, especially in hot weather. Quinine also appears to reduce the likelihood of cramps, but it must be prescribed by your doctor. (There's not enough quinine in tonic water to have any beneficial effect.)

Relief. Though medication is sometimes used to alleviate calf cramps, your best bet is massage and stretching. To halt the cramp, flex your foot by pointing your toes upward. Lying down and grabbing the toes and ball of your foot and pulling them toward your knee may help. At the same time, massage the muscle gently to relax it fully. Ice packs can reduce blood flow to the muscles and thus relax them. Walking may help, too, particularly if you put your full weight on your heels.

In addition, if you get the cramp during a workout, especially if you are participating in a long athletic event in the heat, drink water. This can help correct any fluid loss from excessive sweating. If a mineral imbalance—too little potassium or sodium, for instance—is contributing to the cramping, a sports drink may help. Don't take salt tablets; these can be counter productive.

Strains and sprains

These are the most common type of acute injury—that is, an injury that usually results from a single, abrupt incident causing sharp pain, often accompanied by swelling. Strains and sprains are especially common among eager weekend athletes who don't know the limitations of their unconditioned muscles and joints.

Strains. Also called "muscle pulls," these occur when muscles or their tendons are stretched to the point their fibers actually start to tear. This can happen when you lift a heavy weight or suddenly overextend a muscle—for instance, when swinging a golf club or stretching to catch a baseball. The most common sites for strains are the hamstring and quadriceps muscles in the thigh and the muscles in the groin and shoulder—all large muscles that are used for sudden powerful movements.

Mild strains are usually only a nuisance; the tears are microscopic and, with rest, repair themselves easily. More severe strains involve a greater degree of fiber destruction and produce not only sharp pain but also loss of power and movement.

Cold, fatigue, or immobilization reduces blood flow and lessens muscle elasticity, increasing the risk of strains. The best way to prevent them is to warm up, then stretch all the muscles involved in your upcoming activity. A full-body warm-up, such as jogging in place or stationary cycling for five to ten minutes, increases blood flow and raises the temperature of large muscle groups. You can also warm up by slowly rehearsing the sport or exercise you're about to perform. A light sweat usually indicates that you've warmed up sufficiently.

Sprains. Whereas strains occur to muscles, sprains damage ligaments (the bands connecting bones) and joint capsules. They are most often the result of a sudden

Myth: You can "run through" pain.

Fact: If you feel pain (beyond mild discomfort), stop exercising and rest.

It may seem that many professional athletes bounce right back after an injury. But they usually have the benefit of care by experts who diagnose and treat their injuries quickly. Moreover, they are usually in better condition than the rest of us and are highly motivated to recover.

The surest way to speed recovery is to treat any recurring ache or pain right away, even if you're able to continue exercising in spite of them.

force, typically a twisting motion, that the surrounding muscles aren't strong enough to control. As a result, the ligaments, which usually wrap around a joint, get stretched or torn. Like strains, sprains can range from minor tears to complete ruptures. But sprains tend to be more serious than strains: not only do they often take longer to heal, but a torn ligament can throw bones out of alignment, causing damage to surrounding tissues. The acronym RICE is the key to treating a sprain: Rest, Ice, Compression, Elevation (see page 423). A ruptured ligament requires medical attention.

Because of its construction and the fact that it must support your body weight, the ankle is the most frequently sprained joint—in fact, a sprained ankle is probably the most common sports injury. The knee, too, is vulnerable because it must absorb twisting stresses every time the body rotates from the hips. You can protect these joints by strengthening and stretching key muscles (see page 416).

Overuse injuries

Also known as chronic or stress injuries, overuse injuries are brought on gradually as a result of wear-and-tear from a repetitive activity such as cycling, running, or playing tennis. Although a weekend athlete can experience overuse soreness, it is far more of a problem for people who do the same exercise repeatedly and/or often. In one survey of athletes, overuse injuries outnumbered acute injuries in all activities except basketball and skiing. In two of the most popular activities, running and tennis, almost 80 percent of all injuries were of the overuse variety.

Whereas you can almost always pinpoint the incident that caused an acute injury, an overuse injury may have no obvious cause. For instance, you suddenly increase the intensity or duration of your normal workout and feel a dull pain. Over the next few days, the pain recurs intermittently, but isn't bad enough to stop you from exercising. In effect, you have pushed your body beyond its ability to absorb the force of exercise effectively. As a result, muscle tissue has gradually developed microscopic tears that can cause pain, tenderness, and swelling. Initially, an overuse injury may seem less serious than an acute one. But as time passes, you usually feel pain during and after exercise. If you ignore the damage, it can worsen—and you may suffer a strain or other acute injury at the site of the weakened tissue.

Tendinitis. This condition is the problem behind many common overuse injuries. Tendons—the fibrous cords that anchor muscles to bones—are vulnerable, since the force of muscle contractions is transmitted through them. People who exercise regularly are especially at risk because of the strong forces produced by their well-conditioned muscles. These increase tension on the tendons, which can then rub against bones, ligaments, and other tendons, causing irritation. The suffix "itis" means inflammation (characterized by pain, swelling, warmth, and redness).

Tendinitis is deceptive: the pain can be severe when you start exercising, then diminish as you continue—only to return sharply once you've stopped. Perhaps the most common form of tendinitis is tennis elbow (see page 419). In sports and activities that involve running and jumping, tendinitis is most likely to develop in the knee, foot, and the Achilles tendon at the back of the ankle. For cyclists, knees are most vulnerable. Shoulder (rotator cuff) tendinitis can develop from pitching a ball, swinging a golf club, or swimming.

Stretching and strengthening routines can help prevent tendinitis, but equipment and technique may be equally important. For example, an improperly exe-

---

Keys to preventing tendinitis

•Don't overdo it. Drastically increasing the distance you run, for instance, or suddenly working out more strenuously or longer, can produce muscle fatigue and thus lead to an injury.

•Keep muscles flexible.

•Be more careful as you grow older. Starting in your thirties, tendons gradually lose elasticity and become brittle. However, plenty of young athletes injure tendons.

•Develop the right technique. An improperly executed backhand, for example, is often the cause of tennis elbow.

•Compensate for musculoskeletal problems. For instance, if your feet roll inward (overpronate) as you run, you may develop runner's knee. You may need to consult a physical therapist, orthopedist, or other specialist.

•Counter muscle imbalances. If your calf muscles are very strong from running, but you don't strengthen the opposing shin muscles, you increase the chances of injuring your Achilles tendon. Strengthen the key muscle groups for your activity.

cuted backhand is often the cause of tennis elbow, and running shoes with worn-down heels contribute to Achilles tendinitis.

At the first signs of tendinitis—pain and swelling—you should stop your activity. It's usually wise to consult your doctor (who may refer you to a physical therapist), unless it's an injury you've had before and know how to treat. Rest and intermittently ice the area for the first seventy-two hours to reduce inflammation; a compression bandage can help minimize swelling. After that, according to many physical therapists, you should start applying heat—or alternate heat and cold—to increase circulation and speed healing (see page 424). You should also start stretching to restore flexibility, and then gradually add strengthening exercises with light weights to strengthen the tendon and muscle.

Stress fractures. These microscopic breaks in bone, usually in the foot, shin, or thigh are another form of overuse injury. Common among long-distance runners, aerobic dancers, and basketball players, the fractures are caused by the repeated impact of running or jumping. Often the pain is mild at first, occurring during or right after exercising. If you continue to exercise it gradually worsens, but for the first few weeks such fractures are usually too small to be detected, even by X-ray. Fortunately, the fractures rarely break through the bone, so they don't require splints or casts to heal, only rest.

Prevent stress fractures by increasing the intensity of your workouts gradually, not dramatically. Try to minimize impact on your legs: run and jump on soft or resilient surfaces—grass, carpet, mats, or suspended wooden gym floors—rather than concrete. Wear well-cushioned exercise shoes.

Injury Sites

The following pages contain tips and exercises that are aimed primarily at helping prevent injuries to a joint. The exercises can also be used to condition muscles during recovery from an injury. *But if you are recovering from an injury, consult your physician or physical therapist before undertaking any exercises, including those shown here.*

The ankle
In the architecture of the body, the ankles are among the most vulnerable elements. These complex hinges of bone, ligament, tendon, and muscle support your entire body weight and, when you run or jump, may transmit a force of impact equal to three times your weight. Thus ankle injuries, usually the tearing or straining of a ligament called a sprain, are the most common of all joint injuries. Anybody is susceptible to them—from the basketball pro and surfer to the runner navigating an uneven surface and the woman in high heels stepping off a curb.

The great majority (85 percent) of sprains are *inversion* sprains. This happens when the sole of the foot turns inward, injuring the ligaments on the outside of the ankle. *Eversion* injuries occur when the foot turns outward, affecting ligaments on the inner side. Some sprains are minor and can be successfully treated at home, but many do need medical attention, and any sprain can put you at risk for another. This is because when the injury heals, it leaves the tendon weakened, less flexible, and more susceptible to injury.

How do you know if you've sprained your ankle? Your ankle turns and you may

Ruptured tendons

If chronic tendinitis goes unchecked and the weakened tendon continues to be damaged by repetitive activity, there's an increased risk that the tendon will rupture—that is, tear away from the bone or even snap in half. But a rupture can also occur without tendinitis—for instance, if you suddenly put too much force on the tendon, especially from an abnormal direction. Weekend athletes who push their bodies too hard are at greatest risk for such ruptures. If you completely rupture a tendon, such as the Achilles tendon, you may hear a distinctive popping sound. You may feel searing pain—or perhaps little or no pain if the nerves have been damaged.

It's crucial to get medical attention immediately. Many athletes who rupture a tendon eventually play again, but it usually requires surgery and months of rehabilitation.

stumble or fall. You'll have pain, tenderness, and swelling, usually pretty quickly. If you heard a popping sound when your ankle turned, that probably means the sprain is severe. Sprains are graded as *mild* (ligament is strained or stretched), *moderate* (partially torn ligament), and *severe* (a complete tear, meaning that the ligament can no longer control the ankle joint). If you heard a pop, if the ankle looks abnormally bent, or if the swelling is severe and the skin discolored, you should suspect a severe sprain and see a doctor or go to the emergency room. Don't aggravate the sprain by flexing your ankle or putting weight on it.

If you can put weight on the ankle and if swelling and pain are slight, you may not need medical attention right away, or at all. *Icing the injury as soon as you can is essential.* Ice applied for fifteen minutes at intervals of about two hours for twenty-four to forty-eight hours will reduce pain, inflammation, and any bleeding into the ankle joint. (You can apply ice at more frequent intervals if necessary.) Then apply the other steps of RICE. Make sure your foot is elevated slightly higher than your hips. Stay off your feet. Using crutches, even for mild sprains, is advisable in the first few days, as is compression with tape or elastic bandages. Aspirin or ibuprofen will also relieve pain and inflammation. Keep up the treatment for up to seventy-two hours, if necessary.

It takes a mild sprain about ten days to heal and longer for full range of motion to return. Once the swelling has subsided, you can start gentle exercises to rehabilitate the ankle.

But if, after twenty-four hours of self-treatment, you still can't put any weight on the ankle, or are having severe pain or swelling, you should see a doctor to have the injury evaluated. Most sprains, even the most severe, do heal without complications. After rehab, you should be able to resume your full range of activity. But check with your physician first.

Preventing ankle sprains. These tips may help you avoid an ankle sprain:

• Before and after exercising, stretch your calf muscles, as shown below. Tight calf muscles pull on the Achilles tendon, attached to the heel bone, and can cut down the range of motion in your foot, thus sometimes promoting twisted ankles.

Can high-tops help?

For active sports where there is a tendency to roll over on the ankle, most (but not all) evidence shows that wearing snugly laced high-topped shoes is protective. We're not talking about floppy canvas high-tops but the padded, flexible kind worn by basketball players. These stabilize the ankle and protect against inversion injuries. According to the American Orthopaedic Foot and Ankle Society, a study of Israeli army recruits showed that high-top basketball shoes were as effective as army boots in protecting against ankle injuries. A study of basketball players at the University of Washington School of Medicine in Seattle also showed that ankle taping combined with high-tops were good protection.

When shopping for high-top shoes, look for a pair with an ankle collar high enough to support your ankles well.

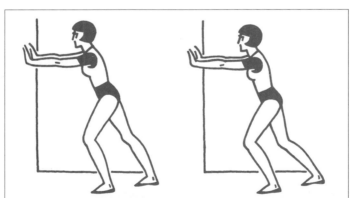

Calf stretches. To stretch the gastrocnemius, stand about two feet from a wall and place your hands against it (left). Extend one leg behind you with the knee straight. Keep your heel on the floor and lean forward until you feel a stretch in the rear leg. To stretch the soleus, assume the same position but keep the back knee slightly bent (right). Hold each stretch for twenty to thirty seconds, then repeat two or three times. Do each stretch in three positions: rear foot pointed straight ahead, pointed in, and pointed out. Keep the front foot flat, and make sure your knee is in line with it.

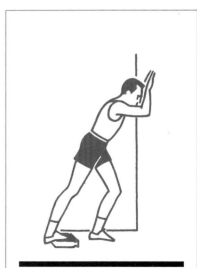

Variation. To further stretch your calf, place the ball of your foot on a book, lean into the wall and slowly lower your heel.

•When you're on your feet, especially if you're walking, wear stable shoes that offer some support. Replace or repair run-down heels and soles.

•Avoid platform soles and high heels, or any shoe that throws the foot off balance. Open shoes and sandals, which are less stable than other footgear, are a poor choice if you're trying to avoid ankle injury.

•Follow a regular exercise program. Sedentary people are more likely to experience a sprain than those with strong muscles.

•Strengthen your ankles. Start with heel raises: stand with your feet comfortably apart. Rise on the balls of your feet as far as possible, hold for a few seconds, then lower. Gradually work up to twenty repetitions. Eventually try this exercise while standing with the balls of your feet on the edge of a step, so that you dip your heels lower than your toes. Alternate these with toe raises: wearing flat shoes with smooth soles, stand on your heels and keep your toes as high off the ground as possible; walk like this, keeping your toes elevated, for three to five minutes. Also try walking on the insides of your feet, then the outsides.

The knee

Your knees are put under a lot of stress, whether you're running, playing basketball, dancing, or simply house cleaning. Just climbing stairs can put pressure on each knee equal to four times your body weight. The result is that an estimated 50 million Americans suffer from knee pain or injuries, or have in the past. At least one out of every four sports injuries involves the knee. In addition, for millions, the knee is affected by chronic, age-associated ailments such as osteoarthritis.

The knee is the largest joint in the body. Functioning simultaneously as a hinge, lever, and shock absorber, the knee is the key to your ability to stand up, walk, climb, and kick. Yet it depends almost entirely on soft tissue—ligaments and tendons—for stability. Because of its complexity and the great forces to which it is routinely subjected, the knee is susceptible to a host of injuries, which can take weeks, if not months, to heal, even with proper rehabilitation. Here are the most common problems:

Sprain (torn ligament). The knee connects the thigh bone (femur) to the shin bone (tibia), and the only things holding these two large bones together are four ligaments, which are strong but not very flexible. If these are stretched beyond a certain point, one or more of these ligaments can be sprained. The sprains can range in severity from minor tears to complete ruptures, in which the ligament tears away from the bone and snaps (often with an ominous popping sound). Most seriously, the anterior cruciate ligament can rupture when you twist the knee in a fall, typically while downhill skiing. Other ligaments in the knee can be injured by a violent blow to the knee or sudden wrenching or twisting, as in hockey or soccer.

Runner's knee (chondromalacia patella). This overuse injury is due to degeneration of the shock-absorbing cartilage (called the meniscus) under the kneecap and covering the ends of the femur and tibia. It is characterized by dull, aching pain under or around the kneecap and is usually most noticeable when descending stairs or hills. Nearly 30 percent of runners eventually develop this disorder. But runners hardly have a monopoly on it—skiers, cyclists, soccer players, and people who participate in high-impact aerobics classes are also prone to it.

Tendinitis. The tendons above or below the kneecap (patella) can become inflamed, usually through overuse—for instance, from dancing, hiking, or cycling.

One frequent complaint is "jumper's knee," a form of tendinitis that afflicts basketball and volleyball players and weight lifters in particular.

Iliotibial band syndrome. If the tendon that runs down the outer side of the knee is tight, repetitive motion (as in running or cycling) can cause the tendon to rub against the bony area at the end of the thigh bone and become irritated.

Torn cartilage. This injury to the cartilage in the knee typically occurs when you twist your knee while putting weight on it. Over the years, frequent squatting can weaken the knee to the point where something as minor as getting out of the car can tear the cartilage.

Arthritis. The knee is a common site for osteoarthritis, which involves the degeneration of cartilage at the joint and subsequent inflammation. It is the result of normal wear and tear over the years. Gentle exercise is a good way to keep arthritis at bay.

You can reduce the likelihood of a knee injury with the following precautions and conditioning exercises:

• Beware of suddenly intensifying or lengthening your workouts. This can create additional friction in the joint and increase the risk of an overuse injury.

• Check your exercise shoes. If they are worn or don't fit well, they may put your knees at risk.

• Check your feet. The knee sometimes pays the price for foot abnormalities (such as flat feet), overpronation (the feet roll inward too much), or poor leg alignment (such as knock-knees), which can put greater stress on the joint. An orthotic device—a custom-made arch support—may help correct some foot or alignment problems. Make sure your knee is always aligned with your foot while exercising.

• When cycling, minimize knee stress by making sure the seat is at the proper height and avoiding high gears. At the bottom of the stroke, your knee should be only slightly bent. If your knee is bent too much, the seat is too short, and you will wobble and lose stroking power. If the knee doesn't bend at all, or if you have to reach for the pedal, the seat is too high, which can stress the knee joint. Cycling in high gear increases the pressure on your knees, so shift to low gears and faster revolutions. You'll get more aerobic exercise with less stress on your knees.

• Strengthen your leg muscles, especially the quadriceps, the large four-part

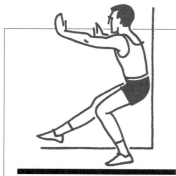

One-quarter knee bends: Holding on to a wall, lift and extend one leg forward and slowly lower yourself by bending the other knee. Don't go more than one-quarter of the way down. Hold for five seconds, then slowly straighten up. Repeat ten times, then switch legs.

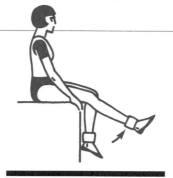

Knee extensions: Sit on a desk or counter and hold onto the edge. Slowly straighten one leg, extending the knee completely. Hold for five seconds, then lower slowly. Repeat ten times, then switch legs. You can also do this with a light weight.

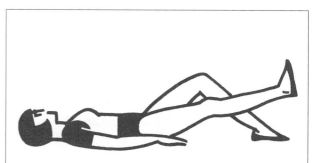

Straight leg lifts: Lie on your back and bend one knee, keeping your foot on the floor. Slowly lift the straight leg about twelve inches off the floor; keep hips and lower back on the floor. Hold for five seconds, then lower slowly. Repeat ten times, then switch legs. You can also do this with a light weight around your ankle. Avoid this exercise if you have back problems.

group on the front of the thigh, which, along with the hamstrings (located behind the thigh), power knee movements (the exercises illustrated on page 416 will get you started). If these muscles are weak and/or tight, extra pressure is put on the knee. Weakness in the quadriceps can contribute to improper tracking of the kneecap and to runner's knee. If you're a runner, your quadriceps are probably much weaker than your hamstrings, so it's a good idea to alternate cycling (an excellent way to strengthen the quadriceps) with running. Walking up stairs or hills also helps strengthen these muscles.

•Stretch your leg muscles before and after exercise.

•If you have knee problems, avoid hills and stairs as much as possible; also don't kneel or do full squats, which can greatly increase stress on the knee. Also avoid "knee-unfriendly" sports such as football, running on concrete, soccer, squash, tennis, and skiing.

The first step in treating most knee injuries is RICE: rest, ice, compress, and elevate. One relatively new rehab technique for controlling a painful kneecap that doesn't track properly in the groove at the end of the femur is called McConnell taping, in which tape is used to pull the cap into the correct position, thus improving muscle balance. A physical therapist will teach you how to tape yourself and perform rehab exercises; eventually you wean yourself off the tape.

The lower leg

The catch-all term "shin splint" refers to a family of overuse injuries causing inflammation of muscles and tendons of the lower leg. Pounding the feet on hard surfaces in aerobic dance class or jogging is a common cause. The pain generally starts during exercise and continues during daily activities, but sometimes begins several hours later. Only a physician can diagnose the exact type of injury and prescribe proper treatment.

Shin splints are referred to as "posterior" or "anterior," depending on the location of the injury. A posterior shin splint is characterized by aching pain on the inner side of the calf due to inflammation of the muscles that roll the foot inward and support the arch. People with flat feet are the likeliest candidates for posterior shin splints. An anterior shin splint causes pain along the outer side of the calf.

To lessen your risk of shin splints:

•Wear well-cushioned running shoes with good support.

•Don't run on hard surfaces.

•Don't suddenly increase the intensity of your workout.

•Stretch calf muscles before running (see page 414).

•Begin a regular routine of stretching and strengthening leg muscles. Do toe raises and foot rolls several times a day; lie on your back and flex your feet; sit on the edge of a table and flex your foot with a weight attached to it.

•Check with a podiatrist to see if you need an orthotic device to improve your posture and gait. If so, wear it in all your shoes.

The shoulder

Unless and until they get a stiff and painful shoulder, most people don't know they have any such thing as a rotator cuff. Golfers, swimmers, tennis players, volleyball players, and baseball pitchers may all have trouble with their rotator cuffs, as may those who install high shelves, work with hand tools, or do anything with a lot of

Don't ignore aches and pains. Studies show that exercising before an injury has healed may not only worsen it, but greatly increases the chance of re-injury. Learn to monitor your body for abnormal sensations, and to apply appropriate treatment as early as possible.

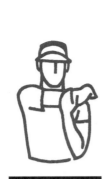

Shoulder stretch: Stretch the back of your shoulder by reaching with one arm under your chin and across the opposite shoulder; gently push the arm back with the other hand. Hold for fifteen seconds. Re-peat five times, then switch sides.

Another stretch: Raise one arm and bend it behind your head to touch the opposite shoulder. Use the other hand to gently pull the elbow downward. Hold for fifteen seconds. Repeat five times, then switch sides.

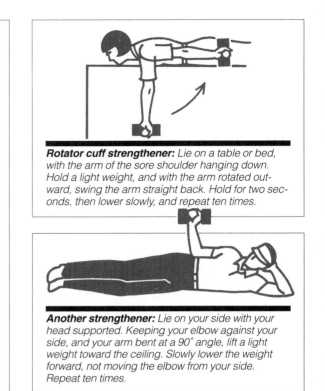

Rotator cuff strengthener: Lie on a table or bed, with the arm of the sore shoulder hanging down. Hold a light weight, and with the arm rotated outward, swing the arm straight back. Hold for two seconds, then lower slowly, and repeat ten times.

Another strengthener: Lie on your side with your head supported. Keeping your elbow against your side, and your arm bent at a 90° angle, lift a light weight toward the ceiling. Slowly lower the weight forward, not moving the elbow from your side. Repeat ten times.

Favoring one sport can cause problems: you are likely to strengthen certain muscles at the expense of others, leaving tendons and ligaments unbalanced and thus vulnerable. Varying your activities is one way to prevent this; another precaution is to strengthen the muscle groups you underuse, and stretch all muscles involved in your workout.

shoulder movement. The rotator cuff is actually four muscles (subscapularis, infraspinatus, supraspinatus, and teres minor) and their tendons; it stabilizes the upper arm in the shoulder socket and allows it its range of motion. Rotator cuff pain may be caused by what's known as an "impingement syndrome." This means that because of exertion or overuse, one or more of the muscles and tendons are impinged upon—that is, compressed and irritated—by the shoulder bone, resulting in inflammation and possibly microscopic or even larger tears. The bursa, small fluid-filled sacs that protect the muscles and tendons from irritation by the bone, are usually inflamed as well.

The first stage of this condition may be tendinitis or bursitis. If you have rotator cuff pain, the important thing is to treat the injury, so that it does not become chronic. A mild case of shoulder tendinitis or bursitis can be treated as follows:

•Rest. If you suspect that a certain activity has caused the pain, stop it for a while.

•Take aspirin, ibuprofen, or naproxen sodium (brand name Aleve). Acetaminophen (such as Tylenol) doesn't counteract inflammation.

•Apply ice during the first day or two. Then try heat.

•Do some gentle exercises, such as those shown above, to restore range of motion and strengthen the rotator cuff.

If you often have pain when raising your arm above your head, or with any activity, it's a good idea to get medical help. Your doctor may send you to a physical therapist or other specialist in body mechanics. Rotator cuff tendinitis usually responds well to moist heat, ultrasound, and gentle exercises, especially stretching. Taking time off from the activity that caused the injury is usually essential. In advanced cases of rotator cuff injury, surgery is sometimes recommended. However, a controlled study of 125 people with severe rotator cuff injuries (age nineteen to sixty-six) found that a supervised exercise program brought about the same significant improvements as surgery. Conducted at University Hospital in Oslo and published in the *British Medical Journal,* the study showed that even in patients whose condition resists treatment, an exercise program is worth trying before any kind of surgery is considered.

For chronic rotator cuff pain, you'll need professional advice in designing an exercise program. The exercises on page 418 will help get you started, but first discuss them with your doctor. Do not continue any exercise that causes pain.

Prevention. If you are a golfer or swimmer, or have other risks for rotator cuff injuries, these same exercises, performed regularly, can help strengthen your rotator cuff muscles and tendons and make them less susceptible to injury.

The elbow

One of the most common stress injuries of the arm is tennis elbow, a type of tendinitis that at some point sidelines about half of all amateurs who play tennis at least three times weekly. Professional players suffer from it, too. And tennis players aren't the only ones at risk—any activity that calls for forceful, repeated contraction of the arm muscles can bring on tennis elbow (the medical term is epicondylitis). Working with carpentry tools, gardening, raking leaves, or even tightly gripping a heavy briefcase are only a few of the activities that can cause tennis elbow. Baseball, golf, bowling, racquet sports, even darts can also bring it on.

The injury occurs when you flex, extend, twist, or contract your wrist or forearm excessively or improperly, and thus strain the tendons that connect muscles to the elbow joint. In time, the overstressed tendons develop microscopic tears, producing tendinitis (painful inflammation of the tendons) centered around the epicondyle, the point at which the tendons attach to the elbow. The pain can radiate down to the wrist and up to the shoulder. Moving your arm or gripping something aggravates the pain.

For most recreational tennis players, the backhand may be the main culprit causing the condition, because during the backhand the muscles that extend the wrist undergo an eccentric contraction—that is, the muscles lengthen during activation. However, the serve or forehand may also promote tennis elbow. The elbow tendons can develop microscopic tears anytime they are exposed to a repeated stress greater than the tissues can withstand. Experts think it's not the vibration that causes the tears but excess torsion—for instance, when the ball hits off center, the racquet twists your arm. Pain on the lateral side of your arm (the side your thumb is on) is ten times more common than pain other (medial) side.

What determines who gets tennis elbow? To some extent it depends on the condition of your muscles and how much they are overused. In tennis, the injury occurs most frequently among recreational players who are thirty-five to fifty years old—when muscles have begun to lose their resiliency—and who play at least two or three times a week. In a study of 2,600 amateurs, almost half of those who played daily got tennis elbow. Occasional players are less vulnerable as they tend not to play often enough or hard enough to overstress their arms. And pros are generally protected by superior conditioning and stroking technique, though they too can develop tennis elbow as they grow older.

Prevention. If you play tennis regularly, here are the keys to avoiding tennis elbow. Beginners should remember that technique and conditioning are far more important than racquet in preventing epicondylitis.

Try a better racquet

•Try a mid-sized racquet, which has a bigger sweet spot and absorbs vibration better than a small one. It plays softer and gives more power, so you don't need to swing as hard. An oversized racquet, in contrast, can increase the risk of the racquet overtwisting if you hit the ball off center.

•Chose a flexible racquet—one that is injection-molded or that contains a high proportion of fiberglass—which will dampen shock well. According to Dr. Howard Brody, professor of physics at the University of Pennsylvania, composite racquets with an increased ratio of nylon matrix, as opposed to epoxy resin, are good shock stoppers.

•An increased grip size can also help. Too small a grip can lead to arm muscle fatigue, from overtightening. But too large a grip may put you at a strength disadvantage.

•Lower your string tension to dampen shock. Higher string tension does give more control, but also increases the shock to your arm after ball impact.

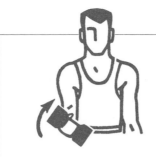 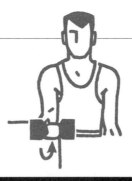 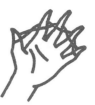

Arm rotation: *Sitting or standing, hold a light weight (two or three pounds) in front of you with your elbow bent at a 90° angle and your palm up. Slowly roll your forearm to palm-down position, then return to the starting position. Repeat twenty to thirty times. Switch arms and repeat.*

Wrist curls: *Lay your forearm on a table with your hand hanging over the edge and your palm up. Holding a five-pound weight, slowly flex your wrist ten to twenty times. Then turn your hand over so the palm faces down and repeat ten to twenty times. Switch arms and repeat.*

Finger strengtheners: *Twist a thick rubber band around all five fingers. Keeping your elbow straight, try to straighten and spread your fingers. Hold for three seconds, then relax your fingers. Repeat until fatigued. Switch hands and repeat.*

Braces may help

In one study of 2,633 tennis players who suffered from tennis elbow, 84 percent claimed an elbow brace improved the condition. The brace recommended by most health professionals is called a counterforce brace. This is different from the elastic braces you may find in sporting-goods stores—elastic doesn't give enough support. The counterforce brace functions as a constraint against muscle contraction and excessive movement of the tendons, thus reducing force and overload on the soft tissues of the elbow.

When a muscle contracts, it tends to expand, and the nonelastic brace controls the expansion and thus reduces the forces developed by the muscle. A counterforce brace, however, won't interfere with your game because it does not prevent motion as does a brace with metal supports (such as a knee brace). You can get a counterforce brace through your physician; some sporting-goods stores also carry them.

•Work on your form. Power your serve and backhand with your legs, torso, and shoulder muscles rather than with your forearm and wrist. During a stroke, your elbow should be almost fully extended but not locked, and your grip should be firm but not viselike, so that force is transferred to your shoulder.

•Some teaching pros recommend that beginners learn a two-handed backhand; players who use this technique seldom develop tennis elbow, since the second hand provides additional support.

•For athlete and nonathlete, the best defense against tennis elbow is to strengthen muscles in the forearm. According to Dr. Robert Nirschl, director of the Virginia Sports Medicine Institute, half the tennis-elbow sufferers he sees have some major strength deficits in the shoulder and upper back. The key therefore is to restore strength, endurance, and flexibility to the arm, shoulder, and back. The forearm exercises above will get you started. (Another forearm strengthener: simply squeeze a ball forty or fifty times with your arm extended horizontally in front of you.) If you're under treatment for tennis elbow, you should consult your doctor before embarking on an exercise program.

If you develop tennis elbow, reduce your playing time or stop completely until the pain lessens. For players persistently troubled by tennis elbow, some sports physiologists recommend the use of an elbow brace, which supports and protects the muscles and tendons of the forearm; this offers some pain relief without restricting movement (see marginal at right).

The wrist: preventing carpal tunnel syndrome

If you put in long hours at a repetitive hand-intensive task—working on an assembly line or in the garment industry, typing or computer keyboarding, or a hobby like knitting or piano playing—you could develop carpal tunnel syndrome (CTS).

In other times this pain in the hand may have been called anything from "writer's cramp" to "washerwoman's thumb." Deriving its name from the Greek karpos, or wrist, the carpal tunnel is the passageway, composed of bone and ligament, through which a major nerve system of the forearm passes into the hand. These nerves control the muscles in this area, as well as the nine tendons that allow your fingers to flex. The wear and tear of repeated movement thickens the lubricating membrane of the tendons, and presses the nerves up against the hard bone. This process, called nerve entrapment, can be caused not only by repetitive strain, but by bone dislocation or fracture, arthritis, diabetes, and fluid retention (as may occur in pregnancy)—anything that narrows the tunnel and compresses the nerve.

CTS usually affects the dominant hand and begins with pain and tingling or numbness. As an occupational injury, it's brought on by repetitive work or movement. Carpenters, dentists, people working with electric drills or other vibrating instruments, sewing machine operators, needlepointers, piano players, and indeed anyone who works with her hands for long hours can get CTS. So can tennis and squash players, aerobic dancers using hand weights, and people who frequently use rowing machines or other exercise equipment. (CTS is part of a larger category of work-related injury known as repetitive strain injury, which has a long history and can be found in many jobs and professions.) Thousands of cases of CTS are diagnosed each year, and women are far more susceptible to it than men because women tend to do the kinds of industrial, office, and domestic jobs that promote CTS. And their carpal tunnel space is smaller to begin with.

What are the signs? The syndrome is much easier to treat and much less likely to cause long-term problems if you diagnose it early. Usually symptoms first occur early in the morning: you waken to burning, tingling, and numbness in your hands, which may also awaken you at night. (Flexing your hand in your sleep or sleeping on it may aggravate the discomfort.) If left untreated, the tingling and numbness can progress to a weakened grip and severe pain in the forearm or shoulder. By all means, get medical advice before this happens. If you have to take aspirin or other painkillers in order to keep working, you should see a physician.

CTS is not difficult for a doctor to diagnose, but you may still need to go to a neurologist for an electrodiagnostic test, which checks the nerve's ability to transmit impulses. If your condition is mild, wearing a splint at night may be all you need. But if that doesn't work, your doctor may suggest anti-inflammatory drugs such as aspirin or ibuprofen, or injections of cortisone. If nerve injury or muscle damage progresses, surgery may prove advisable. Surgery is usually successful in restoring full hand function unless the condition has been present for several years.

Avoiding CTS at home and at work. A few simple precautions can help minimize the risk of CTS:

• When working with your hands, keep your wrists straight. Flexing and twisting them stresses the carpal tunnel.

•Lift objects with your whole hand—or better yet, with both hands—to reduce stress on the wrist.

•Make sure your work station is comfortable. If you're working at a computer keyboard, make sure your fingers are lower than your wrists; don't rest the heel of your hands on the keyboard.

•Take breaks frequently when working with your hands. Working too rapidly may contribute to the problem.

•Type with a soft touch—don't pound the keys.

•If your hands hurt while you're on the rowing machine, for instance, or while playing a racket sport, ease up. Pain is always a signal to stop. If you carry hand weights while running or exercising, make sure they aren't too heavy.

•If the work you do is stressing your hands, see if you can rotate tasks or share work with someone else.

Side stitches

While running or walking briskly, nearly everyone has experienced the sharp pain in the side known as a stitch. No one knows what causes a stitch, though there's no shortage of educated guesses. One theory is that the diaphragm (the large muscle that separates the chest from the abdominal cavity) sometimes fails to receive enough blood during its contractions, and, much like a leg cramp, this results in spasm and pain. Another theory is that a stitch is caused by trapped gas pockets brought on by exercising right after a meal.

To prevent stitches:
•If stitches seem to hit you after a meal, wait thirty to ninety minutes after eating before exercising.

•Warm up before exercising—a good policy in any case.

•Work out at lower intensity for longer periods, rather than suddenly increasing the intensity of the workout. If you are going to increase intensity, do so gradually.

•Well-conditioned runners and walkers don't seem to get stitches as often, so work at increasing your aerobic capacity.

If you get a stitch:
•First stop or slow down, then bend forward and push your fingers into the painful area.

•Breathe deeply and exhale slowly through pursed lips. This should help relax the diaphragm.

•Stretch the abdominal muscles by raising your arms and reaching overhead.

Treating Injuries

Unfortunately, no matter how careful people are, injuries do occur. And injured tendons, muscles, ligaments, and cartilage—the soft tissue involved in most sports injuries—can take a long time to heal, longer in fact than broken bones. What follows are guidelines on the most effective home remedies, which are aimed at assisting the healing process.

Stages of healing

Here is how the natural healing process works:

Inflammation. In this initial response to injury, blood vessels in surrounding tissues dilate and release a variety of substances. White blood cells arrive to remove dead tissue and other debris. These and other vascular changes produce heat, swelling, and redness. The subsequent pain and stiffness has the beneficial effect of keeping you from moving and aggravating the injured muscles or other body parts.

Regeneration. After twenty-four to forty-eight hours, the body begins replacing injured tissue. Damaged cells are flushed from the area, then a network of capillaries forms that allows a greater flow of oxygen and nutrients into the injury site. Two to three days after the initial damage, strands of collagen—a protein that is the major component of connective tissue begin forming scar tissue over the damaged areas, a process that lasts two to three weeks.

Remodeling. If you don't move the injured body part at all, the collagen will grow into a puckered, inelastic scar that remains weak and can cause tightness and discomfort—particularly in muscles, which are normally far more elastic than tendons or ligaments. That's why you should gently stretch and strengthen damaged tissue. When it recovers properly, the affected muscle or tendon usually regains 80 to 95 percent of its original strength within three to six months. (There will always be at least a slight residual loss in strength).

Ice: the first step of treatment

Ice is the most effective, safest, and cheapest form of treating an exercise or sports injury, whether acute or chronic (such as tendinitis). With acute injuries such as torn ligaments, muscle strains, and bruises, *the key is to start icing as soon as possible.* Even if you plan to go to the doctor immediately, icing the injury right away will help speed recovery. Not only does ice relieve pain, but it also slows blood flow, thereby reducing internal bleeding and swelling. (Though inflammation is part of the healing process, too much of it can impede healing). This in turn helps limit tissue damage and hastens the healing process. Follow these steps:

•Apply the ice on the injured area for ten to twenty minutes, then reapply it every two waking hours (or more frequently if necessary) for the next forty-eight to seventy-two hours. Be sure not to go over the twenty-minute limit; longer than that may damage skin and nerves.

•If you start to feel *mild* discomfort when exercising and think it may be the first sign of an overuse injury, such as tendinitis, you may well be able to finish your activity—a set of tennis, for example. But apply ice over tender areas right after you finish, and reapply it several times a day for the next forty-eight hours.

•To minimize swelling, especially in severe injuries, use ice in conjunction with these other measures that are often referred to as RICE:

> **R**est the injured body part;
> apply **I**ce;
> apply **C**ompression;
> **E**levate the injured extremity above heart level.

Resting not only reduces pain, but also prevents aggravating the injury; compression and elevation help keep excess fluids from accumulating in tissues. To apply compression, wrap a towel or an Ace-type elastic bandage around the injury (don't wrap it so tightly that you cut off circulation). You can often combine ice and compression by holding the ice pack in place with a bandage. And for certain injuries, you can combine ice with massage: just wrap ice in a towel and move it gently over the affected area.

Should You See a Doctor?

There is no hard and fast rule—it depends both on the type of injury and especially on how severe it is. A severe acute injury such as a pulled muscle or a sprained ankle may require a cast or surgery. *Call a doctor if any of the following symptoms persist :*

• severe or persistent muscle pain, swelling, or spasm;

• pain centered in a bone or joint;

• stiffness or decreased mobility of a joint or inability to move it at all;

• stabbing or radiating pain;

• numbness or tingling.

If dealt with properly, overuse injuries such as tennis elbow or runner's knee—which are due to the cumulative wear and tear of a repetitive movement—probably won't require a doctor's care. In fact, self-treatment is generally just what the doctor recommends. However, if pain persists for more than ten days in spite of self-care measures, or if it is severe or is growing worse, consult a doctor.

Ice precautions

• *Don't leave an ice pack directly on the skin: either keep moving it or wrap it in a thin towel.*

• *To avoid skin damage, stop icing once skin is numb. Set a timer so that you don't go beyond twenty minutes or fall asleep.*

• *Be careful with refreezable gel packs and self-freezing chemical packs, which may be colder than regular ice. And beware of punctures in the pack, since the chemicals can burn.*

• *Don't use ice on blisters or open wounds, or if you are hypersensitive to cold or have a circulatory problem.*

• *Be particularly cautious when icing the elbow or knee, where the nerves are near the surface and can be damaged by prolonged exposure to cold. Never put an unwrapped ice pack over the elbow or the outside of the knee.*

Remember that icing is not a substitute for seeing your doctor in case of a serious injury and/or an injury that does not respond to self-treatment in twenty-four hours.

When to apply heat

Traditionally people started applying heat to an injury soon after icing it. But heat actually stimulates blood flow and so increases inflammation. Most sports physicians and trainers now recommend that you stick with ice for at least the first forty-eight hours after an injury, and only then, *after swelling has subsided,* try heating. At that point, the increased blood flow caused by heating can speed up healing. Heat can also help relieve pain, relax muscles, and reduce joint stiffness.

You can apply either dry heat (using a heating pad or lamp) or moist heat (a hot bath, whirlpool, hot-water bottle, heat pack, or damp towel wrapped around a waterproof heating pad). There's still debate about whether dry or moist heat is best, and for what type of injury, so check with your doctor about which is appropriate for you. If you have a heart condition or a fever, or if the injury is bleeding, you may be told to avoid using a hot bath or whirlpool. Don't apply heat if you have an infection. If pain or inflammation gets worse after heating an injury, stop.

The key word is "warm," not "hot." Use heating pads on low or medium settings, and keep the water in baths between 98° and 105°F. (It should feel comfortable when you dip your wrist in.) Apply the heat twenty to thirty minutes, two to three times a day. You can also use heat for five to ten minutes before exercising to reduce stiffness. To be safe, wrap a hot water bottle, hot pack, or heating pad (if it doesn't have a cover) in a towel.

Sometimes both help. For some types of chronic pain or muscle spasm, ice or heat may help. For instance, some people with lower-back pain find that ice works, while others can't tolerate the cold and prefer heating. For some chronic or recurrent pain, once the initial ice treatment has brought the swelling down, a doctor or trainer may recommend what's called "contrast therapy"—alternating cold and heat (usually cold and hot water).

Pain-relief medication

Taking over-the-counter pain relievers such as aspirin, ibuprofen (for instance, Advil or Motrin), or naproxen sodium (Aleve) can indeed help ease the pain and reduce inflammation of minor sprains, strains, and tendinitis. The other major over-the-counter pain reliever, acetaminophen (such as Tylenol), is good for relief of muscle soreness, as discussed on page 519. However, it is less helpful for these other injuries since it has no anti-inflammatory effect.

There are more potent prescription medications, widely recommended by athletic trainers, which can eliminate pain and swelling very quickly in many cases. But these drugs—which include cortisone (or its derivatives), the strongest of all anti-inflammatory medications—can produce serious adverse side effects. Another potential problem: they can let you ignore the pain—which is a warning sign that you are doing damage to your body—and allow you to exercise vigorously and perhaps cause permanent damage to the injured tissue. Hence, such drugs should be used only under medical supervision and for brief periods of time.

How long to rest

For most overuse injuries, rest a day or two and then try to exercise the affected area at an intensity that doesn't cause pain. You can try to gradually return to your usual workout routine, initially decreasing your speed, duration, and/or frequency by at least 25 percent. Don't work out, though, if persistent pain returns, and

Ice packs

Although commercial ice packs are available, plain ice is fine: simply put ice cubes or crushed ice in a heavy plastic bag or hot-water bottle, or wrap the ice in a thick towel.

Packs that remain flexible when frozen, such as a gel pack or even a bag of frozen peas, can provide more cooling since they conform to the body. If you have injured a foot or hand, you can immerse it in ice water.

Injury Specialists

Sports medicine is a rapidly growing field. However, there's no board certification for "sports medicine," and so-called "sports doctors" may have varied training and specialties. Your family doctor will be able to treat common sprains and strains, but for more severe or complicated injuries you may be referred to a sports medicine clinic or one of the following:

Orthopedists are MDs with specialized surgical training. They treat injuries to any part of the musculoskeletal system; some specialize in athletic injuries.

Physical therapists administer techniques to enhance recovery, from massage to rehabilitative exercises. A therapist typically has a degree in physical therapy and is licensed by the state as a registered physical therapist (RPT). Seeing a therapist requires a doctor's referral in most states.

Podiatrists deal with foot and foot-related problems, which are among the most common sports-related injuries. Though not MDs, podiatrists receive special training and are licensed by the state.

Sports Medicine Clinics are likely to include some of the specialists mentioned above. Check with your local medical center to see if it has a sports medicine clinic or department or if there's one in the area.

don't resume your full level until you are free of pain both during and after exercise. It's also important to identify the cause of the injury—poor equipment, poor technique, or some other factor—and correct it.

For minor strains and sprains—if you turn your ankle slightly while hiking, for example—staying off the injured part for a day or two is often enough. More serious injuries will require a longer rest period, and you may have to immobilize the injured part—keeping weight off a wrenched knee, for example, or supporting an injured wrist or elbow in a sling. Check with your doctor.

Unless an injury is severe, however, absolute rest should not exceed forty-eight hours. Otherwise, muscles may weaken, joints may get stiff, and scar tissue that forms around the injury may start to tighten. Activity helps prevent this and, by increasing blood flow, also encourages healing.

As soon as the initial pain and swelling of a sprain or other acute injury subside, therefore, you should begin to exercise the injured area gently. (If you have any doubts, consult your doctor). Start with isometric exercises. Then do stretching and strengthening exercises that move the affected muscles through their full range of motion. To maintain aerobic fitness, you can substitute another activity that puts less stress on the injured part. So if you're a jogger with a sprained ankle, for instance, try cycling or swimming until you recover.

Arthritis

Arthritis is not one disease but many, notably osteoarthritis and rheumatoid arthritis. Osteoarthritis is so common that nearly everyone over forty shows some signs of it on X-rays—a gradual loss of the soft, smooth cartilage at joint surfaces, and frequently a compensatory overgrowth of bone at the joints. There are two types of osteoarthritis. Primary osteoarthritis, resulting from normal wear and tear, most commonly affects thumb joints and the end joints of other fingers, the hips, knees, neck, and lower spine. Secondary osteoarthritis can occur after injury to a joint; from disease (such as diabetes); or as a result of chronic trauma (due to obesity, poor posture, or occupational overuse). Unlike rheumatoid arthritis, which is a completely different disease, osteoarthritis causes minimal inflammation.

Because arthritis makes joints stiff and painful, the natural tendency is to minimize movement. Unfortunately, this can simply lead to stiffer joints—and thus more pain—since inactivity weakens the muscles that stabilize joints. Studies have shown that many people with osteoarthritis can maintain flexibility, and even restore it to some degree, through a well-designed exercise program that is gradually implemented and followed regularly. Specialists have devised scores of exercises (such as the ones below) to stretch muscles or strengthen important joints. Exercise may cost you some pain at first, but the discomfort should diminish. Here are some guidelines about the types of exercises that are helpful:

Stretching exercises limber up muscles and help increase joint mobility.

Strengthening exercises tone muscles that support vulnerable joints, making them more stable. If you're having an intense flare-up, isometric exercises—which are static and thus move muscles, not joints—are safest and easiest.

Endurance activities enhance aerobic capacity (the ability of the cardiovascular system to carry oxygen to the muscles) and thereby improve overall fitness, provided they are done at least three times a week for twenty minutes at your training heart rate. Swimming, particularly in a heated pool, is excellent because the water supports the body as you take your joints gently through their full range of movement. Walking is another good choice; if you're able to, gradually work up to a brisk, heart-healthy pace. As a general rule, it's wise to avoid high-impact activities like tennis, aerobic dance, or running, which can overload sore joints.

Exercises must be individualized, depending on the joints involved and the degree of pain. Your doctor or physical therapist will help you develop an exercise program that focuses on your most painful joints and takes into consideration your overall level of fitness. Whatever exercises you do, there are some general rules:

Warning signs of arthritis

You should see your doctor if any of the following symptoms persist:
- *early morning stiffness;*
- *swelling;*
- *recurring pain or tenderness in one or more joints;*
- *changes in joint mobility;*
- *redness or warmth in joints;*
- *unexplained weight loss, fever, or loss of strength in association with joint pain.*

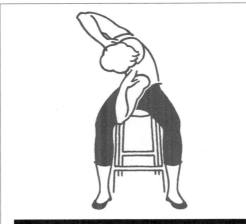

Back stretch: *Sit erect with feet apart. Place fingertips on shoulders with elbows spread wide apart. Gently bend over and twist so that you move one elbow across and down to opposite knee. Straighten up and gently bring both elbows back. Repeat to other side.*

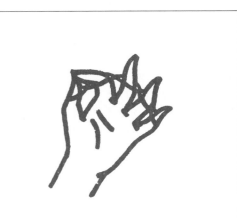

Finger exercises: *1. As shown above, twist a large rubber band around all five fingers of your hand. Gently spread the fingers apart, using the rubber band as resistance. 2. Try to form a letter O with your thumb and index finger, then spread your fingers as wide as you can. Then touch the thumb to the tip of each of your other fingers, spreading your fingers wide after each attempt. If you can't bring the fingers together, use your other hand to help. 3. Squeeze a soft rubber ball.*

Start gradually and never overdo it. Follow the instructions of your doctor or physical therapist. There will probably be some pain or discomfort, but stop that particular exercise if there's unusual or severe pain. Cut back if need be, but don't stop exercising entirely.

Always warm up first. After walking in place for a few minutes, do some gentle stretches. Gently massaging stiff joints may help, as may heat (a warm bath or shower, an infrared lamp). Wear a sweat suit, or leg or arm warmers.

Vary your exercises, so that you work different muscle groups. Don't rely on one long, strenuous (and painful) session a week. Begin with as few as three repetitions of an exercise. Over the course of several weeks try to work up to ten repetitions, or as many as your doctor recommends.

Note: Remember, unless you know you are healthy and have only mild osteoarthritis, talk to your doctor before attempting these, or any, exercises.

Bursitis

Bursitis, that dull misery in the shoulder or knee, can and does strike anybody, from the sedentary to the highly trained athlete. And though the shoulder is a common locale for bursitis, any of the bursae in the human body—there are around 150—can get irritated. Bursae (from the Greek word for wine-skin, and related to the English word purse) are small, closed, fluid-filled sacs that protect muscles and tendons from irritation produced by contact with bones. But if friction gets too great—from over-exercising, hard work, or injury, for instance—the bursae themselves may get inflamed. Occupational bursitis is not uncommon and is known by old, familiar names such as "housemaid's knee," and "policeman's heel." One of the most common foot ailments, the bunion, is a form of bursitis caused by friction: a tight-fitting shoe causes a sac on the joint of the big toe to become inflamed. Older people, especially athletes, are more likely to get bursitis.

Though bursitis may hurt as much as arthritis, it isn't a joint disease. Sometimes it recurs and becomes chronic, but with proper treatment, most attacks of bursitis go away in two or three days.

Prevention tips

Strong, flexible muscles can help prevent bursitis. Also, the measures that protect you from other kinds of overuse injuries, such as tendinitis, may also protect you from bursitis. Whatever you're doing, don't push yourself too hard or too long. If you're in pain, stop. If you're beginning a new exercise program, work up to higher levels of fitness gradually. If you're doing hard physical labor, pace yourself and take frequent breaks. If you're taking up a strenuous new sport, such as tennis or long-distance running or cycling, teach yourself proper techniques—or get professional advice—before you throw yourself wholeheartedly into it. It isn't always possible to avoid the sudden blow, bump, or fall that may produce bursitis. But you can protect your body as follows:

•Keep yourself in good shape with strengthening and flexibility exercises.

•Make sure your technique is correct if you play tennis or golf or any sport that may strain your shoulder. Don't push yourself too long or too hard.

•One common form of bursitis in the elbow is brought on by constantly resting

Diagnostic testing

Women approaching menopause who are at risk for osteoporosis should consult their doctor about getting a bone density study to assess their skeletal status. Several scanning techniques can be used to measure bone density at the hip, spine, or wrist, though many physicians are uncomfortable with the predictive value of wrist bone diagnosis. You can be tested at selected hospitals as well as at specialized diagnostic centers. Your doctor can help you decide whether a test is necessary and refer you to a reliable test unit in your area.

the elbow on a hard surface, such as a desk. If you habitually lean on your elbow, this may be a sign that your chair is uncomfortable or the wrong height. Try to arrange your work space so that you need not lean on your elbow to read, write, or view your computer screen.

•If you have a job that calls for lots of kneeling (for example, refinishing or waxing a floor), cushion your knees, change position frequently, and take breaks.

•High-heeled or ill-fitting shoes cause bunions, and tight shoes can also cause bursitis in the heel. Problems in the feet can also affect the hips. In particular, the tendons and bursae in the hips can be put under excessive strain by worn-down heels. Buy shoes that fit and keep them in good repair. Never wear a shoe that's too short or too narrow or that chafes your foot. Women should wear comfortable shoes for walking and for daily chores, saving their high heels for special occasions.

Osteoporosis

Osteoporosis is a word that's come into common usage, but the condition is by no means a recent discovery. Meaning "porous bones" in Latin, osteoporosis literally is a thinning of the bones, which makes them fragile and brittle, so that they fracture easily. It can affect both men and women, but it's about eight times more common in women. For men and women, however, the chief risk factor is age: the disease usually becomes detectable in people in their sixties, seventies, and beyond. About 1.3 million older Americans suffer fractures each year due to osteoporosis. It can also result in a decrease in height because of the compression of the vertebrae in the spine and also cause the stooped posture known as "dowager's hump." It's a major cause of disability among older women.

There's no cure for osteoporosis, though there are treatments. Like hypertension, osteoporosis has been called a "silent disease." You may not be aware of it until you fall and fracture a bone. Thus prevention is the best line of defense.

Unfortunately, many women think they don't have to start worrying about osteoporosis until menopause. This a myth. Recent research shows that certain lifelong habits are the best preventive for osteoporosis. About 45 percent of a person's bone mass is formed during the teen years. Indeed, young adulthood or even the teen years is the right time to form the health habits that help prevent osteoporosis. Still, it's never too late to begin. Your bones continue to evolve and change throughout your life. Bone tissue constantly "remodels" itself (lays down and then releases and replaces calcium) but for most of adult life there is equilibrium—calcium is laid down and released without apparent change in bone density. However, at about age thirty-five for women and slightly later for men, bone density begins to decrease.

Many factors influence the processes carried on by bone tissue. The sex hormones (testosterone in men, estrogen in women) are a major influence on calcium uptake by bone tissue and thus skeletal strength. Other hormones aid in the release of calcium and the breakdown of bone mass.

Second, nutritional factors—your intake of calcium and vitamin D, as well as other nutrients whose function in bone building is not fully understood—play an important role in bone formation and maintenance, too.

Third, there is physical activity. Bones respond to mechanical stress by becom-

---

Bursitis treatment tips

It may be hard to tell whether you have bursitis or tendinitis—but bursitis is usually characterized by a dull, persistent ache that increases with movement (in contrast to the sharp pain typical of tendinitis). If you do develop bursitis:

•Rest the body part that hurts. If you suspect that one activity has caused the pain, stop it for a while.

•Try aspirin or ibuprofen for easing inflammation.

•Apply ice packs during the first two days to bring down swelling, then heat to ease pain and stimulate blood flow.

•Resume exercising only after you feel better, and start slowly with gentle activities.

Liniments and balms are no help for bursitis. Liniments don't penetrate deeply enough to treat bursitis; they mainly warm the skin and make it tingle, thus distracting attention from the pain beneath. Massage is likely to make matters worse. If bursitis pain is disabling or doesn't subside after three or four days, get medical advice.

ing denser and stronger. This stress comes primarily from weight-bearing activity, in which your legs support your body, and from strength-building activity such as weight lifting). If you walk a lot, for example, your leg bones will respond by increasing their mass. If you regularly use your arms to lift weights or swing a tennis racket, the bones in your arms will grow stronger. Perhaps the most dramatic demonstration of the influence of weight-bearing exercise is found in astronauts who spend several weeks in space. In this weightless environment, even these young healthy men lose significant amounts of bone mass.

Another influence on bone is genetics. Asian and Caucasian women tend to be small-boned, which makes them susceptible to osteoporosis. African and many African-American women tend to have more bone mass throughout life (which is a protective genetic trait), though that doesn't mean they never develop osteoporosis.

Gender may be the most important factor in the bone-maintenance game, and women are at a disadvantage. They begin life with less bone mass, on average, than men. Then at menopause, usually around fifty, a woman's supply of estrogen decreases, and her bone loss is more rapid than a man's. That's why, after age sixty-five, so many women suffer from osteoporosis.

Bone loss does not mean that the bone is diseased or abnormal. It just means there's less of it—and when new bone forms, it's less dense. The body continues to remove calcium from the bone storehouse, but in older people some of this calcium is not replaced.

What Puts You at Risk: A Checklist

- Increasing age.
- Being female. By age sixty-five, the average man still has 91 percent of his bone mass, but the average woman only about 74 percent.
- Being chronically underweight or having a slight frame.
- Being Caucasian or Asian (usually small-boned).
- Having osteoporosis in the family.
- A poor diet, low in vitamins and minerals, especially calcium.
- Being sedentary and lack of weight-bearing exercise.
- Smoking. In women this lowers the estrogen content of the blood, thus weakening the bones. Smoking is particularly dangerous for women who have other risk factors for osteoporosis.
- Heavy drinking. It's not known why heavy drinking weakens the bones—perhaps because heavy drinkers often eat a poor diet.
- Long-term use of certain medications. Some people with asthma and rheumatoid arthritis take cortisone for long periods, which can diminish bone strength. So can long-term use of thyroid hormones, which, although most physicians do not recommend them, are sometimes used to treat obesity.

Prevention: when and how

You can't do much about it if hereditary factors or a small frame size puts you at risk for osteoporosis—but that's all the more reason to take preventive steps. The best time to begin a program of prevention is in childhood and then continue it throughout your life. In your twenties and early thirties, bone density is on the increase. The more bone you build early in life, the better you will be able to withstand bone loss later in life. But if you've waited until your forties, fifties, or sixties, there's still plenty of reason to follow a preventive program.

Make weight-bearing exercise part of your daily life. That means walking, running, cycling, dancing, or weight lifting—or activities such as housework or mowing the grass. Swimming and yoga are not weight-bearing exercises, and thus don't build bones, though they have other benefits. Exercise should be part of your life at all stages, but it's particularly important as you grow older.

Consume enough calcium. Besides building strong bones and maintaining bone density and strength, calcium also plays a role in regulating your heart beat and other vital functions. The daily recommended dietary allowance, or RDA, is 800 milligrams, except for adolescents and young adults (aged eleven to twenty-four) and pregnant or lactating women, who are advised to consume 1,200 milligrams daily; some experts recommend that postmenopausal women consume at least 1,500 milligrams. Many dark green leafy vegetables are rich in calcium. But the best source of calcium for most Americans, who usually don't eat much kale, beet greens, or fish bones, remains low-fat or nonfat dairy products. The vitamin D added to milk and the lactose naturally in milk and dairy products are thought to aid in the absorption of calcium. (For more information on calcium sources and the use of calcium supplements, see pages 138-139.)

If you smoke, stop. Not only for the strength of your bones, but for your general health and well-being.

If you drink, drink only lightly or moderately. Light to moderate drinking is defined as an average of no more than two drinks a day. A drink is defined as 5 ounces of wine, 12 ounces of beer, or 1.5 ounces of 80-proof liquor (all contain about half an ounce of pure alcohol).

If you are menopausal, consider hormone replacement therapy (HRT). This consists of low-dose estrogen and progesterone treatments that can unquestionably slow bone loss and prevent fractures as well as reduce hot flashes and other common menopausal symptoms (see page 404). The added progesterone also reduces the risk of endometrial cancer. HRT probably protects against heart disease, though the evidence remains controversial. (It's estrogen, not the combination of estrogen with progesterone, that's known to be protective.) HRT, if used to prevent osteoporosis, should be started at menopause for maximum effect.

But menopause is not a medical condition that automatically requires drugs. Some women do very well without HRT, which has its downside, too. It may increase the risk of breast cancer, though the evidence isn't yet clear. Still, women who have had breast cancer should not undergo HRT. Those with migraine headaches, diabetes, and other disorders are sometimes advised against it. All women should be informed about HRT and, at menopause, should discuss the pros and cons with their physicians.

In particular, if you have one or more risk factors for osteoporosis, you should consider HRT. But whether you opt for it or not, you should modify the risk factors that you can modify: begin an exercise program if you're sedentary, increase your calcium intake, don't smoke, and limit your alcohol intake.

If you are taking oral contraceptives, you'll be pleased to learn that recent studies have shown that their use has a notable positive effect on bone density, independent of other factors such as calcium intake and exercise.

Back Care

About 80 percent of all Americans will have at least one backache during their lifetime. Every year articles and books about back pain appear, espousing new and old theories about its causes and how to treat it. However, there's room for controversy because the back is such a complicated, sophisticated structure, and while we can name all the bones, joints, nerves, muscles, and ligaments that comprise it, the sum total remains something of a mystery. Fortunately, most backaches aren't serious and generally go away in a few weeks, with or without medical attention. And they are usually preventable.

Dealing with Back Pain

Back trouble is so common because the human spine hasn't evolved to the point where we can walk upright without some risk. Being erect puts extra pressure on the vertebrae of the lower back, or lumbar region, where the back curves most and where pain most often strikes. Backache becomes more common between the ages of thirty and fifty, as the disks—the fibrous pads that cushion the vertebrae—start to lose water and elasticity and thus some of their ability to absorb shock. In middle age, too, people tend to become less active and their muscles grow lax, contributing to back instability.

Sprain, strain, or spasm

A small portion of all backaches do have clear causes—for instance, a ruptured disk or some underlying disease. But in the great majority of cases the exact diagnosis isn't known. Is the cause of your backache that sudden movement yesterday when you bent to pick up the newspaper, or is the problem that you get too little (or too much) exercise? Or could it be your poor posture, or just everyday wear and tear? In fact, it's probably a combination of all these. A backache can range from mild discomfort to excruciating pain. Usually X-rays show nothing wrong despite the pain—yet in some cases there's dramatic damage to disks but no pain whatsoever.

The terms back strain or sprain are often loosely applied to a broad spectrum of back disorders. *Strain* is generally used when a muscle is overstretched, and *sprain* when a ligament is partially torn. However, it is seldom clear whether it's a muscle or ligament that's been damaged, let alone whether it has been torn or not. Two other terms, muscle spasm and ruptured disk, are more clearly defined.

Muscle spasm. The most common form of spasm is a sudden onset of sustained, painful, involuntary contractions of muscles in the back. This may serve to immobilize irritated back muscles, thereby protecting them and spinal nerves. A spasm usually results from a back injury, but may also be caused or aggravated by poor posture, lots of sitting in the same position, tense back muscles, and weak abdominal muscles. Many researchers claim that psychological stress can also trigger muscle spasms.

Disk problems. These are actually relatively uncommon. Only 2 to 4 percent of back ailments are due to what is commonly called a "slipped" disk. The term "slipped" is a misnomer, since the disk actually bulges (herniates) from between two vertebrae and may eventually rupture. If a displaced disk presses on a spinal nerve, the nerve can send shooting pains to the legs or arms, or create a tingling or sensation of numbness in them. If, as is common, the affected nerve is the sciatic, the condition is called sciatica (see below).

Underlying diseases and structural problems. A small percentage of all backaches are related to identifiable medical problems such as kidney disease, cancer, arthritis, osteoporosis, or spinal infection. Sideways curvature (scoliosis), sway back (lordosis, or excessive curve in the lower back), or other structural defects may also be at the root of back pain.

When sciatica strikes

One common kind of back disorder that may strike, especially in middle age, is sciatica, so called because it involves the sciatic nerve. This is actually a group of nerves (the body's longest) bound in one nerve sheath, which runs from the lower back through the buttock and thigh to the knees (where it branches) on down into the foot. Thus, besides back pain, an irritated sciatic nerve also produces pain in the thigh that may radiate all the way to the feet. Weakness and numbness in the legs are other common symptoms.

Though sciatica often affects people in their fifties, it's not age that causes it but probably a complex of other factors: work that requires repetitive lifting, constant exposure to mechanical vibrations (for example, long hours behind the wheel of a car or truck). Severe low back-pain (including sciatica), according to a report in the *New England Journal of Medicine,* also shows a high correlation with job dissatisfaction and depression—though whether depression aggravates back pain or is the result of it is hard to determine. Some studies have also suggested that cigarette smoking may be a risk factor.

But you can have sciatica even without any of these risk factors. You may be a healthy, happy person who never lifts anything and yet, for no apparent reason, suffer a sudden attack when you bend or turn slightly.

Some experts blame herniated disks that press on the sciatic nerve. Muscle spasm, resulting from a fall or injury, can also irritate the nerve. Some researchers blame the piriformis muscle of the buttocks—the muscle that allows you to lift your leg sideways. If inflamed by injury or over-exertion, the piriformis muscle can press against the sciatic nerve. Overall, there's no consensus; indeed in most cases, an exact diagnosis may not be necessary. Sciatica often gets well with the simple measures described below.

Self-treatment for a backache

The great majority of backaches (less serious strains, sprains, or spasms) usually don't require a doctor's attention. For soreness and minor pain in the back, avoiding physically demanding activity may be sufficient. But if the pain is more severe, lie down and rest. Reclining may relieve the pain, and takes mechanical pressure off the stressed back during the first day or two of injury. Allowing the inflamed tissue to repair itself can prevent a chronic cycle of back injury. According to research by the Swedish orthopedist Alf Nachemson, compared to standing, reclin-

---

Treat yourself to back-pain relief

In a recent study in the Annals of Internal Medicine, doctors at a large HMO who routinely prescribed bed rest and prescription drugs for treating back pain were significantly less successful with their patients than those who taught patients how to deal with their own back problems through exercise and life-style changes, and who prescribed drugs less frequently.

In addition, patients seemed to benefit from being told that back pain is amenable to self-care, that it usually goes away in a reasonable time, and that even though it becomes chronic in some cases, it's manageable. Patients taught self-care did better and were also better satisfied.

Wellness Body Atlas

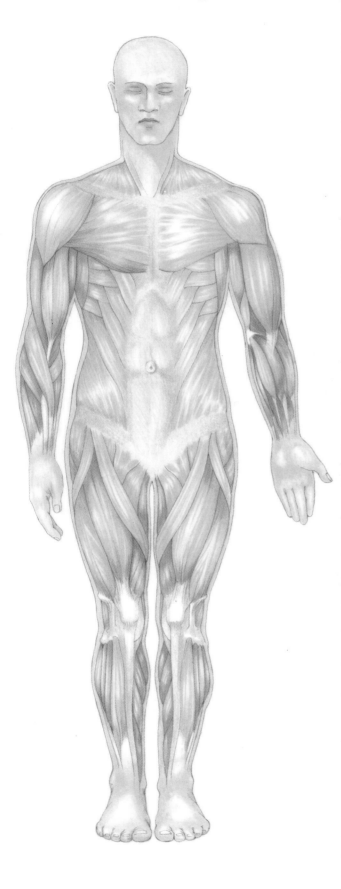

Knowing how joints and muscles operate can help you safeguard them. Basically, joints permit movement, while skeletal muscles create and control movement. Aided by fibrous bands called ligaments, joints bind two or more bones together in a variety of ways to give your limbs, torso, and neck flexibility. Muscles, which are attached to bones by tendons, operate around a joint in a seesaw pattern, working in pairs to pull the joint in one direction or another. By virtue of the body's sophisticated nervous system, many muscles can be coordinated to perform complex actions—for example, consider the variety of movements in a tennis game, which involves almost every area of the body.

The following seven pages illustrate principle joints and muscle groups, explain how they function, and indicate some of the ways in which these body parts are vulnerable to injury.

The Back

The mainstay of the back is the spine (illustrated below). Forming an S-shaped curve from the base of your head to your pelvis, this mechanical marvel is sturdy enough to support the upper body, yet pliable enough to allow the trunk and neck to bend, stretch, and rotate. The spine is involved in almost every movement you make, from walking to serving a tennis ball to opening a door. It must also provide adequate stiffness and stability to protect the bundle of nerves that makes up the spinal cord.

The spinal column, or backbone, is composed of twenty-four separate spool-shaped bones called vertebrae, plus the sacrum (a triangular bone located between the hipbones), and the tailbone (coccyx). These are all stacked like a flexible tower with three curves—in the neck, chest, and lower back. The vertebrae are connected and held erect by ligaments and muscles that act much like the guy wires that hold up a ship's mast. In addition, much support for the lower back comes from the muscles in the abdomen. (When you lift a heavy weight, your abdominal muscles tighten.) Sandwiched between the vertebrae are gel-filled pads of tough connective tissue called discs, which act as shock absorbers. Discs contribute to the spine's flexibility, as do facet joints, which help stabilize the spine while contributing to spinal movement.

A healthy spine is capable of great strength: a single disc in the lower back has been shown to bear loads in excess of 2,500 pounds. While wear and tear on discs and joints can cause back pain, as can a number of structural problems, most cases of pain in the lower back stem from sprains to ligaments. These are usually aggravated or even caused by muscular weakness, particularly in the abdominal muscles. Strengthening this supporting musculature (illustrated on the next two pages) is the best way to spare yourself back pain and strain. When well conditioned, these muscles act like a protective girdle to keep the spine properly aligned and to distribute stresses placed upon it.

Cervical vertebrae
Slender, highly flexible section of seven vertebrae that allows movement of the head.

Thoracic vertebrae
Larger, more rigid section of twelve vetebrae that is partially supported by the ribs. This part of the spine helps anchor the chest and protect the lungs.

Lumbar Vertebrae
Largest, sturdiest vertebral section that acts as the pivot point for most movements of the trunk and supports heavy loads.

Sacrum
Triangular bone that holds the pelvic arch in place with a network of ligaments. The sacrum serves as the base for the spinal column.

Coccyx
Four small segments of bone that fuse together to form the tailbone.

Trapezius
Triangular muscle covering the upper part of the back that moves your head and shrugs your shoulders. Along with the latissimus dorsi, the trapezius also distributes the efforts of the arm and shoulders along the back.

Erector spinae
Overlapping muscles that run the length of the spine and are connected to the vertebrae and ribs. Also called back extensors, they extend, rotate, and stabilize the spine, and absorb much of the stress of everyday movements.

Latissimus Dorsi
A wide flat muscle attached along the lumbar and lower half of the thoracic spine. The latissimus provides support for the torso, moves the arm, and assists the trapezius.

The Midsection and Upper Body

Several sets of muscles support and propel your torso and arms. The abdominals (illustrated below) help transfer force between your upper and lower body, and they also protect your internal organs. But their most crucial function is to support your back. Running in several directions, these muscles help maintain your posture and aid your spinal muscles when you bend, twist, and perform other everyday movements. Most activities do little to exercise the abdominals; hence, if these muscles are not toned and strengthened regularly, they will weaken, and the result can be increasingly "swaybacked" posture and chronic lower back pain.

Muscles also play a key role in the functioning of the shoulder (illustrated opposite). Compared to a joint like the knee or elbow, the shoulder is highly mobile. Indeed, it is the body's most flexible joint, allowing you to throw a ball, swing a golf club, perform a backstroke, or swing your arm in a full circle. But whereas the knee and elbow are secured by their ball-and-socket structures and by a network of strong ligaments, the shoulder's socket is more like a shallow dish upon which the ball rests—an arrangement that makes it comparatively unstable. Moreover, the ligaments that keep the shoulder in place are weak, and it depends for stability on muscles and tendons running across the joint. If some of these muscles are weak or out of balance with other muscles, the risk of strains or sprains increases. Hence, to safely meet the demands of swimming, rowing, golf, and other activities that involve throwing, lifting, pulling, and stroking, it is important to strengthen this array of musculature, which includes the biceps, triceps, deltoid, latissimus dorsi, and pectoralis major as well as a deeper layer of four small muscles (and their tendons) called the rotator cuff.

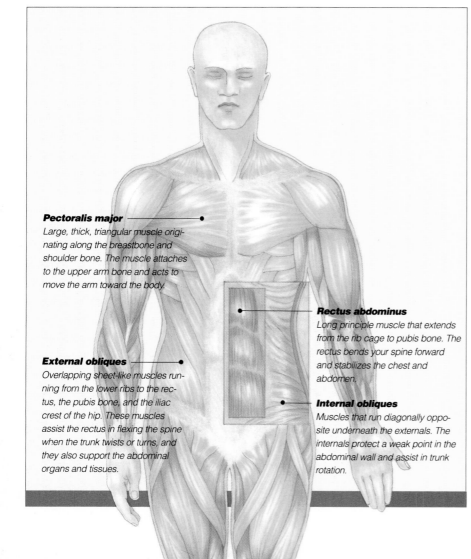

Pectoralis major
Large, thick, triangular muscle originating along the breastbone and shoulder bone. The muscle attaches to the upper arm bone and acts to move the arm toward the body.

External obliques
Overlapping sheet-like muscles running from the lower ribs to the rectus, the pubis bone, and the iliac crest of the hip. These muscles assist the rectus in flexing the spine when the trunk twists or turns, and they also support the abdominal organs and tissues.

Rectus abdominus
Long principle muscle that extends from the rib cage to pubis bone. The rectus bends your spine forward and stabilizes the chest and abdomen.

Internal obliques
Muscles that run diagonally opposite underneath the externals. The internals protect a weak point in the abdominal wall and assist in trunk rotation.

Biceps
Two-part muscle that runs along the top of the shoulder to the base of the forearm. Its primary functions are to lift the forearm and flex the elbow.

Deltoid
A thick, triangular muscle that covers the shoulder and gives it a rounded appearance. In addition to stabilizing the shoulder, the deltoid helps control the motion and functioning of the upper arm bone.

Brachioradialis
Forearm muscle that originates on the outside of the elbow joint and extends to the wrist. It helps stabilize and bend the elbow.

Triceps
Three-part muscle on the back of the arm that opposes the biceps and the brachialis. The triceps extends the forearm and protects the shoulder joint.

Brachialis
Slender muscle in the lower half of the upper arm. The muscle protects the elbow, and helps bend and rotate the forearm.

Extensor digitorum
A slender muscle along the back of the forearm that runs from the outside of the elbow to the wrist. The muscle works with two smaller extensor muscles to extend the hand and fingers.

The shoulder forms a base for the arm, the most versatile, mobile part of the body. In the upper arm, the biceps and triceps are arranged to give the forearm power to thrust and bend. The two muscles join at the elbow, a hinge-like joint that allows you to bend and straighten your arm, and also rotate your wrist and hand. Forearm muscles transmit power to the wrist, hands, and fingers. The wrist, despite its vulnerable location and delicate structure, is a relatively sturdy joint due to strong interlocking ligaments and tendons that run through the forearm. Unlike the shoulder, the wrist is rarely dislocated, but both it and the elbow may be strained by performing activities that involve repetitive or excessive use of the forearm.

The Thigh and Knee

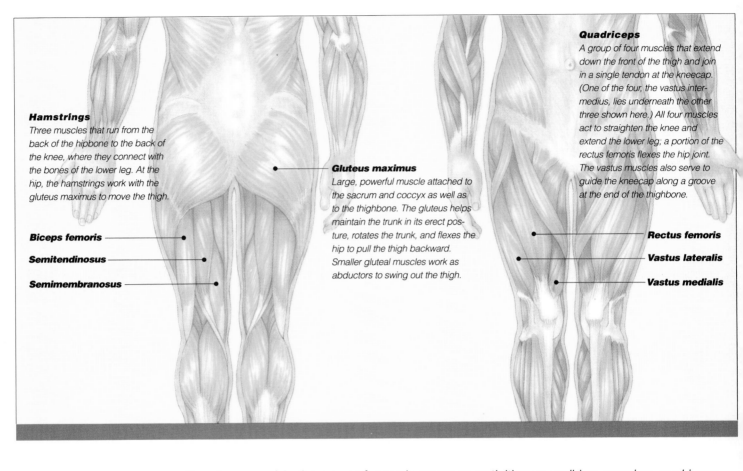

Hamstrings
Three muscles that run from the back of the hipbone to the back of the knee, where they connect with the bones of the lower leg. At the hip, the hamstrings work with the gluteus maximus to move the thigh.

Biceps femoris
Semitendinosus
Semimembranosus

Gluteus maximus
Large, powerful muscle attached to the sacrum and coccyx as well as to the thighbone. The gluteus helps maintain the trunk in its erect posture, rotates the trunk, and flexes the hip to pull the thigh backward. Smaller gluteal muscles work as abductors to swing out the thigh.

Quadriceps
A group of four muscles that extend down the front of the thigh and join in a single tendon at the kneecap. (One of the four, the vastus intermedius, lies underneath the other three shown here.) All four muscles act to straighten the knee and extend the lower leg; a portion of the rectus femoris flexes the hip joint. The vastus muscles also serve to guide the kneecap along a groove at the end of the thighbone.

Rectus femoris
Vastus lateralis
Vastus medialis

Your legs provide the power for such common activities as walking, running, and jumping, they absorb the cumulative impact of those activities, and they also bear much of your body weight. Not surprisingly, then, the leg's muscles and joints are strong and relatively stable. The thigh consists of the body's largest bone—the femur—which is girded on all sides by sets of powerful muscles that allow it to bend and straighten (also referred to as flexion and extension) as well as move outward and inward (or abduction and adduction). Some of these muscles are relatively long and participate in more than one type of movement—for example, the rectus femoris, a quadriceps muscle, flexes the hip and also extends the knee.

The hip is an exceptionally solid joint held intact largely by a round ball that is form-fitted into a deep socket. The knee stands midway between the hip and the shoulder in terms of stability. Although its ball-and-socket arrangement is not as secure as the hip's, the knee is held together by an elaborate system of strong ligaments and tendons that function like stays and pulleys. They not only allow the joint to twist, bend, and push, but also keep the kneecap properly aligned during these movements, and help the knee withstand the pressure of running and jumping.

By virtue of its engineering, the knee is the most complex joint in the body and also the one most frequently injured during exercise and athletic activities—mainly because it is subjected to a good deal of stress and because there are so many places where it is vulnerable. Strengthening the muscles in the thigh, particularly in the quadriceps, goes a long way toward preventing these problems.

Hip flexors and adductors
A diverse group of muscles, only some of which are indicated here, that extend from the hip to the lower spine or the thighbone. (The rectus femoris forms part of the hip flexors as well as the quadriceps.) In various combinations, the hip flexors bend and extend the hip, raise the thigh, and flex the knee (as when you move your knee toward your torso). The adductor muscles running along the thighbone also act to pull your legs in toward one another (as when you ride a horse).

Iliotibial band
A long thick tendon running down the outside of the thigh and connecting to the tibia, or shinbone. Acting almost like a ligament, this tendon helps mainly to stabilize the knee joint, but also acts in flexing and extending the knee.

Hip Joint

Tensor fascia latae

Abductor magnus

Adductor longus

Femur (thighbone)

Knee Joint

Patella (kneecap)

The Lower Leg

The calf, ankle, and foot are controlled largely by a series of muscles and tendons that function as a single biomechanical unit. Acting like a sling and lever system, the calf muscles, Achilles tendon, heel bone, and plantar fascia—which runs from the heel bone to the toes—work to lift or lower the heel for virtually any activity that involves locomotion. All of these parts in the lower leg are interconnected: for example, when you stand on your toes, you can feel the muscles in back of your calf doing most of the work. If you flex your foot, muscles along the front of the calf are brought into play.

Because of its structure, and because it absorbs the impact from activities like running and jumping, the lower leg is subject to more exercise-related injuries than any other area of the body. These problems range from bunions and blisters to stress fractures—microscopic cracks in bone—to sprained ankles, the most common sports injury of all. The construction of the ankle is straightforward compared to the knee or shoulder—the main ankle bone (the talus) fits into the concave surfaces of the lower leg bones (the tibia and fibula), and is held in place by a set of ligaments. But the borders of the leg bones are not parallel, which allows the ankle bone to roll more easily toward the outside of the joint. Moreover, the musculature around the ankle is relatively weak, affording minimum stability. Therefore, if you turn or twist your ankle, the ligaments often cannot withstand the stress, and they stretch or tear. An excellent defense against an ankle sprain is to strengthen and stretch the muscles in the lower leg.

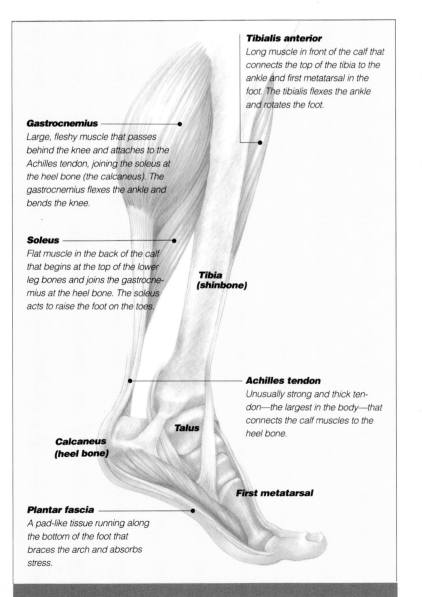

Tibialis anterior
Long muscle in front of the calf that connects the top of the tibia to the ankle and first metatarsal in the foot. The tibialis flexes the ankle and rotates the foot.

Gastrocnemius
Large, fleshy muscle that passes behind the knee and attaches to the Achilles tendon, joining the soleus at the heel bone (the calcaneus). The gastrocnemius flexes the ankle and bends the knee.

Soleus
Flat muscle in the back of the calf that begins at the top of the lower leg bones and joins the gastrocnemius at the heel bone. The soleus acts to raise the foot on the toes.

Tibia (shinbone)

Achilles tendon
Unusually strong and thick tendon—the largest in the body—that connects the calf muscles to the heel bone.

Talus

Calcaneus (heel bone)

First metatarsal

Plantar fascia
A pad-like tissue running along the bottom of the foot that braces the arch and absorbs stress.

ing reduces pressure on the lumbar disks by 70 percent, while unsupported sitting increases it by 40 percent.

The current trend in treating common backaches is to get people out of bed as soon as they can get up comfortably. While doctors traditionally recommended a week or two of bed rest, a study at the University of Texas Health Science Center at San Antonio found that two days in bed were usually sufficient for run-of-the-mill backaches and suggested longer bed rest only for disk problems. Moreover, shorter periods of bed rest tend to reduce the potentially adverse effects of prolonged bed rest, such as weakening of muscles from inactivity, that can lead to further back injury. (As patients bedridden for other reasons often discover, a couple weeks of bed rest can actually produce a painful back.)

Aspirin or ibuprofen will help reduce the intensity of pain and inhibit inflammation. It's also a good idea to begin walking as soon as possible. If you are overweight, try to lose weight by cutting calories from your diet and exercising more.

Seeing a doctor: be conservative

If the pain from backache or sciatica is severe, or it doesn't improve after two days, see a doctor. In addition, call your doctor if you have any of the following symptoms: pain, numbness, or tingling that radiates down an arm or leg; back pain that continues unabated when you're lying down; back pain after a fall or car accident; vomiting or fever associated with back pain; or backache in an elderly person or child. *Any of these may indicate a more serious problem.*

On your first visit, the doctor probably won't perform any high-tech tests but will simply examine you and take a history. The first thing physicians try is bed rest and painkillers. Your doctor may prescribe a stronger painkiller than aspirin and ibuprofen. Cold packs help some people, while a heating pad may feel more comforting to others. If your back improves, it's all right to sit up and begin to move around, so long as you avoid bending and any strenuous activity. Let your own discomfort level be your guide.

If you don't get better, your doctor may need to find out whether your problem comes from a herniated disk, an inflamed piriformis muscle (which can trigger sciatica), or other causes. X-rays may be called for, along with magnetic resonance imaging (MRI), a relatively new diagnostic technique that uses magnetic fields and radio waves. An MRI reveals spinal architecture accurately and in much more detail than an X-ray. But what may look like a trouble spot often is not. Abnormal-looking disks in the lumbar spine are almost as likely to show up in people with no back pain as in those with pain—that is, abnormalities that show up in MRIs are not necessarily related to back pain. Dr. Richard Deyo of the University of Washington, who heads a five-year study of back-pain treatment, has urged doctors not to rush to use MRIs to diagnose patients with sciatica or uncomplicated acute low-back pain (that is, pain not due to underlying illness or injury, and not involving nerve damage or paralysis).

Whatever the diagnosis, *opt for the most conservative treatments—rest, exercise, painkillers, and physical therapy.* Surgery may be an option in some persistent cases, but it is expensive, and requires a long period of recuperation. It is also frequently unsuccessful. Before considering surgery, you should exhaust all other forms of treatment. If your doctor suggests surgery, always get a second opinion.

Don't consent to traction, which has not been shown to be beneficial for low-

One reason protracted bed rest may be counterproductive for relieving low-back pain is that people tend to sit up in bed rather than lie flat. Unfortunately, pressure on the spinal disks is greater when sitting than when lying down or even standing. In addition to limiting bed rest to a day or two, most back experts also recommend that people begin to walk as soon as the acute pain subsides.

Exercises for a Better Back

The key to a pain-free back is strong, supple abdominal and lower back muscles, which can be developed through calisthenics and stretching routines. The following exercises can form the core of a back-strengthening program. They should be done at least four times a week. Start any exercise program slowly, especially if you have ever had back pain. Stop if you feel any pain. Avoid exercises that increase the stress on the spine, such as straight-leg toe touches or backward bends. And always warm up and stretch before working out.

Begin an exercise routine *before* you feel any back pain. If your back currently hurts, do not do these or any other exercises. What type of exercise is best for people with back pain remains controversial, so before beginning an exercise program you should first consult a therapist.

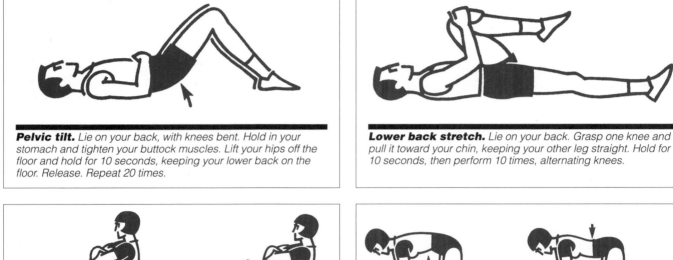

Pelvic tilt. *Lie on your back, with knees bent. Hold in your stomach and tighten your buttock muscles. Lift your hips off the floor and hold for 10 seconds, keeping your lower back on the floor. Release. Repeat 20 times.*

Lower back stretch. *Lie on your back. Grasp one knee and pull it toward your chin, keeping your other leg straight. Hold for 10 seconds, then perform 10 times, alternating knees.*

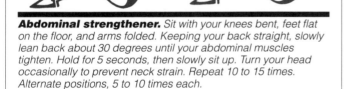

Abdominal strengthener. *Sit with your knees bent, feet flat on the floor, and arms folded. Keeping your back straight, slowly lean back about 30 degrees until your abdominal muscles tighten. Hold for 5 seconds, then slowly sit up. Turn your head occasionally to prevent neck strain. Repeat 10 to 15 times. Alternate positions, 5 to 10 times each.*

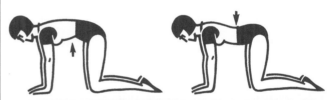

Cat stretch. *Start on all fours, with hands and knees shoulder-width apart. Slowly curve your lower back downward, pressing your stomach down and lifting your head. Then gently arch your back and lower your head. Hold each position for 5 seconds. Alternate positions, 5 to 10 times each.*

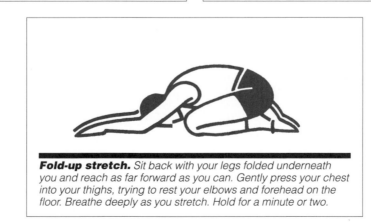

Fold-up stretch. *Sit back with your legs folded underneath you and reach as far forward as you can. Gently press your chest into your thighs, trying to rest your elbows and forehead on the floor. Breathe deeply as you stretch. Hold for a minute or two.*

back pain. Some studies have shown short-term benefits of chiropractic care for acute low-back pain (see page 436). If you decide to consult a chiropractor, ask your doctor for a referral.

Remember, any resumption of activity must be gradual, since your back needs time to heal completely. Once the pain is gone, take it easy for a week, and avoid heavy chores and sports for at least two weeks. If you wish, continue taking aspirin or ibuprofen to reduce pain. However, do not use a corset or back brace unless your doctor prescribes it.

Back Pain and Sports

Regular exercise is essential for maintaining a strong back and protecting it from injury. Exercise also promotes weight control and good posture, and helps reduce muscle tension —important factors in maintaining a healthy back. Sports can be excellent back conditioners, too, but some forms of physical activity carry high risks of back injury, particularly if carelessly performed. The best way to avoid back injuries is to play regularly and stay within your physical limits. Begin any new activity gradually, and supplement it with exercises specifically for strengthening the back. Remember, always warm up, stretch, and cool down to minimize any risks to your back.

Good for the back

The following sports reduce stress on the back and, in some instances, help tone and stretch key muscles.

Walking. This is the perfect exercise for promoting a healthy back. According to Swedish back expert Dr. Alf Nachemson, walking puts less strain on the spine than does unsupported sitting, and only a little more than plain standing.

Swimming. Since the water supports the spine, thus relieving pressure on it, swimming is the best activity for relieving back pain. The back stroke and side stroke are best for the back; avoid the butterfly and breast stroke, which cause you to arch your back.

Cycling. This is an excellent aerobic exercise if you have back problems, provided you maintain an upright posture.

Jogging. The great impact running places on your body is normally absorbed by your shoes, feet, legs, and spinal disks. Jogging with poorly cushioned shoes, on hills, or on hard surfaces increases the jarring impact on the back. If you are in good condition and have a smooth stride, jogging will probably not put your back at risk. Still, runners with bad backs should swim and/or do exercises to strengthen muscles in the back and abdomen.

Rowing. Proper posture is vital, since rowing places great stress on the lower back. If done correctly, rowing can strengthen muscles in the lower back. Always keep your back straight; avoid hunching over or swaying.

High-risk sports

Activities that involve lifting, twisting, arching of the spine, sudden starts and stops, and falls or collisions with other players are most risky for people with back problems.

Golf. One survey found that 25 percent of golf pros suffer from lower back injuries. If you have a weak back, you may have to learn to minimize the twisting movement of your swing. Teeing the ball, removing the ball from the cup, and prolonged putting practice all involve bending forward at the waist, which strains the lower spine. When bending, keep your knees bent and try to keep your back straight.

Tennis and racquet sports. These activities can strain the back because of their twisting and quick stop-and-go movements. Work with a pro to modify your serve and backhand if you are straining your back.

Bowling. Lifting a heavy weight while twisting and bending your upper body can easily aggravate back problems. Try to develop a smooth delivery, and don't use too heavy a ball.

Football, basketball, baseball. Because they involve twisting, jarring movements, jumping, bending, and, often, contact with other players, these sports are potentially hazardous for a weak back.

Weight lifting. If not done properly, this can put immense stress on the lower back. The worst thing you can do to your back is to bend over with your legs straight, twist to one side, and pick up something heavy like a dumbbell or bag of groceries. Keep your back as straight as possible when hefting a weight, and bend your knees so that your legs help you lift it. Avoid jerky movements. A weight lifting belt may help maintain correct, back-preserving posture when hefting a heavy load.

Chiropractors

According to one estimate, about 5 percent of Americans see chiropractors regularly, and the majority like what they get. Yet many lay people and physicians think chiropractic is worthless, fanciful, or even harmful. Indeed, chiropractors and the medical profession have waged verbal and economic war on one another for many years.

Chiropractic (a noun derived from Greek *cheir*, meaning "hand," and *praktikis*, meaning "practical") was founded in 1895—about the same time that modern medical schools came into being. Chiropractic was based on the theory that subluxations (that is, minute misalignments of the vertebrae) are the source of all illness, and that spinal manipulation can therefore prevent or cure all illness. However, many chiropractors no longer endorse this "single source" theory or base their practice on it.

Indeed, one problem in sorting out the claims and counterclaims about chiropractic is that chiropractors now represent such a wide range of practices and treatments. Within the profession, there are the "straights," or old-line practitioners, whose theoretical base is subluxation and who may obtain frequent X-rays and perform manipulations. The "mixers" may adopt other approaches. Some promote health fads like iridology and hair analysis, as well as prescribing and then selling vitamin supplements and "glandular" treatments of dubious value. Some look upon themselves as family doctors—and as the only health provider you'll ever need. Others work with medical doctors, referring patients and taking referrals.

Some newer-minded chiropractors have voiced criticisms of older theories and practices. The most progressive new group, the National Association for Chiropractic Medicine (NACM) has disavowed the subluxation theory. NACM members limit themselves to treating low-back pain and are likely to work in tandem with medical doctors—considering themselves partners of the medical profession rather than competitors or antagonists.

Recently, the RAND Corporation reviewed all existing scientific evidence and found that chiropractic can be effective in treating acute back pain when no serious neurological symptoms are present. But these findings were limited—in the RAND study, for example, only patients with acute low-back pain did better with chiropractic treatment. Those with chronic low-back pain, sciatica, or neurologic involvement did not do so well. Another review published in the *British Medical Journal* found that evidence supporting chiropractic treatment was not conclusive.

Evaluating practitioners. Chiropractic, like other professions, is evolving. One reason people like chiropractors is that they seem to take more time with patients, and the treatment is usually hands-on. If you have acute low-back pain and wish to see a chiropractor, here are a few pointers to keep in mind:

• Be wary of any chiropractor who claims that subluxations are the root of most illnesses. Similarly, be wary of practitioners—and there are many—who claim to cure everything from bedwetting, chronic fatigue syndrome, and migraines to menstrual cramps, cancer, and heart disease. A recent promotional piece from one New York chiropractor, for instance, claims that by "correcting spinal nerve stress" he can "turn on your inner doctor" and cure any of these ailments and more. The ad goes on to say, though, that chiropractors don't "treat disease." This is double talk.

• Be wary of any chiropractor who sells you the supplements and nutritional treatments he prescribes. Physicians are not allowed to sell the medicines they pre-

---

Ice or heat?

Though icing is best for many types of injury, there is some disagreement when it comes to the back. Most physical therapists now recommend icing immediately after a sudden, wrenching back injury that causes localized pain. This can both relieve a spasm and minimize swelling. Ice for ten to twenty minutes several times a day during the first forty-eight hours. On the other hand, for a widespread backache that gradually sets in hours after an injury, or for chronic back discomfort, a hot bath or moist heat may be soothing and can promote healing. The ultimate criterion is what works for you: if cold therapy feels uncomfortable or doesn't offer relief, try heat. (For more information on ice and heat, see pages 423-424.)

scribe, and for good reason. Such regulations were designed to protect patients.

•Don't agree to full-spine or full-body X-rays. According to the chiropractors who now work with the National Council Against Health Fraud (a California-based physician group), full-spine X-rays have little or no diagnostic value and expose patients to unnecessary and potentially dangerous amounts of radiation.

•When dealing with chiropractors, as with any practitioner, it pays to be well informed and to protect yourself. As you would with a medical doctor, question a chiropractor about treatments. Don't believe anybody who promises miracles, or who asks you to sign a "treatment contract" obligating you to show up every week or every month to "maintain" your health.

Preventing Back Pain

Because most backaches are due at least in part to excessive strain or to weak or tense muscles, there is much you can do to prevent them. In more than half of all cases back pain eventually recurs, so it's a good idea to consider the following preventive measures, especially if you have a history of back problems:

Extra weight. A paunch can strain back muscles, distort posture, and overly compress the disks in the lower back. Not surprisingly, then, most obese people have chronic back problems. Excess weight, particularly if it has been recently gained, puts increased strain on back muscles and ligaments. Being pregnant can have a similar adverse effect because it alters your center of gravity.

Poor posture. Sitting and standing puts considerable pressure on the lower back. Correct posture keeps the head and chest high, neck straight, pelvis forward, and stomach and buttocks tucked in.

Sleeping. Don't lie on your stomach, since that makes the stomach muscles sag and increases sway back. Instead, lie on your side with your knees bent to relieve pressure on the disks. For the same reason, if you lie on your back, keep your knees slightly bent by putting a pillow under them. For most people, the ideal mattress has firm inner support but adequate surface cushioning. If your mattress is too soft, insert a board under it.

Exercise. Regular exercise is vital to the health of your back. Calisthenics and stretching routines (such as those on page 434) can help strengthen the back. In addition, low-impact activities like walking, swimming (but not the butterfly or breast stroke, which can put excessive strain on the lower back), and cycling (with an upright posture) are good for the back. For information on the effect of other sports on the back, see the box on page 435.

Lifting and carrying. Bending to pick up an object puts maximum strain on your back and is probably the number-one cause of backaches. When you lift, bend at the knees, not at the waist, making your leg muscles do most of the work. To pick up something heavy, squat with your legs apart, tighten your stomach muscles, keep your back straight, and hold the object close to your body. Better yet, push a heavy object instead of lifting it. Pulling is more likely to injure your back. When carrying a heavy load, don't arch your back or twist your body—try to let your arms and abdominal muscles bear the weight. Because a heavy purse or briefcase can pull your back out of alignment, alternate the load from side to side.

Dress. Prolonged use of tight pants and girdles may induce weak abdominal muscles and result in back trouble. Avoid high heels since they tend to increase the curvature of the back and increase the risk of a fall.

Good Posture

Sitting and standing put considerable pressure on the lower back; standing exerts five times more pressure than lying down, and sitting, surprisingly, is even more strenuous. So posture is not just a matter of appearance—though good posture does indeed improve appearance, as well as helping you project self-confidence and dignity. Not only will good posture help you mentally and psychologically, it can also help prevent back and neck problems. Good posture is worth achieving, just for the aches and pains it may prevent.

As long as people aren't actually in pain, they tend to forget how delicately their backs are engineered. The three spinal curves (neck, upper, lower) need to be kept in balanced alignment, and for this, strong, flexible muscles are important. Poor posture can strain both muscles and ligaments, making you more vulnerable to injury—as well as complicating such everyday tasks as carrying groceries or even sitting at a desk. An improperly aligned spine may narrow the space between vertebrae, thereby increasing the risk of compressed nerves.

Poor posture may be caused by many factors, including previous injuries, disease, poor muscle tone, and emotional stress. A sedentary lifestyle can reduce muscle tone and strength and lead to bad posture. Sore, aching feet have a negative effect on posture, too. (Foot pain may mean simply that you're choosing the wrong shoes. Or you may need special supports—orthotic devices—in your shoes and an evaluation by a podiatrist. For more about foot care, see page 444.) One very important factor is habit. Contrary to what some people believe, "straightening up" now and then isn't enough. Retraining postural habits takes time and effort.

Standing. Take a look in the mirror for these signs: a protruding abdomen, slumped or rounded shoulders, or swayback (an excessive forward curve in the lower back). Any of these could be putting extra pressure on the muscles and ligaments of your spine. *A slight* hollow in the lower back is natural and desirable; in fact, good standing posture maintains this and the two other natural curves that are visible from a side view—a gentle forward curve in the neck area and backward curve in the upper back. The goal is to avoid exaggerating these curves. The "military" stance, with chest thrust forward and shoulders and derriere pushed way back, isn't desirable, since it creates a sway back.

•Think tall. Simply stand with your

Bending and lifting

Lifting a heavy object from the floor puts enormous strain on your back, but good posture while you're lifting can prevent injury. Always bend your knees, so that you reduce your distance from the ground (and hence the load on your back). You can squat or go down on one knee, as well. Hold the object close to your body, and lift it only chest high. Rise slowly. Use your legs to help with the lifting rather than your back. Avoid twisting your torso while lifting any object. If you must turn while holding something heavy, turn with your feet.

Standing Tall

A simple test can make you more aware of what constitutes good posture and help improve your spinal flexibility. Stand in a normal, relaxed posture with your back against a wall—upper back and buttocks touching the wall. Slip your hand into the space between your lower back and the wall; it should slide in easily and almost touch both your back and the wall. If there's extra space, you may have a sway back. To correct it, imagine that a string is tied to the top of your head and is pulling you straight up; then tuck in your abdomen and tilt your hips so that the space between your lower back and the wall is lessened. When you walk away from the wall, try to maintain the stance and the mental image of the string.

head held over your shoulders, your chin parallel to the floor, and your neck straight. Your shoulders should be level without any slumping, and in front your chest, waist, and hips should all line up.

•Practice tightening your abdominal muscles and flattening your stomach. To locate the muscles you're trying to exercise, clasp your hands and press against the abdomen as you slowly draw in the muscles, flattening them as much as possible. Hold the position for a few seconds, then relax. Repeat three or four times, and also on occasion throughout the day. Without the hand movement, this is an almost invisible exercise that you can do anywhere.

•When standing for long periods, minimize stress on the lower back by putting one foot on a low stool or other stable object. Frequently shift your weight from one leg to another. To relax, bend over and let your head, neck, shoulders, and arms hang down briefly.

•Don't stand too long in one position.

Sitting. The extra pressure that sitting exerts on your lower back comes from the upper body shifting forward, forcing the back muscles to strain to hold you upright. Slouching increases the pressure on your lower back to about *ten to fifteen times* as much as when you're lying down. And hunching over tenses the muscles in the neck and upper back. Good sitting posture involves the same slight forward curve in your lower back that's also the key to good standing posture. The following steps can help improve your sitting posture:

•Choose a chair that firmly supports your lower back (for long periods of sitting, choose a straight chair). The chair shouldn't be heavily padded, since that can cause excess curving of your back. It should fit under your desk or table so that you maintain your upright posture (see illustration, page 440). Chair armrests are a plus, too, since you can support some of your weight on them, especially when you shift positions in the chair. Propping up reading matter also helps.

•Sit firmly back in the chair (rather than on the edge) with your shoulders against the chair back, your chest lifted, and your upper back straight. A rolled up towel or small lumbar pillow can provide extra support. When working at a desk or table, bring your chair close enough that you needn't lean over. Your feet should touch the floor comfortably—if they don't, rest them on a small stool or telephone book. Sitting with your knees slightly higher than your hips can reduce excess curvature in your lower back. Crossing your legs occasionally can be a good idea, too. Change sitting positions frequently, and get up to stretch and move around every half hour, if possible.

•If you're typing or working at a computer, make sure any work you're copying is at a comfortable level. Looking up or down for long periods can put stress on your neck, shoulders, and upper-back muscles.

•When sitting, as when standing, remember the string pulling up on the top of your head. Sit tall. It's also a good idea to practice the pelvic tilt from time to time and to tighten your abdominal muscles occasionally, as recommended for standing.

•For driving, position your seat so that you can easily reach the wheel and get your foot on the brake and accelerator. Many seats adjust for height, so try to have your knees slightly higher than your hips. Change the seat position occasionally (tilting slightly forward or back) if you're driving for long periods. Stop every couple of hours and stretch or walk around. If your seat provides inadequate support for your lower back, try a rolled up towel or lumbar roll. A seat pad may also help.

Frequently repositioning your hands on the wheel can take some strain off your upper back and neck muscles.

•When driving, too, remember the string on top of your head and practice good sitting posture. Avoid slumping forward or sitting in a twisted position (for example, with your elbow resting heavily on the window sill or armrest). Maintaining good driving posture can have positive effects on your back, as well as on the way you drive.

Desk Stress

Anyone who sits at a desk or computer terminal all day is subject to the physical stress induced by static as opposed to dynamic muscular effort. Static effort, in which muscle groups are contracted for long periods in an unvarying position, may obstruct blood flow, possibly inducing fatigue in oxygen-deprived muscles. It generally constrains the way you hold your back, arms, head, and shoulders—encouraging overall poor posture. Think a moment about the position in which most desks and chairs force you to work: perched on the edge of your seat, leaning forward, your neck bent as you scrutinize documents, your shoulders hunched as you type. All of this requires strenuous static effort, and causes office workers to complain about back, knee, neck, and shoulder pain, usually in that order.

A properly chosen chair and desk or work table can go far to alleviate aches and pains due to the strain of static effort. Much of this misery is due to poorly designed office furniture: desks and work surfaces that are too low or too high, chairs that are at the wrong height and whose backs fail to offer support where it's needed. Adjustability can provide the first line of protection against static-effort fatigue. A study of AT&T operators showed that switching to easily adjustable tables and chairs resulted in a significant decrease in reported discomforts, particularly in the shoulders, back, and legs. The table used in the study could be adjusted for both computer-screen and keyboard height; chair heights could easily be adjusted while the occupant remained seated. Similarly, a study of computer operators showed that adjustable terminal heights and flexible backrests helped reduce pressure on the spine.

If you often feel discomfort or muscle strain after long hours at your desk and chair, measure their dimensions and compare them to those illustrated below. Adjust them where possible. If you are shopping for a desk or chair designed to minimize stress, look for these features and optimal dimensions.

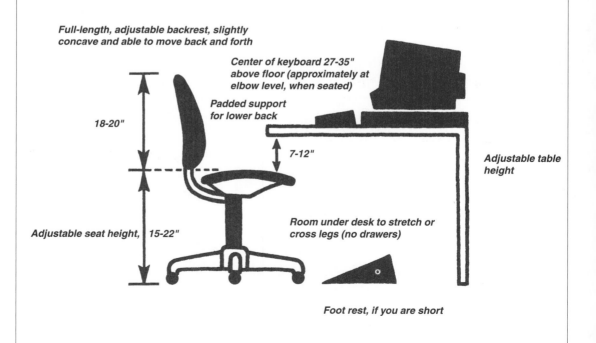

Full-length, adjustable backrest, slightly concave and able to move back and forth

Center of keyboard 27-35" above floor (approximately at elbow level, when seated)

Padded support for lower back

18-20"

7-12"

Adjustable table height

Adjustable seat height, 15-22"

Room under desk to stretch or cross legs (no drawers)

Foot rest, if you are short

Other tips and strategies

•Choose a firm mattress to support your spine. Try to avoid sleeping on your stomach—it's better to be on your side with your knees bent. But if you do sleep on your stomach, choose a large pillow that gives your shoulders some support. Whatever your customary sleeping posture, make sure your pillow supports your neck in a straight position. This may prevent neck pain and the sore muscles that can interfere with good posture when you're awake.

•Maintain a healthy weight. Obesity is hard on the muscles in your back and abdomen and can cause bad posture.

•Avoid high-heels and platform shoes, except for short periods. For daily wear, especially when you're on your feet, make sure your shoes fit and offer good support. For exercise, including walking, invest in a shoe that not only fits but supports your foot. High heels throw the back out of line and adversely affect posture.

•Get regular exercise. Besides promoting weight loss and better general health, exercise tones and strengthens the muscles that are important to good posture. Walking is one of the best ways to improve posture.

•Consult your physician or an orthopedist if you have chronic neck or back pain caused by poor posture, and your own efforts to correct bad posture don't succeed. Physical therapy, as prescribed by a doctor, can be helpful. Many kinds of movement therapies focus on posture.

Posture and back-care products

One way people try to improve their posture and/or protect their backs is by using one of a variety of backrests, special pillows, and other devices now available in orthopedic-supply stores and catalogues. (Certain back products, especially those that immobilize the spine, should be prescribed by your doctor or other qualified practitioner and must be specially fitted.) Choosing an off-the-shelf back-care product is largely a matter of personal preferences and comfort. There's no scientific research showing, for instance, that a lumbar roll is better than a larger backrest, or vice versa. In fact, there's a great deal of disagreement among back experts (such as orthopedists, physical therapists, chiropractors, and product designers) about what's best for backs in general. Since backaches tend to be idiosyncratic, no single piece of advice or gadget will work for everyone, and for some backache sufferers no device will help.

Backrests. Sitting actually puts more pressure on your spinal disks than standing; slumping or hunching over in a chair is particularly straining. A chair that supports your lower back is essential. Backrests can also help encourage good sitting posture, especially when the chair is not adjustable. Backrests come in many sizes and shapes. Some contoured models are made for use in cars; others are inflatable and can be conveniently taken into planes, trains, or theaters.

Lumbar rolls. These cylindrical foam pillows (4 to 5 inches in diameter) are placed directly in the small of your back for support when seated. Many have straps for attaching to a chair.

Seat wedges. When placed on a seat, one of these fabric-covered pieces of foam can tilt you forward and prevent you from sinking into an unsupportive chair. You can also place it behind your back to adjust the angle of a chair's backrest.

Neck supports. These pillows wrap around the neck and thus help keep your head upright and your cervical disks properly aligned. There are inflatable models.

Back schools

Some of the best places to learn self-care for your back are the hundreds of "back schools" that have sprung up around the country. They range from classes set up by hospitals, corporations, and YMCAs to post-surgical rehabilitation groups at leading spine centers. Most are run by a physical therapist, often in conjunction with a physician. The general concept gets high ratings from back specialists, since such programs are inexpensive, safe, and, when complied with faithfully, can be highly effective.

The typical back school includes three or four weekly sessions plus a follow-up meeting. You'll learn how the back works and analyze your living, sleeping, and work habits and their effect on your back. Most important, the program should help you design an exercise program suited to your physical condition and lifestyle. For information on back schools near you, check with your doctor, a local hospital, or an orthopedist or physical therapist in your area.

Slant boards. These angled boards, when placed on desks, help prevent neck strain and slouching while you read or write. Most are adjustable.

Pillows. Bad sleeping position is a common cause of aches and pains. If you have a stiff neck or shoulder most mornings, try a different pillow. New pillows can be expensive, and no one pillow is going to answer everybody's needs. Ideally, your neck should be straight most of the night. Some foam pillows are too high and firm, or too bouncy. Some down pillows are too soft and flat. If you generally sleep on your back or side, you might benefit from a "cervical roll," a small round pillow for neck support. This can be used by itself or in addition to your regular pillow. If your mattress is very firm and you sleep on your side, you may need a thicker pillow than you would on a mattress that allows your shoulder to sink into it. If you sleep on your stomach most of the night, try a soft, oversized pillow that goes under your chest but supports your head and neck. Try sleeping with different pillows or combinations of pillows. Or simply try a rolled-up towel as a cervical pillow. Some people prefer no pillow at all.

Bed wedges. These help you stay comfortable while reading or watching TV in bed. You can also use them to elevate your knees to relieve pressure on the disks in your lower back if you sleep on your back.

Bed boards. You can firm up a sagging mattress (a frequent contributor to back pain) by placing a board between it and the box spring. Lightweight folding models are available for travel.

"Back-saving" tools. One type of snow shovel or rake has a bent handle that allows you to stand nearly upright while working, thus reducing stress on the lower back. Lightweight shovels can also help. Some shoehorns have an extra-long handle so you don't have to bend over when putting on shoes.

Shopping tips:

• If you have chronic back pain, discuss your options with your doctor, who may direct you to sources of back-care products.

• Try out different devices, models, and sizes in the store, if possible. Lumbar rolls, for instance, come in various sizes and degrees of firmness.

• Expensive isn't always better. Some of these products are really quite simple, and low-tech substitutes may work just as well. For instance, you can try a rolled-up towel instead of a ready-made lumbar roll, or a piece of foam rather than a fancy car seat or seat wedge.

Relieving neck tension

The head of an adult weighs ten to twelve pounds, and it's the job of the neck and shoulder muscles to hold it upright as well as allow it easy movement. No wonder these muscles sometimes develop kinks and become painful. Poor posture is the most common cause of neck pain. If you habitually thrust your chin forward or tilt your head to one side, your muscles may start aching under the strain. But many daily activities can also stress your neck and shoulder muscles. How to avoid neck stress? One key is to work on your posture. Here are some other corrective actions you can take:

• Whether in a movie or an airline terminal, don't stare for long periods at screens above eye level. Avoid the first few rows of a movie house or theater. When you watch television, make sure the screen is at or below eye level.

• When you sleep, on your back or side, use a small synthetic or feather pillow

Neck Stretches

If you are prone to neck pain, start a regular routine of neck stretches and exercises; those below will get you started. If you feel pain when exercising your neck muscles, cut back on repetitions and resistance. Stop if you feel any sharp pain or one that radiates down your arms. If you've had any serious injury to your neck, such as a whiplash, or if you have persistent neck pain, consult your doctor before beginning a neck-exercise program.

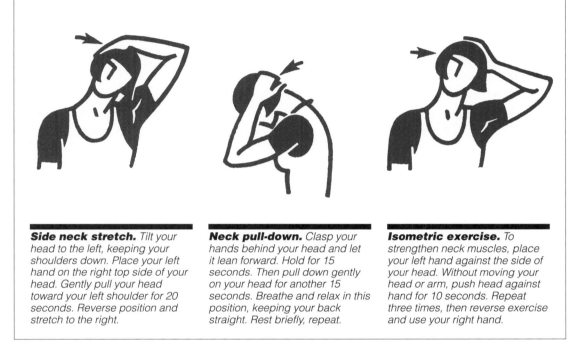

Side neck stretch. *Tilt your head to the left, keeping your shoulders down. Place your left hand on the right top side of your head. Gently pull your head toward your left shoulder for 20 seconds. Reverse position and stretch to the right.*

Neck pull-down. *Clasp your hands behind your head and let it lean forward. Hold for 15 seconds. Then pull down gently on your head for another 15 seconds. Breathe and relax in this position, keeping your back straight. Rest briefly, repeat.*

Isometric exercise. *To strengthen neck muscles, place your left hand against the side of your head. Without moving your head or arm, push head against hand for 10 seconds. Repeat three times, then reverse exercise and use your right hand.*

under your head and neck. When sleeping on your back, make sure your head is not pushed forward toward your chest by your pillow. You can use a rolled-up towel instead of a pillow, if you prefer. Keep your neck and shoulders covered when sleeping in a drafty or chilly room. Feeling cold may cause you to hunch up and the resulting muscle tension can produce a neck ache.

•Don't read or write with your chin on your chest, or your neck tilted backward. If you watch TV in bed, don't lie on your stomach.

•When cycling, make sure your bike helmet fits. A helmet that slips back and forth can cause neck strain. See that your handlebars are at a comfortable distance—if they're out of reach, you'll assume a neck-straining position. You can move your seat forward to correct this or you can get a repair shop to install a different handlebar stem.

•When doing any kind of activity that puts stress on the neck—cycling, driving, or typing—for long periods, stop at intervals to stretch.

•Don't use your shoulder to cradle the telephone receiver, especially during long conversations.

•Routinely perform the neck exercises in the box above.

Protecting Your Feet

The foot is a structural marvel, consisting of some twenty-eight bones laced together with many layers of ligaments, tendons, and muscles. It functions as a stable structure when we stand on it, yet adapts to any kind of terrain as we walk. The foot is built to absorb shock. Like a suspension bridge, the arching bones of the foot (the metatarsals) distribute weight from the heel bones toward the toes. The sole is designed for protection: it is thicker than other skin, and beneath it lies a thick pad of fat and fibrous tissue known as the plantar fascia.

The average person takes 5,000 to 10,000 steps a day, mostly on hard surfaces; over a lifetime, that's equal to several hikes around the earth. The impact of each step you take exerts a force about 50 percent greater than your body weight upon your feet. Running or jumping more than triples this impact.

It's no wonder that three out of five adults have painful feet, and accept it as a fact of life, according to a Gallup survey. Many common foot problems develop as a result of foot abnormalities (such as flat feet and idiosyncrasies of gait and stance) that are often inherited. Some medical conditions such as obesity, poor circulation, arthritis, or diabetes can cause or intensify foot problems,

At the same time, much of the everyday agony people experience stems from ill-fitting shoes, socks, and stockings, or from footgear that is not appropriate to the activity it is being used for. This kind of foot pain is preventable. Moreover, many problems of the feet that do develop can be treated effectively at home.

Proper footwear: the key to healthy feet

Your first line of defense is to buy shoes that fit; ill-fitting shoes, it is thought, cause 80 percent of all foot problems. Besides causing corns, bunions, nail deformities, and other problems, painful shoes can alter your gait.

Yet a good fit can be hard to find, and the problem has gotten worse because about three quarters of all shoes sold in the United States today are imports—often from countries where the ethnic mix is not as diverse as it is here. While American-made shoes, in their heyday, offered the largest selection of sizes and widths found anywhere in the world, the range of available lasts (the metal, wooden or plastic forms over which the shoes are made) and sizes are not as varied in imported shoes. Inexpensive imports in particular tend to be made in one wide width.

Another complicating factor is that feet are as individual as fingerprints, and no two (not even your own two) are exactly the same. Your feet continue to change throughout your adult life. Your shoe size may change when your weight or your pattern of activity changes. The pads on your feet get thinner as you grow older.

While numerical sizes can serve as a guide, they aren't what matter most. More important to your foot and to your comfort is the shape. Sneakers, loafers, moccasins, and most men's shoes are made on a straight last (a shoemaker's mold), by far the most comfortable. Many shoes, however, are shaped for style. Elegant as they may look, these can cause problems if worn over a long period.

As well as fitting your foot, your shoe should fit your life. If you stand up several hours each day, or if you walk or run on hard surfaces, you need shoes with a thick sole and a soft upper. If you run for exercise, you need a running shoe. But practicality need not rule every shoe decision. Most people also want dress shoes, which is fine, so long as they fit.

Because stylish shoes for women are often high-heeled and pointy-toed, women have far more foot problems than men. If you wear high heels, save them for special occasions or times of day when you know you'll be sitting down—at your desk, for example. Then change into walking shoes for other activities. If you wear high heels most of the time, your calf muscles may ache when you do put on low heels.

Finally, if you buy a pair of shoes that prove painful, don't wear them. Throw them out and buy another pair. And if the heels of your shoes wear down, replace them or throw away the worn shoes. Unevenly worn heels can decrease foot stability and make you tired.

Shopping tips

• Ask to have both feet measured (the metal Brannock device is more accurate than a wooden ruler) and always put your full weight on the foot being measured. Try the size that fits the larger foot. Remember, sizes indicate very little: size 8½ C in one brand may be a 9 B in another. Imported shoes are likely to run small.

• Try to shop for shoes in the middle of a normal day, not early in the morning, since your feet swell as the day progresses due to friction, heat, and use.

• Wear the kind of socks or stockings that you intend to wear with the shoes. Avoid socks and stockings that constrict your feet or that bunch up.

• When testing new shoes, stand on one foot at a time. Wiggle your toes. Stand on tiptoe. The shoe should bend where your foot bends.

• Never buy a shoe with the idea of breaking it in. Your foot may alter in an uncomfortable shoe, but the shoe won't.

• Check to see that you have one-half inch of space between the end of your big toe and the tip of the shoe.

• Make sure the widest part of your foot—the metatarsal joint—fits comfortably in the widest part of the shoe.

(See page 242 for information on choosing athletic shoes.)

Common Foot Problems

Ingrown toenails

Perhaps the most common of all foot afflictions, ingrown toenails usually occur on the big toe. The edge of the nail cuts into the soft toe tissue, causing swelling and redness. Besides being painful, ingrown toenails can lead to infection. They have two causes: tight shoes or stockings that press the nail into the tissue and improper trimming of the toenail. When trimming toenails, follow these directions to avoid ingrown toenails:

• Use heavy long-handled scissors or nail clippers to cut the nail neatly.

• Never try to tear away the nail with your fingers.

• Always trim the nail straight across—the end of the nail should be a square, not a half moon. Don't trim too close. Finish the edge with an emery board or nail file, and clean the grooves with an orange stick.

If you've got flat feet and they don't bother you, there's certainly no reason to think of them as disadvantageous in any way. A low arch or the absence of one does not mean you're a clumsy walker or that you'll necessarily suffer if you take long hikes or engage in vigorous exercise. Feet, like hands and noses, come in all shapes and sizes. Whatever the height of your arches, make sure your shoes fit your activities as well as your feet. If you do suffer chronic discomfort or pain in your hips, legs, knees, or feet, you should consult your doctor or a podiatrist.

Contrary to myth, making a V-shaped cut in the middle of your toenail won't make it grow toward the middle and thus won't prevent an ingrown toenail.

Treatment. If you have an ingrown toenail, try to determine and eliminate the cause. Soak the toe in warm water to soften the nail, and then press a few strands of absorbent cotton under the nail to keep it from cutting the skin. Do this several times a day, if necessary, until the nail grows out. Wear open shoes, if possible. If pus, bleeding, or painful swelling occurs, get medical advice.

Athlete's foot

Prevention is the best treatment for athlete's foot, which basically means keeping your feet clean and dry, especially in hot weather. Despite the popular name for this usually harmless infection, it can develop in places other than locker rooms or gym showers. The fungus that causes it thrives best in warm, moist, enclosed environments: snug, poorly ventilated shoes and damp, sweaty socks provide an ideal breeding ground. (Your chances of catching athlete's foot from another person is slight, but the fungus can be spread by shed fragments of affected skin.) .

You'll know when athlete's foot strikes. Your toes, soles, or sides of your feet will itch, tiny blisters may appear, and there may be red scaling in these areas and between your toes.

Treatment and Prevention. The usual treatment is one of the over-the-counter antifungal preparations. Things should clear up in a week or two. If they don't, or if the area turns red and swollen, see your doctor.

Some people are more susceptible to the fungus than others. If you are susceptible, follow these commonsense rules, especially when you're very active and your feet tend to perspire:

•Keep your feet clean. Daily washing with soap and water is a good idea, but be sure you dry thoroughly, especially between the toes (you can use a hair dryer on low heat).

•When you can, go barefoot. Next best thing to bare feet is sandals. But when you wear shoes, wear socks, too—preferably ones that "wick" away moisture and keep your feet dry. Change your socks daily.

•Choose shoes that let your feet breathe and don't wear the same pair every day. Air them between wearings.

•Cornstarch or baking powder can also help keep feet dry; if you already have athlete's foot, try an antifungal powder. An antifungal solution or ointment may also help against athlete's foot.

Toenail fungus

The same fungus responsible for athlete's foot or other related yeastlike fungi can grow under and within a toenail given the right environment—such as sweaty socks, shoes with poor ventilation, or a bandage worn around a toe for an extended period of time. Less commonly, trauma to the nail may also increase the risk of fungal growth. The fungus may cause the toenail to thicken and become brittle, discolored, and distorted.

Treatment. There is no sure way to prevent the growth of toenail fungus, but keeping your feet dry and clean may help. The same guidelines for preventing athlete's foot apply here: dry your feet completely after bathing, and wear dry socks and well-ventilated shoes.

Plantar warts

Plantar warts—so named because they grow on the sole, also called the plantar surface of the foot—are flat and light-colored with tiny dots inside. Like all warts, they are caused by a virus and are slightly contagious. They can be painless or quite painful.

If a wart is small and doesn't bother you, just leave it alone. Such warts usually disappear by themselves, typically within two years. If your wart stays small but doesn't go away, you can try an over-the-counter wart remover, usually containing salicylic acid. But again, follow directions carefully and avoid getting it on the surrounding skin. If that doesn't work, or if the wart grows or spreads, consult a podiatrist or dermatologist. Never try to cut a plantar wart yourself.

Curing chronic toenail fungus is difficult, or, in many cases, impossible. To control it, file or sandpaper the thickened nail and apply an antifungal product (over-the-counter or by prescription); the solution form can cover the nail more thoroughly. If you can't control the fungus, or if your nail becomes red or painful, seek medical attention.

Blisters

Friction or pressure from ill-fitting shoes, socks, or stockings—either too big or little—causes blisters. Going without socks or stockings in normally well-fitting shoes can also blister heels and toes, particularly in hot weather, when feet are likely to swell and sweat. Sandals and other shoes with straps are particularly likely to blister bare skin.

Treatment. If it's a small blister, it will heal by itself—just make sure it stays clean. To take pressure off it, cover it with a moleskin pad with a hole cut in the middle. If the blister breaks, wash it with soap and water, and protect it with a light bandage. However, if you have a large blister that hurts when you walk on it, you may want to puncture it. First wash it, then make a small hole near its edge with a sterile needle (hold it in flame for a few seconds). Then gently squeeze out the liquid and cover it with a tight sterile bandage; try to keep it dry. See a doctor if any blister shows signs of infection (reddening, swelling, or pus).

Corns and calluses

Corns and calluses are thick, hard growths of skin formed in response to excessive pressure and chafing. People with flat feet are particularly susceptible to them. Corns, which usually appear on the toes, are thickenings of skin around a core, whose apex points inward. Most hard corns appear on the little toe; soft corns appear on the web between toes. Calluses are thickened pads of skin, usually on weight-bearing portions of the sole.

Treatment. The best way to treat corns and calluses at home is to soak the foot in warm (never hot) water until the hardened skin softens, then gently apply a pumice stone or callus file; don't rub the area raw. It may take several treatments. Afterwards, protect the area with a light pad or bandage. Moleskin comes with adhesive and can be trimmed to fit the spot and relieve pressure. Many over-the-counter corn remedies are available, most containing salicylic acid. Though the Food and Drug Administration (FDA) has approved these products, most doctors advise using them only with caution; they can burn the surrounding healthy skin and result in additional discomfort.

Bunions and hammertoes

When the large metatarsal bone angles outward at the big toe joint, thus forcing the toe inward, pressure over this distended joint can cause swelling and eventually a bony outgrowth. This is a bunion, which is not only disfiguring but painful, and can seriously interfere with standing and walking if neglected over the years. (Smaller bunions—bunionettes—may occasionally appear on the fifth metatarsal bone and the little toe joint.) The tendency to develop bunions may be hereditary, and flat-footed people are more likely to get bunions than others. But poorly fitting shoes—especially those with high heels and narrow toes—are undoubtedly the worst bunion-makers. Thus women are more prone to bunions.

Special insoles, sold in shoe stores and sporting goods stores for up to $20 a pair, won't significantly increase the shock-absorbing ability of good athletic shoes, according to recent studies. Your best bet is to concentrate instead on choosing shoes that provide sufficient cushioning by themselves. Once the shoes' own cushioning ability wears out, it's time to replace the shoes, not add insoles.

Treatment. If you think you are developing a bunion, switch to shoes with a low heel and ample toe room; avoid any shoes or stockings that put pressure on the big toe joint. Wearing open shoes, if practical, may be a good idea. Soaking your feet in warm water and gentle massage may also relieve some symptoms.

Hammertoes and mallet toes are deformities of the toe bones, usually of the second, third, or fourth toes, whereby the toes grow in a bent position. This can be painful and even disabling and can keep shoes from fitting properly. Shoes, particularly high-heels with pointed toes, are almost always to blame for these deformities. Well-fitting shoes are often the best treatment, and corrective pads can help as well. If the deformity is painful or hinders walking, seek professional advice. Both bunions and hammertoes can usually be corrected by surgery.

Painful heel syndrome

Runners and other athletes get painful heels, but it can happen to anybody. The pain may originate in the plantar fascia, which is the thick connective tissue under the skin on the bottom of your foot and the sides of the heel, and in this case the condition is called plantar fasciitis. The plantar fascia, which acts as a kind of bowstring for the arch of the foot, can develop small, painful tears under repeated stress. Other sources of pain may be minute breaks in your heel bone, or in a heel spur, which is a bony growth on the underside of the heel bone. Tendinitis or bursitis (inflammation of the tendons or bursae) may also be part of this syndrome.

The first symptom is usually discomfort in the heel first thing in the morning when you put pressure on your foot, and it may ease off as the day goes on. If this happens to you, you may try the remedies listed on the next page and experience gradual and complete improvement. But if the pain is severe and doesn't improve, you may need the advice of a doctor, a podiatrist, or a specialist in body mechanics to figure out what's causing it. Rarely, infections, arthritis, gout, diabetes, and other ailments can be part of the problem, and if you suspect any of these, you should see a doctor. More commonly, the following factors promote heel troubles:

Orthoses

In theory, the human foot is a perfect piece of design, but in practice some people's feet don't hit the ground in quite the right way. The resulting condition can be painful for the knees, hips, and the feet themselves, and the pain may be particularly noticeable for those embarking on a fitness program.

To correct for abnormal foot motion and alignment, many people buy devices called "orthoses," popularly (but incorrectly) known as "orthotics." Made of foam, leather, plastic, fiberglass, graphite, or some combination thereof, orthoses are foot supports that fit in your shoes. A podiatrist or orthopedist should prescribe and fit them, since they must be specially cast or designed. Improperly constructed orthotic devices can do more harm than good. They are expensive—they can cost up to $600 for the examination, casting, X-rays, and lab fees. Fortunately, some medical insurance plans cover them.

Orthoses can't change the shape of your foot, but they can make its motion more efficient and can correct certain structural imbalances that may lead to pain in the hips, knees, back, or feet. Some athletes—for example, certain runners, cyclists, and skiers—have been shown to benefit from them. And for people with alignment or imbalance problems, orthotic devices can relieve discomfort and reduce the risk of foot injury. They are, however, an aid, not a cure; If you need therapy for structural foot problems, orthotic devices can be one part of the total treatment program.

Bad biomechanics, which is another way of saying abnormalities in your walking or running gait that stress your heel bone and the tissues attached to it. Your heel should be the first part of your foot to hit the ground when you are walking, and ideally the arch distributes your weight toward the outside of your foot and then toward the ball of it. But if your feet roll inward or outward too much, the weight isn't properly distributed, and the plantar fascia and heel bear excess stress.

Being overweight or habitually carrying heavy things puts pressure on heels.

Growing older. Although no scientific study shows that older people are more prone to heel pain, it's probably true that they are. As you grow older, the pads that protect the heel from injury, like pads under a carpet, can wear down and thus not provide the shock absorption they once did.

Frequent running, walking, tennis-playing or other vigorous weight-bearing exercise. Athletes, like older people, may be prone to heel pain, especially if they also have excessively pronating feet or other biomechanical problems.

Ill-fitting, thin-soled shoes, or worn-down shoes, as well as wearing the wrong shoes while exercising.

Prevention, treatment

Heel pain, in most cases, is something you can prevent and something you can treat successfully yourself. As with many other injuries, prevention and treatment overlap to some extent.

•Buy shoes that fit and have shock-absorbent soles, rigid shanks, and some extra padding in the heels. Good ankle counters are important, too, so your foot doesn't slip up and down. If you must wear dress shoes for work, wear athletic shoes to and from work and at home. Women should avoid both thin-soled flats and high heels.

•Discard or repair shoes with worn-down heels and soles.

•If you are overweight, try to trim down.

•Pace yourself in exercise and athletic activities. If your feet hurt, take a break. Find out why they hurt: are you overdoing it, and do your shoes fit?

•If your heel does begin to hurt, rest is the first line of defense. Limit your activities for a few days. If possible switch to swimming, indoor cycling, weight-training, or sit-ups for exercise.

•Over-the-counter pain relievers (aspirin and ibuprofen) should help.

•Try heel cups or soft plastic inserts in your shoes.

•Tight calf muscles can tighten the fascia and contribute to heel pain, so do some calf stretches (see page 414).

•Cold provides relief. Massage your heel with a small jar or paper cup filled with ice.

•If your heel does not improve with home treatment, see a doctor. (Heel pain often persists for several months.) There's a great deal that can be done—taping and strapping of the foot, orthotic devices, medication, and special exercise, depending on what your diagnosis is. But according to the American Podiatric Medical Association, surgery is seldom necessary except in some cases for removal of a spur. If your doctor suggests surgery, try other treatments first and, as with any surgery, get a second opinion.

When you can't treat it at home

If you have any medical or inherited problems—or if any of the problems described in this chapter do not respond to home treatment—you need professional advice. Two kinds of medical professionals specialize in foot care. Orthopedists *are MDs trained to treat all types of bone and muscle disorders, both medically and surgically.* Podiatrists *(DPMs, doctors of podiatric medicine) treat foot disorders and in some states can prescribe for ankle disorders as well, but they are not MDs. Like orthopedists, they can perform surgery and prescribe medications, but only for problems of the foot and ankle.*

Once you've seen a doctor, a physical therapist *can also check your gait and stance, and develop an exercise program for alleviating and preventing foot pain.*

Most insurance plans, including Medicare, cover medical treatment for feet.

Stress

Stress has never been adequately defined, beyond such vague generalizations as "stress is how people respond to demands." Once stress became a popular concept, old terms such as "worry," "anxiety," "fear," "impatience," and "anger," gave way to "stress" and its offshoots, "stressful," "stress-related," and "stressed-out." "Stressors" have been defined as everything from war and famine to job loss, family arguments, and encounters with the IRS. Further complicating matters is the fact that different people react to the same "stress" in unpredictable ways.

Then there is the issue of the impact of stress on health. It may seem quite reasonable to think that states of mind affect health and that extreme emotional distress can damage the body's immune system and bring on illness. However, it has been hard to scientifically demonstrate that specific attitudes lead to specific illnesses, as explained on pages 453-456.

In fact, according to some experts the psychological concept of "stress" (as something originating in a person's mind) should be retired. The idea that emotional anguish arises from personality or individual flaws beclouds the fact that many physical and psychological problems come from social conditions not always within an individual's control. Many problems arise specifically from problems relating to a person's occupation and financial security—or the lack of them. (Not having a job at all can be at least as painful as having the wrong one.) Of course, the workplace is not the only source of human happiness and misery: we all live within society and with our friends and families. Still, most of the important research on stress so far has been conducted in the workplace, and the theory that has developed there may apply to other situations.

The Control Element

Most of us dread intense demands in the workplace, but sometimes such demands can lead to a sense of control and indeed exhilaration. Many occupations (including even some that are unpaid, such as raising children or doing community work or playing an instrument for pleasure), can, under ideal circumstances, provide great challenges and intense satisfactions—a sense of cohesion, accomplishment, and control. A sense of personal control may, in fact, be critical in maintaining health. The evidence is strong, and growing, that *people whose lives or jobs make high demands on them but allow little latitude for decision-making have higher rates of many diseases.*

Indeed, the risk of illness for such people is two to four times what it is for others, independent of all other risk factors. Though it's not known exactly how unsatisfying jobs and unhappy lives might make people sick, one possibility is by interfering with some general integrating system of the body—the nervous or hormonal or immune system. But there is solid evidence that social support (i.e. involvement with family, friends, and community) can buffer social stress.

Researchers Robert Karasek of the University of Southern California and Töres

Theorell of Sweden's National Institute for Psychosocial Factors and Health, divide occupations into four categories:

Active jobs. Heavy pressure to perform, but leeway allowed for problem solving. Examples: doctors, engineers, farmers, executives, other professionals. Hours may be long, but are partly at the worker's discretion. Job provides chances to advance and to learn new skills. Initiative is part of job description.

Low-strain jobs. Self-paced occupations. Examples are tenured professors, carpenters, repairmen, successful artists, naturalists, or any occupation with low demands and high decision latitude. (This idyllic category seems somewhat underpopulated in this research, no doubt because few such jobs exist in an industrial society. Professors, carpenters, artists, and others can certainly experience high strain.)

Passive jobs. Low demands on skills and mental processes, little leeway for learning or decision-making. Examples: billing clerks, nightwatchmen, janitors, dispatchers, key-punchers. These jobs offer almost no latitude for innovation; sometimes worker skills actually atrophy.

High-strain jobs. Heavy pressure to perform but little control over decisions. Examples: assembly line workers, waiters, waitresses, nurse's aides, telephone operators. Includes any job where hours and procedures are rigid, where the threat of layoff may loom, where no new skills are learned from day to day, and where it may be difficult to take time out, or off, for personal needs.

Who is subject to stress

Studies in the United States and Europe have consistently shown that people in high-strain jobs (that is, those at the bottom of the job ladder) have the highest rate of heart attacks, while those in active jobs have the lowest. Passive jobs and low-strain jobs were in between. Those in high-strain, low-echelon jobs also exhibited the highest levels of psychological stress (including depression and exhaustion), and they took the most medications for depression—while those at the top of the job ladder were by far the best off in this category. In short, though "executive stress" exists, it's the bossed, not bosses, who experience the most stress on the job.

A study conducted at the Volvo plant in Goteborg, Sweden, showed that those who saw themselves as influential (usually managers, men, and white-collar workers) were much more highly motivated and less subject to stress-related medical complaints than those who saw themselves as cogs in the wheel (nonmanagers, women, and blue-collar workers). In another area, studies of older people living in nursing homes indicate that a sense of self-management (expressed even in such small ways as the ability to choose one menu over another) can strongly contribute to psychological as well as physical well-being.

Driving a big-city bus fits every criterion for a high-strain job (that is, one with high workload demands but little sense of control): pressure to meet a schedule, physical discomfort, high noise levels, unruly or hostile passengers to be dealt with, heavy traffic, the risk of a crash or breakdown. According to a paper by Gary Evans of the University of California at Irvine, over twenty studies of bus drivers in various cities reveal that they have excess rates of death from heart disease, and are more prone to suffer from gastrointestinal disorders and musculoskeletal disorders, such as bad backs. They retire earlier than other civil servants, too, usually because of medical disabilities. A study of 1,428 San Francisco bus drivers (male, mostly non-white) supplied one puzzling piece of information: those who scored low on the

Researchers at the University of Massachusetts Center for Health and Fitness found that after subjects worked out by taking brisk forty-minute walk, they experienced a 14 percent average drop in anxiety levels.

stress scale—that is, who perceived their jobs as unstressful—tended to have high blood pressure more often than those who recognized the strain they worked under.

But a growing body of evidence shows that job strain by itself may contribute to hypertension. In a 1990 study, researchers monitored 200 people in different occupations in New York City with a twenty-four-hour blood pressure device; some subjects were hypertensive to start with, some not. Those who worked in high-strain jobs, such as bus drivers and air-traffic controllers, not only had higher blood pressure, but were also likely to show a thickening of the wall of the left ventricle of the heart.

Stereotypical "high stress" jobs such as manager, electrical engineer, and architect have proved not to be associated with health risks, because professionals get to make more of their own decisions and thus feel more in control. Even when such risk factors as age, race, education, and smoking were factored into the equation, those in the bottom tenth of the job echelon have turned out to be in the top tenth for stress. They have four to five times the risk of heart attack as those at the top tenth of the ladder whose jobs gave them a high sense of control.

Since there are still few occupations with large proportions of both sexes, much of this type of research has focused on men. Nevertheless, according to Karasek and Theorell, "women's average level of decision latitude is markedly lower than men's." Women fill more than their share of high-strain jobs, less than their share of active ones. Many of the high-strain jobs for women are newly created clerical jobs (such as computer operators in highly automated offices). This might have some impact on women's health in the future.

Regaining control

In the workplace, supervisors are recognizing that people do better work if they have some say over what they do. If your job is managing others, you can reduce the stress of your own responsibilities by asking others to share them. If those who report to you seem bored, uninterested, and all too willing to vanish at quitting time, remember that powerlessness is a bad motivator. Provide some on-the-job training and some real responsibilities that lead to a sense of control.

If you feel that your job does not provide you with enough input, try either to change the way you feel or change the situation. For a start, try to analyze what bothers you and come up with one or two possible solutions. Then see whether you can discuss these matters with a co-worker. Next, try to talk to your supervisor. If you can spot problems and discover solutions, your supervisor may like your suggestions and give you more responsible work to do. Work toward the goal of being an active participant at your job, rather than a passive observer.

At the same time, be willing, if necessary, to conclude that you're in the wrong place. Some bad work situations can't be changed. If you know you're in the wrong job, consider improving your skills in your leisure time and looking for something new. You can also try to improve your life outside the workplace. Some people dissatisfied with their jobs can find a sense of effectiveness and control by becoming more active outside their jobs—in community organizations for instance.

The benefits of social support

Support of co-workers and supervisors may be one of the most important factors ameliorating workplace stress. Social support at work acts as a palliative, mitigat-

---

The ideal job

According to researchers Robert Karasek and Töres Theorell, a satisfying job provides:

Skill discretion. The job requires maximum use of skills and offers chances to increase them.

Autonomy. Workers are in control of machines; they can participate in long-term planning; flexible hours are available.

Psychological demands. Routine demands mixed with new but predictable challenges. Workers have some say-so over magnitude of demands.

Social relations. Workers can collaborate.

Social rights. Democratic procedures rule the workplace. Some way exists to settle grievances.

Meaningfulness. Workers understand what they are producing and for whom. Feedback from customers is provided.

Integration of family and community life with work. Working men and women are able to share family responsibilities. The job also allows time and energy for activities outside of work-related ones.

ing the bad health effects of even high-strain jobs. A variety of circumstances can provide social support on the job: a comradely atmosphere among co-workers and between workers and management; a boss who treats his staff with respect; and the feeling of making a creditable contribution in a team effort. Labor unions and other kinds of employee organizations also provide social support. Indeed, depending on the circumstances, some high-strain jobs (in restaurants or factories or hospitals) can have some support built in—a good supervisor, regular job breaks, or a sense that customers or patients appreciate the service rendered.

If a job is lonely or a person's colleagues are unhelpful or even actively hostile, there is some evidence that social interactions with family and friends, as well as with the community can be a factor in maintaining health. Studies have shown that people who enjoy the companionship of friends or family live longer and are healthier than people who are socially isolated. Dr. Leonard Syme of the University of California at Berkeley and Dr. Lisa Berkman of Yale University followed the health and social habits of 7,000 individuals for nine years. They found that lonely women have nearly three times greater risk and lonely men a doubled risk of illness and death than people who can count on family or friends. Earlier studies indicated that married people are healthier and live longer than single people, but this study suggested that marriage per se is not essential for health but that the companionship and emotional support associated with marriage are. However, a study of Swedish workers did suggest that in some circumstances "the psychosocial situation at work appears to have a greater impact on psychological well-being than do family situations." Nevertheless, since high demand coupled with a low sense of control appear to create the most damaging strain in the workplace, it's reasonable to wonder whether the same principle wouldn't apply to family life and to many situations outside the workplace.

Mind/Body Links

More than two decades of research into the relationship between personality and disease has found little of significance, and indeed has created a lot of confusion. People who get ulcers have a wide range of personalities and habits. Some appear to live under extreme emotional stress; others are calm and contented. Optimists and pessimists, extroverts and introverts get cancer—and recover from it (or do not). For many years, scientists have looked for links between emotional states, particularly anger, and heart attack, stroke, and high blood pressure, or between chronic hostility and cancer. Scores of studies have been carried out—some leading to dead ends. Nevertheless, some plausible theories have begun to emerge

Hostility and the coronary arteries
The idea that personality and heart disease might be linked was formalized in 1969 with the concept of "Type A." Two California cardiologists, Dr. Meyer Friedman and Dr. Ray Rosenman, presented evidence that men with a certain kind of hard-driving, aggressive, competitive, tense, and hostile personality were at risk for chronic chest pain or angina (a word with the same root as anger) and for heart attack. The Framingham Heart Study, an important and large-scale investigation of the risk factors for heart disease—and one of the few that included women—also

According to one Swedish study, commuters who board a train twenty miles outside of their destination were found to have significantly higher stress levels than those traveling twice the distance. Apparently the more control the commuter has over his surroundings (such as being able to get a seat), the less stressful the journey. This suggests that commuters may be better off trading a short, stressful ride for a longer but calmer one.

Stress and the Immune System

Do stressful states deplete the body's complex defense mechanism against infection known as the immune system? The science of mind and immunity, psychoneuroimmunology, is relatively new (having been named only in 1974), and has turned out to be a more difficult area of study than anticipated. One problem is that the immune reaction seen in a single experiment may not reflect the action of the whole system. For example, an experiment may show that extreme grief depresses human T-cells, a type of white blood cell that switches on (and off) various aspects of the immune response. But we don't know if the rest of the system is harmed. And nobody knows whether temporary boosts or reductions in certain immune system cells are of any significance. In healthy people, immune cells fluctuate regularly, according to time of day, recent exercise or infections, and other variables.

It's known that immune cells and nerve cells interact. For example, when fighting an infection, immune cells are able to stimulate the brain to transmit the impulses that produce fever. Receptors for many of the chemicals released during stress, such as epinephrine and norepinephrine, have been observed on the surface of lymphocytes found near nerve terminals in the lymph nodes and spleen. This suggests that what goes on in the brain can interact with the immune system to suppress or, conversely, enhance it.

Yet the jury is still out on whether you can worry yourself sick, or cheer yourself on to recovery. Several studies of students have shown that acute stress—taking academic examinations, for example—can temporarily suppress immune cell activity and make them less resistant to illness. But nobody knows whether it is the stress alone that produces the effect (maybe the students also lost sleep, or ate a poor diet).

In a much talked-about study of 400 people published in the *New England Journal of Medicine* in 1991, "highly stressed" people were somewhat more likely than others to catch cold when exposed to a cold virus. But the increased risk was small, only 20 percent, and it wasn't certain that stress was the only factor. In any case, most of us don't have the option of skipping school or work when we're highly stressed in order to avoid cold viruses. Furthermore, not everybody under stress gets sick. According to a review published in the *Psychological Bulletin* some research even shows that acute stress can briefly stimulate immunity.

Still, reports of increased illness and even death among the recently bereaved are common. One laboratory study showed that the husbands of women with terminal breast cancer showed significantly lower response to a lymphocyte-stimulating chemical in the two months after bereavement than before their wives' deaths (though other immune system components did not alter). There's also evidence that cancer patients with a "fighting spirit" live longer than those who are despondent, but this may or may not prove something about immune function.

Lack of "scientific evidence" does not mean there's no connection between mind and immunity. The ways of measuring immune response may not yet be sensitive enough to show the complex interactions and effects, if any, of emotional stress. It may require not only more years, but also new ways of inquiry, before we can assess the nature of the effects and know how best to deal with stress to achieve health.

---

provided evidence that Type A personality put a person at risk, not only men in white collar jobs, but women as well.

But to the surprise of many researchers, subsequent studies were contradictory and failed to confirm the link between Type A behavior and heart disease. Careful study stripped away aggressiveness, tenseness, and competitiveness as risk factors for heart attacks. A recent twenty-two-year follow-up by Drs. David Ragland and Richard Brand of the University of California at Berkeley indicated that Type A behavior was not related to heart attack deaths. Smoking and high blood pressure were far more important risk factors than personality or behavior.

Thus more than twenty years after Type A was introduced, most investigators have given up on it. What does continue to interest many of them, however, is just one component of Type A—anger, or more specifically the tendency to look at the world with cynicism and hostility. A recent study conducted by Dr. Redford Williams at Duke University Medical Center returned to the subject of heart attack and anger. It found that those identified as hostile personalities when they were nineteen had significantly higher levels of total cholesterol and lower levels of beneficial HDL cholesterol at age forty-two and were thus at higher risk for heart attack.

Dr. Williams and his colleagues hypothesized that hostility can actually affect blood cholesterol levels, or—a very different thing—that it simply leads to bad health habits. Other researchers, too, have conjectured that hostile people may adopt a "why bother" attitude: "Why be careful about my diet, why exercise, why take care of myself when things are so rotten anyhow?" And yet this line of thought hasn't panned out either. Williams's new evidence for a link between hostility and heart disease is called into question by equally good new evidence that no such link exists. For example, a new study led by Dr. Dianne Helmer at the University of California at Berkeley found no significant link between hostility (as measured by standardized psychological tests among 158 people hospitalized for coronary angiograms) and heart disease. Hostility, the study concludes, does not predict heart disease. Other studies have had mixed results.

Expressing anger: does it help?

Some studies have suggested that suppressing anger is what endangers health. For example, Dr. Mara Julius of the University of Michigan, has reanalyzed the data from a long-term study of a Michigan community (the Tecumseh Community Health Study). How men and women in this study coped with anger had been measured by such questions as this: "If your spouse or an authority figure such as a policeman yelled at you for something you hadn't done, how would you react?" Possible answers ranged from "I wouldn't feel annoyed" to "I'd get angry and protest." Women—but not men—who suppressed their anger in such confrontations had a higher mortality rate over time. In fact, women who suppressed their anger in confrontations with their spouses had twice the mortality risk as other women, even when other factors such as high blood pressure and smoking were considered. Among couples, if both husband and wife suppressed anger, mortality rates went up among women but not men. Among men, only those who suppressed their anger and had high blood pressure had a higher risk of dying.

Thus Dr. Julius concluded that suppressing anger was a risk factor for heart disease and cancer in women. Her work also suggests that women may handle anger differently from men and thus be affected in special ways by suppressing it.

But venting anger may not be any better than suppressing it. At the University of Tennessee, a small study of eighty-seven middle-aged women investigated anger levels, and found that angry women tended to be pessimistic about themselves, to lack social support, to be overweight, to sleep poorly, and to lead sedentary lives. They also believed that they could not control their problems and could do nothing about them. The angriest women were also more likely to have health problems already. It's not clear, of course, whether the anger results from this unhappy lifestyle, which is definitely not conducive to good health, or is simply another symptom of unhappiness.

Researchers noted that many of the issues that made these women angry were not easy to modify. They also found that "contrary to popular wisdom, which rec-

Watching television is a favorite relaxation method of 34 percent of American adults, but studies show that time spent watching television programs with a violent theme does little to reduce anxiety. One study found that heavy television watchers tend to express mistrust of others and to view themselves as living in a hostile world.

Supporting Friends in Times of Crisis

It is hard to say which is the more difficult position: to be needing reassurance and support, or to be trying to help a friend or family member and not know what to say. Perhaps you grope for the right words and end up saying nothing, or manage to say exactly the wrong thing.

Most of us (including many doctors) are convinced that grief always follows the same patterns: the bereaved person first experiences deep distress and depression, then begins to "work through" and adjust to the new situation, and finally resolves the loss and resumes functioning. All this is supposed to happen pretty quickly—and any deviation is generally interpreted as "bad."

But according to some researchers people don't always conform to this pattern. Those who don't mourn openly may find themselves accused of "denial." Those who can't recover quickly may be categorized as morbid or self-indulgent. But, in fact, there are really no definitions for "normal" grieving or "working through." Even health-care professionals have been known to recommend "a pat on the back and kick in the pants" for people who seem to be grieving too deeply or too long. But given how little is known about grieving, pats and kicks may not be appropriate at all.

Because mourning is so personal, comments on a person's method of dealing with loss may do more harm than good. Thus when you offer support to someone who's having a hard time, it's always a good idea to stop and think about what you would want to hear yourself, or how you would want to be listened to. Though much depends on the individual you're dealing with, a few general pointers may apply:

•Make sure there's no implicit criticism in any suggestions you make. Instead of "you're brooding too much," try "I wish you'd be our fourth for bridge" or some similar invitation.

•Compassionate listening can often accomplish more than talking. Allow the other person to take the lead in conversation. Instead of making assumptions about how he is feeling, find out what is really on his mind. If your widowed aunt still needs to talk about her husband two years after his death, you can help by listening sympathetically.

•On the other hand, remember that people who are bereaved or ill don't want to talk about their problems all the time. It's all right to bring up other subjects. It may be the most helpful thing for them.

•Just be there. A report by psychologists Gayle Dakof and Shelley Taylor of UCLA, who asked fifty-five cancer patients what they perceived as helpful support, has a similar theme. Love, emotional support, and calm concern turned out to be the most helpful contributions from family members and friends. Such acts of service as coming along for a doctor's appointment, providing transportation to and from treatments, or other kinds of practical aid were also cited. "Just being there" turned out to be the strongest supportive factor for a spouse.

ommends ventilation of anger," the women whose health seemed most adversely affected by anger were not suppressors of anger, but those who "directed it outward." In other words, blowing your stack may merely make you feel worse. And as a rule—no matter how justified the outburst—it doesn't promote social ties, or provoke sympathetic reactions.

Thus for these women at least, the choice between suppressing or venting anger may be irrelevant. It may not be anger that makes people sick, or even the way they express it, perhaps, but the inability to deal effectively with the situations that anger them.

Managing anger: easier said than done

In his book *The Trusting Heart*, subtitled *Great News About Type A Behavior*, Dr. Redford Williams of Duke University Medical Center has written that Type A behavior is not "toxic," but claimed that hostility is. He suggests several stress-management techniques to cope with anger, among them:

•Monitor your cynical thoughts by keeping a log of situations that stir you up.

Attitude and Cancer

The idea that a positive attitude can help keep you from getting sick has been studied in individuals with cancer. Some researchers have suggested that patients with a positive attitude are likely to get well. For example, a study conducted in London showed that a "fighting spirit" as opposed to helplessness and hopelessness, may help women with breast cancer survive, but only if the disease has not spread. These people, of course, have the best prognosis, whatever their mental state. However, studies by Dr. David Spiegel at Stanford University's School of Medicine show that group therapy has doubled life expectancies and increased quality of life of people with more advanced cancers. Other studies, though, have been unable to find a relationship between attitudes and cancer survival.

Still, many doctors believe that a strong desire to stay alive and well is an asset to anybody. If nothing else, it will give you the incentive to take care of yourself. In cancer patients, a courageous attitude and a willingness to follow a prescribed course of therapy is an advantage, not only for them but for their doctors, friends, and families.

- Try stopping cynical thoughts.
- Put yourself in the other person's shoes.
- Instead of yelling angrily, try to be assertive, calm, and clear about what's bothering you.

Of course, a person who can do all that is probably not too bad off to begin with. It's hard to develop a "trusting heart" if you have reasons not to be trustful. Whether to suppress or express anger, and how best to express it, depends inevitably on the circumstances and the other people involved. Managing uncontrollable angry outbursts in oneself or in a family member may require counseling, meditation, lifestyle changes, or other kinds of long-term psychological help.

Some suggestions for managing anger from the Institute for Mental Health Initiatives (IMHI) in Washington, D.C., may be helpful. A few years ago, recognizing that "people who have some skill at managing their anger are less likely to. . .suffer from emotional disorders such as depression, or grow up to be early victims of heart disease or stroke," IMHI undertook a study of how anger is handled on daytime TV soap operas. These shows have an audience of 20 million people, most of them women. In 1986 researchers analyzed how anger was presented on twelve daytime dramas on the three major networks. Finding that anger too often resulted in violence on the soaps, they drafted guidelines for producers and writers about healthier ways of portraying anger. No one knows just how effective these efforts have been, but according to surveys completed in 1990, IMHI found that anger has increasingly been portrayed not as an emotion felt by "bad" people but as a normal emotion that even likeable people may exhibit and can deal with constructively. In addition, women have been increasingly portrayed as effective at handling anger. These ideas could conceivably be helpful for some viewers. Out of this research IMHI developed anger-management techniques that emphasize such tips as these:

- Recognize your own anger, and that of others.
- Empathize with a person expressing anger.
- Always listen carefully to what an angry person is telling you.
- Try to express respect along with the anger.
- Notice your own reactions, especially your physical reactions.
- Focus your attention on the present problem, and avoid thinking of old grudges or wounds.

Personality and health habits

According to researcher Suzanne Kobasa of the City University of New York, some people weather adversity with fewer side effects than others. She terms these people "hardy" personalities. According to her surveys, the hardy enjoy better physical health as well as more satisfying personal lives.

One way to spot the hardy personality is in the workplace. For example, Kobasa studied middle- and upper-level executives at a large Illinois corporation, which was undergoing upheavals at the time. The men who coped best with the strains were likely to:

•Consider new developments and problems to be exciting challenges rather than threats.

•Display a sense of commitment to work.

•Find a sense of control in the job, and take part in outside activities (perhaps community affairs) which offer other responsibilities.

•Accept change optimistically and see it as a normal life process, rather than interpreting it as a source of stress.

A person who exhibits such qualities will probably also be "hardy" in personal relationships. Interesting as this research may be, its value as practical advice applicable to the individual is probably limited.

If you aren't hardy, it's difficult to alter your personality (as any one knows who has ever tried). However, Kobasa suggests that the hardy are likely to do the following and perhaps those who are "unhardy" could make some gains by following similar polices:

•Maintain good health habits, such as exercising and eating a healthy diet.

•Engage in open discussion with others, particularly when crises arise.

•Seek social support.

So called "stress vitamins," which claim to help you deal with emotional stress, serve no purpose. Although your body may need more vitamins during periods of physical stress (after surgery for instance), there's no evidence that these special formulas (usually vitamins C, E, and B-complex) will help you if you're facing psychological stress.

Learning to Relax

Although it is not clear what effect your emotional state has on your health, it is clear that when some people are anxious, angry, or tense they experience physiological effects such as increased blood pressure and heart rate, muscle tension, and intestinal upset. These physical responses to emotional situations seem to be the result of the "fight or flight" response—your body's reaction to a perceived threat. This response seems to be a holdover from the time when man had to deal with physical threats to his well-being either by staying and fighting or running away. In order to give man the extra energy and alertness needed, the body responded to emergency situations by releasing two hormones—epinephrine (also known as adrenaline) and norepinephrine (also known as noradrenaline)—which caused the heart to beat faster (thereby pumping more blood to the muscles and brain), increased respiration rate and blood pressure, and activated blood-clotting mechanisms to prepare for physical injury. In today's modern world, this response is rarely needed, but is activated frequently by emotional upsets—arguments with friends and family, excessive demands on your time, irritation with traffic, long lines, and rude people.

It has been a truism in western civilization for centuries that we can control all sorts of physical functions that are under our conscious influence—walking, swal-

Quick Relaxation Techniques

Here are four ways to relax in twenty minutes or less. They require only a little practice and aren't seriously disruptive.

Countdown. With eyes closed, count backward from ten or twenty, saying each number silently as you exhale. You must concentrate and call your imagination into play. Imagine you are going down a stairway, or past the floors in a building as an elevator descends. Count down from your age, and imagine that you are traveling briefly into your past. When you have reached zero and want to resume your normal routine, inhale and count to three.

Imagery. Stop what you are doing and close your eyes. Imagine a beautiful scene, perhaps something you saw on your last vacation. Spend five minutes examining and enjoying every detail of the picture. If you are by a lake, listen to the water lapping. Count the trees and flowers. See, hear, and smell things.

The turtle. This simple exercise, adapted from a yoga practice, is designed to relax the muscles of your neck and back. Sit up straight and let your chin fall to your chest as you exhale. Inhale and move your head back slowly as though trying to touch the back of your neck with your head. Then pull your shoulders up as though trying to touch them to your ears. Then release. You can do this anytime, anywhere. It doesn't even look all that odd.

Scanning. At your desk, during your coffee break, or even while you are riding a bus or waiting at a traffic light, inhale and slowly "scan" your body. Think about each muscle group—face and neck, shoulders, arms, abdomen, legs, and feet—and seek out tense muscles. As you exhale, relax all the muscles that are tense. It may help, as you scan your body, to recite silently some phrase that has a calming effect.

A study at Pennsylvania State University suggests that people who identified themselves as chronic worriers were able to reduce anxiety by setting aside a "worry period" everyday. Subjects set aside a half-hour a day to worry and when they caught themselves worrying at other times during the day, they postponed it.

lowing, writing, even crying—but that we cannot control that wide range of involuntary functions that go on in our bodies without our conscious thought: the regulation of our bodies' temperatures, our heart rate, our blood pressure, or even the tension in our muscles Yet eastern mystics have long studied and practiced control of autonomous functions—not necessarily for health, but in order to achieve a certain composure conducive to meditation and spiritual communion.

Among the western scientists to study just how eastern mystics went about achieving this composure were Herbert Benson, of the Harvard Medical School, and his colleagues. Benson's group focused on transcendental meditation—a simplified version of several eastern meditation techniques (see page 462). In TM, as it is popularly called, a subject is given a mantra—a personal, secret word, sound, or phrase—by his instructor. The subject then sits in a comfortable position and repeats this mantra over and over again to drive out all distracting thoughts and to think about nothing at all. Subjects are advised to meditate in this way twenty minutes every morning and evening.

The Benson group monitored several bodily functions of volunteers trained in this technique, and then before, during, and after meditation. The experiments showed that during meditation there was a marked decrease in the body's oxygen consumption and a corresponding slowing of metabolism. At the same time there was a marked increase in alpha waves, the slow brain waves associated with relaxation. Also there was a sharp decrease in blood lactate—a by-product of metabolism in the skeletal muscles that is associated with muscle tension and physical activity. And finally, both heart rate and respiration rate slowed down. What did not change in these volunteers was blood pressure. And, indeed, later research has shown that blood pressure is lowered only in people who have mildly elevated blood pressure to begin with.

The relaxation response

These results led Benson's group to the next step of their experiments; what if volunteers were taught simple physical relaxation techniques that were stripped of any mystical or religious aura or purpose? Benson outlined four elements necessary to achieve what he called the "relaxation response" and had his subjects learn and practice these techniques over four consecutive days:

A mental device. There needs to be a constant stimulus of some sort—a word, a sound, a phrase repeated silently or audibly, or fixed gazing at some stationary objects—to shift the mind from logical, externally oriented thoughts.

A passive attitude. If distracting thoughts do intrude they should be disregarded, and attention redirected by repetition of the word or phrase, but redirected without worry about how well one is doing.

Decreased muscle tension. The subject should be in a comfortable position so that minimal muscle work is needed.

A quiet environment. The subject should choose a quiet place, with few environmental distractions. A place of worship or a quiet room is good; sometimes closing your eyes helps.

Using these four simple guidelines, Benson's group was able to measure the very same alternations in bodily functions among untrained volunteers that they had measured among those schooled in Transcendental Meditation. In short, though some experienced meditators may use these techniques as avenues toward spiritual experiences, the techniques can be used for simple physical reduction of some symptoms of tension as well.

Benson and his associates used the relaxation response in numerous and varied studies. In one, they showed that people with mildly elevated blood pressure were able to significantly reduce pressure by regular practice of the relaxation response. In quite a different study, Benson found that a group of subjects dramatically reduced their alcohol intake. The alcohol they had used to reduce anxiety and tension had become a problem in itself; invoking the relaxation response reduced general stress levels as well as the need for alcohol.

Progressive muscle relaxation

Benson's technique for achieving the relaxation response is not, however, the only stress reduction technique. Another technique known as progressive muscle relaxation seems especially well suited to reducing muscle tension—and so alleviating the pain of some forms of headache and backache as well as high blood pressure. This simple technique was developed back in the thirties by Dr. Edmund Jacobson, a physiologist/physician. Subjects are instructed to lie down in a quiet room and let their minds drift into as passive a state as possible. Then, one by one, muscle groups are singled out—tensed to their ultimate extent and then relaxed. A subject works his way from toes to head in this way, several times if necessary, until he has achieved deep relaxation, particularly in the muscles of the face and eyes. Coupled with this training, subjects are instructed to tense a muscle halfway, or a quarter of the way, or as little as possible—so that they recognize even the slightest evidence of muscle tension in their bodies. Eventually subjects are instructed to relax their muscles without going through any of the tensing routines at all. A study at the Utah Medical Center found that progressive muscle relaxation can reduce blood pressure in some hypertensives by 8 or 9 percent.

Biofeedback

The most "scientific" of all relaxation techniques—or in any event, the most technological—is biofeedback. The technique of biofeedback could not be more direct and simple. A subject is brought into a laboratory and hooked up to a machine that measures systolic blood pressure, the temperature of the fingers, and the tension of the muscles in the forehead. The measurements taken by these machines are then continuously displayed on a monitor—either as numbers or as the sound of high or low pitch. The subject is then told to relax, be quiet, and lower the number, or change the pitch. The subject, using whatever sensations, thoughts, or feelings work for him, is not told how to lower the number or pitch—just to do it. One well-designed study found that biofeedback successfully lowered mild hypertension, and other studies have confirmed these findings.

Meditation

Meditation is an age-old religious practice, an end in itself or a path toward spiritual benefits to many who meditate, as well as a way to divorce the mind from the problems of daily life—and inducing such potentially beneficial changes as lower blood pressure and reduced heart rate. Accomplished practitioners, it's been shown, can also lower their oxygen consumption and body temperature. Thus meditation is sometimes recommended to people with heart disease or other medical problems, as well as to anybody who's trying to control emotional stress. For them, meditation may serve less as a religious experience than a practical measure—relaxation therapy, stress control.

But what does it mean to meditate? Does the use of disciplined meditation techniques produce greater physiological effects than just sitting quietly? These questions are hard to answer with "scientific precision," because states of mind and spiritual effects can't be measured. At the same time, there is no dearth of clinical studies. In a book called *In The Mind's Eye,* the National Academy of Sciences reviewed the evidence about meditation and came to some surprising conclusions. Among other things, they observed that the benefits of meditation are hard to prove—and yet meditation may be "a complex and powerful system" that lies beyond scientific analysis.

The word "meditation" means many different things. Most commonly it requires sitting or lying quietly in a prescribed position, usually with the eyes closed, so that attention is withdrawn from the outside world and from customary activity. Some—not all—forms of meditation involve concentrating on breathing in and out, and repeating a word or phrase (called a mantra) aloud or silently. Disciplined meditation is a part of every major religion—Buddhism, Hinduism and Yoga, and certain mystical branches of Christianity, Judaism, and Islam. The Buddhists, especially, seek "stillness of mind" and "mindfulness" (heightened focussing on thoughts and psychic processes through meditation. Eventually, by understanding the imperfect nature of worldly things, they hope to attain a state of serenity, abandonment of self, and enlightenment called Nirvana.

According to a recent report in the *American Journal of Psychotherapy,* brain-wave studies have shown that Yogic meditators are oblivious to what is happening around them, while Zen Buddhist meditators are "keenly attuned to the environment." Not all meditation involves sitting motionless, however. Hasidic Jews and some Moslems (the Whirling Dervishes, for example) may dance, whirl, or chant

Pet Therapy

Studies suggest that pets can be a significant source of comfort for the ill, the elderly, and the very young. If nothing else, animals provide a sense of normalcy in what otherwise might be a frightening or a depressing situation. In one experiment conducted at the University of Pennsylvania School of Veterinary Medicine, children were brought into an unfamiliar room and interviewed by a stranger—a situation designed to make them nervous. Researchers found that the presence of a friendly dog helped put the children at ease, as indicated by a slight decrease in their blood pressure. Other investigators have reported that pets have been effectively used to allay the fears of children undergoing psychotherapy and of nursing home residents.

Nevertheless, despite some extravagant claims made for the health-enhancing potential of pets, no pet can lower the blood pressure of a hypertensive or otherwise take the place of preventive health care. The real therapeutic usefulness of pets may be as an adjunct to psychotherapy, particularly with disturbed children or people recovering from illnesses. Pet therapy reinforces what many people want to believe anyway—that pets are intrinsically good for people. If walking your dog makes you happy, or you love coming home to your cat, the health benefits are self-explanatory. No scientific studies are necessary. As one researcher in the veterinary field has written, "pets are active members of human social systems." The benefits they bring to normal life at home may be translated into therapy for those whose normal life has been interrupted.

in order to achieve an altered consciousness. The form of meditation most familiar to Americans over forty, perhaps, is transcendental meditation (TM), which swept the country in the 1960s, after being introduced in the late 1950s by the Maharishi Mahesh Yogi, an Indian sage or teacher who captured the attention of the world, or at least the world press. What the Maharishi taught didn't require a religious conversion or a renunciation of one's worldly goods and was less a search for contact with a deity than a means of controlling emotional stress, or achieving a kind of spiritual "high."

Any kind of meditation can serve as a distraction—you learn to shut out disturbing thoughts, and as you meditate, your blood pressure, heart rate, and breathing rate may drop. But is it the meditation that does it? When meditators are compared with control groups who simply sit quietly, the control groups usually achieve the same beneficial results. It's hard to prove, the Academy concludes, that meditation is any better than just sitting (or lying) serenely. Other forms of relaxation training (biofeedback, or techniques of progressive muscle relaxation), may be just as useful in reducing blood pressure and emotional stress.

Nevertheless, the National Academy of Sciences review concluded that some forms of meditation have not been carefully studied—specifically certain techniques (Kundalini Yoga and others) from India and China. Moreover, the editors said, it's claimed that no one can really evaluate religious meditation "unless one experiences it in a deep and thoroughgoing way." And, they conclude, "Contemporary science is but one way of knowing."

If you already meditate and find it helpful, you should certainly continue. It's not for everybody. Some people find that meditation actually increases anxiety. If you don't want to meditate but would like to relax, find a few minutes each day to be alone without any distractions at all. It may be that for many people, lying or sitting quietly, taking a long walk, or listening attentively to music—whatever works to produce a feeling of serenity—may be just as good as meditation.

Pros and cons of relaxation techniques

Just how to evaluate the relative merits of all these techniques is difficult to say. While all these phenomena of lowered respiration and metabolic rates are interesting, it is not clear just what significance they have for the health of any individual. The principal clinical benefits of meditation, relaxation, and biofeedback techniques would seem to be in the reduction of headaches, muscle aches, and hypertension. In people who conscientiously practice biofeedback techniques over a long period of time, such maneuvers seem to help headaches. However, it is wrong to look at biofeedback as the new health panacea. There are no licensing guidelines for biofeedback personnel and it can be very expensive. The American College of Physicians concluded in a position paper that there was no evidence that biofeedback was more effective than less expensive types of relaxation techniques.

Muscle relaxation techniques clearly help muscle tension. Whether any of the techniques has a sufficient impact on blood pressure, however, and whether patients will sustain their biofeedback or relaxation techniques for a long enough duration to make the sort of difference that drugs demonstrably do is still an open question. In the treatment of mild hypertension, these methods are most likely to be effective when they are combined with a change in lifestyle—that is, with weight reduction, sodium reduction, exercise, cessation of smoking, and moderation in the use of alcohol.

At the same time, some studies have indicated that some people even have increased anxiety as a result of relaxation training. Evidently, the varieties of individual response to such forms of psychological manipulation are a reflection of individual temperament. For some people such techniques may be of profound and lasting benefit; for others they may be a mere escape mechanism from the normal strains of daily life; for others they may be misleading substitutes for proven medical drug therapies.

For most people, though, relaxation techniques rarely harm and may help. If you are under a doctor's care for hypertension, heart disease, or headaches, you can try adding relaxation techniques to your daily routine, but certainly don't discard medication without your physician's approval. If you are healthy, you may want to try relaxation techniques to reduce daily tension.

Memory

All people—even young adults, adolescents, and children—forget things. The names of new acquaintances. Possessions. Phone calls they meant to make. When this happens, they and their elders may joke about "selective memory." But for the older adult, the very same lapses can provoke intense anxiety.

If you're over forty-five, you have no doubt experienced annoying delays in recall. You can't remember the name of your high-school chemistry teacher, but later the name "Mrs. McCoy" floats into your consciousness. Or maybe it never surfaces. Or you find yourself standing in the middle of the kitchen and can't recall what you came in there for.

"Am I losing it?" you wonder. "Is this going to get worse?" Or you may worry that you are experiencing the first symptoms of "Alzheimer's." This disease is better understood and more readily identified by doctors today, even though it remains incurable. But only a small percentage (anywhere from 5 to 10 percent) of people over age sixty-five suffer from Alzheimer's disease. For the majority of healthy people, some degree of memory loss, especially after sixty-five, is a normal part of aging.

Yet even as you search everywhere for your car keys, do remember this: many people can and do retain a very high level of mental functioning as they grow older. There's no uniform pattern of age-related changes in mental abilities for adults—it's a very individual matter. Declines, when they do occur, happen gradually, over many years.

How memory works

Our senses are continually bombarded with stimuli—all potential memories. Fortunately, we do not keep every item on short-term recall. The S-shaped ridge called the hippocampus (from the Greek for "seahorse," which it resembles) appears to play an important role in registering this sensory data and screening it for discard or storage.

Yet memories can't be said to be "located" in the hippocampus or in any other easy-to-pinpoint part of the brain. Research indicates that they are also stored throughout the cells of the cortex, the mass of wrinkled tissue that forms the surface of the brain, and in the cerebellum, a structure situated beneath the cortex at the rear of the brain, that coordinates movement and balance. Electrical stimulus of specific brain areas can occasionally provoke vivid "you-are-there" memories (childhood scenes, music) almost like switching on a radio. But the exact storage points of more abstract memories (stories, mathematical formulas) have yet to be determined.

Prior to storage, sensory information passes in the form of patterns of electrical impulses into your short-term memory, which processes it for immediate use, then discards or retains it. It allows you to remember a number, for instance, just long enough to make a phone call. If you rehearse it—repeat and memorize it because you know you'll need it again—the number is processed for long-term storage.

Memorization and studying are forms of rehearsal, but so are more casual moments when you ponder something you've just read in the newspaper or seen on television. Items that are rehearsed or that carry emotional impact win a secure niche in our long-term memories.

This stored information is received through the interaction of recognition and recall. Both depend on the mind's power to make associations. Recollections of your high-school prom may surge into consciousness unbidden when someone describes the gardenias you wore. Even the scent of gardenias on its own could summon up such memories.

Multiple-choice tests are largely based on the faculty of recognition. Other tests, and daily life, ask for answers to direct questions, answers that depend on the employment of recall, a more conscious scanning of memory files. "Who was in the White House during the First World War?" "How did you make that delicious stew you served last night?"

If you've trained your memory by developing a solid system for associating one memory with another, the answers may pop into your head immediately. On the other hand, in your search for Woodrow Wilson you may have had to consider and reject Theodore Roosevelt and William Howard Taft. As you go through the list of ingredients for your stew, you might forget to include turnips if you've always relied on a cookbook and have never rehearsed the recipe.

The processes involved in short-term memory and storage and retrieval depend on a chain of electrical, chemical, and physical changes to some of the brain's more than 100 billion nerve cells, or neurons. Under the stimulus of incoming sensory information, received as electrical impulses, projections called axons (transmitters) and dendrites (receivers) branch out from each neuron to form electrical circuits with neighboring neurons. The axons and dendrites transmit the information they carry through synapses, the junctions between the cells. In addition, chemicals called neurotransmitters are produced at neuron junctions to facilitate the passage of these impulses. They also stimulate an increase in the size of the cell bodies and the number of their smaller dendrites. Training increases the amount of neurotransmitters and synapses. But the impulses rapidly disappear from the neuron circuits unless they are reinforced by repetition or rehearsal.

Memory and aging

Because an aging brain produces smaller amounts of neurotransmitters (and because neurons die), growing older affects our ability to process incoming information rapidly, and in the case of long-term memory, to retrieve the appropriate recollection as quickly as we used to. Our store of memories expands enormously with the passing of time. An obvious example is our vocabulary. At college age most of us have command of 20,000 words or so; by age sixty our vocabularies have doubled. Access to that stored information remains unblocked. It is the act of remembering—the process of retrieval—that may slow down with age, but the fact is that age usually enhances "intelligence," in part because our store of memories has become so vast.

In terms of short-term memory, some psychologists suggest, however, that we may institute a kind of unconscious screening process as we get older: at fifty or seventy we may discard facts and observations that would have been retained as fresh and new at an impressionable eighteen or twenty-five. Selectivity could be one factor in short-term memory slowdown, but the aging process looms larger. Even so, studies repeatedly show that older people who make a poorer showing than college students on timed tests actually do as well or better than the students when they are allowed to pace themselves. It's not so surprising, given their far larger stores of experience.

Forgetting is not necessarily a sign of senility. According to the National Institute on Aging, senility "is not even a disease," and the term should not be used, as it commonly is, to cover everything from Alzheimer's disease to more widespread and reversible conditions that mimic symptoms of Alzheimer's such as memory loss. Memory problems are eminently treatable when triggered by minor head injuries, high fever, poor nutrition, adverse reactions to medication, or the emotional problems common to old age—depression, loneliness, boredom.

Memory loss in Alzheimer's disease is irreversible, however, though it is benign in the early stages—when victims begin to forget appointments or friends' names. As millions of brain cells die, it worsens inexorably to a malignant state in which sufferers don't even remember that they have friends. While only a small percentage of the population over sixty-five will come down with true Alzheimer's, it is the apparent triviality of those early symptoms that provokes anxiety among the not-so-silent majority of the "normally" forgetful.

It's true that, despite continuing research, the outlook at the moment is bleak for the victims of Alzheimer's and those who care for them. But most people don't get the disease. Even among Americans over eighty, only one out of every four or five get Alzheimer's or another form of dementia. For the majority of healthy people who, according to one estimate, do suffer a degree of memory loss after the age of sixty-five, the culprit is simply the normal aging process.

The fear of any slowdown as a symptom of degenerative brain disease can often provoke a self-defeating attack of the very forgetfulness we dread. Fortunately, there is little for most of us to worry about, and plenty we can do to improve our memory. Studies have shown that, like physical exercise, we can take steps to train our memories even late in life.

Attitude and self-awareness

The research of Dr. K. Warner Schaie of Penn State University has shown that people in their seventies and eighties are quite capable of learning and can even reverse mental declines. As part of the ongoing Seattle Longitudinal Study of Aging, Dr. Schaie tested a group of over 800 people whose mean age was sixty-eight initially (the range was twenty-nine to ninety-five). He found that many of them were sharper than they thought. Though verbal abilities generally remained stable into the mid-seventies, many people were overly pessimistic about their verbal abilities by the time they were tested again seven years later. Women also tended to underestimate their ability to visualize and to deal with objects in space. Dr. Schaie emphasized that some of this is reinforced by cultural stereotypes that people buy into. It helps just to know that you can expect to retain your verbal abilities and your sense of spatial orientation.

Being realistic about your abilities and assessing your strengths accurately can help. Self-aware people are able to adapt more readily. Staying aware could include anything from getting a checkup (to rule out any physical causes of forgetfulness) to simply forming the habit of writing things down.

What about the happy majority who maintain high levels of functioning into their seventies and eighties? The Seattle Longitudinal Study, underwritten by the National Institute on Aging, has followed 5,000 people, some for as long as thirty-five years. A summary of findings that appeared in *American Psychologist* cited some predisposing factors: good health, good educational backgrounds, keen interests, positive attitudes, and job satisfaction—as well as living with a smart spouse. Yet even if you have not led a charmed life and don't fit into this profile, there is plenty you can do to keep your confidence level up and your mind supple as you grow older:

Know your health status. Untreated high blood pressure, for example, can mildly impair memory and lengthen recall time. If you have high blood pressure, this is one of many reasons to treat it and keep it under control.

Be patient with yourself. Don't worry if your short-term recall slows down, or if it takes you longer to rummage through your memory bank and come up with the fact you want. All this is perfectly natural and no big deal. The average sixty-year-old has a vocabulary of twice as many words as the average twenty-year-old. That's one reason it takes longer to do the sorting. The process of retrieval may slow down, but age usually enhances "intelligence" and may even result in "wisdom," in part because our store of information has grown so much.

Give yourself credit for all you do remember. Prospective memory—remembering to keep a dentist's appointment for next week, for example—usually does not decline with age. Compare yourself to young adults you know: are you really so much more forgetful than they?

Stay active mentally. Pursue old interests and cultivate new ones. Play Scrabble or bridge, work on puzzles. Read the newspaper. Take a course in some subject that interests you, or learn a craft or skill. All these are good exercises for improving memory and maintaining intellectual function.

Be physically active. While there's no proof that physical fitness goes along with intellectual fitness, regular exercise confers a sense of well-being and may help control or ward off health problems.

Exercising your memory

Mnemonics, the art of improving short-term recall and ferreting out stored facts, depends on strong visual images and meaningful associations: it's a system for cross-indexing stored information in arresting ways. These methods take only a little time to master. They work because they seize the attention and demand concentration. The more outrageous the connections you set up, the better.

Use "loci" (Latin for "places"). Take a string of facts to be remembered: for instance, points you want to cover in a talk. Match each one to a specific site you can visualize easily—your living room, perhaps, or your street. If you're giving a talk on substance abuse, make a tour of the living room, stationing your introductory remarks on drug cartels on the table left of the fireplace. On the mantel, store what you're planning to say about government policy. To the right of the fireplace, in the bookcase, situate drug education, and beyond that, on the television set, leave your notes on police enforcement—and so forth, around the room. When you give your talk, make another mental tour of the room and "pick up" your notes. Adopt the same loci to something more innocuous, like a grocery list: pasta on the table, tomatoes on the mantel, lettuce in the bookcase, dressing on the television.

Make up rhymes. Nobody ever forgets the useful "I before E, except after C." But to remember home chores, make up your own rhymes: "Skitty, skat, let in the cat," for instance. The cornier the better.

Compose mental pictures, particularly when you're trying to remember a name: Helen Decker, say, might conjure up a vision of Helen of Troy on shipboard.

Repeat or rehearse new facts. "How do you do, Helen," you say when introduced at a party. A few minutes later you say to yourself, "That's Helen Decker." And a minute or so after that, "Can I get you anything to drink, Helen?" You probably won't forget Helen's name.

Make up acronyms or sentences. "Maple" could help an out-of-towner in New York remember the order of Madison, Park, and Lexington Avenues. "The postman at Sutter's Mill was bushed from pining for California" could help a visitor remember the order of five San Francisco streets, Post, Sutter, Bush, Pine, and California.

Chunk or regroup clusters of data to give them a pattern. Telephone numbers are already partially grouped, but you can give them further meaning. Helen's three-number exchange, 744, is easy to remember, but you won't forget the rest of the number either, 4591, when you reflect that she looks to be about 45, almost halfway to 91.

Write things down. Writing notes and making lists will fix things in your mind. You may not even have to refer to your notes or lists.

Structure your life. The hook for the house keys by the back door is a mnemonic device: you'll always look there first. For example, keep your checkbook in the third drawer of your desk, or park your reading glasses on the night table.

Headaches

Headaches are one of the most common human ailments. For most people a headache is merely an infrequent annoyance, a passing discomfort that results from lack of sleep, sitting in a smoky room, or having an argument with someone. With aspirin, rest, and maybe a gentle massage, the pain goes away.

But for millions of others the pain does not go away; they suffer from chronic headaches. Americans spend upwards of $400 million a year on headache remedies, leading researchers to estimate that as many as 45 million Americans suffer from chronic and/or severe headaches that seriously interfere with their lives.

Like the common cold, headaches are not completely understood by medical science, and researchers have advanced numerous theories to explain them. Tension, personality traits, heredity, and diet are a few of the factors that may play a role in chronic headaches. There appear to be various types of headache, but any hard and fast classification is open to debate, in part because the types often overlap—both in their symptoms and their response to medication. Moreover, triggering factors and modes of relief vary from person to person.

Still, the great majority of primary headaches (that is, those not due to underlying disease) fall into three categories, according to the International Headache Society: tension, migraine, and cluster.

Tension headaches

Also called a muscle-contraction or stress headache, this is the type almost everyone gets occasionally. The dull, steady pain—mild compared to migraine or cluster headaches—may be felt in the forehead, temples, back of neck, or throughout the head. A feeling of tightness around the scalp is typical; muscles in the back of the upper neck may feel knotted and tender to the touch. It's not known whether it's the sustained muscle tension itself or the subsequent restricted blood flow that causes the pain.

Tension headaches are associated with stress (often the pain actually comes after the stress has ended), fatigue, or too much or too little sleep. Assuming a posture that tenses your neck and head muscles for long periods, such as holding your chin down while reading, can trigger such headaches; so can gum chewing, grinding your teeth, or tensing head and neck muscles during sexual intercourse. Men and women are about equally likely to suffer tension headaches.

Depression headaches. Some people who have daily headaches have been found to be suffering from depression as well. Usually they are muscle-contraction headaches. Persistent headaches accompanied by lethargy, insomnia, or suicidal thoughts are signs of clinical depression. Researchers do not understand the connection between depression and headaches, though some have suggested that the depression and the headaches may have a common biochemical cause. In some cases it may be the persistent headaches that cause the depression. And in some cases treating the depression makes the headaches go away.

Migraines

The word migraine, derived from the Greek, means "half a skull"—an apt description of the pain, which usually occurs in only one side of the head. Migraines appear to involve the abnormal expansion and contraction of blood vessels in and around the brain. In some people, migraines start with distorted vision, called an "aura"—generally characterized by zigzag patterns of shooting lights, blind spots, and/or a temporary loss of peripheral vision. The throbbing, pulsating pain can be incapacitating. It can last anywhere from a few minutes to several days; if it lasts longer than that, it's probably not a migraine. Migraine sufferers may also experience nausea, vomiting, and sensitivity to both light and noise.

About 80 percent of migraine sufferers having a family history of the ailment; women are nearly four times more likely to be afflicted. The typical sufferer is young (under thirty-five), and had her first attack during her teens or twenties. With age, attacks usually become less severe and less frequent. Hormonal changes can play a role: thus susceptible women may have more attacks if they take oral contraceptives or around the time of menstruation; they may have fewer attacks during pregnancy and after menopause. Attacks can also be instigated by certain substances in foods, emotional factors, and environmental changes (such as glaring light, strong odors, and changes in weather).

It may seem that a headache causes your brain to hurt, but actually brain tissue contains no sensory nerves—it's immune to pain.

Feeding a Headache

Researchers estimate that food plays a role in anywhere from 10 percent to 40 percent of all headaches, especially migraines. But proving a definite link between diet and headaches is often difficult, and no single food affects all sensitive individuals. Most of the suspect foods and beverages contain substances that may constrict or dilate blood vessels in the brain. One major culprit is tyramine, a chemical that occurs naturally in many foods. Nitrites, used in cold cuts and frankfurters, can also dilate blood vessels. Although a variety of foods may provoke headaches in sensitive people, these below have been most commonly implicated:

Aged cheeses
Alcoholic drinks (especially red wine)
Nuts and peanut butter
Yogurt
Sour cream
Cured or processed meats
Caffeine-rich drinks
Freshly baked yeast products
Chocolate
MSG (monosodium glutamate)
Hydrolyzed vegetable protein
Aspartame (artificial sweetener)

Cluster headaches

These strike in a group or "cluster" for up to a few hours, and recur daily for days, weeks, or even months on end. There may be months of freedom between attacks. Some researchers consider cluster headaches a variant of migraines, largely because the excruciating pain is centered on one side of the head, as in a migraine. But unlike the throbbing of a migraine, this pain is steady and piercing. There are other notable differences: typically cluster headaches strike at night or early morning, and the pain is located around or behind one eye or in one temple. Cluster headaches are about six to nine times more likely to strike men than women; the first attack usually comes in a person's twenties or thirties. They are sometimes misdiagnosed as a sinus disorder (because stuffy nose or sinus congestion is a common symptom) or even an abscessed tooth. There's no clear cause, though heavy smoking and drinking are possible contributing or triggering factors.

When to See a Doctor

Most people who suffer from migraines or cluster headaches need to consult a doctor about treatment. In addition, in a small number of cases, severe headaches may be a warning sign of a more serious disorder, such as very high blood pressure, stroke, bleeding in the brain, or even a brain tumor. The following signs should send you to your doctor right away:

•You suddenly start having severe headaches—especially if they're your first ones and you are over thirty-five.

•You have a severe headache during or immediately after physical exertion or straining. Some activities, including sexual intercourse and strenuous sports, may lead to "exertion headaches," which are fairly common and usually harmless. But to rule out internal head injury, it's prudent to see your doctor.

•A headache with a fever and neck stiffness.

•A headache accompanied by confusion or loss of speech—especially after a blow to the head, even one that occurred several weeks earlier.

•A headache accompanied by inflamed, clogged sinuses. Occasionally, a severe headache results from infection and the build-up of pus in the sinus passages.

•Any increase in the intensity or frequency of headaches.

Exertion headaches. Some physical activities, including sexual intercourse and strenuous sports, have led to so-called exertion headaches. Football players and joggers are the athletes most frequently struck by them. These attacks are probably vascular, caused by abrupt dilation or constriction of blood vessels, but researchers have not been able to pinpoint the exact cause of pain. The headaches often hit just after exercise and are so painful that some sufferers have been rushed to emergency rooms. This is a prudent precaution in sports such as football, where a head injury is possible. But in nearly all cases exertion headaches are neither harmful nor symptomatic of other ailments. With rest the pain goes away.

Treatment: drugs

The most common headache medications are sold over-the-counter—aspirin, ibuprofen (such as Advil or Motrin IB), or acetaminophen (such as Tylenol). It's impossible to predict which will work best for you. Remember that just because a drug is sold over-the-counter, that does not mean it is harmless. No one should take a pain reliever for long periods without consulting a doctor.

If over-the-counter pain relievers aren't sufficient, you'll have to work with your doctor to find the right prescription drug for you. A wide variety of such drugs are available—from narcotic pain relievers and antidepressants to beta blockers and muscle relaxants. Most of these medications are meant to get rid of the headache, but for people whose headaches are very severe or frequent, there are drugs designed to prevent attacks.

Many migraine sufferers find that it's essential to nip the pain in the bud—that is, take medicine at the first sign of an attack. However, the long-term frequent use of certain medications may actually result in drug-related headaches. Most of the prescription drugs have unpleasant and sometimes dangerous side effects, so it's always best to rely on nondrug treatments when possible.

Prevention and treatment without drugs

If you have recurrent headaches, try to find out what triggers them. Keeping a diary may help—it can show you that a certain activity, circumstance, food, or

Other causes of headaches

The most common disease that causes persistent headaches— often as the only symptom—is high blood pressure. If you suffer from frequent headaches, get your blood pressure checked, especially if you are over forty. A lot of people think first of a brain tumor as an important cause, but that is very rare. Of all the people who seek treatment for headaches, less than one-half of one percent have been found to have a brain tumor.

The sudden onset of severe headaches in a person who previously had been free of headaches can indicate a serious disorder.

Eyestrain can cause a headache but it will go away as soon as you rest your eyes. Poor lighting or posture may also lead to a headache.

medication is associated with the attacks. Treatments like the following may allow you to get by without drugs:

Relaxation training. Learning how to relax and cope with stress sometimes helps relieve headaches and other kinds of pain—in part by reducing muscle tension, in part by shifting attention away from the pain. One common technique is progressive muscle relaxation. It calls for tensing and then relaxing specific muscle groups, working from the feet to the head, while focusing on deep, regular breathing. Another technique, called the relaxation response, is a form of meditation, and requires you to repeat a word or phrase until the mind is free of distracting thoughts and the body relaxed.

One study published in the journal *Headache* found that migraine sufferers who were taught relaxation training had 30 percent to 40 percent fewer attacks over the course of three years. The twenty four subjects were also better able to cope with the attacks they did have and required less medication.

Biofeedback. This high-tech relaxation method calls for hooking a subject up to a device that continuously measures a physiological variable—muscle tension, for instance, or skin temperature. Meter readouts or tones tell whether the variable is increasing or decreasing—this is the "feedback." The subject then tries to lower the number or change the pitch by focusing on whatever sensations, thoughts, or feelings work for him. When biofeedback is successful it relaxes muscles, reduces anxiety, and most important, produces an increased sense of control, all of which may contribute to pain relief.

Ice packs. Reusable gel packs—kept in the freezer and then wrapped around the neck during a headache—may provide relief, in lieu of medication or as an adjunct to it. A study, published in *Postgraduate Medicine,* found that of ninety headache sufferers, 70 percent experienced some relief from such gel packs. Running cold water over your head may have a similar effect.

Heat. You may find that heat, rather than cold, helps relieve your headaches. A hot shower or bath, or moist heat applied to the back of the neck (use a wet towel wrapped around a waterproof heating pad), may relieve some tension headaches.

Massage. Many people find that massaging muscles in the neck, forehead, and temples promotes relaxation and offers some relief, especially for tension headaches.

Headbands. A recent study published in *Headache* found that a headband (with two small rubber disks to apply pressure over areas of maximum pain) provided at least partial relief in sixty out of sixty-nine migraine headaches. The band provides more consistent pressure on the temples, scalp, and forehead than finger pressure.

Exercise. In some people, regular exercise helps relieve tension and thus may prevent some headaches. Neck, back, and shoulder stretches may also help.

Improved posture. When working at a computer terminal, for instance, adjust your seat and table so that you don't have to bend your neck for long periods.

Get to the source. You may discover that your headaches disappear only when you resolve some underlying stressful problem in your life—a troubled marriage, for instance, or a major upcoming exam.

The advertising industry virtually invented the notion of sinus headache. Persistent headaches due to chronic sinus problems or allergies are very rare. The congestion and swelling that come with these ailments can touch off a headache, but sinusitis or allergies are almost never the cause of frequent headaches. One sign of a real sinus headache is that it gets worse if you bend over.

Sleep

Everyone needs to sleep, and a sound sleep can leave us feeling wonderfully refreshed. For many people, going to bed is among the day's most pleasant experiences. At the same time, there are many others who worry about not getting enough sleep. Yet how much sleep is optimal, and whether getting less than this amount is harmful in any way, remain unclear. The truth about sleep's relationship to health has been difficult for scientists to trace: for example, we still do not know why sleep is necessary. However, researchers have uncovered a great deal about what takes place during sleep, what disturbs sleeping patterns, and how to improve sleeping habits.

The sleep cycle

A person's sleep alternates through two phases of sleep, which researchers have called REM (Rapid Eye Movement) and non-REM. Non-REM, the first phase, is called "the quiet sleep"—there is a general absence of body movement, brain activity is slow and regular, and the five senses shut down. The non-REM phase moves through four stages as sleep gets progressively deeper and the sleeper becomes more difficult to arouse. The deepest sleep—called delta sleep—appears to be the most restorative stage. People deprived of sleep will spend more time in delta sleep during subsequent nights.

About seventy to ninety minutes after falling asleep, having moved through the non-REM stages, the brain switches into the second phase of sleep, REM. Abruptly the sleeper's eyes begin to dart behind closed lids; heartbeat and metabolism speed up; and breathing gets faster and more irregular, as do the brain waves. Toes and fingers twitch, yet large muscles are practically immobile. And the sleeper dreams, often vividly.

The first episode of REM ends after about ten minutes, completing a sleep cycle of about ninety minutes which will recur four or five times during the night. The first few hours of sleep are dominated by deep sleep; in the final sleep cycle, REM can last thirty to forty minutes. An adult who sleeps seven and a half hours will spend one and a half to two hours in REM sleep.

The benefits of sleep

There seems to be little doubt that sleep rests and restores our bodies. Delta sleep is the time for releasing most of our growth hormone, which some researchers credit with the renewal of worn-out tissues. More specifically, researchers at the University of Goteborg in Sweden found that growth hormone enhances bone synthesis, while a study at the University of California School of Medicine linked it to the formation of red blood cells.

The most important benefit of sleep may be that it restores us mentally. Without it our minds seem to suffer more than our bodies. A person kept up twenty-four hours, studies have shown, feels fatigued, is easily distracted, and has difficulty performing simple routine tasks. The psychological effects are even more

Napping for Energy

About half the people in the world take a nap each day—the afternoon siesta is part of life in most tropical and subtropical regions. And in our own society, those who have the time to nap indulge in it: one study of college students found that 55 percent of them nap one or more times a week.

For most of us, the urge to nap strikes in the afternoon. We tend to attribute this drowsiness to eating and digesting lunch, or in warm climates, to the heat of midday. But in fact our bodies experience a slight drop in temperature—part of our internal biorhythms—that probably promotes sleepiness.

If you want to try renewing your energy and reducing everyday stress by taking a nap, bear the following in mind:

• The ideal nap time is mid-afternoon, between 2:00 and 3:00 p.m., when body temperature is at a low point
• Afternoons are also optimal because napping early or late in the day can interfere with your nighttime sleep. It's all right to use a nap for catching up on lost sleep—but naps shouldn't become a substitute for sleep.
• Afternoon naps also give you just enough deep sleep to feel refreshed. Morning naps are mainly light sleep, while evening naps put you into an overly sound deep sleep; either way, you end up feeling fatigued or groggy after the nap rather than invigorated.
• Keep your nap under an hour—more than that won't increase the benefits, and is likely to result in intense grogginess.

dramatic. In a study at Walter Reed Hospital, volunteers who stayed up beyond sixty hours experienced distortion, mood shifts, headaches, and blurred vision.

Yet in spite of such consequences, the ability to perform complex tasks—such as taking examinations—does not diminish significantly with short-term sleep loss, nor is physiological performance impaired. In an Indiana University study, researchers tested subjects who stayed awake for thirty hours and then exercised. They found that heart rate, oxygen intake, carbon dioxide production, and other measures of physical exertion were not affected by the sleep loss. However, subjects perceived that their exertion was greater after sleep loss than after a period of sleep. Perhaps most remarkable is how efficiently we make up for drastic amounts of lost sleep. Studies have confirmed that, even after being awake for days, most people need only one long night's sleep to recover.

How much sleep do we need?

The notion that we all need eight hours a night—or any other fixed amount—is nonsense. A good night's sleep is whatever allows us to feel refreshed, alert, and in good spirits the next day. And there are wide individual differences in how much sleep people need to achieve that. Some need nine or ten hours, others only six.

But how solidly you sleep is as important as the amount of sleep. Most people feel more rested when they consolidate sleep than when they parcel it out over five or six periods in a day.

Sleep and age

Age is the most important trait affecting sleep. Infants sleep roughly twice as much as adults, slumbering fourteen to eighteen hours a day. After six months, sleep time dwindles and increasingly takes place at night. By age twelve, sleep patterns approximate those of adults.

The next dramatic shift appears in the elderly—though what changes are sleep patterns, not the need for sleep. In about 80 percent of people over sixty, sleep

Circadian Rhythms

Science has discovered that human beings—indeed all living things on earth—operate according to an inborn circadian (from the Latin words *circa* and *dies,* meaning around the day) rhythm. This inner body clock regulates practically all physiological functions including your hormone levels.

But, human beings are out of sync with the turning of the planet: the human internal "day" does not last twenty-four hours, but twenty-five. Experimental subjects confined for several days to a clockless room and given no clues about the actual time of day tend to go to bed an hour later each night and wake up an hour later each morning.

Thus it is easier for us to lengthen our days than to shorten them and we feel all right after a plane flight westward across two or three time zones, but exhausted after flying the same distance eastward. That's also why we happily adapt to a new bedtime in the fall when we switch to standard time and gain an hour but complain about the springtime switch. This may also help explain why it's hard to get up on Monday morning, since on the weekend you may have drifted toward your natural twenty-five hour cycle.

Circadian rhythms and work

These circadian rhythms can have major economic and health consequences. It is estimated that some 27 percent of American working men and 16 percent of working women rotate between day and night shifts. These people work in round-the-clock manufacturing, in the military, on airlines and other forms of transportation, in radio and television, or as health care professionals. According to a study in the *New England Journal of Medicine,* over 80 percent of these people have serious sleep disruption (insomnia at home and sleepiness at work), which lowers their productivity as well as the quality of their lives. The study also cites a higher risk of cardiovascular and digestive tract diseases among these workers.

Adjusting circadian rhythms

These problems, however, can be alleviated by applying our knowledge of the circadian rhythms. In one experiment at a Utah potash mine and processing plant, workers had been advancing from day to evening to night shifts on a weekly basis, a grueling procedure that would have affected them rather like flying eastward around the world in three hops, departing every Monday. But when they were allowed to stay on one shift for three-week periods and to rotate in the other direction— night to evening to day—their circadian rhythms were disrupted less. Productivity improved and so did health.

Can light help?

Another study has suggested that light affects the inner clock independent of its influence on our sleep/wake patterns. Researchers were repeatedly able to readjust the biological clocks of fourteen men (age eighteen to twenty-four) by exposing them to light (equal to sunlight in brightness) for three five-hour sessions at various stages of their circadian cycles over the course of three days. Circadian rhythms were reset by as much as twelve hours, backwards and forwards.

These findings may have practical applications. For instance, after a jet trip across many time zones, or after a sudden change from a daytime to nighttime work shift, it may take as long as nine days for the body to fully readjust. (As a rule of thumb, for each one-hour time zone you cross, it takes roughly one day to recuperate.) But properly timed exposure to bright sunlight and/or artificial light may be able to reset the biological clock much more quickly.

While this research is encouraging, more studies will need to be done before scientists can prescribe specific amounts of light for people with circadian disorders. Meanwhile, after a long jet trip, try to get some sunlight during the first few mornings and afternoons. Just walk around, sit, or even run outside; wearing sunscreen won't cancel out the beneficial effect of the light.

If you travel on business and will have to spend all your daylight hours indoors, try to arrive a day early so that you can recover from your flight by getting some light. Despite tiredness or wakefulness, try to go to sleep and awaken at the usual local times.

becomes more fragmented. They tend to wake up more often (and for longer periods) during the night, and earlier in the morning, with generally less deep sleep and more light sleep. Though the amount of time in bed stays fairly constant, sleep time usually lessens—averaging six and a half hours a night. And older people sometimes compensate by daytime napping.

According to a review article in the *New England Journal of Medicine,* aging does not explain insomnia, even though sleep problems may increase. A study of healthy women in their sixties, published in *Psychology and Aging,* suggested that emotional distress is a significant factor in disrupting sleep. People who are aging successfully—that is, who are in good health and leading an active, involved life—seem to preserve a more youthful pattern of sleep.

While increasingly fragmented sleep in many older people may be normal, it can also also result from a specific sleep disorder. For instance, sleep apnea—a potentially dangerous condition in which you stop breathing temporarily and then snore loudly as you struggle to recover—can prevent restful sleep (see box on page 477). In addition, the elderly consume an abnormally high proportion of sleeping medications—drugs that often do not improve sleep and may be harmful (see page 478).

Nightmares are most common among children aged three to seven. But some adults are also prone to them. Researchers have isolated the characteristics of these chronic nightmare sufferers— sensitive, open, and vulnerable. Creative people, who are in touch with imagery and fantasy, seem to have more nightmares than others.

Troubled sleep

The elderly are not the only ones with sleeping problems. An estimated 20 to 40 percent of all adults complain about insomnia—a general term that refers to difficulty falling or staying asleep. In one survey of some 7,000 San Francisco residents, 30 percent across a broad age range reported insomnia-related problems. And according to a review in the *New England Journal of Medicine* of more than a hundred studies of insomnia, 17 percent of the sleepless consider the problem serious.

Insomnia is not a disorder but a symptom with many causes. For example, temporary insomnia can be caused by jet lag, which upsets the body's biological clock, or by some specific stressful situation like a divorce or change in job. Once these situations have been resolved, sleep returns to normal.

Persistent insomnia is more difficult to diagnose. The Association of Sleep Disorders Centers has suggested causes ranging from psychological and medical conditions to environmental factors like noise and room temperature. There have also been many studies to determine if personality differences make one a good or poor sleeper. Some researchers found that poor sleepers are more anxious, depressed, and introspective, and tend to internalize psychological conflicts. But other studies have found no personality differences between the two groups.

Many experts are convinced that in the majority of cases, the original cause becomes secondary; instead, the insomnia persists because of behavioral factors that reinforce it, such as excessive time in bed, drug dependency, and napping. Also, the harder you try to fall asleep, the more anxious you become, which makes success all the more difficult.

The effects of sleep loss

It's not unusual to lose sleep the night before an important event—an exam at school, a presentation at work, or a crucial race. You may worry that this loss of sleep will impair your performance, and this worry may in turn make it even harder to sleep. As research has accumulated in recent years, it has become increas-

Snoring

Over 100 million Americans snore, which can seriously disrupt sleep or annoy a sleeping partner. Snoring occurs mostly during non-REM sleep and is caused by the rattling of the walls of air passages, which can happen when nasal passages dry out or when the sleeper lies on his back. If you are getting a good night's sleep, your snoring is probably harmless. But if it annoys your bedmate, try these techniques to stop it.

• Attach a rolled up sock to the back of your sleepwear to keep you from lying on your back when you sleep.

• Check the bedroom's humidity level. Low humidity dries out mucous membranes, so consider getting a humidifier.

• See a specialist to determine if you have a nasal obstruction, adenoids, a deviated septum, or enlarged tonsils, all of which can cause snoring.

Snorers who are chronically sleepy may have sleep apnea, a potentially dangerous condition that afflicts 50,000 or more Americans. Sleepers with apnea stop breathing temporarily and snore loudly struggling to recover. New surgical techniques have been used to treat apnea. if you suspect you have it, visit a sleep disorders clinic.

A nightcap might lull you to sleep, but it won't be a sound sleep. Alcohol typically produces light, unsettled sleep, and often the sleeper will suddenly snap awake.

ingly apparent that the effects of sleep deprivation depend not only on the amount of sleep you've lost and the type and length of your activity, but also on your age, personality, and even the time of day. It may help you sleep better to know that under most circumstances a night or two of poor sleep will put you at little or no disadvantage for moderate physical performance. But it may impair some types of mental activity.

Athletic performance. Most studies have found that simple physical exertion is not significantly impaired by lack of sleep or poor sleep for a night or two. Changes in cardiopulmonary function in sleep-deprived people at rest and while exercising have varied greatly from study to study, and from subject to subject. Many subjects perceived that their exertion and fatigue were greater than after a period of normal sleep. However, their actual performance usually suffered little or not at all.

Most studies of sleep deprivation have focused on repetitive exercise (such as running, cycling, or swimming), so there are still questions about sports that require vigilance, cognitive skills, and a high degree of coordination (such as baseball, tennis, or fencing), which are more likely to be affected by sleep deprivation. And few studies have looked at the effects of sleep loss on elite athletes, for whom a difference of a few seconds in a race may be crucial. In addition, the "rush" of competitive activity and the cheering of a crowd can more than compensate for any possible effects of sleep loss. In any case, for recreational exercise or the physical demands of the average workday, moderate sleep loss should not be a problem.

Mental performance. Studies bear out the fact that the loss of even one night's sleep is likely to result in fatigue, irritability, inability to concentrate, and mood shifts. But long repetitive tasks are more likely to be affected by sleep loss than short interesting tasks. Most research has focused on pilots, industrial workers, radar operators, resident physicians, and other people whose sleep habits may increase the risk of accidents, and has found that the longer people are deprived of sleep, the greater the possibility of accidents. Thus the federal government regulates how long pilots can fly without sleep, for instance, and the states regulate how long resident physicians can work without sleep.

Some other findings about sleep loss and mental abilities:

•Creativity may suffer. Work by the English researcher J. A. Horne has suggested that loss of a night's sleep undermines creative thinking (characterized by spontaneity, flexibility, and originality) and the ability to deal with unfamiliar situations. Yet the loss of one night's sleep had little effect on less creative endeavors, such as solving familiar problems using well-established skills.

•An internal "clock" sets the body's daily, or circadian, rhythms—and it may affect mental performance as much as, or even more than, the amount of lost sleep (see page 475). One Israeli study of sleep-deprived people found that the degree of

The average man in his twenties awakens ten times during the night. By the time he reaches forty, the number of wakenings increases to fifteen. By age sixty, it may be as many as twenty-two times. Sleep interruptions among women follow a similar upward curve, though frequency is somewhat less at every age.

Sleeping Pills

Prescription sleeping pills and other sleeping aids are among the most frequently taken medications in the United States. But how effective and safe are they—and what, if anything, should you take?

Over-the-counter sleeping pills. Most such drugs are antihistamines (just like many hay-fever remedies, which may also induce drowsiness) and at the suggested dosage are probably harmless. It won't hurt to try them for occasional sleeplessness—they may work for a night or two—but studies show that they quickly lose their effectiveness.

L-tryptophan. This so-called "natural" sleeping pill, once sold in health-food stores, is an amino acid (one of the essential building blocks of protein). The body converts tryptophan to serotonin, a neurotransmitter or brain chemical that helps regulate sleep. Most studies show that, in large enough doses, tryptophan does help induce sleep. But when isolated and manufactured as a supplement, and then taken in large doses, it may pose several health risks. Tryptophan was taken off the market in 1989 when a contaminated batch was shown to cause a rare blood disease. In addition, animal studies have found that even pure tryptophan poses risks, such as severe scarring and inflammation of the pancreas and changes in the immune system. If tryptophan is at all effective against insomnia, it is a drug like any sleeping pill, and studies should be done to prove it safe and effective before it is marketed as either a prescription or nonprescription drug.

Seconal, Nembutal, and other barbiturates. Though once widely prescribed as sleeping pills, these drugs are no longer used for this purpose. They proved to be highly addictive and are almost always fatal in an overdose.

Halcion and other tranquilizers (benzodiazepines). Marketed under such names as Valium, Klonopin, Xanax, Dalmane, Restoril, and Halcion, these prescription-only antianxiety drugs really do act as sedatives and are very widely prescribed for people suffering from insomnia. They are less likely than barbiturates to be lethal in overdose, or to create physical dependency. But long-term users do experience some dependency and will usually have withdrawal symptoms when they stop taking the drugs. And many side effects have been reported for all benzodiazepines—disorientation, confusion, "hangover" the next day, blurred vision, nightmares, and daytime depression. The drugs cease to work if you take them every night.

Halcion, a short-acting benzodiazepine (that is, its sedative effects last about three hours), has recently been under fire for causing serious psychiatric side effects and was taken off the market in the United Kingdom. Canada did not ban it but placed restrictions on the strength of the dosage that could be prescribed and the duration of use (fourteen days maximum). In this country the FDA did not take Halcion off the market but did require the manufacturer to provide more explicit information to consumers about the risks and benefits of the drug. The FDA has said it still believes that the benefits of Halcion outweigh the risks, but "in no sense should this suggest that Halcion is free of side effects." It may be no more dangerous than other drugs in this category, but since it is more widely used, more side effects are reported.

If, for some reason, you and your doctor decide you need one of these drugs, try a low dose first, and don't take it for more than three nights in a row. Never combine it with alcohol. A physician who's truly interested in your welfare will not automatically renew your prescription, but will want to find out if your problem has cleared up. Your goal should be to reestablish normal sleeping habits without any drugs.

sleepiness they felt was influenced more by the time of day (that is, the phase of the circadian cycle) than by the amount of sleep loss. Like everyone else, sleep-deprived people are likely to function best in the early evening and mid-morning, typically the high points of the circadian cycle.

•Older people may be more alert. A study at the University of Pittsburgh School of Medicine found that sleep-deprived people in their eighties were able to concentrate better and maintain more stable moods than people in their twenties. Perhaps older people were less affected because their normal sleep was lighter and more fragmented to begin with.

Getting a good night's sleep

In a study reported in the *American Journal of Psychiatry,* one group of insomniacs was treated with the prescription sleeping pill Halcion, while another learned to do some muscle relaxation exercises and to follow the kind of advice outlined below. At first the Halcion group got more sleep, but by the second week, the other group had caught up. By the fifth week the members of the behavior-training group were falling asleep faster and sleeping better than the Halcion group.

1. If your sleeplessness arises from worry or grief, try to correct what's bothering you. If you can't do anything about it right now, try confiding in a friend, joining a support group, or finding a qualified counselor.

2. Don't drink alcohol before bedtime—and don't smoke. Alcohol can disrupt sleep patterns and make insomnia worse. Nicotine makes you wakeful, too.

3. Avoid reproaching yourself. Don't make your sleeplessness a cause for additional worry. Insomnia is not a crime. Nobody needs exactly eight hours sleep. You can feel well—and be quite healthy—on less. Don't worry that you have to "make up" lost sleep. One good night will repair the fatigue.

4. Avoid eating a heavy meal in the evening, particularly at bedtime. Don't drink large amounts of liquids before retiring.

5. Eliminate caffeinated beverages except in the morning or early afternoon.

6. If you're unable to fall asleep after twenty minutes, get up and do something rather than lying there trying to fall asleep. But don't bring work to bed. If you wake up and can't fall asleep in the middle of the night, try reading for a short time. Counting sheep (or flowers or whatever appeals to you), or reconstructing a happy event or narrative in your mind may lull you to sleep.

7. Don't watch the clock at night. Turn it to the wall if you can't help looking at the time and worrying.

8. Avoid daytime naps, even when you're tired.

9. Spend an hour or more relaxing before you retire—read, listen to music, watch TV, or take a warm bath.

10. Go to bed and get up on a regular schedule, no matter how much you haven't slept.

If these commonsense tips don't work the first night, they may start working over a week's time. If you continue to suffer from chronic or severe insomnia, you should also visit a doctor or sleep disorders clinic to see if there is an underlying medical condition.

If you find that out-of-the ordinary sleep loss is taking its toll on you, remember that all it takes to regain mental acuity is one—or at most two—good nights of sleep.

Travel Health

Leisure travel is one of life's greatest pleasures—but only if you stay well. Illness cuts into vacation time, and several large surveys of international travelers have indicated that, depending on destination, 25 to 75 percent of them had one or more symptoms of illness. In a foreign country, not knowing what is safe to eat or drink or where to turn for help with medical problems is especially upsetting. Some health risks may be encountered only in exotic locales, while other problems, such as motion sickness, can occur virtually anywhere. But wherever you wander, the key to a healthy trip is planning ahead.

Coping with flying

As anyone who flies is aware, traveling by jet can be stressful. Conditions on board the plane disrupt your system, as does flying across time zones. The resulting symptoms are such that, after a flight of, say, ten hours, it can take days to recover your sense of well-being.

One potential problem is the cabin atmosphere. While air quality is regulated in airport buildings and ground facilities, federal regulations do not apply to the air in planes—and provisions to ensure air quality can be lacking. According to a report from the National Academy of Sciences, basic design standards for ventilation in airplane cabins are minimal. Allowable levels of carbon monoxide in airplanes are, according to the Academy, much higher than standards for other confined environments. Cabins are tightly sealed, and fresh air is drawn inside and then conditioned by an "environmental control unit"—at great loss in fuel efficiency. Ironically, because of efforts to achieve greater fuel efficiency in aircraft, newer planes are likely to have the worst ventilation, especially wide-body jets. When the plane is on the ground, there is little ventilation; in the air it may not be much better. Moreover, cabin airflow and air quality are seldom measured once the aircraft is in service.

The main contaminant of cabin air is cigarette smoke (when smoking is permitted). According to the Academy's report, the concentration of smokers in airplane cabins and their patterns of smoking result in higher concentrations of cigarette smoke than other public places where smoking is permitted. These concentrations occur all over the cabin, not just in the smoking sections. Fortunately, smoking is now banned on domestic commercial flights in the United States as well as on many international flights, and it is quite possible that, in the near future, all flights will be smoke free.

How can you assure yourself of better air quality in the plane? Ventilation is five times better in first class than in coach, if you can afford the fare. Anywhere you sit, you can ask the flight attendant to ask the captain to increase the airflow. Because maximum ventilation consumes additional fuel, fresh air is expensive; still, the crew can improve air quality to some extent.

In addition to air quality, there are other cabin conditions that can cause discomfort and fatigue, and things you can do to alleviate them:

Altitude Adjustment

Travelers coming by plane from sea level to such high elevations as Denver, Aspen, Mexico City, or Yosemite National Park may suddenly experience shortness of breath, fatigue, headaches, nausea, and other symptoms resembling flu. This disablement, called Acute Mountain Sickness (AMS), is usually mild and, at levels around 5,000 feet, likely to last only a day or so. As mountain climbers know, it results from a lack of oxygen. Barometric pressure decreases as you go higher—that is, the air gets thinner—and you inhale less oxygen per usual breath. Trying to compensate for this, you breathe more deeply.

Not everyone feels sick at increased altitudes, and there is no way of predicting what a person's highest comfortable altitude is. Being physically fit is not necessarily a protection. Indeed, athletes accustomed to working out daily at low altitudes may be the first to get ill if they continue intense workouts at high altitudes. Susceptibility to AMS is greater in those under forty.

Skiers, hikers, and others who go above 8,000 feet risk getting more severe symptoms of AMS and at higher altitudes may even develop a serious condition known as High-Altitude Pulmonary Edema (HAPE). This life-threatening condition is due to an accumulation of fluids in the lungs. Those afflicted must immediately descend at least 2,000 to 3,000 feet. People with chronic lung or heart ailments should avoid extreme altitudes, and anyone planning to travel to altitudes of 8,000 feet or more should seek medical advice in advance. Acetazolamide, a diuretic, may reduce the incidence and severity of AMS, but this drug is not recommended in place of acclimatization.

If you are going to the Rockies or other mountain regions (see chart below), you can probably avoid high altitude symptoms—or get rid of them quickly—by simply taking the following precautions:

1. Spend your first day at high altitudes relaxing. Avoid even moderate exercise until you get used to the new heights.

2. Drink extra water and avoid alcoholic beverages. The fast, deep breathing you must do at higher altitudes will tend to dehydrate you—an effect that alcohol intensifies.

3. If your destination is above 8,000 feet, spend a day acclimatizing at a lower level, or climb to a new level at a rate of 500 to 1,000 feet daily with an occasional day of rest.

An Altitude Sampler	
Albuquerque, NM	4,950 ft
Denver, CO	5,280 ft
Lake Tahoe, NV	6,200 ft
Aspen, CO	7,930 ft
Yosemite National Park	4,000 to 8,850 ft
Banff, Alberta	4,540 ft
Mexico City	7,440 ft

• Aircraft aren't perfectly pressurized, so the air is thin, like that at about 5,000 feet. At that altitude the effect of alcohol is almost twice as great, so have one drink at most. When descending, ease sinus and ear discomfort by pinching your nostrils, closing your mouth, and trying to blow out slowly (a procedure called the Valsalva maneuver).

• Cabin air is much drier than normal air. Relative humidity at flight altitudes falls into the 5 to 10 percent range—a desert climate that can cause dryness of the eyes, mouth, and throat. Consuming fluids will help counteract the dryness, so drink plenty of nonalcoholic fluids, even if you are not thirsty. Saline nose drops are also helpful. Dryness is yet another reason to avoid smoking, which further dries out sinuses and depletes oxygen intake.

• Long periods of sitting can hamper digestion, circulation, and flexibility, and cause feet to swell. To loosen up, walk around the cabin once an hour and do some light stretching.

Overcoming jet lag

Fatigue, insomnia, and general malaise are common problems that may affect anyone who crosses more than three time zones in a flight. Jet lag is caused by a disruption of sleep/wake patterns: your biological clock is disrupted. Flying westward lengthens your day, and flying eastward shortens it. Because it compresses the day/night cycle, the eastward flight is most likely to produce jet lag.

•One preventive is to start shifting your sleep/wake cycle to the new time in advance. If traveling east to west, go to bed—and get up—an hour later each day for three days before departure. For a west-to-east trip, move your sleep time an hour earlier each day. If traveling great distances, schedule a stopover if you can.

•Changes in diet may also be helpful. The principle behind the so-called "jet lag diet" is to eat high-protein meals when you are trying to stay awake and high-carbohydrate meals when you want to sleep. A study of U.S. military travelers found that this system alleviated jet lag. Start this diet three days before departure, alternating feast days (high-protein breakfast and lunch, high-carbohydrate dinner) with fast days (salads, soup, fruits in small quantities). If you don't want to upset your dietary habits in this manner, you may do as well by getting plenty of rest before the trip, and by assuming local eating and sleeping times as soon as you arrive.

•Sunlight may help reset your biological clock. Try to spend some time outdoors your first few days after arrival.

Individuals vary greatly in how they respond to time changes, and these procedures may not be especially helpful. Thus far, the most reliable aid in adjusting to a new time zone is simply the passage of time.

Traveling abroad

Medical standards and practices can differ in other countries, sometimes dramatically. Before you travel abroad, review your medical records and insurance. If you have not had recent medical or dental checkups, see your doctor and dentist before you leave—particularly before a long trip. Pregnant women, people on prescription medications, those recovering from illnesses, and those with chronic health

What you can do about airline food

Airlines are required to offer special meals. Usually you need only place your order twenty-four hours before your flight. You can often get low-calorie, low-cholesterol, low-sodium, vegetarian, diabetic, kosher, Hindu or Moslem meals—just ask what's available. On some airlines you can get a "healthy heart" meal developed in cooperation with the American Heart Association. It is also perfectly all right to bring your own low-fat meal on the plane; pack it in disposable cartons or plastic bags. And ask the flight attendant for low-fat milk in your coffee. The nondairy powdered creamer routinely handed out has more saturated fat than milk.

Easing Motion Sickness

In a ship's cabin during rough weather, your eyes may not register much movement, but your inner ear does. Such conflicting sensory input often leads to motion sickness. *Mal de mer*, or seasickness, can strike the traveler by land and by air as well. The principal symptoms are nausea and vomiting, as well as dizziness and a cold sweat. Once you are seasick, there is no relief except getting away from the cause. But if you act in advance, you may be able to prevent it. Experts recommend the following steps:

•Avoid eating heavy meals and drinking alcohol before traveling.

•On a boat or in a car, focus on the horizon or some other fixed point in the distance.

•At sea, stay amidship and topside.

•Small children who get carsick in the back seat may be helped by being elevated on a car seat or cushion (rather than by being moved to the front seat). This will allow them to focus on distant points. Make sure their seat belts are in place.

•If you always suffer from motion sickness, the best plan is to head it off with medication. Some over-the-counter antihistamines (such as Bonine, Marezine, Dramamine, and Benadryl) have been approved by the Food and Drug Administration for motion sickness. Start taking them thirty to sixty minutes before you leave, but remember, they may cause drowsiness. If simple remedies don't help, ask your doctor for a prescription. Scopolamine (sold under the name of Transderm Scop) is highly effective. Administered via a skin patch, which is usually placed behind the ear, scopolamine is not likely to produce any side effects beyond dry mouth.

problems should discuss their travel needs with a doctor. If it seems likely that you'll need medical attention during your trip, your doctor may wish to give you a letter of explanation. If you do fall ill or have an accident abroad, the nearest U.S. Embassy or Consulate should be able to refer you to reliable medical care.

Carry a written summary of your health history with your passport: an immunization record (the Government Printing Office or local health department can supply a form for this); a list of current medications by brand and generic name; a list of all medical problems; a list of any drug allergies; and your doctor's telephone number. Heart patients should bring a copy of their latest electrocardiogram (ECG). Anyone with serious allergies or special conditions such as epilepsy or diabetes should have a health identification bracelet giving the diagnosis and medical precautions in case of an emergency.

You might also wish to find out whether your regular medical insurance will cover illness and hospitalization abroad. Many policies, including Medicare, do not. Blue Cross/Blue Shield is good worldwide, but most hospitals abroad won't bill them: you will have to pay cash and save receipts for reimbursement. If you decide you need additional coverage during a long or hazardous trip, start by consulting the latest edition of *Health Information for International Travel* (available from the Government Printing Office in Washington, D.C.), an indispensable reference for foreign travel. Credit card companies also offer medical insurance abroad. And for travel information of all kinds, get in touch with the International Association for Medical Assistance to Travelers (IAMAT, 417 Center Street, Lewiston, N.Y. 14092). This organization provides a number of excellent traveling aids, including a world immunization chart, world malaria charts, and a world-wide directory of physicians, many of them English-speaking.

Immunization

If you are traveling outside the "developed" world, get proper immunization. Since the risk of disease changes around the world, so do requirements for immunizations. Check with your doctor or local health department, or, better yet, consult *Health Information for International Travel,* which annually lists immunization requirements for all countries. You can also check with the Centers for Disease Control and Prevention (CDC) in Atlanta, Georgia. (You can call 404-332-4559 for recorded information on immunization schedules and other health information pertaining to overseas travel.) Typhoid immunization is not legally required anywhere, but many countries suggest it. Vaccines for cholera and typhoid are not entirely effective, so you should be sure to observe strict sanitary precautions as well (see next page).

Allow six weeks minimum before your trip for immunizations. (If you have to make a trip on short notice, the process can be speeded up, but the risk of unpleasant side effects from the vaccines increases.) Some countries require an "International Certificate of Vaccination" to prove that you have had yellow fever and cholera immunizations (available from the Government Printing Office).

There's no immunization against the types of hepatitis transmitted by food or drink, but a shot of gamma globulin may be useful if you're going to areas with poor sanitation for any length of time. While there is no vaccine against malaria, anyone who might be exposed—the disease now infects parts of about 100 countries—should start taking chloroquine, the most common antimalarial drug, two

Don't rely on the embassies

Don't count on the embassies in developing countries for up-to-date information about which shots you may need to enter those countries. Researchers from the University of Iowa Travel and Tropical Medicine Clinic surveyed 151 embassies and consulates and found that they often supplied poor advice. For instance, while twenty-seven embassies said their countries required yellow fever vaccinations, in fact only thirteen did.

Thirteen embassies also said that a cholera vaccination was needed, while none of their countries actually required one. Cholera is rarely a risk for travelers, and the vaccine is only 50 percent effective and commonly causes side effects. Thus the vaccine is not recommended by the Centers for Disease Control and Prevention in Atlanta— which is the most up-to-date source for medical recommendations.

weeks before entering a malarial area. In some part of Latin America, East Africa, India, Southeast Asia, and the South Pacific, chloroquine must be supplemented with another drug, Fansidar, because chloroquine-resistant strains of malaria are increasing. A traveler must continue taking the medication for six weeks after leaving an infected region. And wherever you are going, make sure your booster shots are up to date, especially for polio and tetanus.

Unfortunately, no immunization exists against AIDS. This disease is not transmitted casually: not by ordinary human contact, by swimming pools, or via food handlers. However, infection may be a risk anywhere hypodermics and other medical equipment are reused without sterilization. To be safe, follow these precautions when traveling:

- Don't get tattooed, have your ears pierced, or undergo acupuncture.
- Avoid injections, immunizations, or vaccinations in underdeveloped regions.
- Except in life-or-death situations, refuse blood transfusions and blood products.
- Wherever you are—here or abroad—remember that casual sex can be dangerous. If you do take a new sexual partner, use all precautions to prevent sexually transmitted diseases (see pages 389-392).

Food and drink

Water and food are generally safe in most of Europe, Australia, New Zealand, Canada, and Japan. Elsewhere—even in rural areas of southern Europe—haphazard refrigeration and poorly regulated water supplies may expose travelers to parasites and bacteria. Contaminated water and food can cause traveler's diarrhea as well as more serious diseases such as cholera and hepatitis. Take the following precautions when you are in a rural or undeveloped area:

- Don't drink hotel or restaurant water, brush your teeth with it, or eat raw foods that were washed in it. Be prepared to purify water in one of two ways. Boil it for two or three minutes (take along an immersion heater for this purpose). Or, add purifying tablets such as Halzone or iodine to the water. Tincture of iodine can also be used, three drops per quart if water is clear, six drops if cloudy; let water stand thirty minutes before drinking.
- Safe beverages include coffee and tea (provided that the water for them has been boiled), bottled wine and beer, and canned soft drinks. Beware of locally bottled waters, since they may just be unpurified tap water, and bottled soft drinks. Drink only beverages kept in closed containers. Wipe the top well and, if possible, use a straw that has a paper wrapping. Avoid ice cubes as explained at right.
- Since raw vegetables may be contaminated, don't eat them. Vegetables are safe when cooked. Eat fresh fruits only if they are intact, with no breaks in the skin. Wash them with soap and water, rinse them with boiled water if possible, then peel them.
- All meat and fish dishes should be thoroughly cooked and eaten hot to avoid bacteria or other contamination. Unless it is refrigerated, fish should be cooked and eaten within two hours of being caught. Don't eat large predatory fish (sharks and barracuda) or fish liver or roe. Shellfish anywhere in the world may carry hepatitis, so don't eat it raw.
- Be cautious about milk and dairy products. When in doubt, avoid them.
- Don't eat custards, pastries, cold cuts, meat salads, or other perishables that are sold unrefrigerated.

Drinking water

"Don't drink the water" is a warning usually heeded by travelers in Mexico and other developing countries. In addition, though, studies suggest that ice cubes made from contaminated water be treated with equal caution. When contaminated cubes are allowed to melt in a variety of liquids—alcoholic and otherwise—enough bacteria survive to cause traveler's diarrhea.

Therefore, it's best to avoid any ice cubes you are offered. If you are making your own ice cubes and safe water is unavailable, boil tap water for two to three minutes.

Traveler's diarrhea

Traveler's diarrhea, long known by such names as Montezuma's revenge, is something of a misnomer. Though it has been defined in the pages of the *New England Journal of Medicine* as diarrhea that occurs when a person living in an industrialized region travels to a developing or semitropical country, some people get traveler's diarrhea when entering the United States or other industrialized countries. Any change of locale and eating habits can make you more vulnerable to it. Also, imported melons, fruit, and other produce, which occasionally are contaminated, have caused rare outbreaks of diarrhea in the United States. Nevertheless, traveler's diarrhea is still more common among travelers from low-risk to high-risk areas—40 to 60 percent of Americans traveling to developing countries are laid low with diarrhea, although of course that doesn't mean you can't get the same bug in Kansas City, Palo Alto, or Utica, New York.

Causes, treatments. Up to 80 percent of traveler's diarrhea is bacterial—the ubiquitous *E. coli* found in fecal matter, plus some others, which are also transmitted via contaminated food or water. Less common agents are viruses and such parasites as *Giardia lamblia.* In many cases, it's impossible to identify the exact culprit. Besides loose, watery stools, symptoms may include vomiting, stomach cramps, nausea, fever, and blood in the feces. The condition is uncomfortable, but seldom life-threatening, and usually improves in two or three days. If fever lasts more than twenty-four hours and there is no improvement in your condition after forty-eight hours, you should see a doctor. If the cause is bacterial, antibiotics can help.

Meanwhile, the most important thing is to replace lost fluids as soon as you can keep them down. Bottled water, flat soft drinks, sports drinks, or tea will help. For a sick child, try sweetening water with honey, and add a pinch of salt. Salted crackers are a good way to begin eating again—and their salt helps restore fluid balance.

If you're traveling in out-of-the-way places, beyond the reach of a druggist, you'll probably have been advised to carry some diarrhea treatments along. Imodium and Lomotil are "antimotility" drugs that work against loose stools. Bismuth subsalicylate (Pepto-Bismol, which is also sold as a generic) is good, too. But people who are aspirin-sensitive or take aspirin for other reasons, as well as children under twelve, should not use it. Moreover, you should not take any of these drugs if you have high fever and bloody stools; these two symptoms can be signs of a serious infection that requires immediate medical attention.

Avoiding it. When traveling in developing countries, take these precautions:

•Drink only bottled or canned beverages, and be sure you're the one who breaks the seal. Or stick to hot drinks such as tea or coffee made with boiling water. Bottled wine and beer are all right. In some areas, locally bottled water and soft drinks may not be safe. If in doubt, stick to tea and coffee.

•Never use tap water, even for brushing your teeth.

•Pass up ice cubes.

•If need be, take along an immersion heater and boil your own water or add a purifying tablet such as Halzone to it.

•Don't eat anything raw, particularly not salad greens. Raw fruit is okay only if it can be peeled and if you do the peeling. Be certain not to wash the fruit in tap water. Avoid rare meats, undercooked eggs, and all dairy products, since it's hard to be sure they've been pasteurized.

•Don't buy food from street vendors.

Watch where you swim

In some countries, water for swimming as well as drinking can be hazardous. In Africa, the Philippines, parts of the Caribbean, and much of Asia, freshwater lakes often contain a parasite that penetrates the skin and causes schistosomiasis, a serious worm infestation that is second only to malaria as a worldwide health problem. Since it is difficult to treat, stay out of fresh water in the tropics—don't even wash your face in it—unless it has been purified.

Before you set out. Some travelers take antibiotics or Pepto-Bismol before they leave home in order to ward off traveler's diarrhea. But antibiotics can have side effects, and any of these drugs can give you a false sense of security. Do carry antibiotics with you, along with instructions on how and when to use them. If you are traveling to developing countries and are pregnant or nursing, are accompanied by infants or small children, or have chronic health problems, it's a good idea to get a doctor's advice before you go. And it's especially important to follow health precautions carefully.

Traveling with medications

You'll travel lighter if you pack medications in pill or capsule form rather than as liquids. On any trip, be sure to pack a full supply of any prescription drug you take; abroad, you may not be able to obtain the identical drug. But in case of need, take along an extra prescription. Ask your doctor to print or type it, and to specify brand, as well as the generic and/or Latin name of the drug. Pack a supply of any contraceptives you may use. A small kit of over-the-counter medications will also be useful, particularly for a long or potentially trying journey. Be sure to include a pain-reliever such as aspirin, an antihistamine, and an antidiarrheal such as Pepto-Bismol in tablet form. Pack an extra pair of glasses or contact lenses, and if you are traveling far and wide or plan to be away for a long period, take along an extra eyeglass prescription from your optometrist or ophthalmologist.

Pack at least a small supply of needed medications in a carry-on bag; checked luggage may not always arrive when you do. Be sure to take everything in the original pharmacy containers. This may save delay and trouble at customs. To protect pills from breakage, keep (or replace) the wad of cotton in the top. A small medicine cup can be a handy addition to the kit.

Using the Health Care System

This chapter provides information that will enable you to become a working partner with a doctor or other health care professional. It will help you take an active role in your health care by becoming an informed patient. And it will help you understand and evaluate preventive services available in the health care system.

No matter how much attention you pay to your health, there comes a time when you need to seek professional advice, either for a specific medical problem or for a medical checkup. But what should your doctor be doing for you, especially when it comes to preventive services? Many people are unsure what a medical checkup consists of—and how often they need one. The annual or biannual "complete physical," once regarded as a necessity, has now been discarded, since it didn't pay off in terms of better health and longer life. Over the long run, the head-to-toe physical exam for symptomless people doesn't play a decisive role in keeping them healthy. Furthermore, it has proved to be too expensive for patients and insurers alike. But should you get a checkup every so often, even though you're feeling fine? And are there certain tests that are essential?

Some years ago, at the request of the government, a committee of physicians known as the U.S. Preventive Services Task Force reviewed all available evidence about preventing illness and concluded that it's pointless for all people to have the same battery of tests routinely, regardless of their age, sex, or symptoms. For example, if you have no symptoms of diabetes or no risk factors (such as obesity or family history of the disease), there's no point in your being screened for the disease. Similarly, for most people there's no point in having a routine chest X-ray. People should receive preventive services and seek screenings based on their personal risk factors and symptoms. The task force conclusions about what makes sense are summarized in the chart on page 489. (Please note that recommendations on the chart *do not apply to pregnant women, infants, and children,* who need ongoing surveillance by a physician or other health professional.) The key tests are covered in detail beginning on page 497.

Health care without doctors, checkups, or tests

Besides the tests listed on the chart, there are other important preventive measures, the kind of commonsense prevention that could save millions of medical dollars and prevent injury, illness, and premature mortality—the kind of preventive self-care that is covered throughout this book. These include avoiding smoking; keeping alcohol consumption moderate; preventing sexually transmitted diseases; getting regular exercise; eating a diet low in fat and rich in fruits, grains, and vegetables; taking proper care of your teeth; driving soberly and defensively, with seat belts fastened; and keeping your home environment safe.

None of theses measures is expensive, and the only ones that require professional services are contraception and a dental checkup.

The U.S. Preventive Services Task Force strongly recommends that doctors talk with patients about all these issues, though it recognizes that doctors often lack the time—or simply don't take the time—to explain the basics of a healthy diet, for example, or to urge patients to stop smoking or change their sedentary habits. As a rule doctors don't get paid for counseling.

According to the task force report, if prevention is to work, people must assume greater responsibility for their own health. The physician's most important job is to treat illnesses and injuries, while the patient's most important job is to take every possible step to keep them from occurring. This requires an activist attitude on the part of the patient—and close cooperation with the doctor.

CHOOSING A HEALTH CARE PRACTITIONER

Doctors

Everyone should have a good, reliable doctor for the ordinary medical problems that come up from time to time. Using a specialist such as a gynecologist or a cardiologist for basic medical care is a mistake—and can be costly. Going to an emergency room is also a mistake, since emergency rooms will not have access to your medical records and are, in any case, oriented to handle emergencies, not ordinary medical problems. A primary care physician ought to be competent to recognize and handle the full range of problems that individuals usually encounter, know your medical history, and keep your records on file. For adults, there are three basic types of such physicians to choose from:

General practitioners. At the turn of the century, most doctors were general practitioners—able to deliver a baby, set a broken bone, and even perform surgery. Then the age of specialization hit, and the number of general practitioners (GPs) fell from 112,000 in 1910 to just over 24,000 in 1988. Yet, there are still some general practitioners in business—usually older men who went into practice after only a year of postgraduate training, and who often make up in clinical experience for what they lack in formal education. General practitioners still treat the full range of medical problems, though they usually refer patients to specialists for consultation and sometimes ongoing care for such conditions as heart disease, diabetes, arthritis, asthma, cancer, and most surgical procedures. They are usually associated with community hospitals.

Family practitioners. Because of the decline in the number of general practitioners, the American Medical Association in 1969 recognized family practice as a specialty. To qualify, a physician must complete a three-year residency that covers certain aspects of internal medicine, pediatrics, obstetrics, and orthopedics, and then pass a comprehensive examination. Family practitioners handle a wide range of problems for people of all ages, treating most acute and chronic illness, and even offering psychological counseling for such family problems as alcoholism. For complicated ailments and diseases, they refer individuals to appropriate specialists.

Internists. These doctors specialize in adult medical problems. Internists must take a three-year residency after medical school and pass a rigorous examination to receive specialty certification. They have more advanced training in the diagnosis and management of such common medical problems such as heart disease, diabetes, arthritis, and cancer. Some internists will take further training in one of

Staying Well: A Checklist of Preventive Services

Most Health Maintenance Organizations cover these services; fewer Preferred Provider Organizations and even fewer traditional insurers pay for them. Pregnant women need care not described in this chart.

Service	Who Needs	How Often	Average Cost
Blood pressure measurement (to detect hypertension, which may lead to stroke and heart disease)	Everyone	Periodic measurements after age 3; every 2 years for normal adults	Usually part of office visit; also offered at community screening programs
Cholesterol screening (to detect high blood cholesterol levels and low HDL "good" cholesterol)	Every adult; most important for women over 55, those with high blood pressure, those with a family history of premature heart disease, diabetics, and smokers	At least once every 5 years; more often if your total cholesterol level is high or HDL low and/or you have other risk factors for heart disease	$20 plus office visit to check total cholesterol level, more for HDL profile
Pap smear (for early detection of cervical cancer)	All women beginning at age 18 or at onset of sexual activity if earlier	Every 1 to 3 years, depending on risk factors such as smoking or the presence of genital warts	$20 to $50
Mammogram (X-ray for early detection of breast cancer)	All women 50 and older (women in their forties at risk for breast cancer should seek professional advice on screening)	Annually after 50	$100 to $125, with a range of $50 to $200
Professional breast exam (plus monthly self-exam)	Women over 40	Annually	Usually combined with other exams
Sigmoidoscopy (for early detection of colorectal cancer)	Everyone over 50; earlier if you have a family history of colorectal cancer before age 55 or a personal history of precancerous polyps	Every 3 to 5 years; more often for those at high risk	$100 to $200
Digital rectal exam (to detect colorectal cancer and gynecological problems)	Everyone over 50	Varies according to age, other factors	Usually part of office visit
Prostate-specific antigen (PSA blood test to detect prostate cancer)	Any man over 50 when advised by physician	On professional advice	$80
Eye exam	Everyone over 50, especially anyone with a change in vision or eye problem	Every year, or on professional advice	$60
Glaucoma screening	Everyone over 65; earlier if at high risk (severely nearsighted, diabetics, African Americans, and those with a family history)	On professional advice	Usually part of eye exam
Tetanus/diphtheria vaccine	Everyone	Every 10 years	$15 to $20
Influenza vaccine	Everyone over 65, nursing-home residents, and others at high risk	Annually	$15 to $20
Pneumococcal vaccine	Everyone over 65	Once	$15 to $20
Dental exam	Everyone	Every six months for evaluation and cleaning; more often for treatment of specific problems	Variable; about $50 to $100 for evaluation and cleaning

A Glossary of Specialists

The following are some of the most common types of specialists:

Anesthesiologist. Decides which type of anesthesia will be used, administers it during surgery, and monitors its effects after surgery.

Cardiologist. Specializes in diagnosing and treating abnormalities of the heart and the blood vessels.

Dermatologist. Diagnoses and treats disorders of the skin, hair, and nails.

Emergency medicine specialist. Practices emergency medicine in a trauma center.

Gastroenterologist. Diagnoses and treats disorders of the digestive system and liver.

Geneticist. Specializes in diagnosing and predicting inherited disorders, such as some forms of mental retardation, cystic fibrosis, hemophilia, and many metabolic disorders.

Hematologist. Diagnoses and treats disorders of the blood.

Internist. Specializes in the nonsurgical treatment of adults. Some internists obtain sub-specialities, such as cardiology, gastroenterology, hematology, and oncology.

Neurologist. Diagnoses and treats disorders of the brain and nervous system as well as of the muscles.

Neurosurgeon. Specializes in operating on disorders of the brain and the blood vessels that supply it, the spinal cord, and the peripheral nerves.

Obstetrician/gynecologist. Specializes in the treatment of the reproductive systems of women. A gynecologist can treat diseases of the reproductive organs with or without surgery. An obstetrician specializes in the treatment of pregnant women and delivering babies.

Oncologist. Diagnoses and recommends treatment for cancer.

Otorhinolaryngologist. Specializes in the ear, nose, and throat.

Pediatrician. Specializes in treating children and adolescents. Like internists, pediatricians may choose to develop subspecialties, such as pediatric cardiology.

Physiatrist. Specializes in physical medicine and rehabilitation.

Psychiatrist. Treats behavior disorders. Psychiatrists often use psychotherapy in helping patients, but as medical doctors they are also able to prescribe medications.

Radiologist. Administers multiple imaging technology, such as X-rays and ultrasound. A diagnostic radiologist uses radiology to diagnose medical problems. A therapeutic radiologist uses radiation for the treatment of certain forms of cancer.

Surgeon. Specializes in the diagnosis and the surgical treatment of a wide range of diseases. A general surgeon may choose to specialize further, choosing, for example, to be a thoracic and cardiovascular, pediatric, colon and rectal, or plastic surgeon.

Urologist. Diagnoses and treats disorders of the urinary-tract organs, and in men, problems in the reproductive system.

---

these or other subspecialties. A general internist may refer a patient to a subspecialist for evaluation, but will usually continue to see the patient for supervision of treatment.

When you need a specialist

Primary care physicians (except GPs) are, in effect, specialists. But since the whole science of medicine has become so complex, many doctors specialize even further. Specialties in medicine can range from the broad—for example, a pediatrician, who treats only children, or an obstetrician, who provides care during pregnancy and delivers babies—to the very narrow, such as a gynecological oncologist, who treats cancers of the female reproductive system. When you have a specific problem or condition that your primary care physician is not equipped to handle, a specialist's experience and knowledge in that area can be invaluable. The most common types of specialists are listed in the box on page 490.

How do you know if you need a specialist? The best way is to ask your primary care physician. If he or she says you have a particular medical problem, ask if there is anyone who specializes in that area, and if you would benefit from a consultation. How narrowly specialized the specialist should be depends on the nature of your problem. It's important to remember that many insurance companies will not completely cover the cost of visits to very specialized physicians, which is why it's not a good idea to see a specialist for routine problems. In addition, some carriers require that you get prior authorization before seeing a specialist.

If you have determined that you need to see a specialist, remember that any doctor can legally use the title specialist without having completed any official training or gaining certification from the American Board of Medical Specialties. (Certification guarantees minimum competence, and shows that the physician has had the requisite training.) Therefore, you should ask for a referral from your primary care physician. Other good sources include local hospitals and professional organizations such as the American College of Surgeons. The reference department of a local public library or the library of a large hospital or medical school should have a copy of either the *AMA Directory of Physicians* (which lists all licensed doctors and indicates if they are board certified) or the Marquis *Directory of Medical Specialists* (which lists only board certified physicians).

Selecting a doctor

Whether you're choosing a primary care physician or a specialist, you should do some investigating before selecting one. In making your choice, you will want to consider the following factors:

•The most difficult—and yet most important—task is to make some judgment of a physician's technical abilities. Check educational background and professional associations, including hospital privileges and board certification. Ask friends and other physicians for recommendations.

•Is the physician easily available? If you have an emergency, he or she should be able to make time to see you the day you call, as well as be available to talk to you by phone and return your calls promptly.

•Is the doctor in a solo or group practice? If alone, are there other doctors available who will cover when your doctor is away—and who will have access to your medical records? If in a group practice, does the group represent a range of subspecialists? Do you have confidence in these associates?

•What is the physician's medical philosophy? Does he dismiss all your problems—or prescribe medication every time you have a complaint?

•What kind of payment is required? Do you have to pay the fee directly, or will the doctor's office bill the insurance company or accept Medicare.

•Finally, do you feel you can confide in the doctor completely and can you expect an informed and considered opinion?

Improving communication

Competence, knowledge, and expertise are important qualities in a physician, but the rapport between doctor and patient also plays a crucial role in the quality and effectiveness of treatment. Surveys have indicated that many people are dissatisfied

Your medical records

In the past, many doctors and health-care providers argued against patients' right of access to medical records, since these files are often highly technical—and possibly confusing and alarming. However, in recent years, thanks in large part to lobbying by consumers' groups, about half of all states now guarantee access to medical (and often mental-health) records. To obtain a copy of your records, simply contact your doctor's office or the hospital where tests or procedures were done. Even in states without full guaranteed access, most doctors and hospitals will honor requests for copies. There may be a charge for photocopying and mailing. A good way to keep records up to date is to regularly request copies of test results and notes from your doctor after each visit.

Emergency Rooms

In case of accident or sudden illness, most people don't call a doctor. Instead, they head for the nearest emergency room. It makes sense to investigate emergency rooms in your area beforehand, particularly if you have small children in the house or anyone with a chronic condition that might require attention in a hurry. You can't always judge the quality of an emergency room by the reputation of a hospital. A certain hospital in your area may have a good reputation, but it doesn't necessarily follow that its emergency room is the best, since many emergency rooms are operated on a contract basis.

Obviously, if there's a fine hospital nearby, you should investigate its emergency services as part of your research. For starters, it's a good idea to ask your doctor and your neighbors about local emergency rooms. You can also write or phone the local health department. And keep the following criteria in mind:

Location. Pick a nearby facility and check how long it takes you to get there by car or taxi. If you are driving, notice where the entrance is and where you can park. Go inside the hospital and look around.

Service. By phone or in person, find out what the hours are, whether there's always a physician on duty, and whether there's a surgical team that could treat severe injuries.

Cost. Are they willing to bill you or do they want immediate payment? Would they bill your insurance company? Would they accept a credit card? Would the physician's bill be included in the emergency room fee, or should you expect a separate charge?

Transportation. In some emergencies (if you or the person you are caring for has chest pain, severe bleeding, or some other condition that rules out driving), you'll need to call your local paramedics, who may not be able to allow you a choice of facilities. You may want to keep the number of a private ambulance service close to your telephone, so that you can be taken to the hospital of your choice. But in any life-threatening situation, you should, of course, go to the nearest hospital. (If you're not satisfied, you can always arrange for a transfer later.)

What is an emergency?

Emergency rooms should not be used for nonemergency situations or in place of routine medical care. In fact, many insurance companies will not pay for nonessential visits to emergency rooms. The following is a list of what doctors generally consider emergencies:

- severe chest pain
- difficulty breathing or shortness of breath
- severe abdominal pain
- slurring or loss of speech
- convulsions
- unconsciousness
- uncontrollable bleeding
- bullet or stab wounds
- broken bones
- head injuries
- eye injuries, sudden loss of vision, or foreign substances in eyes
- poisoning
- drug overdose
- choking
- smoke inhalation
- gaseous fume inhalation
- heat stroke or dehydration
- hypothermia
- temperature over 103 degrees
- prolonged vomiting or diarrhea
- snake or animal bites
- insect stings resulting in shortness of breath

with their physicians, not because they doubt their medical expertise, but because they are unhappy with their "bedside" manner.

The time to establish a relationship with a doctor is before you need treatment. Opening lines of communication with someone you see infrequently and usually only in times of stress isn't easy. Here are some guidelines for getting the most from your visit to the doctor.

Prepare for your appointment. An analysis by the American Society of Internal Medicine concluded that 70 percent of correct diagnoses depend solely on what you tell your doctor. Be as detailed and specific as possible when describing your condition—jot down your symptoms and concerns if it will help you. If it's your first visit to a doctor, be well versed in your own and your family's medical history. Bring along any medications you are taking, and mention any treatments you are undergoing. Try not to leave anything out; what you think is a minor detail could be important.

Become an educated patient. No question is a dumb question. You are entitled to a diagnosis given in terms you understand. You should also get a full explanation of treatments, expected outcomes, as well as the risks and benefits of the various alternatives. Your doctor should encourage you to make an informed decision about your treatment. If you want details about your condition, ask the doctor to recommend reading material. If there is a medical school nearby, you can do research in their library.

Take part in your own health care. Your doctor's advice can only help if you follow it. Listen attentively to instructions and ask when would be the best time to call if you have additional questions. If lab tests or X-rays are required, have them done promptly, and be sure the doctor reports the results to you—by telephone, mail, or in person.

Of course, communication is a two-way affair. Realizing that physician/patient communication is important to patient welfare and can enhance the outcome of treatment, experts are now recommending an empathetic or "affiliative communication style" for doctors, rather than an authoritarian approach. "Affiliative" is a ten-dollar word for "friendly, interested, and respectful." Patients, certainly, are better satisfied with this approach, whatever the outcome of the treatment. And a satisfied patient is more likely to comply with medical advice as well as to be honest about symptoms and personal habits. A study at Wayne State University School of Medicine suggests that doctors who interrupt patients instead of hearing out their opening statements are more likely to miss essential information. In the classic example cited in the paper, only when the office visit concludes and the patient heads for the door does he mention that he's been having chest pains.

Medical schools do try to train doctors to be empathetic and compassionate, but the lesson doesn't always sink in. Patients, too, need training in effective communication and "physician-management"—but such training is hard to come by. Keep these pointers in mind:

•Ask your doctor questions. One of your rights as a patient is access to information, including your medical records.

•Doctors are human, too, and often work under great pressure. Keep your remarks to the point. Before you go, give some thought to your concerns. If you're afraid of forgetting something, make a brief list.

•Be as well informed as possible.

•If you have a symptom you're uneasy about, don't put off mentioning it.

You may decide to put up with a crusty manner if the physician is truly skilled. But if a physician is rude, dismissive, or intimidating, you are justified in looking for another. Make sure your records, including X-rays and lab work, are forwarded to your new doctor. Don't stay with a doctor just to protect his or her feelings, or because you were referred to the doctor and think you can't make the decision to switch on your own.

When to seek a second opinion

It's common for patients facing surgery to seek a second opinion. Many insurance plans now require you to get a confirming opinion before some kinds of elective surgery—for example, surgical repair of a hernia or removal of tonsils, uterus, gall-

What if You Need a Transfusion?

Although the risk from contracting a disease such as AIDS or hepatitis is small it still makes sense to think ahead about how you might want to deal with the need for blood replacement in the event of surgery.

When you know in advance that you'll need blood, you can donate autologously—that is, for your own use. The surest way to avoid infection from donated blood lies in storing your own blood for delivery to the operating room on the day you need it. It will remain usable for a maximum of forty-two days, but at the rate of one unit a week, you could safely build up a supply of six units. (The average amount of blood needed for a transfusion is two to three units. Exceptions include heart and blood vessel surgery and some plastic, orthopedic, and gynecologic procedures.) To allow your body to replace lost fluid, you will be asked not to give blood for three days preceding surgery.

Planning ahead this way really works only for people facing elective surgery. But, in emergency surgery a surgeon can resort to "intra-operative salvage"—a variation on the autologous-transfusion technique. The surgeon simply recycles blood lost during an operation. It is filtered, cleaned, and fed back into the patient's circulatory system on the spot. It helps solve the problem of the need—as in open-heart surgery—for many more units of blood than can safely be donated ahead of time. Another advantage: the apparatus used to do the job can recycle three units in nine minutes, and that's less time than it takes in emergency situations to identify the type of donated blood and cross-match it to the blood type of the recipient.

Caution on transfusion alternatives

There are two alternatives to traditional blood banks and autologous transfusions that may at first sound like good choices. But on closer examination, they prove not so smart after all.

The first is called "directed" donations. You ask friends and relatives to donate blood. But is their blood safer than anonymous donations from a blood bank? Not necessarily. A friend or family member will find it hard to turn down a request to give blood—but might find it harder to admit to a high-risk lifestyle.

The second alternative is having your own blood frozen and stored for future use. But there are two serious drawbacks to this alternative: expense, for one. It costs a lot to store frozen blood that you may never need. It must be thrown out after three years anyway. Time is the other disadvantage. If your stored blood is in a San Francisco deep freeze, and you face emergency surgery in New Orleans, considerable time (and more expense) is involved in rushing it to the surgeon—who must then wait another ninety minutes while it thaws. Chances are that in an emergency, even with a large supply of your own blood in cold storage somewhere, you'll have to rely on the public blood supply anyway.

This may all sound discouraging, but you should remember that blood transfusions are life-saving measures. Compared to the risks of not receiving blood, the risks from transfusions are negligible.

bladder, or enlarged prostate. Medicare and Medicaid may require a confirming opinion, too.

There are many strong arguments for seeking a second opinion. Even though the second surgeon may only confirm the opinion of the first one, the patient can benefit. Sometimes it's the only way a person can be reconciled to having surgery. And someone who is more confident that the procedure he's undergoing is the right one will be a better patient and more likely to comply with instructions. Finally, although it may be rare for the second surgeon to disagree with the first, it does happen, and thus some unnecessary surgery can be avoided. If this occurs, you'll be happy you took that extra step. Keep these pointers in mind:

•Consultation has always been part of good medical practice, and no competent doctor should be insulted if you decide to get a second opinion, even if your insurance company does not require you to do so. Be tactful about it, however.

•Seek out the most highly qualified consultant available. At the very least, make sure that the second physician has been certified by the American Board of

Medical Specialties. If you are uncomfortable with asking direct questions about a doctor's qualifications when you make the appointment, ask your family doctor, a local medical society, or the surgical department of your nearest medical school.

•A consultation allows you to compare medical opinions about how an operation will affect the quality of your life, the risks involved, and which treatments might be available. It gives you a chance to ask additional questions that might occur to you. Perhaps the most important reason to seek a second opinion is that it puts the final decision in your hands.

Nurse-Midwives

Most pregnant women are at low risk for complications during childbirth: for them, a birth is not a cause for medical intervention. For such women, there's an alternative to relying solely on an obstetrician: the certified nurse-midwife. Midwifery, the art of assisting at childbirth, is an ancient practice that has seen a revival. Qualified nurse-midwives (they may be women or men) are always registered nurses and must have advanced training in midwifery as well. They work as colleagues of an obstetrician and offer up-to-date prenatal care as well as attended childbirth in a relaxed setting that will appeal to many prospective mothers and fathers. In addition, because nurse-midwives use fewer hospital facilities and make less money than doctors, their bills will run 30 to 40 percent less than standard obstetrical care.

About 85 percent of nurse-midwives currently practice in hospitals and 11 percent in independent birthing centers, with ready and quick access to nearby hospitals should an emergency arise. In either setting, nurse-midwives usually work in birthing rooms, which are combined labor and delivery rooms that make moving from one room to another unnecessary. A nurse-midwife stays at the mother's side during labor and may encourage the mother to walk around, sit, stand, curl up, or otherwise make herself comfortable. The rooms are usually furnished to create a pleasant, homelike atmosphere, and family members are usually encouraged to be present. If labor proceeds normally, the woman may be able to avoid electronic fetal monitoring and other high-tech procedures, as well as anesthesia.

Nurse-midwives are licensed by state boards of nursing or medicine; many states require certification by the American College of Nurse-Midwives.

If the idea of a nurse-midwife appeals to you, remember the following:

•Make arrangements with the person you select as early in your pregnancy as possible. Choose one who has been licensed by your state and certified by the American College of Nurse-Midwives.

•Choose a person with whom you feel comfortable. The nurse-midwife will supervise your prenatal care as well as your labor. Choose someone with whom you are able to talk freely, who is able to answer any questions you may have, and can address your special needs.

•Find out what the backup system is in case you need medical help at any time during pregnancy or childbirth. Where would you be taken and who would take charge if an emergency should arise? Will pain relief be available should you need it? Which kind would it be? Be sure to meet the obstetrician who will be on call.

•If you want to give birth in a hospital rather than in a birthing center, choose a nurse-midwife who practices in one. If you prefer a birthing center, that's fine, but be sure it has hospital access.

•Although nurse-midwives have become popular (and deservedly so) in many areas, don't feel pressured to use one if you'd really prefer an obstetrician and a regular hospital delivery room. The point is to feel confident about the kind of care you choose.

Pharmacists

Drugstores no longer double as social centers and ice cream parlors, and friendly pharmacists may seem to be an endangered species. But if you need prescriptions fairly often, try to have one pharmacist fill them all. A good pharmacist should get to know you. A conscientious pharmacist will keep your "drug profile" on record: a confidential rundown of medications prescribed, food and drug allergies, and your doctor's name and address. If you're seeing more than one doctor, the pharmacist can spot drug incompatibilities that they, or you, may not be aware of. Even if you're only buying aspirin, you may need expert advice.

Shop for a pharmacist who's willing to keep records for you and also is available—not only for filling prescriptions but for answering questions. Suppose you didn't quite understand what your doctor said. Are you sure you know whether to take the drug before, with, or after meals? If you miss a dose, is it advisable to take two the next time? Should you take all the medication, or quit when you feel better? Your pharmacist may know the answers to the questions, or at least be willing to telephone your doctor to find out.

Keep the following points in mind:

Professional qualifications. Pharmacists must be registered with the state pharmaceutical board; a certificate should be prominently displayed.

Generic drugs. These can often be substituted effectively for brand-name products and will usually cost less. Your pharmacist should stock them and be willing to use them. (Laws on generics vary from state to state. First, ask your doctor about using them.)

Customer services. Find out whether your pharmacist offers such conveniences as charge accounts, home delivery, and yearly statements for tax and insurance purposes, and whether these cost extra. Some drugstores offer discounts to senior citizens and other groups.

Emergency services. A phone number for after-hours and weekend emergency service should be displayed.

Packaging. Lots of adults can't deal with child-proof containers; don't be shy about asking for a different kind of cap, as long as there are no children in your home. If the print on the label is hard to read, say so. A good pharmacist will package the prescription to suit you—for example, by providing different-colored containers for multiple medications so that you don't confuse them.

Health aids. If the store stocks such items as crutches or braces, the pharmacist should be qualified to give advice on their use and fitting.

Even at a large chain or discount drugstore, it's worthwhile getting acquainted with the pharmacist. Find somebody with the time to get to know you. Relaxed, informed advice can save time, complications, money, and possibly even your life.

Nutritionists

Chances are, you don't need a nutritionist. Still, if you are overweight and unable to lose pounds on your own, or if you have some medical problem—such as diabetes, elevated cholesterol, hypertension, or a high-risk pregnancy—requiring a special diet, your physician may suggest that you get a specialist to design a diet for you.

Since there is no licensing requirement, anyone can hang out a sign saying "nutritionist." Thus, it pays to choose carefully. Ask for a referral from your doctor, the dietician at a local hospital, the department of nutrition at the nearest university, your local health department, local chapters of the American Heart Association or the American Cancer Society, or your state dietetic association.

The nutritionist to whom you will be referred will probably have "R.D." after his or her name—identifying a registered dietician, certified by the American Dietetic Association—although many competent nutritionists are not registered. A registered dietician has at least a bachelor's degree in nutrition or a related science, has done an internship at a hospital or other professional setting and has passed a comprehensive examination. He or she is likely to be a member of the American Dietetic Association; nutritionists who are PhDs or MDs may also be members of other professional groups, such as the American Society of Clinical Nutrition, the American Institute of Nutrition, and the Society for Nutrition Education.

A nutritionist should review your medical history provided by your doctor (with your written permission), and consult with you about your food preferences, level of physical activity, and general lifestyle. He or she will help you translate basic nutritional advice into customized menus and provide follow-up support to make any needed adjustments in your diet. This could involve as few as two visits; fees vary depending on the area of the country and whether a computer-based dietary analysis is used.

When consulting with a nutritionist, be wary of anyone whose dietary recommendations lean heavily on "special" foods or megadoses of vitamins or minerals, unless it has been medically established that you have a deficiency. Don't trust a nutritionist who guarantees results or who recommends hair, nail, or saliva analysis—procedures for which there is no proven merit.

COMMON DIAGNOSTIC TESTS

Although many people think of diagnostic tests being performed only when there is a suspicion that something is wrong, many of them are conducted as part of a physical exam or as screening procedures. The tests that are listed below may be done on healthy individuals as part of routine examinations.

Blood Chemistry Tests

The following tests are conducted to determine the levels of circulating chemicals in your blood to detect whether you have higher or lower levels of substances normally present. They are simple procedures done in a doctor's office that involve drawing blood either from a vein or by a finger or ear-lobe prick. Although you can have each test performed individually, the tests listed below are often done in panels—a group of different tests taken from one sample of blood—because it is generally less expensive than conducting each test separately.

Blood glucose. Blood glucose tests determine the amount of glucose, or sugar, in the blood, which can help a physician diagnose diabetes or hypoglycemia (low blood sugar). It is usually performed if an individual experiences any symptoms of diabetes (such as excessive thirst or urination), hypoglycemia (such as light-headedness or unexplained loss of consciousness), or it may be part of a routine physical exam. Blood glucose tests are also performed by diabetics themselves to test the

---

Assessing Test Laboratories

The labs that your doctor sends your tests to should either be accredited or licensed. The difference between the two categories is that accreditation is voluntary whereas licensing is mandatory, although the requirements may vary from state to state.

Accreditation. A lab that wants a professional society's seal of approval must have certain prescribed personnel on staff and must pass whatever tests and inspections the organization specifies. But this can be an expensive process, and many labs may not be able to qualify. This does not mean, however, that the lab is not reliable.

Licensing. Most states usually call for proficiency tests and conduct on-site inspections. In addition, the Clinical Laboratories Improvement Act passed by Congress in 1967 provides that any lab receiving samples of biological material from out of state must be licensed by the Department of Health and Human Services. Such licensing requires a quality control program and proficiency testing by the Centers for Disease Control and Prevention (CDC) in Atlanta. Amendments to this act—to be implemented over the early 1990s—require labs to be federally certified, either directly by the Department of Health and Human Services or by approved accrediting agencies except in states where licensing laws are at least as stringent. In a state with strict licensing requirements, accreditation may not matter. California, Connecticut, Florida, Illinois, Maryland, New York, and Pennsylvania are all known as stringent states, but this does not mean that labs in other states are inferior.

Does licensing then assure you of accurate test results? Licensing and/or accreditation means that the lab may be doing high-quality work, but there are no guarantees. And even though the new laws—once they are in widespread practice—should markedly improve the quality of laboratory procedures, at least in the mean time, you still may want to consider the following:

•Talk first to your doctor or the health practitioner doing the test. Ask if the lab is licensed by the state or the Department of Health and Human Services, and if it is accredited. It's likely that the doctor knows about the lab's quality control program and the results of the lab's proficiency tests.

•Lab work done in the doctor's office on his own patients does not have to be licensed. Studies have generally shown that the results of such tests aren't as accurate as those of licensed labs.

•You might also ask whether the lab ever returns specimens as being inadequate. Well-run labs will occasionally ask for a redo. Lab work can be only as good as the specimen sent out.

•Ask your doctor about previous experiences with the lab. Some doctors will test labs by dividing a sample in two and sending them off under different names. If the results are significantly different, a doctor will know that the lab isn't accurate or well controlled. Or the batches can be sent to different labs and then the results compared.

•Check with your state health department for information about licensed labs.

•If you are especially concerned you can contact the lab directly. Large ones publish their credentials and are willing to supply the results of proficiency tests and to provide tours—but usually only to physicians and hospital representatives.

•There isn't necessarily anything suspicious about a physician sending a sample to an out-of-state lab. Some complicated tests can be done only by specialized labs.

effect of their treatment. Generally, the blood is drawn in the morning after a twelve- to fourteen-hour fast to determine the basal levels—that is, those not influenced by food or activity.

If the results show that a blood sugar level is abnormal, a more extensive test called a glucose tolerance test may be performed. This determines the cause of high or low blood sugar and also offers insight into how the body deals with an overload of sugar. The individual being tested eats a high carbohydrate diet for several days, and then drinks a concentrated sugar solution before the test. Blood glucose levels are then measured at regular intervals over the next several hours.

Blood creatinine. This test measures kidney function. Creatinine is a waste product of muscle metabolism; kidneys that are working properly adequately filter creatinine from the blood. A high level may indicate kidney damage.

Blood urea nitrogen (BUN). This is another test to evaluate kidney function. Blood urea is an end product of protein metabolism. An excess amount in the blood may indicate kidney disease, impaired kidney function, or a very high protein intake.

Blood electrolytes. A test for blood electrolytes—sodium, potassium, chloride, and bicarbonate—is not usually ordered individually unless there is an indication of an electrolyte problem, such as water retention or weakness. In addition, tests for blood electrolytes are routinely performed in diabetics or individuals who have a history of heart, liver, or kidney disease, since these conditions can lead to electrolyte imbalances. This test may also be performed if a person is are taking diuretics or experiencing such symptoms as dehydration or excessive vomiting or diarrhea that may deplete the body of electrolytes.

Complete Blood Count

A complete blood count is safe, inexpensive, and practically painless, and it probably provides you with more information than any other single laboratory screening procedure. Less than two teaspoons of blood are necessary for a complete blood count. Although the blood sample is analyzed in a number of ways, four measurements—hemoglobin concentration, red blood cell count, hematocrit, and white blood cell count—are the most important ones. Here is the information each of these tests reveals to a physician.

Hemoglobin concentration. Hemoglobin is the chemical substance that transports oxygen through the bloodstream to all the cells of the body. It imparts the red color to blood and is normally contained within the red blood cells. This measurement determines the level of hemoglobin per unit of blood.

Red blood cell count. The primary function of red blood cells is to carry oxygen to all parts of the body. The presence of too few red blood cells often indicates simple anemia, usually the result of a diet deficient in iron. But it may also be an early clue to a more serious problem such as leukemia, kidney malfunction, internal bleeding, or inherited forms of anemia such as sickle cell anemia. Too many red blood cells may indicate that the body is having a difficult time supplying itself with oxygen and is an early clue to the existence of congenital heart disease, respiratory disease, or polycythemia vera, a disease in which there is an overproduction of red blood cells.

Hematocrit. The hematocrit essentially measures the ratio of red blood cells to plasma in the blood. It is also a sensitive indicator of the blood's capacity to carry oxygen to various parts of the body. Abnormal hematocrit readings indicate the presence of the same disease that abnormal red blood cell levels do. Although hemoglobin, hematocrit, and red blood cell counts all give similar information, and any one may be used to determine anemia, the combination of all three measurements aid in diagnosing the specific type or cause of anemia, if it exists.

White blood cell count. White blood cells are the body's primary defense against disease, so their presence or sparsity tells a great deal about health. An elevated white blood cell count indicates the presence of an infection, stress, a major injury, or even leukemia. A depressed level may be a sign of poor diet, certain infections (especially viruses) that have begun to overwhelm the body's defenses, or a failure of the body to produce enough white blood cells (another type of leukemia).

White blood cells are analyzed in two ways: one method is to count the total number present in a given amount of blood; the other is to look at the percentage of different kinds of white blood cells. An increased number of the kind that kill disease-causing organisms can indicate an infection. A greater than normal number of monocytes could suggest the presence of a chronic disease such as arthritis.

Electrocardiogram

The electrocardiogram (also known as an ECG or EKG) is a diagnostic tool that measures heart activity by detecting electric current flowing in the heart. The procedure is simple, safe, and takes five to ten minutes to perform. Ordinarily, you receive a resting ECG: you lie on your back, and your doctor or a technician places metal sensors at your wrists, ankles, and various parts of the chest. The sensors detect the heart's electric impulses, which are recorded as tracings on strips of special graph paper. There is no discomfort, since the current is always coming only from the patient.

A normally beating heart produces basically the same pattern of waves in all people. Variations from this pattern can indicate a number of potential problems: dysrhythmias (irregular heart rhythms), which may or may not be a sign of heart disease; damage to the heart muscle; enlargement of the heart's chambers; mineral imbalances in the blood; and whether the patient has had, or is having, a heart attack. For most people with signs of heart disease, an ECG can help reveal the source of trouble.

However, the electrocardiogram is far from perfect. Some people with normal ECGs have heart trouble, and the graph may also show abnormalities where none exist. The resting ECG doesn't necessarily reveal atherosclerosis—the buildup of fat in artery walls that causes blocked or narrowed coronary arteries—because the heart at rest is receiving enough oxygen. For this reason your physician may want to evaluate the status of your heart vessels with a stress ECG, which is taken while you are exercising on a treadmill or stationary bicycle. (For more information on stress ECGs, see page 511.)

ECGs are usually a routine part of a physical checkup after age forty; before forty, have at least one ECG to use for later comparison.

Should you be concerned about extra heartbeats?

Perhaps as many as 75 percent of us experience occasional extra heartbeats, which usually go undetected but sometimes are felt as a brief flutter in the chest. They may also show up on ECGs, and the discovery often causes alarm for the patient, even though the physician may say that nothing is wrong.

One group of scientists studied extra heartbeats—"ectopic beats," as they are called—in seventy-three people in good health without symptoms of heart disease. The subjects experienced anywhere from seventy-eight extra heartbeats per hour to a high of almost 2,000. However, not one of these people developed heart disease, and the group had a lower mortality rate than the general population. It's worth getting a checkup if you begin to feel extra beats, but if your physician tells you not to worry about it, take the advice.

Mammogram

Mammograms, which are X-rays of the breast done to detect breast cancer, are one of the most valuable diagnostic tests available. It is estimated that yearly mammograms for women over fifty could lead to a one-third reduction in the number of deaths from breast cancer. This procedure is a highly reliable way to detect breast cancer in its earliest, most treatable stage—long before tumors can be felt during a clinical breast examination. Yet only 15 to 20 percent of women over fifty have annual mammograms.

Here are some of the (misguided) beliefs behind why more women don't get this test—*and the reasons why they should:*

"I don't need a mammogram. Breast cancer doesn't run in our family." In the great majority of cases of breast cancer, heredity is not a factor. The role of heredity in breast cancer has been overstated. Most researchers think that fewer than 10 percent of all breast cancers are inherited, and one recent study of over 2,300 women found that only 6 percent of their breast cancers could be attributed to family history. The main risk for breast cancer is simply growing older: most women who develop it have no identifiable risk factors except their age; breast cancer didn't run in their families. After age fifty, every woman should have a mammogram annually (see below). From age forty on, all women need professional breast exams annually, too, and should practice monthly self-exams (see page 502).

"My doctor has never said a word about mammograms." Indeed, many doctors don't mention mammograms, but that doesn't mean you shouldn't get them. A recent study showed, for example, that male doctors were less likely to tell their patients about this important screening test than female doctors. But you should bring up this important matter with your doctor yourself and request a referral.

"Scientists have discovered the breast cancer gene, so a blood test and a cure are on the way." A number of researchers, including a team at the University of California at Berkeley, have made progress toward finding the gene that may transmit a susceptibility to breast and ovarian cancer in some families. However, they haven't found what they're looking for yet, and even if they do, it is unlikely to be of any immediate therapeutic use. Inherited breast cancer is a rare disease. It may be many years before there's a reliable test for susceptibility, let alone a cure.

"Having a mammogram exposes you to dangerous X-rays." It's certainly reasonable to avoid excess X-rays, which can cause cancer. The possibility that a mammogram could promote breast cancer is very remote indeed. The new dedicated machines (that is, used only for mammograms) deliver very low dosages of radiation. Make sure your radiologist uses a dedicated machine located ideally at a facility accredited by the American College of Radiology, which sets strict qualifying standards.

The who, when, and how of mammograms

Any woman fifty or over should be on an annual schedule for mammograms. What about women under fifty? This one is harder to call. The American Cancer Society recommends a single base-line mammogram (for later comparison) between ages thirty-five and forty, and a screening mammogram every one to two years between ages forty and forty-nine.

However, accumulating evidence has failed to show that the base-line mammogram saves lives. Furthermore, although it's clear that mammograms over fifty save

Myth: Mammograms are painful.

Fact: It's true that a breast compression device—trays that hold the breasts and compress them for one second—is crucial: if the technician doesn't use compression, the mammogram will be inaccurate. (Ultrasound scans are an adjunct to mammography; they can help to refine a diagnosis in some cases. But ultrasound is not a substitute for mammography).

Because each breast must be compressed in order to X-ray it, you may feel pinching or unpleasant pressure. However, most women report only temporary discomfort, or none at all. If your breasts become tender before your period, try scheduling your mammogram just after.

Self-Exams

Although many diagnostic tests are performed in a doctor's office, there are examinations that you can do at home to check for cancer. In fact, individuals—not doctors—more often find their own cancers. Therefore, regular self-examination is one of the best preventive measures you can take to significantly increase your chances of detecting cancer at an early stage. Below, are instructions for the most common self-exams.

Breast Exam

One out of every eleven women will get breast cancer in her life—it's the second leading cause of death in women after lung cancer, and it kills more women in their forties than any other illness. But if breast cancer is diagnosed early enough, women have a much greater chance of recovery.

Since 90 percent of all breast tumors are discovered by women themselves, it's a good idea to develop the habit of examining your breasts. The key is being able to detect changes in your breasts. Regular examination is necessary to familiarize yourself with what your breasts are normally like.

Monthly exams are recommended; any more often can be confusing, since your breasts change throughout the month. Do the exam at the same time each month—within a week after your menstrual period, since that is the time when breast swelling is at a minimum. Follow these steps:

1. Begin with a visual exam. Stand in front of the mirror with your arms at your sides. Familiarize yourself with the appearance of your breasts and nipples, including their shape, texture, and any normal asymmetry. Lean over to see breast contour in that position. After learning what's usual for you, look for any of these changes: bulging or flattening in one breast but not the other; puckering or redness of the skin; or reddening, crustiness, or unusual hardening or inversion of the nipples.

2. Raise your arms over your head and check for the same signs. Inspect your breasts while pressing your palms together over your head, and then again with your hands on your hips. Both of these positions contract chest muscles and may make it eas-ier to spot any changes in your breasts.

3. Gently squeeze each nipple to check for any blood-tinged discharge.

4. The next part of the exam—feeling, or "palpation"—can be done while lying down, or in the shower or bath. Water and soap make it easier to slide your fingers over your breasts, but to examine the lower half of them, you should be lying flat. Lie down on your back with your right hand under your head. You can put a small pillow under your shoulder to help flatten your breast against your chest. Using the flat part of the fingers of your left hand, start pressing the right breast lightly against the rib cage. Begin at the outside edge of the breast, and rotate in a spiral toward the nipple, without lifting your fingers, until you have covered the entire area of the breast.

5. Then move your arm down to your side and feel the upper and inner part of your armpit, the area between your armpit and your nipple, and finally between the outer lower part of your breast and the nipple.

6. Repeat these steps for your other breast, using the opposite hand to examine it.

7. Expect to feel many normal lumps and textures; try to get to know these so you can detect changes, such as thickening or hardening of tissue, or pea- to grape-sized lumps. At first, you may want to make a chart recording where normal gland tissue is found. Any changes should be reported to your doctor, but they don't necessarily mean you have breast cancer. Studies indicate that 80 to 90 percent of all breast lumps are benign.

Keep in mind that self-exams are not a substitute for regular examinations by your physician and mammograms (breast X-rays). Mammograms are still the most effective method for early breast cancer detection. The American Cancer Society recommends a mammogram when a woman reaches thirty-five, then repeated mammograms as needed, depending on such risk factors as family history, until age fifty, when they should be performed annually.

Men can get breast cancer, too. Although they get it much less frequently than women, it's fatal more often, since it's not usually detected until it's in an advanced stage. It's a good idea for men to examine themselves occasionally, too.

Testicular Exam

Testicular cancer is rare, accounting for only 1 percent of all cancers, but because the early symptoms of testicular cancer often go undetected, more than one third of all cases have spread by the time they are diagnosed. Although it can strike at any age, it is one of the most common forms of cancer in young men; in fact, it's the leading form of cancer in men between the ages of twenty and thirty-five. Fortunately, the cure rate approaches 95 percent if the cancer is detected early enough. Otherwise, the survival rate drops dramatically.

A monthly self-exam is the best way to detect it in its earliest stages. After a warm bath or shower, when the scrotal skin is relaxed, gently roll each testicle between the thumb and fingers of both hands. Make sure you cover the entire area of each testicle. Feel for lumps, nodules, swelling, or a change in consistency. Be sure to examine the ropelike part called the epididymis.

Each man is different and it may take a few examinations to know what is normal for you, but if you feel anything unusual, consult your physician right away—even though the odds are that it's not cancer. Symptoms of testicular cancer include a slight enlargement of one of the testes and a change in its consistency. There may be no pain, but often there's a dull ache in the lower abdomen and groin area.

There is evidence that men with an undescended or partially undescended testicle have a greater risk of developing testicular cancer. Normally, the testes descend soon after birth; male infants should be checked to make sure the testes have descended properly. An undescended testicle is easily corrected; boys or men with this condition should be checked by a physician.

Skin Exam

Skin cancer is one of the most prevalent forms of cancer. Fortunately, it's also one of the easiest types to detect and treat. Examining your skin is primarily up to you, since most doctors do not perform an overall check of patients' skin regularly. A skin exam is a simple process that should take no more than fifteen minutes, and should be performed monthly.

When you examine your skin, you are looking for any change from what's normal for you. Spend some time looking at your skin, noticing where you have moles or birthmarks and the color, shape, and size of them. Then each month, perform the following steps:

1. Undress completely, and look at yourself in a full-length mirror in a well-lit room. Scan your skin overall (have a hand mirror handy to check places you can't easily see; you may also wish to have a friend or spouse help you examine these areas). Look for any changes in color, size, or shape of moles and birthmarks, or the appearance of new ones; any rough or waxy-looking patches; or any sores or scabs that are crusting, oozing, or bleeding or have not healed within a week or two. Pay special attention to areas where you have been sunburned in the past.

2. Begin a head-to-toe examination of your skin. Run your fingers over your scalp feeling for any bumps or rough or scaly spots. Lift your hair and visually examine the skin underneath. Pay special attention to bald spots.

3. Closely examine your face and the front of your neck in the mirror. Be sure to check your ears and the skin underneath your jaw line and chin. Men with facial hair should be sure to check the skin underneath. These areas are very susceptible to damage from the sun.

4. Look at your hands and arms, turning them over so that you can examine ever side. Look for dark spots under your fingernails, which may be an early sign of melanoma. Run your hands across your arms and shoulders to feel for any rough spots you cannot see. These are also high-risk areas.

5. Use a hand mirror to examine the back of your neck and shoulders, also areas that are susceptible to sun damage.

6. Examine your back, buttocks, and the backs of your legs with a hand mirror.

7. Examine your chest and your abdomen in the mirror.

8. Look carefully at the fronts of your thighs, legs, and feet. Be sure to check the bottoms of your feet and between your toes. As with your fingernails, check for dark spots under your toenails.

(For more information on skin cancer, see pages 298-301.)

Despite a 50 percent increase in the incidence of testicular cancer in the United States since 1973, there has been a 60 percent drop in the mortality rate, thanks to advances in treatment, which usually entails surgical removal of the affected testicle, followed by chemotherapy or radiation. The surgery doesn't affect sexual response or fertility (one testicle is sufficient), but chemotherapy may reduce fertility, at least temporarily.

lives, several recent studies have failed to show that women in their forties really benefit from regular mammograms. This may be because younger breasts are denser, and thus the mammograms are harder to read accurately. Or it may be that breast cancer in younger women tends to be more aggressive, and if it grows fast, an annual mammogram is less likely to catch it at a curable stage.

For women in their forties, mammograms are more likely to result in false positives and thus unnecessary biopsies, with all the expense and emotional upset that may entail. Some people use cost as a reason not to advocate mammograms for women under fifty, but an analysis of the new data would not support them even if mammograms were free.

When you turn forty, discuss your risk factors for breast cancer with a physician. On that basis, decide whether it's advisable to begin mammography. In any case, begin having annual professional breast exams at fifty, and perform monthly self-exams.

A mammogram can be expensive (up to $175, usually on the spot) but many insurance plans cover at least part of the cost. Medicare also provides partial payment for a screening mammogram. Low-cost and even free screening is available in some communities. Phone your local health department, public library, or chapter of the American Cancer Society for more information.

Your physician or radiologist should keep all your films on file, so that each new mammogram can be compared with previous ones. (You may need to carry your films from the doctor's office to the radiologist and back again.) You are entitled to copies if you want them (there may be a charge); the films must be accessible for at least five years. If you move or switch doctors or radiologists, remember to take your films with you or have them sent to your new doctor.

Other tips

•Choose a center accredited by the American College of Radiology or, if there's not one near you at least ask if they use up-to-date, dedicated machines. The recently passed Mammography Quality Standards Act requires that all facilities be government certified and inspected by October 1994. You can get a list of centers in your area by calling your local American Cancer Society or the National Cancer Institute at 1-800-4-CANCER.

•At an accredited center, a breast exam is usually part of getting a mammogram. If not, you should get a professional exam elsewhere.

•The day you go, it's more convenient to wear a two-piece outfit. That way you won't have to undress completely. *Don't use an antiperspirant that morning.* The aluminum in these products can make your film hard to read. You may have to wash and repeat the procedure. Talcum can also interfere with an accurate picture.

Occult Blood Test

Colon cancer is the second most common form of cancer in the United States; about 166,000 people in North America are diagnosed annually with the disease (actually cancer of the colon and rectum, thus more accurately called colorectal cancer). More than 63,000 of these cases are fatal—and yet, the American Cancer Society estimates that 87 percent of colon cancer patients and 79 percent of those with rectal cancer could be saved by early diagnosis and treatment.

Remember that for the great majority of women, the results from a mammogram will be good news. If something does show up on your mammogram, you may need a biopsy, but you still may get good news. If a malignancy is discovered early, you'll have the best chance to overcome it.

504

Unfortunately, the screening tests are unpleasant or embarrassing to varying degrees, since they require a direct examination of the bowels or stool. Thus many people are reluctant to follow the screening guidelines, and the cancer is often detected relatively late. In addition, there has been a great deal of disagreement about which tests are most effective at detecting tumor early enough to save lives.

Blood in the stool is often a symptom of colorectal cancer. Tiny amounts of hidden, or "occult," blood from a premalignant polyp or early tumor may be detected by testing the stool. This inexpensive test calls for smearing cards with stool samples collected over several days; the samples are then tested by your doctor or a lab for the presence of hidden blood. If blood is detected, further diagnostic testing, notably a colonoscopy (a visual exam of the entire colon), will be done.

Besides the difficulty some people have in collecting the samples properly, the stool test often yields incorrect results. First of all, some colorectal cancers bleed only intermittently. Intestinal bacteria can alter the blood so that it doesn't show up on some tests. Moreover, many other factors besides cancer can result in traces of blood in stool, such as hemorrhoids, ulcers, or diverticulitis, or the consumption of red meat or aspirin. Other foods (such as broccoli, canteloupe, and radishes), as well as vitamin C or iron supplements can interfere with the test. As a result, there are many false-positive results, requiring unnecessary colonoscopy. False-negatives, in which a malignancy is missed, are another problem.

Experts have long debated the usefulness of occult blood tests. The controversy heated up in 1993 with the publication of two major studies that had very different findings. One study, published in the *Journal of the American Medical Association*, found that the test missed 70 percent of cancers and 90 percent of precancerous conditions. And 92 to 95 percent of people who tested positive did not have cancer. The researchers concluded that there is no evidence that the stool test saves lives.

In marked contrast was a second study published in the *New England Journal of Medicine*. This study of 46,000 people in Minnesota concluded that those who underwent a stool test annually for eleven years reduced their risk of dying from colorectal cancer by one-third. But of the 33 percent of people who tested positive over the course of the study, only 2 percent were found by colonoscopy to have cancer (another 30 percent had intestinal polyps, which sometimes develop into cancer). Thus many people underwent unnecessary colonoscopy, which not only must be done by a gastrointestinal specialist and is thus expensive, but it is also uncomfortable and poses a small risk of perforation of the colon. It is possible that just doing that many colonoscopies on a randomly selected group, without first testing their stool for hidden blood, would have detected a similar number of cancers and thus would have resulted in a similar decline in cancer deaths.

Our recommendation

Thus the controversy about occult blood tests goes on—and will likely continue until a reliable, inexpensive, noninvasive test for colon cancer is available. The American Cancer Society, among other groups, recommends an annual occult blood test for everyone over fifty. But the editors of the *Wellness Encyclopedia* do not believe that the evidence supports the use of occult blood tests. Instead, we recommend periodic sigmoidoscopy (see page 510) for people over fifty. If you have a family history of colorectal cancer, you should be screened earlier.

Pap Smear

The Pap smear was developed by Dr. George Papanicolaou in the 1940s as a simple, painless, and inexpensive screening device to detect cervical cancer. About 2 percent of all women over forty will develop cervical cancer, but the cure rate nears 100 percent if the cancer is detected early. This is because cervical cancer generally develops far more slowly than most other cancers, progressing through a long "pre-invasive" stage of ten to fifteen years, during which it grows but does not invade healthy tissue.

The test—which consists of cells obtained from the vaginal walls and the cervix that are placed on a slide and examined under a microscope for abnormalities—is a great lifesaver. It has reduced deaths from cervical cancer by at least 70 percent over the past fifty years. In countries where the Pap test is in widespread use, death from cervical cancer are relatively rare. Elsewhere, cervical cancer remains the major cancer killer of women.

How often should you be tested?

The American College of Obstetricians and Gynecologists (ACOG) recommends that when a woman turns eighteen or becomes sexually active (whichever occurs first), she should have Pap smears for three consecutive years. According to the U.S. Preventive Services Task Force, if tests are negative for three consecutive years, she can then be tested less frequently (generally every three years) at the discretion of her doctor. However, many authorities, including ACOG, think that women should have annual tests throughout their lives, particularly if they have any special risks for cervical cancer. Risk factors include the presence of genital warts or other sexually transmitted diseases, frequent sex with many partners, early sexual activity, and cigarette smoking.

The other advantage of annual screening is that Pap tests can also detect many noncancerous conditions, such as infections. And women who go for annual screenings are likely to get breast exams and other kinds of health care that they might otherwise forgo. The fact is, about one-third of all American women do not get Pap tests regularly.

Can you trust the results?

The results of a Pap smear are a description of what the cytologist—a physician specializing in studying cells—sees while examining the cells under a microscope. He then prepares a report that provides the doctor with his interpretation. One problem with the Pap test is that, under some circumstances, it can yield false negatives—that is, a normal reading for someone who actually has the disease. Fortunately, because cervical cancer is slow to develop, a single false negative is usually not disastrous, provided you have annual screenings, which should yield accurate results over time. (If you screen every three years, six years could pass between accurate screenings.)

In addition, worries surface from time to time that the laboratories evaluating Pap test slides are not doing a good job. New technologies may eventually eliminate human error, but evaluating the test still depends on the human eye. You should certainly take an interest in the quality of the lab and in the quality of the smear—which can be hard to put into practice. You may not be able to tell if a practitioner is doing a good job, but it won't hurt to express interest and concern. Fortunately, labs are doing a better job now than in the past, thanks largely to the passage in 1988 of the Clinical Laboratory Improvement Amendment, which provided for more stringent rules and inspections by the Health Care Financing Administration. The following will also help ensure accurate results:

- Select a physician, nurse practitioner, physician's assistant, or certified nurse midwife who has the training to do a good smear and takes time to do it.

- Express your concern about the lab. If the slide is being sent to a lab out of town, ask why. Are the lab's charges reimbursable by Medicaid? Whether or not you are on Medicaid, this means that a lab takes part in a quality-control program. (Another question: does the lab have experience doing the "thin-prep" technique, which is new and more accurate.)

- Having the slide sent to two labs may be overkill. More important, have regular Pap smears. If a problem is missed one year, it will be picked up the next.

PSA: Screening for Prostate Cancer

For men over fifty, cancer of the prostate is the most common cancer and the second leading cause of cancer deaths after lung cancer. The number of cases diagnosed annually has risen dramatically during the past five years, partly due to the availability of a new and relatively simple blood test called PSA, which measures blood levels of the prostate-specific antigen—a protein produced in the prostate that may be elevated when cancer is present. The American Cancer Society estimates that some 200,000 new cases of prostate cancer are diagnosed annually, and that 38,000 men die of the disease.

Yet nobody knows the underlying cause of prostate cancer, and thus there is no known way to prevent it. Age increases the risk—about 98 percent of prostate cancers are diagnosed in men over fifty-five—and so does a family history of the disease. For reasons not yet understood, black men are at higher risk than white men, and married men at higher risk than unmarried.

Other possible risk factors—among them, smoking, sexual behavior, socioeconomic status, and diet—have been investigated in a number of studies in recent years. A review of these risk factors in the *Annals of Internal Medicine* concluded that a diet high in dietary fat may be one of the most likely candidates, and a subsequent study by Harvard researchers in the *Journal of the National Cancer Institute* bears this out. Some studies have also shown a link between vasectomy and prostate cancer, though the connection is slight at most, as explained on pages 387-388.

Moreover, detecting prostate cancer at an early stage is difficult—there's no equivalent of the mammogram, which can detect tumors before they are palpable. Doctors disagree not only about effective methods of screening, but also about treatment, which is costly and carries with it a number of possible complications and side effects.

The prostate gland, located between the bladder and the rectum, secretes seminal fluid, in which the sperm is carried. For unknown reasons, prostates enlarge as men age and they can also develop growths or nodules. Usually, these growths are benign—a condition called benign prostatic hypertrophy, or BPH. At other times, the growth is cancerous. The cancerous cells can develop at different rates, and often they are so small and develop so slowly that most men who have the disease will actually die of something else before the cancer becomes advanced. But if prostate tumors do reach a certain size, they grow out of the prostate, spread to the lymphatic system, and move on to other, vital organs.

Based on autopsies, researchers estimate that about 10 percent of American men age fifty, and 70 percent of men age eighty, have small prostate cancers that haven't spread and are not clinically significant. For a fifty-year-old man, the lifetime risk of developing any type of prostate cancer is about 42 percent. In approximately 23 percent of these men with "latent" cancer, the disease will develop to a point where it is clinically significant; about one in three of these men will die of prostate cancer. Hence, for any American man, there is a 10 percent lifetime risk of developing clinically significant prostate cancer—and a 2 to 3 percent lifetime risk of dying from the disease.

It is this fact of prostate cancer—that many more men have it than will die from it—that explains why screening for the disease remains controversial. In addition, there is no universal agreement on the best treatment for prostate cancer, or whether treating the cancer saves more lives than not treating it.

Three screening methods

The standard screening method is the *digital rectal exam,* or DRE: a doctor inserts a gloved finger into the rectum and feels the lower part of the prostate for abnormal growths. This is not a high-tech procedure involving lab tests and equipment, nor is it painful for patients, though most men dread the probing and some try to avoid it. But DRE is not reliable: two thirds of all suspicious findings that lead to biopsy turn out to be noncancerous, while many cancers go undetected. DREs are usually part of a general physical exam—and yet the annual or biannual physical exam is no longer recommended routinely either. (It proved too expensive for patients and insurers, and did not pay off in terms of better health and longer life.)

Another diagnostic tool is *ultrasound,* but detection of tumors by ultrasound is even less accurate than by DRE, because the ultrasonic appearance of cancer is very similar to that of benign inflammations. Ultrasound is also more time consuming than either a DRE or the PSA test, and it is more costly. Thus, it is usually used after the other two screening methods reveal abnormalities.

The *PSA blood test* was introduced in 1986 as a means of evaluating the progress of cancer in men who had already been diagnosed as having the disorder. But urologists and other doctors began using it to screen apparently healthy men, and the test has come into wide use, especially for men over fifty—even though interpretation of the results for routine screening is far from settled. In 1994, the test received FDA approval as a screening tool.

Preliminary studies in both the *New England Journal of Medicine* and the *Journal of the American Medical Association* were optimistic about the potential benefits of PSA screening. One of these studies found that measuring PSA concentrations in the blood, when done along with a conventional DRE, increases the chance of detecting the cancer by 34 percent compared to the DRE alone. The other study concluded that elevated PSA levels might be a "sensitive and specific early clinical marker for the development of prostate cancer."

A more recent review article in the *Mayo Clinic Proceedings* concluded that measuring PSA levels was just as effective in detecting prostate cancer as a DRE—and sometimes more effective. However, "the two methods do not always detect the same malignant tumor." Therefore it is not advisable to substitute PSA for a conventional exam.

The PSA dilemma

PSA levels can vary even in healthy men, and although a high PSA level does indicate cancer nearly 90 percent of the time, the tumors that are detected at this level are most often large and have spread outside the prostate. By this time the cancer is not usually curable. A normal PSA level, however, may not mean there's no cancer—because some cancers will not cause a rise in PSA. While intermediate elevations in the PSA level can be caused by other diseases of the prostate, it's in this range—where cancers are most curable—that most false positive or false negative test results occur. According to an evaluation of the PSA test in the *Annals of Internal Medicine*, only 30 percent of the time does a positive test correctly identify prostate cancer. Yet if the PSA value is falsely positive, it most likely results in further diagnostic procedures, which can be painful and expensive.

Then there's the matter of treatment. If cancer is diagnosed, it may be treated with aggressive surgery or radiation, which can result in severe complications such as impotence, incontinence, and complications from extensive surgery. Yet if the cancer is slow-growing and symptom-free, the benefit is questionable—and especially so if the man is older, since his chances of dying of something else may be greater than the chances of dying of prostate cancer.

There has also been much debate about whether initial screening can distinguish between cancer that is likely to spread—and so should be treated promptly—and cancer that will cause no trouble and so should be left alone. A study published in the *Journal of the American Medical Association* in 1995 provided the first strong indication that the test can reliably detect a significant majority of cancers that will later spread. Yet, according to other studies, elevated PSA levels may not provide information about how aggressive a particular prostate cancer is. Nor does a normal PSA level with diagnosed prostate cancer mean that the tumor is nonthreatening. Furthermore, "normal" PSA values vary from man to man (though any change in an individual's PSA level deserves attention). There is also considerable overlap in PSA levels in men with benign prostatic hyperplasia and men with cancer that is confined to the prostate. PSA levels also increase with age.

Currently, there is no consensus about the effectiveness and cost benefits of universal PSA screening. Still, both the American Cancer Society and the American Urological Association recommend yearly screening (and a DRE) for all men over fifty. Meanwhile, the National Cancer Institute is conducting a large study to assess the benefits of PSA screening, but it will be years before the results are available.

Should you be tested?

For now, if you are a man over fifty and if any of your immediate relatives—father, brother, even an uncle—has been diagnosed with prostate cancer, or if you are an African American, be sure the digital rectal exam is part of your checkup. You and your doctor may also wish to do the PSA test. It's still too soon to recommend routine PSA testing for all men. If prostate cancer is detected, there is no standard recommendation for treatment, so discuss all options with your physician. If you're still uncertain, another medical opinion may be useful.

Sigmoidoscopy

A sigmoidoscopy is a screening procedure to detect colon cancer and other abnormalities of the lower ten to twelve inches of the large intestine and the rectum (where the majority of cancerous polyps occur). Although a sigmoidoscopy may be uncomfortable, it should not be painful when one of the newer flexible scopes are used (about 50 to 60 percent of colorectal cancers are within reach of the device). The test costs about $140 and is done in a doctor's office. Sedation is not necessary, but a person can request a mild tranquilizer to help induce relaxation. Since a clean intestine is essential for accurate results, people will probably be asked to prepare for the test by following a special diet—frequently an all-liquid diet—for a few days prior to the test, followed by laxatives the night before and an enema on the day of the test.

During the test, a thin, lubricated tube is gently inserted into the rectum and slowly advanced along the large intestine. This tube contains optical filaments through which light can pass and transmit an internal image to a microscope or monitor for a doctor to view. It may also contain small instruments that enable a doctor to take tissue samples. Air may be forced through the tube to expand the large intestine to make viewing and insertion easier. This may cause an uncomfortable feeling of gas or fullness, or simulate the urge to defecate. If a doctor sees any abnormalities as the tube travels through the intestine, he may take a tissue sample; if any polyps are present, they will be removed with the scope for analysis. Once the examination is complete, the tube is slowly withdrawn. The whole process takes about fifteen minutes to a half hour.

Who needs it?

There has been a growing consensus that *everyone fifty or older* should undergo a sigmoidoscopy using one of the newer flexible scopes. In the past, sigmoidoscopy was recommended only for people with a family history of the disease or certain precancerous conditions. But now the widespread use of the flexible sigmoidoscope has made the exam far more effective and much less uncomfortable for the patient than the rigid instrument that used to be the only means of doing the exam. In addition, a major study conducted at the Kaiser Permanente Medical Care Program in California and published in the *New England Journal of Medicine* in 1992 found that people who underwent sigmoidoscopy were 60 to 70 percent less likely to die from colorectal cancer than those who did not have the exam.

For these and other reasons, the American Cancer Society, National Cancer Institute, and American College of Physicians all recommend periodic sigmoidoscopy, preferably with a flexible scope, starting at age fifty. If you're at high risk (because of a personal history of colorectal cancer or precancerous polyps or a family history of colorectal cancer before age fifty-five), they recommend that testing begin earlier, at age thirty-five or forty. Most experts suggest having the test every three to five years, but the Kaiser Permanente study concluded that testing once every five to ten years is sufficient for most people. The U.S. Preventive Services Task Force, which many insurers and health care providers use as a guide to coverage, has recommended sigmoidoscopy only for people at high risk because of a personal or family history. However, the task force is now considering recommending the test for everyone over fifty in light of this study and other recent research.

Periodic sigmoidoscopy with a flexible scope makes sense for people over fifty (earlier if you are at high risk)—far more sense than occult blood tests. Also recommended is a digital rectal exam, in which your doctor uses a gloved finger to feel for tumors in the lower portion of the rectum. About 10 percent of colorectal tumors are within reach of a digital exam, which can also detect some potential prostate problems in men and gynecological problems in women.

And don't forget preventive measures: there's strong evidence that a high-fiber, low-fat diet may reduce the risk of colorectal cancer, as may regular exercise and physical activity in general.

Stress Test

An exercise stress test is one of several techniques used for uncovering cardiac problems. It is frequently used as a screening device for older people about to begin an exercise program; if the test indicates a heart disorder, an appropriate program can be designed. The procedure is usually done in a physician's office or a local hospital, but some health clubs provide them as well. During the test, your heart's activity is monitored on an electrocardiograph while you work out on an automated treadmill or stationary bicycle, usually for ten to fifteen minutes.

The test is a trouble-shooting procedure designed to reveal problems that a resting electrocardiogram (ECG) does not. At rest, an ECG may indicate that the heart is receiving sufficient oxygen; but with exertion, as the heart's workload increases, the ECG may reveal signs of an inadequate oxygen supply to certain areas of the heart muscle. The most common cause of this condition is a narrowing of coronary arteries due to a buildup of plaque. Thus, the stress test can help identify an abnormality that might otherwise go undetected until a person is exercising and unexpectedly experiences chest pain.

Who should have a stress test?
You should undergo a stress test before starting an exercise program if you are included in the following categories:

•You are forty-five or over. (Even if you have been exercising for years, its wise to have a stress test when you turn forty-five.)

•You are between thirty-five and forty-four and have at least one risk factor for coronary artery disease. These include an immediate family member (parent, brother, or sister) who developed coronary artery disease before age fifty, smoking, obesity, and an elevated blood pressure or cholesterol level.

•You have cardiovascular or lung disease at any age, or a metabolic disorder such as diabetes or hyperthyroidism. Since the test itself may entail some risk in these cases, you should first consult your physician.

According to the American College of Sports Medicine, you don't need a stress test if you're under forty-five, are in apparently good health, and have no risk factors for coronary artery disease. Even if you have risk factors, if you're under thirty-five and have no symptoms of coronary artery disease, you don't need this test. Even when a stress test isn't required for health reasons, some people wish to have it done; the information is useful for an exercise physiologist in designing an individualized workout program for them.

How the test works

Before the test begins, sensors are placed on your chest to transmit signals to the electrocardiograph; generally, the more sensors the better, with twelve "leads" being preferable. While your pace on the treadmill or exercise bicycle gradually speeds up, the ECG monitors the changes that occur in the rhythm and electrical activity of your heart; your blood pressure and pulse are also monitored continually. Generally, in a stress test, you exercise until fatigue prevents you from continuing, or until warning symptoms show up. (These may include abnormalities of blood pressure, heart rate or rhythm, or the onset of chest pain, shortness of breath, dizziness, or nausea.)

Administered correctly by a physician or another trained professional, a stress test poses few risks. But the results can be inaccurate, largely because of procedural problems. About 10 to 20 percent of stress tests result in false positives (erroneously indicating heart disease). Even more disturbing, false negatives also occur, and in much higher proportions: 20 to 40 percent. Thus, the results of a stress test shouldn't be analyzed in isolation; they must be evaluated in relation to your age, sex, and medical history.

Urinalysis

Routine urinalysis is a simple, yet very important test in terms of overall health screening. It provides vital information about an array of bodily functions and, most importantly, helps diagnose kidney disease, diabetes, and infections of the urinary tract. The procedure for routine urine testing—the type usually included in a complete physical examination—is performed quickly and easily. A fresh sample collected at any time of day is adequate for the test, and the patient need not take any special steps beforehand. Your doctor will probably instruct you to discard the specimen from the beginning of the urination and to collect a "midstream" sample, which yields the most accurate data. The specimen is then tested with a chemically coated strip of paper, which performs up to ten tests simultaneously. An instrument called an urinometer is used to measure concentration (specific gravity). And the sample is usually examined under a microscope for bacteria and other visible signs of kidney disorders.

Potential signs of kidney malfunction that may be indicated by urinalysis include excessive or diminished acidity and the presence of abnormal particles, protein, blood cells, or crystals. The presence of glucose (sugar) and/or ketones (chemicals that are the result of the breakdown of fatty acids) in the urine are likely indications of diabetes; a sweet or fruity odor may be another warning sign. Bacteria or a high level of white blood cells in the urine are often indicators of urinary tract infection.

Many of these and other findings from urine testing can be attributed to any of a number of diseases or dysfunctions, or even to temporary, harmless conditions. A reddish color, for instance, may simply occur because the tested person ate beets the night before, not because of internal bleeding. In general, the color, odor, and concentration of urine are strongly affected by the foods and liquids consumed before the sample was taken. For these reasons, the discovery of abnormal results from urinalysis almost always calls for further testing.

X-rays

Diagnostic X-rays have been one of the real lifesaving tools in medicine. These "pictures" allow a doctor to see the inside of your body without actually cutting you open. X-rays are performed to detect abnormalities in all parts of the body, including the bones, brain, gastrointestinal tract, and lungs.

How X-rays work

You are placed between a machine that beams X-rays—which are a form of electromagnetic radiation—and an X-ray film. The machine is pointed at the area to be X-rayed and the radiation passes through your body; as this occurs, different types of tissue absorb different amounts of radiation. Tissues that absorb the least, like bone, show up as white on the X-ray film, while tissues that absorb the most, like the lungs, show up as black. X-rays of areas that have a lot of bone, such as the skull or teeth, expose your body to very little radiation; X-rays of fleshy areas, such as the lower back, expose you to relatively high amounts of radiation.

Safer X-rays

X-rays account for about half the estimated lifetime exposure to radiation for the average person (the other half comes from natural background sources). While each individual X-ray is not harmful by itself, exposure to radiation is cumulative; thus a series of X-rays over a lifetime can result in an increased risk of cancer. Aware of the problems caused by excess exposure to radiation from X-rays, physicians have sharply limited their use. And radiologists have adopted the concept of "as low as reasonably achievable" with regard to doses. Although you should never refuse an X-ray that can provide essential medical information, the following steps will help you maximize your benefits from X-rays while minimizing radiation risks:

•Keep a written record of all X-ray exposures—what was done and when, and where the film was stored. This may keep you from having to repeat an X-ray.

•If the X-ray is being done in your doctor's office, ask if the X-ray technician has an appropriate license, and if the equipment has passed an annual inspection.

•See that the parts of your body not involved in the X-ray are shielded. For example, if you are getting a dental X-ray, you should be given a lead apron and collar to wear.

•Ask if the procedure is being done with "state-of-the-art" equipment—that is, high-speed cassettes using the lowest-possible dosage. Many dentists, for example, have switched to E-speed film, which reduces your exposure significantly.

•Try to avoid unnecessary diagnostic X-rays. A routine chest X-ray is a good example; while these may be useful for examining workers exposed to asbestos or pulmonary irritants, as a routine procedure to detect lung cancer and heart disease—especially in an individual with no symptoms—it is of little value.

•When scheduled for a mammogram, ask that it be done on a "dedicated" machine, which means that it's not used for any other kind of X-ray.

X-rays are not the only types of imaging procedures. New techniques of examining the interior of the body have been developed, among them sonograms and magnetic resonance imaging (MRIs). These are noninvasive and do not appear to have any potential adverse effects. They cannot substitute for X-rays in most cases, but can complement them, and often be as good or better diagnostic tools.

In this century, immunization with vaccines has had greater impact on contagious diseases than all other health services available to us. Smallpox, once the most widespread disease in the world, has been virtually eradicated. And in the United States and other developed countries, diseases such as diphtheria, tetanus, polio, and whooping cough—which fifty years ago were killing or crippling hundreds of thousands of people—have been largely been brought under control. Yet as long as even a few cases of disease occur within a population, people who are not immunized are at a risk of catching it. Moreover, when immunization coverage drops, diseases can return with a vengeance, as has happened with whooping cough.

How does immunization work? It prevents diseases caused by microbes— bacteria and viruses—that for the most part cannot be effectively treated. The body builds immunity naturally when it catches some infectious diseases and responds by forming antibodies, which kill the invading microbes or render them harmless. Vaccines create immunity artificially—and more safely—because they contain modified microbes or toxins that aren't strong enough to cause diseases, yet can still stimulate the system to produce antibodies. Once a person is vaccinated with a particular microbe for which there is a vaccine, he will fend off a particular infection by the same microbe with an immediate outpouring of antibodies.

American children are supposed to be routinely immunized against the leading contagious diseases—and for the most part they are. According to recent estimates, 90 percent of preschoolers have now been immunized. However, this makes many adults complacent about immunization, which is dangerous because they need to maintain certain types of immunity. For example, even if you were immunized against tetanus and diphtheria as a child, you need to receive booster shots periodically to remain fully protected. Yet nearly half of American adults are not up to date on their boosters.

Some 40 million adults should get a flu vaccine each fall. Outbreaks of influenza occur virtually every year, usually in winter, and can cause thousands of people to be hospitalized. But only about 20 percent of the people who should be receiving flu shots are getting them. The same figures apply to a new bacterial pneumonia vaccine. Also, adults in certain occupational and lifestyle groups, such as college students and health care workers, may be at high risk and should be immunized.

Along with being complacent, many adults are skeptical about the effectiveness and safety of the vaccines intended to protect them. For example, the influenza vaccine, although advocated by health officials, has never been widely accepted by the public. Resistance to it was especially strong after the winter of 1976-77, when a vaccine for combating swine flu was associated with about 500 cases of a rare paralytic condition called Guillain-Barre syndrome. Because of the wide publicity this received, the safety of the flu vaccine was seriously challenged—even though nearly 48 million people got vaccinated that winter without serious consequences. What is most reassuring is that the influenza vaccines used since have not been associated with Guillain-Barre syndrome or other substantial side effects. Yet a majority of the people who could benefit from the flu vaccine ignore it.

Based on a wide number of studies, however, modern vaccines have been judged to be extremely safe and effective by the American Academy of Pediatrics, the American College of Physicians, and the Centers for Disease Control and Prevention in Atlanta. This does not mean that the adverse effects from vaccines have been eliminated. But the chances of a severe reaction occurring in a healthy adult are extremely slim. For most individuals, as well as for the society at large, there is no doubt that the benefits of immunization far outweigh the risks.

Guidelines for Immunization

Because of the confusion concerning adult vaccinations, the American College of Physicians has issued a set of guidelines on the subject. Their key recommendations are given below. To determine whether you should obtain a vaccination, you need to review your immunization history. If in doubt about whether you have been sufficiently immunized, the safest bet is to assume that you haven't and to consult your doctor for the appropriate vaccine. Be sure to keep a record of current and future vaccines.

All vaccines produce some side effects, though not every time and not in all people. Most of these reactions are temporary and relatively mild, ranging from local soreness and redness to fever and discomfort in the joints. Unusual adverse reactions can take the form of convulsions and paralysis, but these are extremely rare. Individuals with allergies may be hypersensitive to a vaccine, so discuss any allergies with your physician beforehand.

Diphtheria. A disease that typically produces a severe sore throat, diphtheria is spread by airborne bacteria that release toxins that in turn can attack the heart and other internal organs. Because of widespread immunization with a toxoid vaccine, diphtheria has almost disappeared in the United States, but a few cases appear yearly. Most adults received primary immunization during childhood; if you did not, do so without delay. To remain immune, all adults require a booster shot every ten years, which is ordinarily combined with tetanus toxoid in a vaccine called Td. Since many students receive a booster by age fourteen or fifteen, try to establish a mid-decade birthday (twenty-five, thirty-five, etc.) as the time for boosters.

Tetanus. The bacteria that cause tetanus enter the body through a contaminated wound that can cause painful muscular contractions, which may prove fatal. Despite a dramatic decrease, there are still about 100 cases a year, most of them in older people. After primary immunization, adults should receive a tetanus booster (combined with diphtheria) every ten years. If you sustain a heavily contaminated wound, see a doctor: a booster may be appropriate if you have not received one within the preceding five years.

Influenza. To be effective, the flu vaccine must be administered yearly: strains of influenza constantly shift and are never the same from year to year, so the vaccine is adjusted annually to contain viruses that are expected to be prevalent. The vaccine is strongly recommended for anyone sixty-five and over, since severity and risk of death increase with age. Anyone with chronic pulmonary, heart, or kidney disease or with diabetes is also at high risk and should get annual flu shots. Those at high risk of exposure, such as health care workers and college students, should also be immunized annually. (Flu shots are not recommended for healthy adults under sixty-five, for whom influenza is almost never fatal.)

Pneumococcal pneumonia. A vaccine is now available that offers protection against the twenty-three strains that cause about 80 percent of pneumococcal diseases in this country. The same groups immunized for influenza should be immunized with pneumococcal vaccine, but only once. Yearly or booster doses should definitely not be given.

Measles and mumps. Most adults are likely to have been infected naturally with these diseases. But a substantial number of young adults born after 1957 have not been vaccinated and have not had the diseases, so they may be susceptible. (In the first half of 1985, 18.5 percent of reported cases of measles were among college students.) Furthermore, people vaccinated for measles between 1963 and 1967 may have gotten a short-lasting vaccine and should be revaccinated.

Rubella. Injury to a fetus and miscarriage are the major consequences of rubella (German measles) in adults, and an estimated 10 to 15 percent of young adults remain susceptible to this disease. Therefore, all women of childbearing age who have no history of vaccination should be tested for antibodies, and, in their absence, be immunized. Following immunization, a woman should wait for at least three months before becoming pregnant. Combined vaccines for measles, mumps, and rubella are available.

Special situations. A person's health status may determine whether a particular vaccine should be taken. Pregnant women, diabetics, cardiopulmonary patients, and people with other chronic diseases are among those to whom special considerations apply. Also, some people are in environments where there is an increased risk of contracting vaccine-preventable infections. These include college students, military personal, health care workers, veterinarians, and community workers such as teachers, policemen, firemen, and sanitation workers. Individuals in these groups should check with their doctors or medical departments on guidelines for the above diseases as well as for hepatitis B, rabies, typhoid, and meningococcal disease. Finally, travelers going to developing countries should check on recommendations for the places they will visit. (For more information, see page 483.)

Children. The principle immunizations for children are: 1) combined vaccines known as DPT for diphtheria, pertussis, and tetanus; 2) a triple oral polio virus vaccine, or TOPV; 3) vaccines for measles, mumps, and rubella, which can be given separately or combined (MMR); 4) a hepatitis B vaccine. For infants who start immunization during their first year, the American Academy of Pediatrics Committee on Infectious Diseases recommends the following schedule:

•DPT and TOPV at two months, four months, six months, eighteen months, and four to six years; MMR at fifteen months; tetanus and diphtheria (Td) booster at fourteen to sixteen years.

•Hepatitis B vaccine is administered in three doses starting either soon after birth or at two months of age (depending on the type of vaccine) and ending between six and eighteen months. (Children born to mothers infected with hepatitis B virus are vaccinated on a different schedule.)

•Pertussis vaccine should be withheld or moderated for children with convulsive disorders or adverse reactions to the first shot of DPT. It's not given to children over six, since fatalities from pertussis occur almost exclusively before that age.

The case for DPT

American children have been getting immunized against pertussis, or whooping cough, since the 1920s. The disease, which causes violent fits of coughing, is especially damaging, even fatal, to very young children. Thanks to immunization, it has declined drastically. But starting in 1982, the media dramatically publicized instances of serious adverse reactions to the DPT vaccine. The reported reactions included convulsions, physical collapse, and occasional brain damage. Some critics contended that vaccination should be halted because the disease itself no longer posed a threat, so the benefits didn't warrant the risks involved.

Health experts have persuasively defended the vaccine. First, attributing serious reactions to the vaccine is complicated, since the same effects often occur in children without vaccinations. Second, in methodical studies of the vaccine's side effects, serious reactions have been rare. In a University of California at Los Angeles study that involved 15,000 injections, only eighteen children had serious reactions, and all recovered. A British study of 310,000 immunizations found only one case of brain damage.

But the most convincing evidence for continued widespread use of the vaccine showed up in the late 1970s, when routine vaccination declined in Great Britain and Japan as a result of vaccine scares. Within two years, 100,000 cases of pertussis (with twenty-eight deaths) appeared in Great Britain and 13,000 cases (with forty-one deaths) in Japan. Even in the United States, the disease has by no means been wiped out; there are still about 1,500 to 2,000 cases (with four to ten deaths) each year. That is why virtually all health care authorities recommend that we keep using this vaccine.

PAIN RELIEF

Pain is an individual matter, involving complex physical and psychological variables. Your backache may be relieved by massage, while someone else's may not be helped by dozens of different kinds of treatments. No single therapy will work for all people, all types of pain, or even for all people with the same complaint or

---

Opiates and Other Drugs

Pain relievers, called analgesics (from the Greek word for "no sense of pain"), vary greatly in how they work and consequently in the type of pain for which they are most effective. In practical terms, there are two general types of pain. Acute pain is short term, may be mild or severe, and is caused by an identifiable injury or disorder, such as a broken arm or surgery. Chronic pain is long term, can be continual or intermittent, and can be of varying severity.

Analgesic drugs are narcotic or non-narcotic: Narcotic analgesics (such as Percodan, Demerol, and codeine) act like morphine—by inhibiting pain impulses in certain centers of the brain. These are useful in treating acute pain, since it is short term, and as a temporary measure in some cases of chronic pain. However, narcotic analgesics (also called opiates, though not all are opium derivatives) are usu-

ally not suitable for chronic pain because the body may develop tolerance to them—that is, experience a diminished effect with prolonged use. Another danger is addiction, the most dramatic component of which is physical dependence. Narcotics also impair physical and mental function.

The main non-narcotic analgesics (discussed on the next two pages) are aspirin, ibuprofen, and other nonsteroidal anti-inflammatory drugs (NSAIDs), as well as acetaminophen. Most of these are especially useful for bone pain (including dental), some types of arthritis, and headaches.

There is a "ceiling effect"—that is, increasing the dose beyond a certain point doesn't result in greater benefit. There's no risk of addiction. Still, continual high doses of non-narcotic analgesics may entail adverse side effects (see box on page 519).

apparent underlying condition. Thus, trial and error is usually unavoidable.

For most physicians and patients, the primary method of pain control is the use of analgesic medications. Unfortunately, some people, particularly those with unremitting chronic pain, go from one pain medication to another with little relief. Others refuse to use any drug over long periods for fear of addiction. When conventional treatments don't prove effective, alternative therapies can offer relief for some people.

Nonprescription Analgesics

In a typical drugstore, you'll find a multitude of over-the-counter (OTC) products for every sort of pain. This seemingly vast choice of pain relievers is misleading: in fact, over-the-counter pain relievers are of only two types—NSAIDs and acetaminophen.

There are three nonprescription NSAIDs (nonsteroidal anti-inflammatory drugs): aspirin, ibuprofen (such as Advil or Nuprin), and—as of 1994—naproxen sodium (brand name Aleve). NSAIDs work by blocking the effects of chemicals called prostaglandins, produced naturally by the body. When certain prostaglandins are present, you feel pain. Naproxen (brand name Naprosyn) and naproxen sodium (Anaprox) have been sold by prescription as arthritis drugs for a number of years. Because of naproxen's good record as a pain reliever with relatively few side effects, the FDA approved naproxen sodium (which works faster than plain naproxen) as an OTC pain reliever.

Acetaminophen (such as Tylenol or Panadol) is thought to affect pain centers in the brain. It is effective against pain and fever but not inflammation.

Keep the following tips in mind

Buy generic. Generics must meet the same standards as name brands. Advertisements strongly imply that you can't "trust" generics, but it's the ads you should mistrust. Exception: there won't be a generic naproxen sodium until the patent, held by Syntex Laboratories, expires in 1997. Aleve costs about as much as brand-name ibuprofen.

Avoid combinations of ingredients. They cost more and provide less of the pain reliever you seek. If you have a cold, buy ibuprofen and a decongestant (if you want one). If you have a headache and an upset stomach, buy acetaminophen or aspirin for the first and an antacid for the second.

Packaging options. Caplets and gel-caps may be easier to swallow. Timed-release capsules offer prolonged relief and may be helpful for muscle soreness or other kinds of low-level continuing pain. Aleve is also long-lasting.

Effervescent tablets with aspirin (for example, Alka-Seltzer) contain a large amount of antacid, which causes the aspirin to be more quickly excreted and thus reduces its effectiveness.

Children under sixteen shouldn't take aspirin, because of the risk of Reye's syndrome, a potentially life-threatening condition in children that can follow a viral infection such as the flu. Although the exact cause of Reye's syndrome is unknown, it may be triggered by the use of aspirin during a viral illness.

Low-dose aspirin taken daily thins the blood and can prevent heart attacks. But this regimen should be undertaken only on medical advice.

Over-the-Counter Pain Relievers

Product	Where Effective	Cautions	Comment
Acetaminophen (Tylenol, Panadol, Anacin-3)	Aches, pain, fever. Useful for children under 16 with chicken pox or flu or those allergic to aspirin. Does not cause gastrointestinal bleeding. Does not prevent blood clotting. Safe after oral surgery.	Rare reactions include skin rashes and painful urination. HIgh doses over long periods may damage liver and kidneys. Should not be used by alcoholics, people with liver or kidney diseases (such as hepatitis). Pregnant and breast-feeding women should check with their doctors.	Will not reduce inflammation, thus not effective for arthritis pain.
NSAIDs			
Aspirin	Aches and pain, fever, inflammation. On medical advice, low dosages daily can prevent heart attack, because aspirin inhibits blood clots. Some evidence for possible preventive effect against colon cancer but more research is needed.	Not recommended for pregnant women (can cause bleeding); breast-feeding mothers; those with known aspirin allergies, ulcers, gout, stomach bleeding; children under 16 with chicken pox or flu, because of risk of Reye's syndrome; people taking anti-coagulants. Frequent use can lead to ulcers. Excessive doses may produce upset stomach, ringing ears.	A highly effective, inexpensive drug. At least 40% of people have some stomach bleeding (usually inconsequential) after taking aspirin. Those who experience stomach upset may be helped by taking aspirin with food.
Ibuprofen (Advil, Nuprin, Mediprin, etc.)	Pain, fever, inflammation. Inhibits blood clotting.	Fewer side effects than aspirin. Those who are allergic to aspirin may experience similar side effects with ibuprofen. In some people, may cause stomach bleeding, like aspirin. May interfere with diuretic and anti-hypertensive drugs. Children and pregnant or breast-feeding women should take only on medical advice.	Less toxic in large doses than aspirin or acetominophen. Better for menstrual cramps than the other two. Some evidence that ibuprofen is better for muscle aches and fever accompanying a cold because it does not promote nasal congestion, unlike aspirin and acetaminophen.
Naproxen sodium (Aleve)	Pain, fever, inflammation. Inhibits blood clotting.	May cause stomach upsets and stomach bleeding in some people, but less likely to than aspirin or ibuprofen. Not recommended for those with · ulcers, asthma, or kidney disease, or heavy drinkers. Children under 12 and pregnant or breast-feeding women should take only on medical advice.	Longer lasting relief than aspirin or ibuprofen; thus good for taking at bedtime. Good for menstrual cramps, postpartum pain. Worth trying if other OTC pain relievers haven't worked. Sold in tablets of 200 milligrams. For those over 12, maximum daily dose is three tablets with eight to twelve hours between doses.

Buffered aspirin contains a small amount of antacid as a buffering agent, but usually not enough to prevent upset stomach. On the other hand, enteric-coated pills are easier to swallow and may lessen stomach distress. The coating does slow the absorption of the pain reliever and thus delays pain relief.

Alcohol. The Aleve label advises caution when combining frequent use of pain relievers with heavy drinking. Soon other pain relievers will carry such a caution. (Combining alcohol with aspirin or ibuprofen may promote gastrointestinal bleeding. Acetaminophen and alcohol may promote liver damage.)

Store your pain relievers in a cool, dry place. The bathroom is not ideal.

Stick with one type of pain reliever at a time.

"OTC" does not mean harmless. As with any drug, read labels and follow dosages. If your pain persists, or if pain relievers become a habit, seek professional advice.

Alternative Treatments

It's safest to think of alternative treatments as adjunct therapy. Don't give up your regular medical care. Even if pain-relieving drugs have failed you, don't stop taking other prescription drugs that you may need. Talk to your physician about the new approaches you're considering, and make sure he or she continues to keep an eye on your condition. There's little potential harm in an alternative treatment for pain relief—unless it keeps you from getting a correct diagnosis of a treatable or curable condition. The effectiveness of alternative therapies has been difficult to demonstrate in controlled studies; evidence about them is frequently based on anecdotes from people who have gotten relief. Each therapy has its advocates and critics among patients, physicians, and researchers.

Painkillers and placebos

In recent years, scientists have discovered that just as body chemistry creates pain, it may also supply a mechanism to control it. They theorize that some methods of pain control, such as acupuncture and electrical nerve stimulation, reduce pain by activating the body's own pain relief system. Opiate-like substances (such as endorphins and enkephalins) produced in the spinal cord and brain appear to operate in the same manner as opiate drugs. Certain sufferers of chronic pain, in fact, may have lower levels of these natural pain relievers.

Another way alternative treatments may work is through what is called (sometimes derisively) the placebo effect. This phenomenon provides fascinating proof that, when it comes to pain, the mind and body work together. A placebo is any substance or procedure having an effect (usually beneficial) on a patient that, paradoxically, can't be attributed to the specific properties or actions of the drug or procedure itself. Typically, it's an inactive substance like a sugar pill that's given as if it were an effective treatment for the patient's pain or disease, but it can be any treatment, especially when the patient expects it to work. Since the 1950s, scientists have consistently found that 30 to 40 percent of all patients given a placebo show improvement for a wide variety of conditions—whether it's coughing or seasickness, dental or postoperative pain, angina, migraine, or pain from an ulcer. Even more surprising, about 10 percent of people given a placebo report side effects normally associated with a chemically active drug, and others even experience withdrawal symptoms when they stop taking the fake drug.

Contrary to myth, there appears to be no "placebo personality." Placebos can work for anybody (not merely suggestible people) in the right circumstances—namely, if the patient believes that someone is trying to help him and thus expects relief, and especially if the helper is an optimistic physician in a clinical setting. But also contrary to myth, the relief of pain or illness by placebo effect does not mean that the problem was feigned or just in the patient's mind.

There are possible biochemical explanations for the placebo effect. Some researchers suggest that placebos may help activate the internal pain-relief mechanism. To investigate this, they have given naloxone (a drug that blocks the effects of opiate painkillers like morphine) to patients whose pain was reduced by a placebo. Just as naloxone reverses morphine's action, so it canceled out the analgesic effect of the placebo and thus increased the pain—suggesting that placebos do indeed cause opiate-like substances to be released into the blood. On another level, the expectation of relief may itself reduce anxiety, and this calming effect can reduce muscle tension and increase the tolerance of pain.

The placebo effect can play a part in the success of any treatment. Your belief, hope or anticipation that a drug or procedure will heal you may add considerably to its effectiveness. While it's important for scientists to know whether the efficacy of a treatment or drug is due solely to a placebo effect (which is why placebos are usually used in clinical trials of new drugs), all that matters to a patient in pain and his physician is that a treatment works. So one goal for physician (or other practitioner) and patient is to maximize the placebo potential of any treatment.

Acupuncture

Practiced in China for some 2,000 years, acupuncture involves inserting needles into specific points on the skin and rotating them; the needles may be left in place for a period of time. Some acupuncturists transmit electrical stimulation through the needles, while others use low-intensity laser beams instead of needles.

How acupuncture may work is speculative. One theory is that it inhibits painful stimuli by activating the body's pain control system. This theory is supported by the fact that in some studies, when patients are given naloxone, the analgesic effect of acupuncture is reversed; others question these results. Or acupuncture may stimulate nerve fibers that compete with fibers transmitting the pain messages.

Acupuncture has been used to treat a variety of kinds of pain—from backaches and headaches to dental problems. In China, it's even used as anesthesia for some patients undergoing surgery. It appears to be effective as a short-term treatment; few studies have looked at its long-term effectiveness. Several studies indicate that 40 to 80 percent of subjects may benefit. Researchers have reported that acupuncture can be effective even for animals in pain. Still, there has been no conclusive, controlled study that rates acupuncture results beyond those of a placebo effect.

Special risks are involved, too. Incorrectly inserted needles can cause tissue swelling or even organ damage. If the needles are not sterilized and the skin not adequately cleaned, infection or hepatitis may result. Because of the risk of AIDS and hepatitis, disposable needles are recommended. Electric stimulation, either from needles or a Transcutaneous Electrical Nerve Stimulation (TENS) device should not be used on a person with a pacemaker, a fever, or irregular heartbeat. Choose a state-licensed, board-certified practitioner (if your state has certification).

Hypnosis

One of the most widespread uses of medical hypnosis is for pain control. Despite popular notions, a hypnotherapist doesn't put a person to sleep and then simply command him not to feel pain. Instead, the therapist establishes a rapport with the subject, promotes muscle relaxation, produces a trancelike state, and through suggestion tries to shift the subject's attention away from the pain. In some people, the pain is tuned out and thus reduced. Individuals vary greatly in their ability to be hypnotized, however; it's estimated that about half of all people can maintain a moderate trance. Temperament, imagination, motivation, and trust in the therapist are vital. With training, some can practice self-hypnosis.

Studies have found hypnosis most effective in lessening acute pain—for instance, pain caused by a dental procedure or burns. In a small number of people, hypnosis has even served as the sole anesthesia during surgery. It may also help control persistent pain, as in certain cancers.

Relaxation techniques and biofeedback

Although typically used to relieve day-to-day anxiety and tensions, relaxation techniques can also play a role in the management of pain. They help reduce muscle tension and, like hypnosis, shift attention away from pain. In one study, patients who were taught relaxation methods required half the painkillers after abdominal surgery compared to a control group, and were able to leave the hospital earlier.

Progressive muscle relaxation, described in 1938 by Dr. Edmund Jacobson, is a frequently used technique. It calls for tensing and then relaxing specific muscle groups, working from the feet to the head, while focusing on deep, regular breathing. Another technique, called the relaxation response, requires you to select a word or phrase and repeat it until the mind is empty and the body relaxed. This method is, in fact, a form of meditation.

The most technical of all relaxation methods is biofeedback. This calls for hooking a subject up to a device that continuously measures a physiological variable—muscle tension, for instance, or skin temperature. Meter readouts or tones tell whether the tension or temperature is increasing or decreasing—this is the feedback. The subject then tries to lower the number or change the pitch by focusing on the painful area, or on whichever sensations, thoughts, or feelings work for him. When successful, biofeedback produces muscle relaxation, reduced anxiety, and an increased sense of control, all of which may contribute to pain relief, particularly for headaches and muscle contraction pain.

Massage

Massage (the word comes from the Arabic *massa,* to stroke) is one of the oldest hands-on therapies, but modern medical researchers have paid it little attention. Few controlled studies of the physical effects of massage have ever been attempted. What massage therapy can accomplish, however, is to relax muscles, relieve muscle spasms and pain, increase blood flow in the skin and muscles, ease mental stress, and induce relaxation. It can also be useful in increasing the range of motion of joints after injuries.

Massage can be done to the entire body or restricted to the back, neck, shoulders, or feet. It typically involves kneading and stroking of the skin, and the application of pressure on tense muscles. The most common technique in America is known as effleurage or Swedish massage, a gentle stroking and kneading, sometimes with tapping, clapping, or similar percussive movements with the hands. Acupressure or shiatsu (finger pressure) are other massage systems that can be used along with or instead of stroking and kneading. There are many other massage techniques involving manipulating and pressing joints, bones, and soft tissues. In order to do you good, massage should feel good. When tense muscles are massaged, you may feel discomfort or even brief pain. But a good massage should not be painful, and should leave you feeling relaxed—not tense and certainly not sore.

Though you can massage your own body, massage is most relaxing when someone else does it for you. Many health professionals practice massage—physical therapists, athletic trainers, nurses, chiropractors, and, of course, qualified massage

Use a lotion or oil when giving or getting a rubdown. It cuts down on potential skin irritation from friction, feels good, and increases beneficial warmth as you work. You don't need special preparations: light vegetable oils, particularly sunflower, safflower, and almond, work very well.

therapists. A number of states have agencies regulating massage practice and requiring professional training (usually a minimum of 500 classroom hours) for licensing. If you are looking for a masseur or masseuse in one of these states, seek a licensed therapist. Elsewhere find a member of the American Massage Therapy Association (AMTA). Members have to graduate from an approved study program and pass an exam. You can call the national office in Chicago for a referral, or you can check with a good medical or sports medicine center. Many doctors can refer you to a qualified massage therapist.

Massage can be comforting and helpful, but is not a substitute for the medical treatment of an injury. If you have an acute injury such as a sprain, tendinitis, or a swollen joint, get a physician's advice. Injuries should not be massaged directly. Because it is relaxing and stimulates blood flow, massage can be helpful for injured or sick people, especially if they are confined to bed.

Pain clinics

For persistent, intractable pain—especially in the lower back—when other treatments haven't worked, the next step may be one of the hundreds of pain clinics now operating across the country. As part of a coordinated program of treatments, a clinic may offer psychological counseling, hypnosis, or acupuncture, along with such traditional medical therapies as surgery, orthopedics, physical therapy, and drugs. The regimen usually includes a program of aerobic exercise. Exercise may help reduce pain by raising endorphin levels, increasing self-confidence, reducing tension, and/or simply distracting people from their pain.

Pain clinics employ various strategies to deal with the self-perpetuating psychological aspects often associated with chronic pain syndrome. A person's lack of self-esteem, sense of helplessness, chronic depression, or desire for attention can all help perpetuate pain and suffering. At a clinic, a patient may be allowed to discuss pain for only a set amount of time; and the staff tries to reinforce the patient's constructive behavior, such as talking about other topics and participating in group projects. The family is taught to understand the needs that the patient's pain may serve and to help him satisfy these needs without using pain as a lever.

MEDICATIONS

According to a survey done for the Food and Drug Administration (FDA), fewer than 5 percent of patients question their doctors about prescriptions. Yet prescription drugs can be ineffective or even harmful when used in the wrong way. Before your doctor prescribes anything for you, be sure he knows about any special restrictions that apply to you, such as the following:

Allergies or dietary restrictions. A prescription drug may contain any number of substances in addition to medicine, such as a binder to hold a tablet together, coloring, or preservatives. Liquid medications often contain alcohol. Be sure your doctor knows about any drugs to which you are allergic.

Health conditions for which the drug could be harmful. Be sure your doctor is aware of all your health conditions, and certainly tell him if you are pregnant, planning to become pregnant soon, or are breast-feeding.

Also ask your doctor—or pharmacist—about the following:

Remember that a bathroom is actually a poor place to store drugs because the high heat and humidity from the bath or shower causes pills and powders to deteriorate quickly. Choose a cool, dry spot instead—a closet shelf might be a good place, for instance. If a drug needs to be kept in a refrigerator, it will be indicated on the label.

What you are taking. Find out the name of the medication. When you pick up the prescription, check the label to first make sure that it is yours, and second that the drug named on the label is the one the doctor prescribed. Accidents do happen.

When you should take the medication. Must you take it during the night to maintain a proper blood level of the drug, or would taking it at bedtime and on awakening suffice? If you miss a dose, should you double up the next time you are scheduled to take it, or simply forget it?

How you should take the medicine (and store it). On a full or empty stomach? With water, milk, or citrus juices? Can you crush large pills and mix them with food? Drugs that are coated to prevent stomach upset or to provide time release must be taken whole. Should you keep the drug refrigerated or away from sunlight?

Swallowing pills

Always stand up to swallow medicine. If you're confined to bed and cannot stand, at least sit as upright as possible. Pills taken lying down or even sitting may lodge in the esophagus and dissolve there producing inflammation or injury. Even if it causes no harm, a stuck aspirin, for instance, can take an hour or more to reach the source of pain. To help the pill along, follow these guidelines:

•Before you put the pill in your mouth, always drink a swallow of water.

•Put the pill or capsule as far back on your tongue as possible.

•Wash it down with at least four ounces of water. If possible, drink another half-glass in five minutes.

•Stay on your feet for at least two or three minutes afterward.

Try drinking your water from a bottle—the sucking action helps. If you think a pill is stuck, eat several bites of banana and then drink some water.

Medicine Cabinet Safety

Most medicine cabinets are far too ample: the point of stocking drugs and medical supplies is to have essential items on hand in case of any emergency. But medicine chests tend to become an elephant's graveyard: out-of-date drugs pile up, making you think that you're better stocked than you really are. Drugs and supplies usually have a limited shelf life, so check expiration dates every few months. Out-of-date drugs may not only lose potency, they may also be dangerous, particularly antibiotics. If a drug doesn't have an expiration date, write the purchase date on the label. Then check with your doctor or pharmacist before using a drug that is more than a year old. Discard old drugs by flushing them down the toilet; children or pets could discover them in a wastebasket.

Downsizing your medicine chest

Consider discarding these items:

•Prescription drugs you didn't use up. Medications prescribed for a specific condition that has since cleared up should be thrown away, not kept around "just in case." Get rid of outdated medications, too. Flush them down the toilet or dispose of them so that children or pets don't find them in a wastebasket.

•Iodine, hexylresorcinol, Merthiolate, Mercurochrome, and similar products. These actually are not effective disinfectants and can burn the skin under a tight bandage. Be wary, generally, of products that claims to promote healing.

•Hydrogen peroxide. This old standby for "cleansing" can actually damage skin and retard healing. Water is better.

•Stimulant laxatives (such as ExLax, Feen-a-mint, and Cascara). A diet high in fruits, vegetables, and whole grains, plus two quarts of fluid daily, will keep you from needing a laxa-

tive. Stimulant laxatives, which work by irritating the intestinal wall, can be habit-forming. If you must have a laxative, use a bulk laxative (such as Metamucil), which is high in fiber.

If you have any questions about the condition or potency of a drug, call your doctor or pharmacist. Since medicines don't last forever, it may be a waste of money to buy large, family-sized bottles of drugs. They may go bad before you use them.

If there are children in the house or coming to visit, be sure that potentially toxic medicines are in child-proof containers or in a locked box. Keeping them out of reach is not good enough—children are remarkably persistent in searching for colorful things to eat and drink.

What to keep

•A pair of tweezers (for removing ticks, slivers, or dirt particles from a wound), plus a pair of special, thin-tipped "tick tweezers" if you hike often in the woods.

•Bandages (assorted sizes), gauze, and adhesive tape.

•An over-the-counter pain reliever. Because no single pain reliever is right for every situation or every person, you might keep more than one type on hand.

•A simple antacid, especially one with calcium, such as Tums or Rolaids.

•A remedy for mild diarrhea, such as Pepto-Bismol or Imodium, which can be bought in generic form.

•Calamine lotion for soothing insect bites or poison ivy.

•OTC hydrocortisone cream (1%) for skin rashes, insect bites, and contact dermatitis. It generally should not be used on any eruption caused by fungi, viruses, or bacteria (such as athlete's foot, ringworm, or cold sores).

•A fever thermometer.

How long you should take the drug. Just until the symptoms stop? Or, as with many antibiotics, should you finish the prescription? The label frequently says whether—and how often—the prescription can be refilled. If it's refillable, should you call the doctor before refilling it? Also, find out how long the drug takes to work, and what effect to expect, so that you can tell your doctor if it's not working.

Possible side effects. For example, should you immediately discontinue the medication if you experience some mild stomach upset? Or is it likely to pass? Will the drug make you drowsy, like some tranquilizers? Should you avoid driving or operating machinery while on the prescription? Are there any side effects that require that the drug be halted immediately?

Interactions between your prescription and other medicine you are taking. Make sure your doctor knows which other drugs (including over-the-counter medications) you currently take. Mixing over-the-counter antihistamines found in cold remedies with tranquilizers, for example, could make you very drowsy. Can you drink alcohol while taking the medication? Some drugs, such as Valium, can be dangerous when combined with alcohol. A good pharmacist will track all your prescription drugs and notify your physician and you of any incompatibilities.

When the drug will expire. If possible, have the pharmacist write an expiration date on the label for you.

Generic vs. brand-name drugs

More than 8,000 generic drugs are currently manufactured and sold with Food and Drug Administration (FDA) approval, and millions of people use them daily. All Veterans Administration hospitals use generics, and when the president gets medications at Walter Reed Hospital, he gets generics. The FDA estimates that 70 to 80 percent of all generics are made by the same manufacturers licensed to make the brand-name drugs. A pharmaceutical company that develops a drug can patent it and sell it exclusively for seventeen years (this may be extended by five years in some cases); after that, any company can make and sell the drug competitively, provided the copy proves as good as the original—that's what a generic is. All drug manufacturers, whether they're producing brand-name or generic products, must comply with the same FDA-mandated standards.

Generics generally retail for 30 to 80 percent less than their brand-name equivalents, so many people ask their doctors to specify them. In 1984, Congress passed a law that eases the approval process for generic drugs at the FDA, and now half of all drug prescriptions filled these days are generics. Many large insurers and health maintenance organizations, as well as Medicare and Medicaid, favor or require the use of generics as an economical measure.

Some professionals question the efficacy and potency of generic drugs, claiming that if one drug is bio-equivalent it doesn't mean it's necessarily therapeutically equivalent to the brand name. But this is simply not true: if a drug is bio-equivalent, it must be therapeutically equivalent. Even brand names may have side effects or occasionally fail to perform as expected.

Of course, the choice of prescription drug is up to a physician's best judgment, and your doctor is the person to consult if you are worried about any drug you are taking. If you do plan to discuss your medication with your doctor, keep taking it meanwhile. It can be dangerous to make changes on your own. Keep the following points in mind:

Should medication be taken on an empty stomach?

It depends on the medication. Certain types of medication are irritating to the stomach (such as aspirin, erythromycin, prednisone, doxycycline, indomethacin, and ibuprofen) and should be taken with meals to diminish or prevent digestive problems. Some other drugs (such as antibiotics) are poorly absorbed in the presence of certain foods, especially dairy products, and thus should be taken between meals—or at least one hour before or two hours after eating. Still other medications (such as diuretics and acetaminophen) can be taken any time. You should check with your doctor or pharmacist each time you receive a prescription to see which conditions apply.

• If you're taking a prescription generic and both you and your doctor are satisfied with your progress, you have no reason to worry.

• Know what you're taking. If your doctor says a brand-name drug is a must, follow his advice but try price shopping. Some pharmacies charge less than others.

• Over-the-counter generics (aspirin, ibuprofen, steroid ointments, and the like) are also safe, and are often much less expensive than brand names.

Over-the-counter drugs

There are over 300,000 nonprescription drugs available in the United States. Medicines that can be obtained over the counter, by law, must be safe for use without the supervision of a physician. They are not addictive if used correctly, and they must have clear warnings and instructions for consumers printed on the labels . And yet, there's a difference between "safe" and "harmless." Over-the-counter drugs can do damage if used incorrectly, and some can lead to physical dependence if overused. Some nonprescription drugs should not be taken by children, pregnant or lactating women, the elderly, or in combination with other drugs.

To use over-the-counter drugs safely, read the label on any product you buy. It's good policy to reread labels on a new bottle or package even if it's something you've taken before. Manufacturers can and do reformulate their products at higher or lower strengths, or there may be new warnings about side effects. Always follow directions to the letter. The rate at which your body eliminates drugs is fixed, and if you take too much, or even take the recommended amount over too long a period, the drug might build to dangerous levels. Four common kinds of nonprescription drugs are especially likely to produce adverse side effects or dependencies.

Nasal sprays. After several days' use, your nose may be more congested than ever. Sprays, which contain a decongestant, work by constricting blood vessels, but with repeated use the vessels no longer constrict, leading to the opposite effect—a rebound of swelling or congestion. If you use one, limit it to one or two days. Don't spray more often than the label recommends.

Laxatives. Their labels remind you that "frequent or continued use may result in dependency." The most habit-forming laxatives are the so-called "stimulants," which work by irritating the walls of the intestine. Laxatives that increase stool bulk (such as Metamucil) are less dangerous, but any laxative can cause dependency. If you feel in constant need of one, consult your doctor. To kick the habit, increase your intake of fluid and fiber. A diet high in fruits, vegetables, and grains, plus two quarts of fluids a day, will almost always alleviate constipation.

Eye drops. These blood vessel constrictors will whiten bloodshot eyes, but like nasal sprays, they can produce a rebound effect. After a day or two, blood vessels may dilate. If your eyes are red for more than a day or two, you may need medical advice. Eye-drop use can mask serious eye infections and other diseases.

Codeine cough syrups. Codeine, a narcotic, works directly on the part of the brain that controls coughing. In about two-thirds of the United States, codeine-containing cough suppressants are available simply by signing a register in the drugstore. The potential for addiction is small, but you should follow dosage limits carefully. In addition, this drug frequently causes constipation. Don't use such cough syrups for more than three days without the advice of your doctor.

When taking liquid medicines, it's best to use a specially marked measuring spoon or other device to measure each dose accurately. Household spoons may vary widely in the amount they hold, and with some drugs, even small variations in dosage can cause problems.

ENVIRONMENT AND SAFETY

Injuries and illness stemming from either accidents or environmental hazards may seem to be beyond the average person's control. Accidents—which are the fourth most common cause of death in the United States—often appear to be a matter of "chance." But in fact, the risks you are exposed to while driving a car, hiking in the woods, or cooking on an outdoor barbecue can be substantially reduced by heeding basic safety precautions. Similarly, many people believe that, as individuals, they have no control over risks to their health due to large-scale environmental problems such as acid rain or industrial pollutants. While it is true that many environmental issues require national or global policies to be dealt with effectively, you can act to control risks in your immediate environment—in your home, workplace, and local community. This part of the book covers potential problems you may encounter, puts these problems into perspective, and provides safeguards you can adopt to protect yourself and your family.

Part 5

Home and Workplace

Familiar surroundings are often viewed as safe havens, yet on average about 350 injuries and three fatal accidents occur in the home every hour in the United States. This section deals with common safety and environmental hazards in the home and workplace and shows you how to guard against them.

Aerosol Cans

Although in 1978 the Environmental Protection Agency (EPA) banned the use of chlorofluorocarbons (CFCs) as propellants in most aerosol sprays because they endanger the earth's protective ozone layer, they are still used in some sprays. In addition—whether they contain CFCs or not—spray cans present potential hazards to individuals using them. The most common injuries result from heated cans that explode, and from misdirected sprays that get into eyes. Symptoms of overexposure to aerosol sprays—including headaches, dizziness, nausea, skin rashes, and shortness of breath—depend on the active ingredients involved.

Aerosol sprays are prepared from substances that are gaseous at room temperature under normal pressure but become liquid when pressurized; such propellants include petroleum or inert gases such as carbon dioxide. The active ingredient is dissolved or suspended in this pressurized material, and when the button is pressed, the liquid vaporizes and is sprayed through a small hole. The particles in the spray are so small that they are easily inhaled into the lungs where they are absorbed into the bloodstream. This can be extremely dangerous. In addition, some ingredients, such as the propane found in many hair sprays, are flammable and thus hazardous when used near a lit cigarette, match, or open flame.

A safer alternative

Manufacturers are increasingly packaging their products in pump spray containers. Compared to aerosols, these are safer for consumers and not harmful to the environment because they do not use pressurized chemicals; instead, their active ingredients are dissolved or dispersed in water and simply sprayed through a pump mechanism. Still, even though the chemical molecules in spray pumps are larger, and therefore not as easily inhaled, and the spray is more precise, be cautious about using spray pumps around the face and eyes.

Hairspray: use it safely if you use it

The cosmetic industry says that hair sprays are safe, and the Food and Drug Administration (FDA) does require safety studies before a product is marketed. However, the companies are not required to make them public, since hairsprays are cosmetics, not drugs. While stating that low-level exposure to aerosols are probably not harmful, the American Lung Association classifies aerosol hair sprays among the products that can cause skin and eye irritation as well as headaches and nausea when they are inhaled and absorbed into the bloodstream in "unusually large quantities."

The lacquers (containing shellac) that used to be standard ingredients in hairsprays have been replaced by synthetic polymers, usually in an alcohol solution. In studies of cosmetologists with long-term exposure to hair spray, it's been found that some of these polymers can cause lung disease. According to the *Health Hazard Manual for Cosmeticians, Hairdressers, Beauticians, and Barbers* (prepared at Cornell University), the lungs heal when exposure to hair spray is discontinued. Still, their long-term significance is not well understood. It appears that any risk to individual users is much less than for occupational use, particularly in salons with poor ventilation.

Do take the following precautions:

•Buy pump sprays instead of aerosols. These dramatically reduce inhalation because the droplets from pumps are larger. They also contain no propellants. If the nozzle is adjustable, keep the droplet size as large as possible.

•If you do use aerosols, look for carbon dioxide propellant sprays rather than isobutane or propane propellants, which are highly flammable and which should carry a warning label. (CFCs, which are not flammable, were banned in 1978.) Never use a product containing isobutane or propane around an open flame, or when smoking. Injuries and deaths have been reported.

•Use water-based rather than alcohol-based sprays. Alcohol tends to dry the upper respiratory tract.

•Avoid the fast-drying sprays, which tend to contain volatile substances in more concentrated form.

•Use spray sparingly and in a well-ventilated area.

•If you have asthma or respiratory problems, consider using a setting gel instead of hairspray.

Art Supplies

Crayons, felt markers, glue, paints, and clay are standard equipment for most children—at school and at home. And it's not just kids who use and enjoy artists' materials. Almost 40 percent of adults use paints, solvents, clay, aerosol sprays, or similar materials in the practice of a hobby or craft. Thousands of people work full-time or part-time as artists.

Yet many parents and teachers, weekend artists, and even full-fledged professionals do not know that some art materials contain toxins that can be absorbed through the skin or lungs—for example, lead and other heavy metals such as cadmium or mercury. Solvents, concentrated acids and alkalis (such as photo chemicals), dry powders for making clays, and especially aerosol sprays may contain hazardous chemicals. Turpentine, a common solvent, can cause skin allergies, nausea, and (if chronically inhaled) even brain damage. Even small amounts of most solvents can be fatal if swallowed.

Because of the tightening of federal regulations and laws (specifically the Art Materials Labeling Act of 1990), efforts on the part of manufacturers, and the work of consumer groups, it is possible to find safe materials—and the dangerous ones now often have more informative labels. But using materials safely requires some

Homemade play-dough

Commercial play-dough may contain preservatives that are not good for children to ingest. For an alternative to store-bought dough, try making a batch of your own—which will keep in the refrigerator in a tightly covered coffee can for a few days.

2 cups flour
1 cup salt
2 tablespoons cooking oil

Mix ingredients in a large bowl. Add water until the mixture feels right for modeling. (It should have a smooth, silky feel, but not stick to your hands.) Then add a squirt of food coloring.

knowledge, forethought, and attentive label reading. How you use a product can be as important as what it contains.

Buying supplies

Read labels carefully. Any product posing acute or chronic hazards must have detailed instructions for safe use, according to the new federal law. Even though lead in house paint is now illegal, some art materials (such as oil-based paints) may legally contain lead and other heavy metals. Avoid them if possible, as well as any product containing benzene, denatured alcohol, methyl alcohol, or carbon tetrachloride. Look for the seals of the Arts and Crafts Materials Institute, or ACMI (see marginal). Consumer groups have sometimes taken issue with the standards of this manufacturers' group. But its AP and CP seals mean that the product is not acutely toxic if used as directed.

Work carefully

•Always work in a well-ventilated area—by an open window, if possible. Use an exhaust fan to set up a cross draft. An air conditioner only recirculates the air.

•Set up your studio in a separate area rather than the kitchen, bedroom, or any room simultaneously used for other purposes. Keep children away from the site.

•Don't eat, smoke, or drink while working.

•Clean up dust and debris in your work area daily. Don't sweep—it stirs up dust. Use a vacuum or wet mop.

•Don't put your brush or pen in your mouth.

•Wear plastic or vinyl gloves.

•Wear special clothes for art work, and wash them separately.

Art Safety for Children

Because growing tissues can be more susceptible to toxins, young artists are in need of extra protection. Rubber cement, permanent felt-tip markers, spray fixatives, powdered clays, and instant papier-mâché are standard equipment in classrooms and playrooms, yet all of these materials contain chemicals that are hazardous if inhaled, absorbed, or swallowed. Children tend not to follow safety instructions consistently. Toddlers, or even older children, may simply not comprehend the dangers and may chew, swallow, suck, and inhale art materials or decorate their hands and faces with them.

There are many safe art materials for children on the market. Follow these pointers:

•Read labels carefully, and don't buy unlabeled products. Children's craft supplies should ideally bear the seal of the Arts and Crafts Materials Institute—your guarantee that the contents are safe, even if swallowed.

•Don't allow a child to use old art materials that may not meet modern standards.

•Remember that "nontoxic" on a label may simply mean "not acutely toxic." The product can still make a child sick if swallowed. Even wheat-based pastes and Play-Doh should not be eaten, since they may contain preservatives or other elements that should not be ingested.

•Use talc-free, premixed clay. Powdered clay may contain asbestos and is easily inhaled.

•When possible, use vegetable and plant dyes instead of powdered tempera colors.

•Choose water-based ink or paints. Use only watercolor markers.

•White glue and school pastes are fine to use. Try to avoid epoxies, instant glues, or solvent-based adhesives.

If your child uses art supplies in school, check with your child's teacher, the school's principal, a member of the school board, or the president of the Parent Teachers Association (PTA) about the guidelines used for purchasing art supplies.

•When using hazardous chemicals, particularly aerosols, use a proper face respirator (available in hardware stores) and wear gloves and goggles. Outdoor spraying is safer, but stay upwind of the spraying.

•Wash your hands thoroughly when you've finished, and clean around your cuticles and under your nails. Never use turpentine, thinner, or other solvents on your hands. Try scrubbing with mechanic's soap or a safe waterless cleaner. Rubbing alcohol or baby oil, followed by soap and water, may do the job. Odorless mineral spirits (the toxic aromatic hydrocarbons have been removed) are also effective and less toxic than turpentine.

•Pregnant women, as well as men and women planning a family, should be particularly cautious about the use of hazardous materials, some of which are thought to decrease sperm count, promote miscarriage, or damage a developing fetus.

Asbestos

Asbestos consists of a group of minerals that readily form into long, flexible fibers that are noncombustible and chemically resistant. Because of its excellent insulating properties, asbestos has been widely used since 1940 in the building construction trades and in some home products. However, the fiber masses tend to break easily into a dust of nearly invisible particles that float in the air, adhere to clothing, and are easily inhaled—to the detriment of human health. Asbestos has been linked with respiratory diseases and some cancers of the lung, lung lining, and stomach. Most vulnerable are people who mine, process, or work with the mineral, especially if they are cigarette smokers. The more asbestos fibers inhaled and the longer the period of exposure, the greater the danger of lung damage. There are also different classes of asbestos compounds, and these appear to differ in their potential for harm.

Because asbestos is bonded with other materials in many home products, asbestos researchers do not consider households to be high-risk environments. But a damaged or loosely bonded asbestos product may release fibers into the air. There is little evidence that a brief or low-level exposure is likely to be harmful, but no one knows exactly how much inhaled asbestos is necessary to cause disease. Certainly it is important to understand the potential dangers from home products and take any necessary corrective measures. At the same time, there appears to be little reason for the near hysteria that developed some years back over asbestos.

Where asbestos is found

Asbestos is used to strengthen materials, as fireproofing, and as heat and sound insulation. Home-related materials that may contain asbestos include vinyl floor tiles and sheet flooring; patching compounds (prior to 1977); textured paint (prior to 1978); ceiling and wall insulation (especially in homes built between 1930 and 1970); oil-, coal-, and wood-burning stoves as well as their door gaskets and surrounding floor and walls; insulation material covering hot water and steam pipes or furnace ducts; fireplace insulation and radiator covers; siding, roofing shingles, and roofing felt typically found on flat roofs; and some appliances—toasters, broilers, ovens, refrigerators. Most such products aren't harmful if intact and not disturbed by sanding, scraping, sawing, drilling, or removal without proper safeguards.

To determine whether a suspect product contains asbestos, contact the installer or manufacturer. If this isn't possible, ask an asbestos-monitoring company or licensed abatement contractor for an evaluation. These companies will inspect and test questionable materials for you at costs ranging from about $50 to $350.

Sealing in asbestos

Most asbestos-containing materials, if intact, are best left untouched. Attempts to rip out or alter insulation, tiles, pipe coverings, etc. may so damage the materials that asbestos is released. When a product is slightly damaged or beginning to show signs of wear, opt to cover over rather than tamper. For example, if you have heating pipes encased with asbestos insulation with small punctures or minor flaking, wrap protective tape around the damaged areas and coat with a latex paint. When possible, lay new flooring over damaged asbestos tiles or sheets, and avoid sanding or disrupting the under layer. In the case of damaged asbestos roofing and siding shingles, spray painting will seal in the fibers. Apply wood, aluminum, or vinyl siding over asbestos-containing shingles; avoid cracking brittle shingles. A high-temperature paint applied to cement sheets around wood-burning stoves will seal in the asbestos.

Asbestos removal

An asbestos-containing material so deteriorated that sections are falling off or crumbling may be releasing fibers into the air. In this case, or if renovation plans will disturb asbestos materials, contact a licensed asbestos-removal contractor. Attempting removal on your own is unwise; safe equipment may be difficult to acquire, and if improperly done, removal may further contaminate the air. Neither should you dust, sweep, or vacuum any collected debris. Leave that to the contractor. Ordinary dust masks (such as those made by 3M) will not protect you from inhaling asbestos dust.

Be sure to screen any contractor you consider. Ask for a work history résumé, insurance certificates, a written proposal with a price quote, a work procedure outline (including locations of removals), references, and a copy of the notification of removal form that is required by some states. The contractor's job is not complete until air-quality tests—that are performed by the contractor after removal—give safe readings.

Many states require accreditation of asbestos-removal contractors. Your state or city environmental agency may provide a list of licensed contractors. If your state lacks a licensing program, contact your Regional Asbestos Coordinator (a branch of the Environmental Protection Agency) for assistance.

Carbon Monoxide

If you live in a cold climate and use storm windows, weather stripping, and sealers to keep your house warm and reduce fuel bills, you should give special thought to indoor air quality. Probably the chief pollutant of indoor air at home is carbon monoxide (CO), a common product of incomplete combustion—meaning combustion (or burning of gas or other fuels) in which not enough oxygen is present, so that CO forms instead of carbon dioxide. Colorless, odorless, tasteless, and thus extremely hard for a person to detect, CO is lethal in large quantities. Small amounts of it won't kill you, but chronic exposure can cause such symptoms as nausea, headaches, sleepiness, and a feeling of exhaustion. You may have a CO problem if 1) you notice excess moisture in the house, particularly condensation on your window panes, which may be a sign of poor ventilation; 2) you have an outside chimney, which may not vent gases the way it should if it is very cold; or 3) you have made your house airtight for winter and keep all windows closed.

Even at levels too low to cause symptoms, CO can combine with the hemoglobin in red blood cells, interfering with oxygen supply for the cells. People with heart disease may experience chest pains (angina) from breathing low levels of CO that wouldn't affect a healthy person. People with lung disease or circulatory problems (as may be caused by diabetes), infants, pregnant women (actually, the fetus is more sensitive to CO than the mother), and the elderly are also more susceptible. But this pollutant is very much under your control—and it shouldn't cost a fortune or require a team of experts to minimize this gas in home air. Often it's just a matter of ventilation.

These may be sources of CO in the home:
- Gas cooking ranges.
- Tobacco smoke.
- Car exhaust from an attached garage.
- A blocked or leaky chimney.
- Furnaces (oil or gas).
- Fuel-burning heaters of any type, especially kerosene.
- Burning charcoal in hibachis or grills.
- Improperly vented appliances, such as gas dryers.
- Wood stoves and wood-burning fireplaces if improperly vented.

How to keep CO out of the house
Take the following steps:
- Vent all fuel-burning space heaters to the outside. If you decide to use an unvented one in some emergency, read the manufacturer's instructions carefully, and then open a door in the room and keep a window open part way. A yellow-tipped flame usually signals CO emissions. If you have a kerosene heater, use only the fuel called for.
- Vent gas ranges to the outside. Run an exhaust fan and keep a window open slightly while you cook. Make sure the flame is blue. If it's yellow, call your local gas company and ask to have the burner adjusted. A pilot light that runs all the time is another source of emissions. A range with a pilotless ignition is a good investment if you cook with gas.
- When shopping for a wood stove, look for one that's certified to meet EPA emission standards, and make sure the doors are tight-fitting and that the gasket is in good shape. Burn aged or dried wood only, and avoid wood that's been chemically treated.
- Make sure that gas-burning furnaces and clothes dryers are vented to the outside and that the vents are clear.
- Don't let your car idle inside the garage, especially if the garage is attached to the house.

If you go to an indoor skating rink, remember that the ice resurfacing machines are usually gasoline-powered and can be a significant source of carbon monoxide. While resurfacing is going on, the rink management should operate an exhaust system and keep rink barrier doors open.

- Have your heating system professionally inspected and tuned up annually. Your local utility company may offer this service.
- Provide ventilation in winter. Open a window part way at night. If you cook with gas, don't weather-strip every window in the kitchen.
- Don't use an unvented grill or hibachi indoors.
- Don't smoke.

Carbon monoxide detectors

If, despite these steps, you feel something may go wrong, you might get a CO detector. Commercial detectors with an alarm that sounds and a gauge that indicates the level of emissions cost several hundred dollars—and for most homeowners would be overkill. Cheaper models are also available, though their effectiveness has never been studied. One unit, about the size of a smoke detector, costs about eighty dollars and will sound an alarm when dangerous levels of CO are reached. Way down the price scale are chemical dots mounted on plastic strip (five dollars or less). When exposed to CO, the dot will turn dark, and then lighten again in clean air. The main problem is that you have to remember to look at it periodically. If your furnace emits CO while you sleep, you won't know it. But if you are particularly concerned, it might be worth mounting one of these near your furnace or heating vents or in your kitchen or garage.

Computer Screens

Computer screens, also known as video display terminals or VDTs, are almost as common as telephones. In 1990, an estimated 70 million people worked at VDTs, and that does not include those who used computers at home or the millions of children who played at them. What are the health effects? According to research conducted by the Food and Drug Administration (FDA), VDTs do not endanger the health of their users. Other researchers, however, offer conflicting results. And many users complain of eyestrain, blurred vision, sore necks and backs, fatigue, insomnia, headaches, nausea, irritability, and tension. Some believe VDTs can even cause cataracts and birth defects. Often, according to the FDA, the problem is not the computer but environmental factors such as poor lighting or seating, and perhaps increased worker tension because of heightened workload.

Concern specifically about VDTs began in the late 1970s, when reports appeared about computer operators having high rates of headaches, miscarriages, and other health problems. Yet over the years, studies on VDTs have yielded contradictory or inconsistent results. And those that have found an increased incidence in cancers and birth disorders, for instance, generally suggest that the risk is statistically small. In Sweden, meanwhile, the government and labor organizations have set up stringent low-radiation standards for VDTs. There are no such standards on low-frequency VDT emissions in the United States, though some researchers are now advocating such guidelines.

The only consensus among scientists is that more research needs to be done. A number of long-term studies are currently underway (including one at the University of California at Berkeley and one at the Mt. Sinai School of Medicine in New York) and may help clarify matters.

Can video display terminals cause birth defects?

One question not yet wholly laid to rest is whether long hours at a VDT may cause miscarriages or birth defects. A study of over 4,000 pregnant women recently conducted at the University of Michigan showed that those who work at VDTs less than twenty hours per week do not increase their risk of miscarriage. Among full-time VDT workers, however, there was a very slight, but not significant, increase in the number of miscarriages, but researchers emphasized that their findings should relieve the concern for many women who currently use VDTs at their jobs.

What to do

Until we know more, it's probably prudent to minimize your exposure if your work involves heavy computer use and you are pregnant or planning a pregnancy. Though the evidence about birth defects and miscarriages remains inconclusive, women who are pregnant in particular should take these steps:

•Sit farther from the screen—in most cases this is all you have to do. A few inches can make a significant difference. Electromagnetic radiation falls off rapidly with distance from the source. Try to work at least twenty-eight inches (about arm's length) from the screen. The fields are almost always considerably stronger at the sides and rear of the machines, so sit at least four feet from your colleagues' monitors. (Magnetic-field emissions pass through partitions, walls, and even lead barriers.) In some offices, it may be necessary to rearrange work stations.

An adjustable computer desk with a shelf that pulls out to hold the keyboard will let you sit farther from the screen. If you have trouble reading the screen at that distance, enlarge the type size. If your computer program can't do this, you can buy a special large-type program, a magnifying screen, or a pair of eyeglasses that will let you focus at a distance of twenty-eight inches or more from the screen (regular reading glasses focus at about eighteen inches).

•Turn off the VDT when you're not using it but sitting nearby. Dimming the screen won't reduce the emissions.

•Don't fall for the ads for anti-glare screens that claim to block "radiation." Though these costly devices can block low-frequency electric fields, a Macworld study found that they don't block the magnetic fields, which worry scientists most.

•Don't trust a bargain-basement EMF meter to give you an accurate reading on your computer's emissions. In any case, if you sit far enough from your VDT, you needn't worry. If you or your employer nevertheless wants to test your monitors, be prepared to spend at least $200.

When shopping for a new computer

If you're thinking of buying a new VDT, look for one with lower electromagnetic emissions, such as the following:

•Models that meet the "Swedish standards." Several American manufacturers are now marketing "low-radiation" VDTs originally designed for sale in Sweden, where there are strict specifications for VDT emissions. Ask the salesperson about them. Thanks to consumer demand, more such models will undoubtedly be available soon in the United States—apparently at little or no added cost.

•Liquid crystal display (LCD) monitors. Nonbacklit LCDs, which contain no cathode ray tube, generate extremely low magnetic fields. They are generally employed in laptop models, but are also becoming available in some larger models.

•Monochromatic screens. These generally give off less radiation than color monitors. A small monitor, however, doesn't necessarily emit a weaker field than a large one; an undamaged old VDT isn't necessarily worse than a new one.

Other concerns

With a mandate from the World Health Organization (WHO), a group of Canadian experts concluded that VDTs are safe. At the same time, they made the following useful points:

Radiation. VDTs emit the same kind of low-level radiation as soil, rocks, fluorescent lights, or electrical appliances in the home. These emissions are not believed to harm humans in any way.

Room comfort. VDTs are a considerable source of heat. You may need to adjust room temperature accordingly. When operating a computer, keep room humidity at 30 percent or more.

Chairs. A stable chair, preferably with a five-legged base, good back support, a footrest, and adjustable seat height, is a necessity. A seat that curves downward at the front edge will help relieve excess pressure on the sitter's legs. A lumbar cushion—a log-shaped round pillow that is placed between the small of your lower back and the chair when you are sitting—may also be worthwhile.

Stress. Although the authors of the review were concerned chiefly with physical aspects of VDTs, they emphasized that the psychological welfare of VDT operators is important, too. People who are satisfied with their jobs are less likely to suffer from VDT-related symptoms. To compensate for the tension that may be caused by working at a VDT, it is important to take breaks every forty minutes or so: get up, walk around, or do simple stretching or relaxation exercises such as deep breathing (see page 458).

Cooking Equipment: Microwaves, etc.

Do your cooking utensils add ingredients—usually unwanted—to your food? Actually, there is a wide choice of excellent, safe cookware available, and few materials are a health hazard. But keep the following pointers in mind when you buy or use cookware:

Microwave

Plastic, glass, ceramics, and earthenware can all be microwave-safe. But all these materials can pose problems, too. Avoid thin plastic containers such as margarine tubs, or any plastic container not identified as "safe for microwaving." They can get too hot to handle or even melt into the food. They may also leach chemicals into the food, and no one knows whether these chemicals are harmful, and at what levels. It's okay to warm foods in microwave-safe plastic, but foods high in fat or sugar should probably not be cooked in plastic at all. In addition, a dish or container may get hot enough to burn you or may crack as the food heats up. So use a glass or ceramic container that you know to be microwave-safe. By the way, it's safe to use plastic wrap in the microwave, but try to keep it from touching the food.

To test a glass or ceramic dish: Microwave it on high for one minute. If it gets hot, don't use it in the microwave. If it feels lukewarm, it's okay for reheating. If it stays cool, it's safe for cooking. Dishes that get hotter than the food may contain metal and/or may eventually break.

Aluminum: not a problem

Over half the cookware sold in this country is aluminum, a very efficient heat conductor that's comparatively lightweight. Some people worry that aluminum in the body may promote Alzheimer's disease. However, the most convincing evidence shows that aluminum cookware is nothing to worry about. Even scientists who believe that aluminum may be somehow involved in the disease don't advise getting rid of aluminum cookware.

Iron

Depending on what you cook in it, an iron pot can add significant amounts of this important mineral to your food. Acidic foods like tomato or apple sauce that cook for a long time absorb the most iron. Spaghetti sauce, cooked for about twenty-five minutes in an iron pot, will have 5.8 milligrams of iron per 3.5 ounce serving, compared with 0.7 milligrams if cooked in another kind of pot. Applesauce cooked in iron may contain up to 7.3 milligrams, compared to 0.28 if not cooked in iron. (Adult men need 10 milligrams of iron daily, adult women 15 milligrams.) And studies have shown that pots continue to add iron to food even after many uses.

Stainless steel

Stainless-steel cookware is durable and easy to clean, but not as good a conductor of heat as aluminum. (That's why some steel pots come with a coating of aluminum or copper on the bottom.) Recently researchers discovered that stainless-steel cookware, when exposed to acidic solutions, leaches nickel, chromium, and iron. The chromium and iron are useful nutritionally, but nickel is not a mineral humans need. (Low levels of nickel, however, are found in many foods.) At the levels detected in the study, the only hazard the metal might present would be to aggravate a nickel allergy: exposure to the nickel produces a rash in some people; usually it's jewelry that sets it off. But critics of the study thought that the levels were still

---

Microwave Leakage

If your microwave is in good repair and you follow the instructions in the manual, leakage should be of no concern. The most important point is not to operate the oven with the door open—an impossibility, surely, since by law all ovens must have a double interlock that keeps them from operating if the door is open. Beyond that, you should inspect the door gasket occasionally to make sure it hasn't corroded or gotten dirty.

Don't try to use a damaged oven, particularly if the hinges, latches, or seals seem to be broken. Keep the gasket clean, but don't use any harsh abrasives when cleaning it.

From time to time, devices to test microwave leakage hit the market—often accompanied by hair-raising advertising copy. Some time ago the FDA tested nine of these (selling for ten to fifty dollars) and found them unreliable. Recently an inexpensive "sensor" has come out (a plastic card with color bands that presumably detect radiation). The price is only four dollars, but preliminary tests by the FDA have not shown that it works. If your oven is in good shape but you're still afraid of leakage, just stay a foot or two away from it while it's on.

too low to set off a reaction, even in the hypersensitive. The FDA does not regard stainless steel cookware as a problem. Once the cookware has been used for a while, it leaches less and less metals when acidic foods are cooked in it.

Nonstick

Nonstick coatings, such as Teflon and SilverStone, are made of fluorocarbon resin, an inert substance that does not react with food. The coatings lose their nonstick qualities with hard use, but there's no health reason to throw away the pan. Even if a particle of the resin flaked into your food, it would pass unchanged through your body. At extremely high temperatures (500°F), some nonstick pans might give off fumes, but at that temperature the chance of fire would be of more concern than the fumes. Nonstick cookware should not, of course, be used for broiling or heated to extreme temperatures.

Glass, enamel, copper

Heatproof glass (such as Pyrex), glass and ceramic combinations (such as Corningware), and enamel-clad metals are quite inert—that is, they don't interact with foods—and are safe to cook in. Copper is an excellent heat conductor and is preferred by many chefs. But beware of unlined copper: enough copper can dissolve in foods or water to cause nausea and vomiting. Copper lined with tin or stainless steel or stainless steel pans with copper bottoms are fine. If the tin or steel wears off your copper pot, it must be relined. Beating egg whites in a copper bowl is okay.

Copying Machines

According to experts at the National Institute for Occupational Safety and Health, a properly designed and maintained copying machine does not pose any health hazard. However, insufficient ventilation and lack of maintenance can cause some health problems.

Air quality

The most significant potential problem is that some photocopiers generate ozone, an irritant gas given off by high-voltage machines. While ozone in the ozone layer is good, ozone in the air we breathe irritates the respiratory system and can cause sore throats and labored breathing. It can also produce biochemical changes in the blood, and several animal studies indicate that ozone may increase susceptibility to infection—but its long-range effects are still unknown.

There are two reasons for excessively high ozone levels: poor ventilation and poor maintenance. You can ensure proper ventilation by following the recommendations of manufacturers, most of whom publish ventilation requirements for their machines. Some companies also offer filters that trap ozone. Maintenance is just as important. In one study of photocopiers, excessive ozone emissions dropped to nondetectable levels after routine maintenance. Workers should also avoid breathing the exhaust of a copier, which could occur when sitting next to the machine.

Avoiding chemical exposure

Because toners contain chemicals that can be hazardous, workers should watch out for toner dust—loose particles of toner either on copies or around the machine. Toner can be a source of eye irritation for people who wear contact lenses. If you spot toner dust, turn off the machine and have it serviced. Also, don't handle the photocopier's drum, another source of toxic chemicals; leave it to a technician who is trained to handle it safely.

Eyestrain and noise

In addition, copiers can cause eyestrain if they are operated with the cover up. All manufacturers recommend that a photocopier's glass be covered during exposures because the light is extremely intense. If you must keep the cover up, avert your eyes. Many large copying machines also produce noise at levels high enough to interfere with speech or telephone use in the area near the machine. This is another reason that, to be on the safe side, or simply in the interest of worker comfort, a copying machine should have its own well-ventilated room or at least ample space to itself.

Electrical Fields

Wherever there's electricity—be it overhead power lines or home appliances such as toaster ovens, hair dryer, or computer monitors—there are low-frequency electromagnetic fields (EMFs). These imperceptible energy emissions, located at the low end of the electromagnetic spectrum, are produced by alternating current as it surges in electric wires. As the term "electromagnetic" suggests, EMFs have two components, an electric charge and a magnetic attraction. Low-frequency EMFs are less blatantly damaging to living cells than higher-frequency forms of radiation such as X-rays, microwaves, or ultraviolet rays, which contain more energy.

Many Americans today are uneasy with electricity—some are downright fearful. Since 1979, when the first study suggested that EMFs might increase the risk of certain childhood cancers, EMFs have been the focus of dozens of studies and have become one of the most contentious scientific issues. Media reports, sometimes sensational, have generated enormous public concern about EMFs and have spawned a new growth industry among researchers, as well as among marketers of EMF monitors. Some houses near high-voltage power lines have become hard to sell, residents are fighting utility companies that want to install equipment in their towns, and some people with cancer have even sued utilities. In some states, legislation has been proposed or enacted to regulate EMFs from power lines, and there has been talk of requiring warning labels about EMFs on ordinary household appliances.

Are power lines and home appliances—like cigarettes—a health hazard?

Unfortunately, despite all the studies, scientists have not really learned that much about EMFs, according to a comprehensive survey by Britain's National Radiological Protection Board, as well as one by a White House committee. The population studies on the health effects of EMFs have yielded inconsistent and contradictory results. Many have found no adverse effects at all. Moreover, those studies that have found an increased risk of cancer (usually leukemia or brain tumors in children living near power lines or people who work daily with power lines) gener-

No dangers from fluorescent lights

Fluorescent lights emit a very small amount of ultraviolet radiation, but this is no cause for concern for most people. The only people who are at risk from fluorescent lights are those who are endangered by sunlight. There are certain rare skin diseases that make people susceptible to skin cancer. One of these is xeroderma pigmentosum, which occurs when the skin lacks the enzyme that repairs DNA in skin damaged by ultraviolet radiation. For most people, fluorescent lights actually offer a health benefit: their ultraviolet radiation helps the body synthesize vitamin D.

ally suggest that the number of additional cases that might have been caused by EMFs across the entire population would be tiny. In fact, since such small numbers of cases are involved, scientists can't be sure that the differences aren't simply chance variations.

Moreover, nearly all the studies have been seriously flawed. For instance, a much publicized Swedish study published in 1993 appeared to show that for children living near high-voltage power lines, the risk of leukemia was doubled. In 1994, in a paper presented to the National Council for Radiation Protection, Patricia Buffler, Professor of Epidemiology and Dean of the School of Public Health at the University of California at Berkeley, highlighted the serious weaknesses of this and similar studies and pointed out how the results have been overblown and misrepresented.

The problem is compounded by the fact that there is still no convincing theory explaining how EMFs—once considered innocuous, especially compared to higher-frequency forms of radiation such as X-rays, microwaves, or ultraviolet rays—could cause cancer or otherwise be harmful. It is hard to explain, since EMFs from power lines and appliances are minuscule compared to those naturally occurring on the Earth's surface, as William Bennett, professor of physics at Yale, has pointed out in a major article in *Physics Today*.

Some scientists have proposed various sketchy theories for the dangers of EMFs, but none of these hypotheses has widespread support. It is very difficult to determine what subtle effects, if any, low-frequency fields may have on cells—and hard to extrapolate from test-tube studies on isolated cells using intense EMFs to human beings living in the real world. And if EMFs are somehow carcinogenic, the exact component and dosage necessary to cause cancer are unknown, as is the time (months, years, or decades?) between exposure and onset of cancer. In fact, everything here is still unknown, unproven, and unclear.

What should you do?

The evidence so far about EMFs certainly does not justify inordinate concern, let alone hysteria. If EMFs pose a risk, it is undoubtedly extremely small. The stress and anxiety caused by the debate about EMFs have probably been "more hazardous to public health than EMFs of any level can have been," in the words of one researcher.

Some experts try to occupy a middle ground by saying that EMFs are probably safe, but that it can't hurt to take some simple precautions (such as sitting farther from computer screens, avoiding certain types of electric blankets, and not sleeping right next to an electric clock). Some call this "prudent avoidance," but others say it is waffling. "Carried to an extreme, this policy could result in spending millions of dollars [passed on to us in higher energy rates and appliance prices] to avoid an unidentified or 'phantom' hazard," according to Patricia Buffler.

The only consensus among scientists is that more research about the health effects of EMFs should be done. A number of long-term studies are currently underway and may help clarify matters. But, realistically, the results are likely to continue to be inconsistent and inconclusive. Meanwhile, try to avoid the numbing "everything-causes-cancer" mind-set, which can distract you from taking the steps that are known to protect your health.

Shock saver

Protect your house or apartment with an electronic device called a ground fault circuit interrupter (GFCI). A "ground fault" occurs when more current is flowing through the circuit than is returning, thus posing the danger of a severe or lethal shock. (This might happen, for example, when a hair dryer falls into water.) In this event the GFCI simply shuts off the current. Millions of GFCIs have been installed since 1973. You can have an electrician install such a device in your circuit breaker or in bathroom and kitchen electrical outlets—a fairly simple process that does not involve rewiring. Or you can buy a portable GFCI that plugs into any receptacle (any hardware store should sell them), then you plug your appliance into the GFCI. If you don't know whether you have them or not, GFCIs in the wall have a reset button at the center; in the circuit breaker box, it's marked as a "test" button.

Each year in the United States and Canada, about 6,000 people die in fires, not counting firefighters, and more than 31,000 are injured. Billions of dollars of property is lost as well. December, January, and February are the leading months for homes fires, and the leading cause of home fires is heating equipment: portable heaters, wood stoves, and fireplaces. Cooking mishaps, arson, and improper electrical distribution are among other causes. Cooking fires are the number-one cause of nonfatal home fire injury.

Smoking is the leading cause of death from home fires (30 percent of these deaths are attributable to smoking). Alcohol is often implicated as well. One study showed that half of all adults who die in fires have blood alcohol levels of .10 percent (that is, if they were driving, they would be considered legally intoxicated in most states). But many of these fires can be prevented, and precautions can be taken to protect yourself in case of a fire.

Preventing home fires

Use the following guidelines to help prevent fires in your home:

Home heating equipment. Purchase equipment that has been labeled and tested by one of the many independent testing laboratories. Check with your fire department to make sure that it complies with local fire and building codes. Have your furnace inspected by a professional annually. Place portable heaters at least three feet away from combustible materials such as paper, clothing, bedding, and curtains. Inspect the cords of electric heaters—do not use the heater if the cords are frayed, split, or overheat when the heater is on. Turn off the heater before leaving the house or going to bed. (See *Space Heaters*, page 566.)

Kerosene heaters. Don't add fuel to a kerosene heater—or to any other heater that uses liquid fuel—when the heater is hot. Let it cool completely first. Use only fuel recommended by the manufacturer with liquid-fuel heaters. *Never* use gasoline.

Wood-burning stoves. These should be installed at least three feet away from a wall and away from any combustible materials. Place approved heat shields under a wood-burning stove to protect the floor from heat and stray hot embers.

Fireplaces. If you use a fireplace, have the chimney inspected annually. Always use a screen with a fireplace.

Electric blankets. Tucking in an electric blanket can cause excessive heat that will start a fire. Don't put anything on top of an electric blanket while it's on, either. This includes other blankets, comforters, and sleeping pets.

Cooking. Never leave food cooking on the stove unattended. Keep stoves and ovens clean; bits of food or grease can catch fire. While cooking, wear clothing with tight-fitting sleeves and avoid wearing frilly aprons. Don't store pot holders on the stove. Heat oil slowly. Never leave oil heating unattended and never heat oil on high—it can catch fire.

Smoking. Keep matches and lighters away from children and teach them that these items are not toys to be played with. Properly extinguish all smoking materials and never smoke in bed.

Home appliances. Check all electrical appliances for broken, frayed, or split wires. Have broken appliances repaired before using. Make sure that televisions and

Beware of vines entangled in your firewood— they may be poison ivy, which can be hard to identify if the distinctive leaves are gone. Touching dried-out poison ivy can cause a rash.

stereos have some space around them. These appliances can easily overheat.

Flammable liquids. Store all flammable liquids—such as kerosene or gasoline—outside of the house in clearly labeled, tightly closed metal safety cans away from heat and other sources of ignition.

Smoke detectors

Deaths and injuries from home fires most often occur at night. Thousands of lives could have been saved if the victims had been awakened in time to flee. Even though most states require smoke-detector installation in new homes, most fire deaths still occur in homes that have no detectors or those that have detectors that are not working. Surveys have found that one-third to one-half of all detectors are not being used, or are not working because of poor maintenance.

There are three basic types of smoke detectors, powered either by house current or batteries:

Ionization devices. The most common type, these contain a trace of radioactive material that produces a continuous flow of electric current between two electrodes. When smoke particles waft across the current, they break the circuit and set off the alarm. Ionization detectors are sensitive to fast-burning fires and react quickly to cooking smoke.

Photoelectric devices. These more expensive detectors emit a beam of light received by a photocell. If smoke interrupts the beam, it triggers the alarm. These react faster to the kind of smoldering fire that begins, for example, in wiring or upholstery and less quickly to cooking smoke.

Combination units. These combine ionization and photoelectric mechanisms, and thus respond to all kinds of fires. If you're buying only one unit, this is the type of unit to buy.

If your house is large or has more than one floor, it may be best to install some of each basic type in order to get the advantages of all of them. For instance, you can put a photoelectric detector in or near the kitchen (it's less likely to scream an alarm every time you burn toast) and combination or ionization detectors in most

Gasoline stored as far as ten feet from an open flame or spark can explode because of escaping fumes.

Fireplace Safety

If you build fires in a fireplace or heat your home with a wood-burning stove, you should check your chimney annually and take steps to keep fumes and fire from entering the room.

Creosote, a black tarlike substance, can build up in a chimney and catch fire. This can crack the chimney or set fire to the house. If you've just moved in, have the chimney checked and cleaned before you use it. In expert hands, it should be a quick, clean, relatively inexpensive procedure.

A cleaner burn

To cut down on creosote build-up, build small, hot fires rather that large smoky ones. Use seasoned woods (stored and dried for at least six months). Hardwoods (maple, oak, elm, or other trees that lose their leaves in the fall) make an even, long-lasting fire. Softwoods (pine, spruce, or fir) burn faster and hotter. If you want to use softwood, combine it with hardwood for a better fire.

Be selective about other things you burn in the fireplace. Colored paper or plastic can produce harmful fumes. Christmas trees make poor firewood because they produce wild sparks. If you use man-made logs, put them on a grate and burn only one of them at a time. Don't poke them apart. They contain wax and coloring agents and thus make a dirtier fire that will clog your chimney faster, possibly contributing to chimney fires.

other areas. Make sure the units you buy have been approved by Underwriters Laboratories (UL) or another testing organization.

All you need to install a smoke detector is a drill, screwdriver, and stepladder. It's not much harder than hanging a picture. Install detectors in the hallway outside bedrooms and on *every level of the house,* basement and attic included. You can install additional detectors inside each bedroom, especially if you sleep with the bedroom door closed or if you smoke. If you're hard of hearing or a heavy sleeper, look for a model with a loud alarm. Since smoke rises, mount detectors high on a wall or on the ceiling, but no closer than four inches from where wall and ceiling meet. Also, don't put one within three feet of a window, door, or vent, since drafts can prevent smoke from reaching the device, as can water vapor, so avoid bathrooms, too.

Vacuum the detectors at least once a year to avoid dust-related false alarms or reduced sensitivity. Replace the batteries yearly (choose a model that emits a beep when batteries are low), and test them regularly, following the manufacturer's instructions. It's also a good idea to plan escape routes in case of fire and discuss them, or even rehearse them, with your family. Set off the detector so that everybody knows what it sounds like.

Some insurance companies will reduce your household premiums if you install smoke detectors — it's worth inquiring.

Fire extinguishers

Every household should have an extinguisher — probably more than one, since they all don't do precisely the same job. Don't count on water to fight a home fire. Because many fires originate in faulty or overloaded wiring, water can be dangerous, due to the risk of electrocution. You should fight a fire yourself only when you've made sure that everybody has fled the house and someone has called the fire department. Then resort to an extinguisher if the fire is still small and your back is to a safe exit. If any one of these conditions isn't met, or you're simply not sure whether you should stay and fight the fire, leave the house immediately, closing the door behind you.

Extinguishers are labeled A, B, or C (or combinations of these), based on the three types of fires defined by Underwriters Laboratories (UL):

Class A. These are effective against fires fueled by "ordinary combustibles," such as wood, paper, cloth, plastic, or rubber.

Class B. These work on fires fueled by fast-burning liquids, such as gasoline, cooking oils, or paints, as well as grease and tar.

Class C. These are extinguishers with nonconducting contents and therefore are used to fight electrical fires.

The UL label should also include a number indicating how big a fire the extinguisher can handle. Thus, a "2" rating means twice as much extinguishing capability as a "1." The higher the rating, the heavier the extinguisher — but it doesn't pay to buy a model too big to handle. The C models have no number rating.

A good choice to hang near the kitchen door is an extinguisher labeled BC. This is better than an "all-purpose" extinguisher (labeled ABC and filled with ammonium phosphate) because the sodium bicarbonate it contains works best against most kitchen fires. All-purpose extinguishers are smart choices for garages, workshops, and basements.

Hotel Fires

Whenever you stay in a hotel, investigate fire-safety measures. In hotels, as at home, smoke detectors are vital. Most people who die in hotel fires die from inhaling smoke or toxic fumes, not from burns. Adequate detection systems can save many lives; more widespread use of fire-resistant materials might save others.

Fortunately, more and more hotels have installed wireless alarms and sprinkler systems. Sensors placed in rooms, corridors, stairways, and all public spaces send radio signals to a central monitoring station, which can then alert guests, fire fighters, and police. Because the sensors are battery powered, they continue to operate even if the hotel's power is knocked out. And more hotels are decorating rooms with wall coverings and fabrics that are highly fire-resistant and, if they do burn, give off low-toxicity fumes.

Realistically, your chances of getting caught in a hotel fire are very small; chances of injury or death, even smaller. But it's only prudent to take certain precautions:

•Know your surroundings. Check the location of the floor's fire alarm in case you need to sound it, and verify escape routes. Make sure fire stairs are not locked or blocked. Count the number of doors from your room to the nearest exit; this will allow you to feel your way there through darkness or smoke. It's also wise to know where the second nearest exit is.

•Pack a small flashlight; keep it and your room key on the night table—if there's a fire, take them along. That way, if flames force you back to your room, you won't be locked out.

•Most important, do not smoke in bed. Half of all hotel-fire fatalities are the result of careless smoking.

If there's a fire, every second may count:

•If you hear an alarm or smell smoke, get out of your room, but not before you've felt the back of the door and knob. If they're cool, open the door slowly and take the nearest escape route. If they're hot, don't open the door; fire is probably raging in the corridor, so you're safer in your room. Call the management and/or fire department to report your location, and seal the door cracks with wet towels. Shut off fans and air conditioners and wait by your window where rescuers can see you.

•If the corridor or staircase is smoky, crawl. The air will be clearer at floor level. If smoke is thick at lower levels, go back to your room. Never try to run for it through heavy smoke—you won't make it.

•If the fire is in your room, get out, close the door, set off the floor alarm, and report it to the management.

•Don't waste precious time gathering your possessions.

•Don't use the elevator.

Most people who die in fires die from smoke inhalation, not burns. If you run into smoke while trying to escape from a burning building, turn around and try to find some other exit. If you must go through smoke, drop to floor level, where the air is cooler and clearer, and crawl under the smoke.

Another type of extinguisher, no longer manufactured but still in use, is filled with halon gas. Halon extinguishers leave far less residue than other types, and are effective against all classes of fires. But halon is much more expensive than dry-chemical models, less effective against kitchen grease fires, and harder to recharge. Even more important, halon (like its chemical relatives the chlorofluorocarbons) contributes to the depletion of the ozone layer—thus, as of January, 1994, the United States banned the production of halon. There may still be halon fire extinguishers for sale until existing supplies run out, but don't buy one for home use.

Make sure any extinguisher you buy will be easy for you and your family to lift and remove from its wall mounting, and simple to aim and trigger without your having to pause to read instructions. It should have some kind of safety catch to avoid accidental firing.

Also make sure there's an easy-to-read pressure gauge—and remember to check it frequently. Most models have a gauge indicating when the pressure has dropped too low. For recharging, check the instructions on the side, or look in the yellow pages under "fire extinguishers."

Formaldehyde

Formaldehyde, a colorless gas with a pungent odor, is so commonly used today that virtually everyone is likely to be exposed to at least small amounts of it, and a significant number of people are developing symptoms due to exposure to large amounts of formaldehyde in their homes or workplaces. It was an integral component of the urea formaldehyde foam insulation (UFFI) that was installed in more than 500,000 homes in the 1970s. (The use of formaldehyde in insulation was banned by the Consumer Product Safety Commission in 1982, but this ruling was overturned by a federal court in 1983.) In addition, it is present in a large variety of consumer products. It is a major part of the resins used as glue in particle board, plywood, and other wood products used extensively in the construction of homes and furniture. Some cosmetics, upholstery, permanent press fabrics, carpets, and pesticides contain it, too. Formaldehyde is also present in the exhaust from some appliances and in tobacco smoke. Thus, it's virtually impossible to avoid formaldehyde entirely.

The worst-case scenario for exposure would be this: to live in a new mobile home whose flooring, cabinets, and furnishings are made from hardwood plywood and other pressed wood products, and to have a closet full of brand new permanent press clothing and permanent press draperies at every window and new carpets on the floor, and to keep the doors and windows closed. Mobile homes tend to be worse than other homes because they not only contain a lot of new pressed-wood materials but enclose them in a very compact space. New products are worse than older ones: emissions lessen with time. High humidity and temperatures can increase emissions.

Physical effects of formaldehyde exposure

A normal level of formaldehyde in indoor and outdoor air is less than 0.03 parts per million and causes no problems. But when it rises above 0.1 parts per million, it may produce skin irritation, watery eyes, burning sensations in the eyes and respiratory tract, coughing, and similar reactions. It affects some people worse than others. It may be hard to tell what's causing these symptoms, which may also be caused by other pollutants or a cold. Formaldehyde exposure has been shown to increase the risk for some cancers, especially of the nose and throat, in workers continuously exposed to high levels. The Occupational Safety and Health Administration (OSHA) has sought tighter restrictions on formaldehyde exposure.

OSHA is not the only government agency that's responsible for trying to reduce formaldehyde: the EPA and the U.S. Consumer Product Safety Commission are implementing changes to reduce human exposure. The U.S. Department of Housing and Urban Development (HUD), which requires building materials to meet certain standards for formaldehyde emissions. Generally, the use of formaldehyde in such consumer products as permanent press fabrics, pressed woods, and floor coverings has been reduced, and products containing more than 1 percent formaldehyde have to be labeled.

Reducing the risk

If you have symptoms that you (and your doctor) believe are related to formaldehyde exposure, you may want to have your home checked. The steps below, which minimize formaldehyde exposure, are worth taking even if you have no symptoms:

•Increase home ventilation, especially in warm weather. In the cold months, don't seal up all the windows and doors. Circulating fresh air is a necessity to control indoor pollution and allergens of all kinds.

•Wash permanent press clothing and sheets before you use them. (These fabrics do contain less formaldehyde than they used to.) If you're installing permanent press draperies that you can't wash, try to air them out for a few days before hanging them.

•When buying hardwood plywood and other pressed woods for home building projects, get materials stamped with the HUD emissions seal.

•If you buy unfinished furniture or other pressed wood products, plan to varnish or paint them. A waterproof finish such a polyurethane will greatly reduce formaldehyde emissions.

•If you already have formaldehyde foam insulation seal it off. Patch any cracks, or cover the walls with nonporous wallpaper. Seal wood paneling with varnish.

•If buying a mobile home, be sure an adequate ventilation system is installed. HUD regulations require a seller to give a buyer an information sheet on ventilation before a sales agreement is reached.

Don't leave a pot of water boiling on a gas flame all day to boost humidity. You don't want to breathe the continuous emission of fumes from a burning gas flame.

Gas Stoves

About 60 percent of American families cook with gas. Although gas appliances are often called "clean burning," they can emit invisible and odorless by-products of combustion—nitrogen oxides and carbon monoxide. These compounds can irritate the respiratory system and may have long-term effects on lung function. Studies have suggested that children living in homes with unvented gas stoves are somewhat more susceptible to colds and respiratory ailments than those in homes with electric stoves.

Although gas ranges are by far the major sources of nitrogen oxides in the home, unvented kerosene and gas heaters can also be major sources if used more than occasionally. Gas furnaces, clothes dryers, and other vented gas-burning appliances usually do not pollute the air unless the vent flue is blocked or broken. If you do have gas appliances or a kerosene heater, follow the steps for controlling carbon monoxide in your home (see page 550).

Hair Dryers

Hair dryers can cause electrocution if a plugged-in dryer falls into a bathtub while someone is bathing, or the hair dryer falls into a full sink or tub and an unthinking person reaches in to get it. These incidents can be fatal *even if the switch is in the "off " position.*

Safety standards, set by Underwriters Laboratories (UL) in October of 1987, require that hair dryers be designed so they won't produce a dangerous shock if they fall in water when the power switch is in the "off " position. Some recent models also have a feature that will protect you from shocks when a dryer that's turned on falls in water.

546

If you have a hair dryer made before October, 1987, you may want to replace it, especially if you have young children. But even if you buy a model with every safety device, no hair dryer is 100 percent safe. Take these precautions:

•Never use a dryer or other electrical device near a sink or tub filled with water.

•After you're finished using it, *unplug it immediately,* and hang or store it in a secure place.

•If you do drop it in water, unplug it—first making sure your hands are dry—before retrieving it.

If you do not already have one, you might also consider installing a ground-fault interrupter outlet in your bathroom. This special outlet contains a circuit breaker that cuts off power if any device produces an electrical surge. It costs thirty to fifty dollars at hardware stores, and you may have to hire someone to install it. But it comes closer than anything else to making you and your family shockproof.

Household Toxins

"Hazardous waste" is a term more readily associated with atomic power plants than with our storerooms and basements. Yet many home projects such as car maintenance and gardening involve chemicals that are extremely hazardous to your health or that of your neighbor. These substances can be hard to dispose of responsibly: if dumped, they can seep into the water supply; if incinerated, they can pollute the air. Many municipalities are tightening the rules on what may be sent to the local garbage dump.

Ideally every community should have collection centers equipped to handle hazardous wastes. (If your community has none, you can inquire about starting such a center through your state's hazardous waste agency.) Meanwhile, remember that it is dangerous—and in many localities illegal—to dispose of liquid wastes by pouring them into storm drains or into sewage systems.

Disposal tips

Here are some examples and suggestions for safely discarding common types of household waste:

Automotive supplies (motor oils, antifreeze, transmission fluids, car wax). Many automotive chemicals are toxic if absorbed through the skin or if their vapors are inhaled. See if your gas station or automotive store will accept labeled containers of old fluids. If not, try to get the address of an oil-recycling station from your state highway department. As a last resort, pour the fluids into a container filled with sawdust or cat litter, seal it, and put it in the trash.

Painting supplies (paint, thinner, turpentine, mineral spirits). Try to give paint to someone who can use it. Latex or oil paint can be allowed to dry out in an open can and disposed of as trash. Thinners and many other painting supplies are highly poisonous, may contain cancer-causing chemicals, and are usually flammable. Seal them tightly in their original containers and hold them for delivery to a hazardous waste collection program.

Asbestos. Inhaled asbestos fibers can cause serious lung disease. Get professional help in removing and disposing of duct-wrapping and other possible sources of asbestos. Deteriorating asbestos materials can release thousands of invisible parti-

Alternatives to Common Cleaning Materials

The average kitchen and bathroom cabinets are filled with assorted cleansers and disinfectants for almost every part of the house, but many home fixtures can be cleaned just as effectively with only six common household ingredients—salt, baking soda, white vinegar, borax,* washing soda,* and liquid soap.*†

Household Product	Substitute
Air freshener	Find the source of the odor and eliminate it. Put small bowls of baking soda in the refrigerator and around the house. Also sprinkle baking soda into the bottoms of trash cans.
Ammonia- or chlorine-based cleaners	Mix 2 teaspoons borax with 1 teaspoon liquid soap in 1 quart water. (This solution can be stored in a spray bottle.)
Carpet deodorizer	Sprinkle baking soda or cornmeal (approximately 1 cup per room) on the carpets. Let stand 30 minutes, and then vacuum.
Disinfectants	Add ¼ cup borax to ½ cup hot water. (This mixture also deodorizes.) Or sponge isopropyl (rubbing) alcohol onto surfaces and allow to dry.**
Drain cleaner and unclogger	*To avoid clogs:* Always use the drain sieve. *To prevent clogs:* Once a week, pour ¼ cup salt, ½ cup baking soda, and ½ cup vinegar down the drain and cover it. Allow to stand for several minutes, then pour a pot of boiling water down the drain. *To unclog a drain:* Use a plunger (or plumber's snake if the plunger is ineffective) to break up the clog, and then flush the drain with the baking soda method mentioned above.
Glass cleaner	Add 5 tablespoons vinegar to 1 quart warm water. (You can store the solution in a spray bottle.) Stubborn spots can be removed with undiluted vinegar.
Metal polish, brass	Make a paste of equal parts flour, salt, and vinegar. Apply the paste, allow to sit an hour, then rub off, rinse, and polish with a soft, damp cloth.
Metal polish, chrome	Apply undiluted apple cider vinegar. Wipe with a soft, dry cloth.
Metal polish, copper	Make a paste of salt and hot vinegar. Rub, rinse, and polish with soft, damp cloth. Or use a paste of salt and lemon juice. Rub, rinse, and polish with soft, damp cloth.
Metal polish, silver and stainless steel	Make a paste of baking soda and water. Rub with the paste, rinse, and polish with a soft, damp cloth.
Scouring powder	Combine equal parts of vinegar and salt, and scrub with a firm-bristled brush. Or sprinkle borax or baking soda on a damp sponge for a less abrasive cleanser.
Shoe polish	Rub any nut or olive oil into shoe leather and buff with a soft cloth.
Wood floor and furniture polish	Use 2 to 3 parts vegetable oil with 1 part lemon juice. Apply a small amount and rub into the wood with a soft cloth.

* *Found in supermarkets or hardware stores.*

** *Use in a well-ventilated area and wear gloves.*

† *Use only those liquid soaps that contain no added artificial fragrance or color.*

cles, which cannot be swept up with a broom or household vacuum cleaner. (For more information, see pages 531-532.)

Insecticides. These can kill pets or people; some contain cancer-causing chemicals. Unless you can get a neighbor to take your unused insecticides and use them up, store them until you can deliver them to a hazardous waste collection program. Rinse empty containers three times before discarding them.

Batteries. Battery acids are corrosive and can burn your skin. Trade in old auto batteries or return them to the battery dealer. Small batteries contain mercury or lead, both highly toxic, and should not be incinerated. If you have a number of those small button batteries that come out of watches or cameras, you may be able to dispose of them at a hospital or a hearing aid center. Keep these small batteries out of children's hands, since they may swallow them.

Outdated medicines. Flush unused medicine down the toilet; rinse the bottles before discarding them.

Household cleaners containing sodium hydroxide (lye) or ammonia. If you have a large sewage system, these can be washed down the drain with lots of water. Rinse the containers well. (Be careful whenever you mix lye with water—it can spatter in your eyes.) Take care not to mix ammonia-containing products with chlorine bleaches when you dispose of them. Combining ammonia and chlorine releases a toxic nerve gas.

Humidifiers

When winter comes and the heat goes on, relative humidity in most homes falls, sometimes to levels that mimic the desert. Lips may chap, skin may roughen, noses bleed, and throats get scratchy—and thus people resort to portable humidifiers. A proper level of moisture in the air—30 percent to 50 percent is what the U.S. Consumer Product Safety Commission (CPSC) recommends—can make you feel more comfortable and may have beneficial effects on furniture and plants.

However, the health effects of dry air have remained controversial—after all, people live perfectly healthy lives in the desert. Plane cabins are notoriously dry, and there's evidence that flight attendants have more colds than others (though there might be other factors involved besides dry air). In 1986, as reported in *Environmental Health Perspectives,* a review of all relevant studies led researchers to conclude that low relative humidity might cause eye irritations, but they found no evidence that low humidity had any direct effects on health. However, they cited evidence that microbes are more "infective"—that is, likely to cause illness—in very dry conditions. At least one small study has suggested that dry air might impede the action of nasal cilia, the small hairs that help clear the respiratory tract of bacteria and viruses. And it may be that some people are more affected by dry air than others. Thus a humidifier might be worth trying if your indoor air is very dry.

There's no controversy, however, about the ill effects of high humidity. Relative humidities above 60 percent promote the growth of airborne fungi, bacteria, molds, and other allergens and may also favor the survival of some viruses.

Furthermore, any humidifier that isn't kept clean—and studies show that most owners don't clean them often enough—can be a source of air pollution.

The best humidifier

Some people swear by an old-fashioned pan of water on the radiator, but it won't really add much moisture to the air. Large humidifier units attached to your central heating system may work well but are very expensive, as well as impractical for apartments and some dwellings. If you decide to use a room humidifier, four basic types are available in tabletop or freestanding models—but each has drawbacks:

•Evaporative humidifiers create mist by means of a moving belt in a reservoir. They are not likely to contaminate the air if kept clean. Their drawback: hard to clean. But there are newer, better models.

•Steamers or vaporizers turn water into vapor by heating it; "warm mist" models are an update that mixes the steam with cool air. Drawbacks: units are usually small, noisy, and use a lot of electricity. They may also pose some danger of burns or electrical shock.

•Cool-mist humidifiers create a mist mechanically by "impelling" water against a screen or other surface. Drawback: they emit bacteria and molds.

•Ultrasonic humidifiers use high-frequency vibrations to turn water into mist. These are now waning in popularity. Drawbacks: they emit very fine mineral particles that show up as fine white dust on furniture. Using a demineralization cartridge or distilled water will correct this—but most people don't. The particles can get deep into the lungs and then into the bloodstream, as well as cause respiratory problems and allergic reactions in sensitive people. The units may also emit whatever pollutants are present in tap water, such as lead or radon, as well as microbes. Ultrasonics are hard to clean.

Prices vary: a small vaporizer or steamer might cost less than $25, warm-mist table-models under $100, ultrasonics from $75 to $500.

A new choice

A redesign of the older evaporative humidifier is the "wicking" humidifier. The CPSC has not yet tested this type, but overall it seems the best. First, it has a filter that's designed to trap mineral dust—an advantage over ultrasonics. Second, it's less likely than other types to emit bacteria and molds, particularly if you add an antibacterial treatment to the water and replace the filter or wick as recommended. Third, it is easier to clean than the older models. Table and freestanding models range in price from about $50 to $200.

•Whatever you choose, the most important thing is to keep your humidifier scrupulously clean. Change the water in a portable every day—that's the advice of the CPSC. Once the unit gets dirty, it's hard to get it really clean again, especially if mineral deposits have built up. Wash the tank thoroughly according to the manufacturer's instructions. Any standing water (even a pan on the radiator) can quickly become contaminated by mold and bacteria. Vinegar or hydrogen peroxide will kill mold; chlorine bleach kills bacteria.

•Because humidity should be kept within the 30 to 50 percent range, it might also be worthwhile to invest in a gadget to measure moisture. Known as hygrometers, they can be bought at hardware stores or ordered by mail.

Indoor Air Quality

There are many substances that can contribute to a decline in indoor air quality both at home and in the workplace. One possible pollutant of indoor air is carbon monoxide, produced by incomplete combustion of a solid, liquid, or gaseous fuel. Gas ranges, furnaces, and automobiles are all possible sources. Breathing small amounts won't kill you, but can make you sick. Some symptoms of chronic exposure are constant headaches, tiredness, and sleepiness. The problem becomes particularly urgent in the winter when storm windows, weather stripping, and sealers are in regular use and windows are rarely opened.

Houseplants and Air

A NASA scientist, looking for ways to cleanse the air in space stations, discovered that houseplants actually remove pollutants from the air. Indoor air often contains carbon monoxide and nitrogen dioxide released from gas stoves or furnaces, formaldehyde from furnishings or building materials, and smoke from cooking or tobacco use. It turns out that houseplants, besides looking nice and adding a bit of oxygen to the air, may actually perform a service.

For some reason, spider plants, one of the hardiest, most ubiquitous of houseplants, actually seemed to do the best job removing three pollutants: formaldehyde, benzene, and trichloroethylene (TCE), which can come from treated wood, furnishings, carpeting, clothing, cleaning chemicals, and other common domestic sources. Not only spider plants but some daisies, chrysanthemums, bamboo palm, English ivy, philodendron, and golden pothos also did a good job removing these chemicals. This additional research was reported in a 1989 study conducted for NASA under the auspices of the Foliage for Clean Air Council, a nonprofit group underwritten by the decorative houseplants industry.

It's also been shown that potting soil itself absorbs pollutants and removes them from the air. Indeed, a study in *Environmental Pollution* in 1989 showed that defoliated spider plants achieved higher reductions of formaldehyde than those with leaves, and that potting soil is effective, too—but not for long. What combats the pollution is not just one element, but the chemical interaction among soil, roots, plants, and the microorganisms in the soil.

There's still a lot of argument, for example, about exactly how many plants it might take to cleanse the air in a room. Some researchers have said you would need a veritable forest to get the job done. Others think one or two might do. Whatever the answer, we say more power to them. But though they might soak up airborne formaldehyde, they've never been shown to do away with carbon monoxide, tobacco smoke, radon, and other hazards. You'll still need to maintain good ventilation and take other measures to keep indoor air free of pollutants (see page 552).

Other potential pollutants of indoor air are formaldehyde (see page 545); radon (see page 564); nitrogen oxides from gas stoves (see page 546); and passive cigarette smoke (see page 561). Pollen, mold spores, and dust mites can also contribute to poor indoor air quality and cause problems for individuals who suffer from allergies.

Do air purifiers help?

Although air purifiers can remove airborne smoke and dust, they're useless against gas molecules that are too small to be trapped by the filters. These gases include paint and chemical fumes, radon, and formaldehyde from insulation. Air purifiers work by using a fan to draw room air past a filter to remove particles, or by electrically charging airborne particles and using polarized metal plates to pull them out of the air. How effective purifiers are depends not only on how much air they can circulate, but also on the type of filter used. The most effective filter is the HEPA (high-efficiency particulate arresting), which was developed during World War II to remove radioactive dust in atomic energy plants. HEPA filters are manufactured to a high standard and are durable, but they're expensive (from $250 to $650). Some electrostatic filters treat more air per minute and so may be just as effective.

The few controlled studies on air purifiers have shown that they have little or no effect on allergens. A purifier is ineffective against these particles because they don't remain airborne for long. Once they settle, even the most powerful air purifier can do nothing to eliminate them.

One study found that the machines were helpful when placed directly above the heads of allergic children while they slept, because the particles did not have a chance to settle. These children experienced some decrease in their symptoms, or at least needed less medication for their allergies. However, not all steps had been taken to make the rooms free of dust; such steps might have done just as much good as the filters.

Eliminating indoor pollutants

Outdoor air ventilation is most effective in alleviating many home and office pollution problems, but it's still worth taking these precautions in your home:

•Have a reputable heating company inspect your furnace, the flue, and the vent connector pipe. Replace any rusted or damaged parts. If converting from one type of fuel to another, get a qualified technician to do the work.

•Make sure your gas range has an exhaust fan vented to the outside. Use the fan every time you cook.

•Vent all fuel-burning heaters to the outside.

•Never use a gas range or oven to heat a room, even in a power outage.

•Do not use a charcoal grill inside the house: burning charcoal generates carbon monoxide. Even in a fireplace, fumes may back up into the room.

•When warming up your car in the garage, keep the outer door open. Carbon

---

Allergies and Car Air Conditioners

Air conditioners are usually a godsend to allergy sufferers, reducing indoor pollens, spore counts, and dust. Sometimes, however, a car's air conditioner (or even one in a home or office) is itself the cause of an allergy or asthma attack. The culprits are fungi that produce airborne mold spores and grow deep within the car's air conditioner, where moisture (from condensation), engine heat, and darkness combine to make a perfect environment for molds. And the close confines of the passenger compartment make matters worse.

A study conducted at Louisiana State University found that one out of five allergy or asthma sufferers experienced a worsening of symptoms (sneezing, coughing, wheezing, difficulty in breathing) because of car air conditioning, despite the continued use of medications. Up to one-third of all auto air conditioners are infected with quick-growing fungi, especially those in hot, humid regions like Louisiana.

Most people don't suffer ill effects from the organisms that hitch a ride in the air conditioner. They just notice an unpleasant musty odor when they first turn on the air conditioner. *If, however, you're allergic to the molds, try the following:*

Air it out. Keep the car windows open partway for ten to fifteen minutes after you turn on the air conditioner; if necessary, wear an appropriate mask (it must not block your vision) until most of the molds are expelled. Don't direct the vents toward your face. And, if your air conditioner gives you the choice, press the button for "fresh air" rather than recirculated air.

The disinfectant route. If these steps don't help, have your car treated with the EPA-registered disinfectant called RenNew-A/C (containing Alcide, a formulation of chlorous acid), available at a variety of outlets, including car dealer service departments, some service stations, and most auto air conditioner shops. The compound, sprayed into the core of the system, is supposed to keep the car mold-free for about six months, though in humid climates it may last only three months. A study presented at the 1988 meeting of the American Thoracic Society found that this disinfectant was as effective as hydrogen peroxide, without that compound's corrosive effect on metals. The treatment must be done by a trained, equipped mechanic. It usually costs $50 to $100 and takes about one hour. Some shops offer it as part of an annual air conditioner checkup.

By the way, do-it-yourself applications of other kinds of disinfectants are unlikely to have any long-lasting effect, since the sprays don't get into the system's core. Deodorizers merely mask the odor—they don't kill mold spores.

monoxide levels can build up quickly, and if your garage is attached to your house, fumes can seep into it.

Controlling allergens

Some of the steps above will help control pollen, mold spores, and dust. What additional steps you take depends on whether you have hay fever, are asthmatic, or merely have a sensitive nose. But here are some commonsense steps:

•In warm weather an air conditioner can help, especially if you have hay fever. Most systems reuse the air already in the room, taking in very little from the outside, thus admitting little pollen and few spores. However, in humid climates mold can grow inside the air conditioner itself. (For information on mold in car air conditioners, see box on page 552.)

•Vacuum, mop, and dust frequently. Remember, however, cleaning may temporarily stir up dust. Use a damp, not dry, mop or cloth, and change your vacuum's dust bag often. Or get someone else to clean for you, and for about an hour try to stay out of a room that's been vacuumed, until the dust has settled. Minimize the dust-collecting clutter in your home. Wood or linoleum floors are easier to keep dust-free than carpet.

•Clean or replace the filter in a forced-air heater every month. You can also cover vent ducts with filters.

•Keep pets out of the bedroom to minimize dander levels while you sleep.

•Use allergen-proof casings for pillows, mattresses, and box springs. Use washable blankets and bedspreads, and wash bedclothes often (use hot water to kill dust mites). Feather pillows create dust, and foam can harbor molds, so use pillows made of Dacron or other hypoallergenic polyester materials.

Ladders

Nearly 100,000 Americans are treated in emergency rooms each year for ladder- or stool-related injuries. Most ladder injuries are caused by falls, though some result from electric shock when a metal ladder touches power lines. While using a ladder is safer than climbing on a chair or counter, it is a risky activity and requires care and caution.

Choosing an appropriate ladder

Not all ladders are alike. Most ladders sold for household use are type III light-duty ladders, which can hold a maximum of 200 pounds (including both user and materials). If you expect to do heavier work—or are heavier yourself—get a ladder with a more heavy-duty rating (type II will hold about 225 pounds; type I about 250 pounds).

Make sure your ladder is long enough for the job. The length of a ladder is not the same as its usable length. The top three rungs of a straight ladder are not meant to be stood on; similarly, the top two steps of a step ladder are not meant to be used. Metal ladders conduct electricity, so if you plan to use a ladder near power lines, with electrical equipment, or to change a light bulb, a wooden or fiberglass ladder is best. If you must use electrical tools on a metal ladder, make sure the tools are properly grounded.

In addition, take the following precautions:

•Never use a ladder in a strong wind, and never put one in front of a door that is not locked, blocked, or guarded.

•Put the ladder on firm and level ground or on a flat wooden board for firm support; best of all, have a helper hold the bottom of the ladder.

•Always check the eaves for wasps nests; you don't want to discover the nest when you are on top of the ladder.

•Always face the ladder when you climb it, and use both hands. Don't lean too far to the side while you are working on the ladder. Carry tools in pockets or in a bag attached to your belt, or have them attached to a rope you can raise and lower. Be sure the soles of your shoes are clean and dry.

•Avoid metal ladders with sharp edges, dents, or bent steps or rails.

•All metal ladders should have slip-resistant rubber or plastic feet and slip-resistant steps.

•On wooden ladders, watch out for cracks and any large, weak-looking knots. The steps of wooden ladders should be reinforced with metal rods or angle braces.

•Never paint a wooden ladder; the paint will hide defects.

The distance between the base of a ladder and the wall should be one-quarter the ladder's usable length. Don't count the top three rungs of a straight ladder and the top two steps of a step ladder—they are not meant to be used.

Lead

The toxicity of lead is not news: some historians think lead poisoning (from cooking pots and water pipes) caused the decline of the Roman Empire. Lead is a natural element with a thousand uses: it's malleable, plentiful, practically indestructible, and resistant to many kinds of corrosion. Lead is combined with other metals to make them "machinable," and it's a component of paints, glazes, bullets, plastic coating for wire, solder, and hundreds of other items. ("Lead pencil" is a misnomer—the material in pencils is harmless graphite.) As a gasoline additive, lead has anti-knock properties and increases fuel efficiency; it was used on a massive scale until the mid-1980s, though the effects of high doses on humans were known. Lead in car and truck exhaust polluted the air and soil, and some of that lead is still around. Deteriorating leaded paints are still around, too, as are lead plumbing pipes that leach lead into our drinking water. In addition, workers in many industries are exposed to lead.

The problem with lead arises when humans breathe or ingest it. Lead can easily contaminate food and water, where it is undetectable to the eye or taste buds. High doses of lead can be lethal, damaging the nervous system, the kidneys, and the bones. Continuous low-level exposure can cause a range of physical and mental problems (including hypertension and learning disabilities) and is particularly dangerous for fetuses and small children. Exposure to lead can cause miscarriage, or damage the nervous system of the fetus and of the infant or small child. The body absorbs lead as if it were a nutrient, storing it in bone. Children, especially if they are deficient in calcium and iron, tend to absorb more lead than do adults. And lead is more damaging to them than to adults.

Yet real progress has been made in reducing the level of lead in the environment through the government's phasing out of leaded gasoline and its ban on lead-based house paint. According to the Environmental Protection Agency (EPA), nationwide data show that blood lead levels have declined—they now stand at approximately 5 micrograms per deciliter of blood—and there is every reason to hope that blood lead levels will decline even further. The phasing out of leaded gasoline between 1975 and 1980 was a major contributor to the decline in blood lead levels. (The United States, Canada, Japan, and Australia led the way in switching to unleaded gasoline in the 1970s. Now many European Community nations have banned or limited it, as well as South Korea, Taiwan, Brazil, and a few others.) Yet lead still finds its way into our bodies, especially from tap water contaminated by lead plumbing materials. Moreover, as testing procedures become more sophisticated, it is becoming evident that even small amounts of lead can adversely affect the body. The "maximum safe levels" of lead may not be safe enough.

Assessing the risks

The myth was that lead menaced only poor children living in substandard housing and perhaps eating chips of lead-based paint. Indeed, poverty is a hazard for children, but any child may be in danger of lead poisoning because lead is so ubiquitous. It's also recognized now that even low levels of lead exposure can be hazardous for adults, too. According to the Centers for Disease Control and Prevention (CDC), the average adult carries about 5 to 6 micrograms of lead per deciliter of blood (about one-third as much as twenty years ago). Levels above 10 micrograms for children are now deemed a matter of concern.

At least eight federal agencies are charged with studying and monitoring lead exposure and trying to reduce it. Among them, the Food and Drug Administration (FDA) monitors lead in food, beverages, cans, and glassware, among other things; the Environmental Protection Agency (EPA) tries to reduce lead in air, drinking water and soil; Housing and Urban Development (HUD) provides funds for removing lead-based paints, while other agencies are concerned with occupational exposure and other issues. Indeed, the government's goal is to eliminate as much human exposure to lead as possible. Blood lead levels in Americans have already dropped dramatically because of measures like these:
- the phasing out of leaded gasoline, once the main source of airborne lead;
- the elimination of lead solder from food cans made in the United States, once a major source of food-borne lead;
- the banning of lead in interior and exterior house paint;
- new requirements for firing ceramic wares to keep lead from leaching;
- the banning of some lead plumbing pipe and lead solder in plumbing.

But there's still a long way to go to get the lead out. Besides possibly being in your tap water or water pipes, or leaching from a brand new faucet, lead can be found in leaded crystal, ceramic glazes, and old tableware made of pewter. It may be in dirt in your garden, in old housepaints, or in artists' materials. Vigilance and knowledge on your part can truly pay off. Here's what you can do to reduce your exposure to lead.

Lead in paint: still the worst lead source for kids

Though lead in both exterior and interior house paints was banned in 1978 (except for trace amounts), an estimated 57 million homes in this country still contain lead-based paints, which are by far the most common source of lead poisoning for children. Water-based paints are usually lead-free, but oil-based paints applied before the ban went into effect were heavily leaded. Eventually the paints may flake and peel, and children may eat the chips. Paints that are in good condition are not a problem, or paints that have been painted over with lead-free paints, unless painted surfaces rub together and create dust (as on window frames). Remodeling that involves removing leaded paint, particularly by chipping or sanding it, can be extremely hazardous.

If you think you have lead paint in your home, particularly if you have infants or small children, the best plan is to call your local health department. Some health departments will test the paint for lead or advise you how to get it tested. You can also call the HUD hotline (1-800-RID-LEAD) or the National Lead Information Center (1-800-LEAD-FYI) for advice on removing paint. Any painted surface larger than about a square foot should be handled by professionals following federal guidelines. While paint removal is underway, children, pregnant women, and people with high blood pressure should stay out of the house. Furnishings may also have to be removed. Workers should wear respirators, and the clean-up should be thorough. For example, a detergent containing trisodium phosphate should be used to clean up lead dust.

Because any kind of dust, especially paint dust, may contain lead, it's important to keep a child's environment as dust-free as possible. Clean windowsills and floors frequently with detergent and water. Make sure children wash their hands before eating. Keep kids from chewing on painted objects. If you're not sure the paint on a toy is lead-free, for example, if it's an old toy, dispose of it.

Lead in water

Groundwater, water in city reservoirs, and water coming out of treatment plants is usually lead-free. Lead comes only from the plumbing: service lines, pipes, soldering, and faucets. The pipes that connect households to the water main are often made of lead, and even if your house has new copper pipes, they may be lead-soldered (lead pipes and solder were outlawed in 1986, though the ban did not take effect in some states until 1988). Currently all metal faucets, even the newest, contain some lead. Unfortunately, water standing in pipes may dissolve minute amounts of lead. Hard water, which carries high amounts of dissolved minerals, is less likely to pick up lead than soft water, which despite its sweeter taste and other desirable properties is more acidic than hard water and thus more corrosive in pipes.

Two reports on lead in municipal water caused widespread concern. Using the results of its own nationwide survey, *Consumer Reports* in 1993 found that households in Chicago and Boston and the northeast generally, where soft (hence acidic) water is common, had high levels of lead; San Francisco, New York, and Washington had more households with high lead levels than most of the country, though not as many as Chicago and Boston. Nevertheless, the survey showed no widespread national problem. Water from each household was tested twice: a first-draw sample (water that had stood in pipes overnight), and a purged-line sample (taken after the water had run one minute). Ideally, according to the standards of the EPA, first-draw samples should have less than 5 parts per billion (PPB) of lead, and purged-line water no detectable lead whatever. In defining "high levels," Consumer Reports used 15 PPB as the maximum safe level in first-draw samples, and 5 PPB in purged-line samples.

Then in May, 1993, after the largest survey ever conducted of lead in drinking water, the EPA reported that over 800 public water systems across the country serving 30 million people had unacceptably high levels of lead. This does not mean that every household served by these systems had high lead levels, but only those known to be served by lead water pipes inside or outside the house. All these systems were required to take immediate action to reduce lead levels, including corrosion control (adding minerals to harden the water so it leaches less lead) and replacement of lead pipes, as well as further monitoring. Problems seemed concentrated in the Northeast: of the ten large water systems with the highest lead levels, five were in Massachusetts (Brookline, Waltham, Medford, Chicopee, and Newton), two in New York (Utica and Yonkers), two in South Carolina (Charleston and Columbia), and one in Michigan (Taylor).

Testing the water

Whether you live in a "problem" area, as defined above, and whether you get your water from a well or a municipal system, and whether your dwelling is old or new, you may or may not have a lead problem. If you or someone in your household is pregnant or if you have an infant or a small child, take these steps:

•Have your water tested. First, call your local health department or water company. It may offer free testing or may test for a small fee ($15 to $30). If it doesn't, ask how to get your water tested or call the EPA (at 800-426-4791). It can give you names of laboratories who will test the water for you. If you look in the Yellow Pages, be sure to find out if the labs are government certified for lead testing.

•If the test shows high lead levels, at least you'll know where the problem is. If high levels of lead occur in first-draw samples, that means the problem is in the faucet or the pipes inside the house. If the lead is coming from the service lines outside, find out what your water company is doing to reduce lead. In either case, if the lead levels are very high (over 15 PPB in first-draw samples, and over 5 PPB in purged-line samples), consider installing a filtering device. A reverse-osmosis system is the most effective and sophisticated device, but costs up to $800. If your problem is less severe, you may be okay with a less expensive filter, even an inexpensive filtering carafe—or with just running the water for a minute before using it. The EPA can also advise you about filters.

•Any time the water hasn't been run for two hours or more, run the tap for at least one minute before drinking or cooking with the water. This will take care of lead that's leaching into water from the faucet or pipes in the house. But if the service lines under the street are leaching lead, running the water could make it worse. Some municipalities can tell you if the service lines are lead or not; some don't have records. To cut down on wasted water, store tap water in the refrigerator for later use.

•Don't use hot water for cooking, drinking, or mixing infant formula. Hot water dissolves lead more quickly than cold.

•You can switch to bottled water, provided you can assure yourself that the bottled water is lead-free.

Lead in food and drink containers

Lead in food and tableware is not as great a problem as lead paint or water, but you can reduce your exposure to lead as follows:

Earthenware. Most American households contain at least one piece of brightly glazed earthenware. Unless you're sure your pottery is lead free, use it only for ornamental purposes and never for cooking or storage. Unfortunately, some lead-glazed pottery imported from Mexico, China, and many developing nations and, much less frequently, from Europe has not been fired at sufficiently high temperatures to keep the lead from "leaching" into foods. Continued use of a defectively glazed object can expose a person to hazardous doses of lead.

Since 1971 American manufacturers have been legally required to fire their earthenware pottery at temperatures that make the lead glazes relatively impervious. European and Japanese wares are also well fired. But there are exceptions: European wares marketed by reputable retailers may also occasionally have lead discharges that violate FDA safety standards. In addition, lead may occasionally leach out of old lead-glazed American wares.

The FDA tests only a fraction of all earthenware imports. Studies have shown that even when pottery has been tested and found to be safe initially, repeated washings can cause the lead glaze to deteriorate and release several times the allowable limit of lead. You don't have to worry about stoneware (usually marked "oven-proof" or "dishwasher-proof") or porcelain, since they are both fired at very high temperatures.

Nearly 94 percent of all cans contain no lead solder, so the risk of lead leaching into foods is minimal.

Earthenware dinner plates aren't likely to pose a health problem. The seepage of lead is most severe when acidic foods—wine, orange juice, coffee, tomato juice, salsa, spaghetti sauce, pickles, salad dressings—are stored, cooked, or served in lead-glazed jugs, mugs, and dishes. For instance, the lead content of one glass of orange juice stored for 24 hours in a defective pitcher can well exceed the FDA's ceiling for total daily intake of lead for an adult. The same dose of lead is more than four times the daily maximum for children.

Cans. Canned goods manufactured in the United States are not a worry, but imported cans may be. The American canning industry, prodded by the FDA, has phased out lead solder, in favor of seamless welding. If an imported can has a vertical seam (you can feel it through the label) with rough patches of silvery metal, it probably contains lead solder. The FDA intends to ban all lead in imported cans.

Wines. The lead content of wines, especially imported wines, may exceed the maximum amount allowed in drinking water. But most people drink less wine than water, so it may not be apt to compare the lead levels of these beverages. Even a glass or two of wine daily would contribute very little lead. Also, those people most at risk from lead exposure—pregnant women and young children—shouldn't drink wine anyway.

The lead comes in part from the foil wrappers covering the cork and neck on many bottles, which leave a residue on the rim. The lead residue on the rim is greatest if wine seeps between the cork and the wrapping, causing the foil to corrode. Yet even without a foil wrapper wine contains varying amounts of lead, which it gets from contaminated soil, water, and air. (This may help explain why imported wines tend to be higher in lead, since leaded gasoline, which is a major source of environmental lead, is still common overseas.) Wine may also pick up lead during production—from lead-soldered pipes and vats, for instance. (The Bureau of Alcohol, Tobacco, and Firearms monitors lead in wine and can prohibit its sale if levels are too high.)

California wineries stopped using lead-containing wrappers in 1992, substituting tin and aluminum. The FDA proposed eliminating them from all wines.

If you drink wine with a foil wrapper, wipe the rim and neck with a moist towel. The FDA recommends moistening the towel with something acidic, such as lemon juice, vinegar, or a few drops of wine. Screw caps do not contain lead.

Glass. Lead crystal is not a major source of lead exposure for many people. However, lead can leach out of it. (You know it's leaded if it is expensive, brilliant, and heavy.) Unless you're pregnant, drinking from a lead crystal goblet is harmless—only tiny amounts of lead would be released in such a short period. But don't store wine or other acidic beverages in lead crystal. If you have a lead crystal decanter, use it only for serving—pour the beverage into it shortly before you plan to use it, and then return it to its original bottle. Similarly, don't store vinegar-based dressings in lead crystal cruets.

Noise Pollution

Excessive noise takes a heavy toll on your total health, not just on your eardrums. If you live or work in a noisy environment, you may be at risk from such tension-related ailments as high blood pressure and fatigue, in addition to possibly suffering some hearing loss. According to government statistics, one out of every ten Americans is exposed to noise of sufficient intensity and duration to cause permanent hearing loss.

Noise does not have to be painful to damage the ears or cause symptoms of anxiety. The EPA defines excessive noise as sounds that force individuals to raise their voices for normal conversation. Round-the-clock noise in a few urban neighborhoods approaches the maximum legal noise level to which workers may be exposed for eight hours (90 decibels). Traffic, radios, passing trains, lawn mowers, sirens, and jackhammers can add up to a nightmare for the inner ear.

Humans have the capacity to adapt to almost anything, and with noise this capability is both an asset and a liability. We can block out the noise consciously; but our bodies don't adapt physically or psychologically. Noise is like an alarm bell to the body—it signals danger and stimulates alertness. When noise is constant, the body is reacting to an alarm we are no longer aware of. In a study at a sleep center in Strasbourg, France, sleepers were bombarded with traffic noises for fifteen nights. After a few nights the subjects said they were no longer bothered by the sounds. Unknown to them, however, their bodies were still responding to the noise with increases in heart rate, blood pressure, respiration, muscle tension, hormone levels, and perspiration. Their bodies did not adjust with time: on the fifteenth night these effects remained identical to those observed by the researchers on the first night. Besides the physiological impact, there's a psychological effect. A Munich study found that after one night's exposure to noise, subjects were irritable for about ten minutes. After additional noisy nights, their bad moods lasted until the late morning or early afternoon.

Researchers at the University of Amsterdam uncovered troubling links between airport noise and hypertension. They compared the incidence of high blood pressure among people who lived near an airport to that of people from a quiet area. They found that among airport neighbors the incidence of hypertension was 72 percent higher. In another study, the Dutch researchers found that in one area, the sale of antihypertension drugs doubled in the six years following the opening of a new airport runway. People who live near airports are particularly endangered, as shown by a study of children living along the air corridor of the Los Angeles International Airport. Compared to children living outside the flight path, they had significantly higher blood pressure and greater difficulty in solving puzzles and math problems.

Reducing noise

There are many ways to reduce noise in your immediate environment: hang overlapping, double drapes over the windows; upholstered furniture will absorb sounds from inside and outside the house; if the kitchen is noisy, put in sound-absorbing ceiling tiles and place a rubber pad under noisy appliances, such as blenders; install wooden cabinets, which vibrate less than metal ones; to protect your neighbors' health, operate loud machinery such as power saws and mowers at reasonable hours; if background noise is intolerable, you can try using earplugs or protective muffs like those worn by people in factories and rifle ranges.

If you are moving into a new neighborhood, find out if the residents have had problems with traffic noise, airplanes overhead, or loud businesses. Restaurants with noisy ventilators or air conditioners are a common source of complaints in cities. If the area seems noisy, check the sound level by using the "walk away" test, developed by the Department of Housing and Urban Development. Stand outdoors with a friend and have him read aloud in a normal voice. You should be able to walk away from him and comprehend his words at least twenty-five feet away for the background sound level to be considered acceptable.

Prolonged exposure to noise levels over 80 decibels can cause hearing loss, and many everyday noises are even higher than 100 decibels. The noise level from a rock concert can reach over 120 decibels; people wearing headphones on the street typically turn them up to about 115 decibels; and customized car stereos with several speakers are often played at their maximum levels—130 decibels, roughly the sound of a jet engine taking off.

Oven Cleaners

Unless you have a self-cleaning oven, you probably resort to oven cleaners from the supermarket. Most do the job well enough, but they require the user to take special safety precautions.

The ingredient to watch out for is lye (sodium hydroxide), also known as caustic soda. Lye-impregnated cleaning pads have recently come on the market, and lye is the active ingredient in most of the aerosols. While it can clean efficiently, it can also irritate and burn the skin and eyes, and, if inhaled in quantity, the nasal passages and lungs. If swallowed, it can cause burns in the esophagus and mouth.

When using an oven cleaner containing lye, read the package carefully and be prepared to follow first-aid instructions if necessary. Always wear rubber gloves, a paper face mask, and goggles. With an aerosol, cover the floor with newspapers and protect surrounding counters. With the cleaning pad—you puncture the pad and apply the cleaner—you still have to wear rubber gloves and long sleeves because the stuff can drip. When finishing the job, be sure that you really have wiped all the cleaner off the oven. Otherwise, unpleasant and unhealthy fumes will occur the next time you turn it on.

There are also some reasonably effective non-caustic, lye-free cleaners available in aerosol form. Usually labeled "fume-free," these are applied to a cold oven and allowed to sit, though some require turning on the oven to activate the cleaning process. Such cleaners are less toxic than those containing lye, though not as effective at cleaning. They, too, require caution because they can irritate skin and eyes.

Most cleaners come scented, usually with lemon, but that does not minimize their danger. Even if the oven cleaner is in a childproof package, it—and other cleaning materials—should be kept in a locked cabinet well out of the reach of young children.

Passive Smoke

Can other people's tobacco smoke take years off your life? Is "passive smoking" really just another form of active smoking? Indeed, experts now rank it as the third leading cause of preventable deaths in this country, exceeded only by active smoking and alcohol. In a 1992 report reviewing years of scientific studies, the U.S. Environmental Protection Agency (EPA) classified environmental tobacco smoke, also called secondhand smoke, as a cause of lung cancer in nonsmokers and of a wide range of respiratory disorders in children.

Virtually every health organization, from the National Academy of Sciences to the AMA, has concluded that secondhand smoke is responsible for the deaths of tens of thousands of Americans each year, mostly from heart disease. Exposure to tobacco smoke accounts for 150,000 to 300,000 serious respiratory ailments each year in children under eighteen months of age and up to 26,000 new cases of childhood asthma each year, and it worsens symptoms in up to one million asthmatic children. A 1994 study in the *Journal of the American Medical Association* concluded that nonsmoking women exposed to a moderate amount of secondhand smoke at home face a 30 percent increased risk of lung cancer; those living with a heavy smoker, an 80 percent increased risk; and those exposed at work, a 39 percent increased risk.

While the EPA report did not discuss passive smoking as a cause of heart disease in nonsmokers, Dr. Stanton Glantz and Dr. William Parmley of the University of San Francisco Medical School have reviewed the evidence for EPA and published their conclusions. Though most people associate smoking with cancer, passive smoking accounts for ten times as many deaths from heart disease each year as from lung cancer.

How nonsmokers smoke

Passive smoking (also called involuntary smoking) works in different ways from active smoking. Mainstream smoke, filtered through the cigarette and inhaled by the smoker, is highly concentrated; the toxins it contains occur in comparatively large particles. Some particles are deposited in the mouth and may be swallowed, others go into the larger airways of the lungs. Sidestream smoke, which is what comes off the end of the burning cigarette, is one component of secondhand smoke, along with exhaled smoke. What comes off the end of the cigarette actually contains higher amounts of the compounds that tend to cause cancer and heart disease than what the smoker inhales. And although the smoke is more diluted, these compounds occur in smaller particles and, though the passive smoker breathes less smoke, the small particles tend to settle deep in the lungs, where it takes longer for them to clear. They dissolve in the lung tissue and then enter the bloodstream and lymph tissue. Nicotine byproducts can be detected in the bodies of passive as well as active smokers. Of course, active smokers inhale both kinds of smoke.

All the compounds in mainstream smoke that damage the heart have been found in sidestream smoke as well. Secondhand smoke contains carbon monoxide, for example, which interferes with the blood's ability to carry oxygen and thus, over time, can decrease oxygen supply to the heart muscle and impair function in this and other tissues. Both mainstream and sidestream smoke directly damage the cells that line heart and blood vessels and thus contribute to atherosclerosis (clogged arteries). Recent research has demonstrated that smoking makes the platelets, which cause blood clots, clump together and thus increases the risk of heart attack. Inhaling smoke seems to have the worst effects on people who already have heart or lung disorders, as well as children, whose bodies are still growing. Even for a healthy nonsmoker, living with a spouse who smokes increases the risk of cancer and heart disease; and there's some evidence that children and adolescents exposed to secondhand smoke may also have a greater risk for these diseases later in life. Passive smoking has also been shown to have adverse effects on the exercise capability of healthy adults.

Nonsmokers need protection from secondhand smoke. Despite the welcome downward trend in tobacco use in this country, about 30 percent of Americans still smoke, lighting up half a trillion cigarettes each year. Domestic airline flights, government buildings, and many other public places have been declared off-limits for smoking. But if you live with a smoker or work next to one, you probably get more than just a whiff of secondhand smoke.

What to do if smoke gets in your eyes

- Don't rely on air filters and so-called smokeless ashtrays. They won't filter out the toxins in smoke.
- Set aside a smoke-free zone in your home and persuade household smokers to respect it.
- Needless to say, it's better to be polite, but don't be afraid to speak up. "Please don't smoke" is always a valid request.
- If you are an employer, consider starting a bonus system for people who quit smoking. Post information about smoking-cessation groups. Set up nonsmoking areas, or declare the whole workplace a nonsmoking zone.

Poisoning

There are nearly three million cases of accidental child poisoning each year, and in the majority of cases, parents were at home or nearby at the time of the poisoning. Almost 69 percent of accidental poisonings occur in children under six. Children in this age group usually mistake household cleaners for beverages, or prescription and over-the-counter drugs for candy. Often they playfully emulate adult drug taking, which sometimes leads to serious or even fatal results.

Nearly half of all accidental poisonings in the U. S. are caused by a limited group of items: aspirin and acetaminophen, insecticides, household bleach, detergents, fragrance products, disinfectants and deodorizers, soaps and cleaners, furniture polish, kerosene, iron and vitamin compounds, lye and corrosives, laxatives.

To determine a pattern in childhood poisonings, researchers at the Karolinska Institute in Sweden interviewed parents of 600 children who had suffered from

Smokers who switch to low-tar cigarettes may actually increase the health risk for their friends and family, according to a recent study from the U.S. Department of Agriculture. The secondhand smoke released from the burning end of low-tar cigarettes proved to contain up to 30 percent more cancer-causing substances than the smoke from high-tar cigarettes.

accidental poisoning. Results showed that most accidents occurred in the kitchen between four and six p.m. This led doctors to speculate that the children eager for lunch or dinner selected a bottle or container they thought held food.

The second most likely site of poisoning is the bathroom. It takes just a moment for a toddler to climb from the toilet seat onto the sink and then open the medicine chest. All medicine, even aspirin, should be kept in childproof containers in a locked cabinet.

Safety precautions

To prevent poisoning, use the following guidelines. (Remember, adults are also susceptible to accidental poisonings.)

•Remove all poisonous substances from the kitchen and dining areas.

•Keep household cleaners and other potential poisons out of children's reach, preferably in a locked cabinet.

•Keep all hazardous substances and medicines in their original containers. Do not store them in food containers.

•When using toxic substances around children, don't leave a child alone with the product—not even for a minute. If you have to leave the room to answer the phone or the doorbell, take the product or the child with you.

•Buy household cleaners and medicines in child-resistant packaging, although you should not rely solely on this packaging. Continue to store these items out of a child's reach.

•Never refer to medicine or vitamins for children as candy.

•Even if no children live in your house, take precautions when they come to visit. More than one-third of all cases of childhood poisoning from toxic prescription drugs involve a grandparent's medication.

•Avoid taking any medication in front of children, since they tend to imitate what adults do.

•Flush all old medications down the toilet instead of throwing them away in the garbage where children or pets may find them.

Toxic plants

According to the Consumer Product Safety Commission, the ingestion of toxic plants in homes and gardens is common, especially among young children. Since many cases go unreported, no precise figures on plant poisoning exist, but in 1989 some 62,000 children were exposed to toxic plants. Fortunately, few, if any, deaths occur. A child tasting a toxic leaf, for example, will usually be deterred from eating a lethal amount by his own adverse reaction. Still, parents and grandparents childproofing their homes should not overlook the dangers of plants.

Philodendron, the green and leafy vine that is probably the most popular indoor plant, is highly toxic when ingested and can also cause skin irritation. Dieffenbachia, or dumbcane, with its pointed, variegated leaves is almost as familiar and can have similar effects. A leaf of either plant, if chewed, produces severe mouth pain, swelling of the tongue, and difficulty in speaking. If you have children, the following points are worth keeping in mind:

•With infants or toddlers in the house, don't keep plants where they can reach them. Don't keep philodendron or dieffenbachia plants in your home at all if you have preschool children.

Children's vitamins and poisoning

According to the National Capital Poison Center, children's vitamins shaped like cartoon characters are among the most common agents of childhood poisonings. By banging and rolling around the supposedly childproof bottle, a small child can open what appears to be a jar of little candies. A bottle of 100 or so vitamin tablets contains enough vitamin A to cause hypervitaminosis A, a vitamin-A toxicity.

Vitamins enriched with iron are even more toxic and can be fatal if taken in large quantities.

•Teach children not to sample plant leaves of any kind, and not to experiment with wild plants for food.

Where to get help

Poison control centers exist in every state. Find the number of your local regional center and keep it near your phone *before* you need it. If you discover that your child has swallowed a poisonous substance, call your poison control center immediately (unless he or she is unconscious or having convulsions; in that case call 911 or your local emergency number). Be ready to tell them: the age and weight of the child, what was ingested (have the bottle or container with you), when it was ingested, how much was taken, how the victim is feeling or acting at that moment, and your name and phone number. If you are instructed to go to a hospital emergency room, bring the container of the poison or a sample of the plant with you.

You should keep a bottle of syrup of ipecac on hand to induce vomiting—it is available over the counter at pharmacies—but you should not use it unless instructed to do so by the poison control center or a physician. Some corrosive chemicals, such as bleach, and petroleum products, such as gasoline, can cause more harm if they are brought up.

Radon

Radon, a colorless, odorless, tasteless gas, occurs as a by-product of decaying radium and uranium in rocks and soil. This process is entirely natural and has occurred since the earth was formed. But radon gas is also often a contaminant of indoor air, water, and building materials. It's been known for almost a century that radon increases the risk of lung cancer in underground miners, especially uranium miners exposed to high levels of the gas. Miners are often smokers, too, and tobacco smoke acts synergistically with radon, multiplying the risk of illness.

But household or indoor levels are lower than those in mines. Are low levels dangerous? How much radon would it take over what period of time to cause cancer, and how many people would it affect? In spite of years of research (at least nineteen more studies are underway) and millions of dollars spent, there's no answer to these questions. Some studies of radon in homes find associations with lung cancer; some have suggested that the lung cancer risk from radon in American homes is low. One problem is that epidemiological studies concerning radon are good at detecting high risk, as in uranium mines, but not sensitive enough to detect low risks, such as may result from exposure in smoke-free homes.

Radon is measured in picocuries per liter; the Environmental Protection Agency (EPA) calls four picocuries per liter of air the "action level"—that is, if you get such a reading in your home, you should do something to reduce it. It's thought that 6 to 7 percent of homes in this country exceed this level. However, critics say there's no evidence that four picocuries is a meaningful figure. The EPA used to say that radon caused 20,000 deaths a year. Now they estimate 14,000 (with a range of 7,000 to 30,000), and many experts question where those numbers came from.

Poisons are not just swallowed

Poisons can also cause trouble if they get in the eyes, on the skin, or are inhaled. You should seek medical help immediately for these episodes as well, but you may have to deal with the situation before going to the emergency room. Here's how to cope with these emergencies:

Eyes. Flood the eye with lukewarm or cold water for at least fifteen minutes. Encourage the victim to blink while flushing the eye, but do not force the eyelid open.

Skin. Remove contaminated clothing without contaminating yourself. Flood the area with water and follow with a mild soap and a final rinse.

Inhaled. Move the victim to fresh air immediately or open all the doors and windows. If the person has stopped breathing, perform artificial respiration; if the heart has stopped, perform CPR (cardiopulmonary resuscitation).

Useless worry, useless tests

According to Dr. Anthony Nero of the Lawrence Berkeley Laboratory, "the EPA has exaggerated and misrepresented the radon question, in regard to both the risks involved and the prevalence of high concentrations. These misrepresentations have led to the universal testing recommendation and that, together with an ill-conceived testing protocol, has put the public in the position of worrying when they shouldn't and getting useless results when they do test."

Dr. Nero estimates, and the EPA has recently confirmed, that perhaps one house in a thousand has levels above twenty picocuries per liter of air, exposures that wouldn't be allowable even for nuclear workers. Since such houses tend to cluster geographically, the first order of business is to identify high-radon areas. A group funded by the EPA and the Department of Energy has undertaken this task. The monitoring of radon, as well as efforts to eliminate it, should be concentrated in those areas.

How to be on the safe side

Already, a number of high-radon areas have been identified through existing monitoring efforts. If you live in such an area, it's worth the trouble of testing. If so, you're probably aware of newspaper publicity on the subject, but if you don't know, you can check with your local EPA office to find out whether your area has been pinpointed. If it has not yet been studied, you might wish to test anyway. But how to test is still a problem, and many scientists disagree with the current EPA recommendations.

You can buy inexpensive testing kits ($50 or less) at home-supply stores. The best choice is an "alpha-track" and "electret" detectors, which are used for more than 90 days. Be sure the kit you buy has a label saying "meets EPA requirements" or is state-certified, and follow all instructions carefully. It's also a good idea to obtain and read two EPA booklets: *A Citizen's Guide to Radon* and *Consumer's Guide to Radon Reduction*. Check at the nearest public library. Reducing the radon levels in your home, if necessary, will require the services of a contractor. Be sure you hire someone who is state-certified or has passed the EPA Radon Contractor Proficiency (RCP) Program. Your state radon office (see lists of such offices in the EPA pamphlets) should be able to help. Repairs and modifications can be expensive: the range is $500 to $2,500.

Whatever you do, beware of "quickie" testing, specifically the radon canisters. Radon levels vary year round, and even a short-term test (days to weeks) will not reveal much. If a first short-term test shows high levels, that certainly indicates the need for further testing. The EPA, in its *Citizen's Guide,* does say that short-term tests are adequate to decide whether or not to take remedial action. But its motive was to satisfy the need for testing when a house is being sold. Critics have said that short-term testing isn't much better than guessing.

If you're selling and want to assure your buyer that the house is radon-free, start testing the year before the sale. Or, your buyer can test during the first year while an agreed-upon sum is held in escrow.

Whether or not you have radon in your home, a cheap and sure way to reduce the risk of lung cancer is for smokers in the household to quit. Smoking *and* radon are an especially lethal combination.

Space Heaters

If you need additional space heating in your home, electrical heaters are better than kerosene or gas—they don't pollute indoor air and are less likely to be a fire hazard, but any portable heater can cause burns or start a household fire if misused. More than most appliances, portable heaters need to be handled with care.

Check your wiring and read the instructions for your heater. Most home electrical circuits (15 amperes) carry 1,500 watts, and a portable heater may use 1,200 watts or more. Check to see that you aren't overloading the circuit. If a fuse blows or the circuit breaker trips when you turn on a heater, or if the lights dim or flicker while it's running, unplug some other appliance. If you aren't sure you've corrected the problem, get help from a qualified electrician.

Avoid using lightweight extension cords to connect a heater. Poorly insulated extension cords can overheat and cause a fire, particularly when powering a power-hungry appliance like a heater. If you must use an extension cord (and it's not a good idea for a heater), be sure it's marked #14 or #12 AWG and bears the label of an independent testing lab. The cord may feel warm while in use and still be safe, but if it's really hot, unplug it.

Check the wall plate occasionally after you plug in a new heater. If it becomes hot or discolors from heat, that's a danger signal. Don't use the heater again until you get the problem corrected.

Have smoke detectors installed in rooms where portable heaters are often in use—especially in areas where people sleep. Choose one that makes a noise to alert you when the battery is low.

Keep heaters at least three feet away from bedding, furniture, and curtains. Don't put them where towels or other flammable things can fall on them. If you need a heater in a bathroom, buy one designed for use in moist locations.

Buy a heater with safety devices, such as a tip-over switch that turns off the heater if it gets knocked over and a thermostat that shuts off the heater if it gets dangerously hot.

Water

The body needs to replace about two and a half to three quarts of water every day to keep functioning. Without a supply of fresh water, we will die in only a few days. Some of this water supply comes from the water in foods. But about six to eight glasses of water are needed to make up the balance. You can fulfill this requirement with juice, milk, or other beverages; however, alcoholic drinks, coffee, tea, and colas have a diuretic effect—they wash water from the body by way of urination. Still, the best source for our bodies is plain, pure water.

Water comes from rain and snow, which runs off into rivers, lakes, and oceans or seeps into the ground to form part of the underground water table. Half of our drinking water comes from the surface water in rivers and lakes and reservoirs, the other half from groundwater.

Americans are even more concerned about contamination of their drinking water than about pollutants in the air, according to several polls. As a result, they spend billions per year on bottled water and water-purifying systems.

Until this century, of course, there was obvious cause for concern about the safety of drinking water. Contamination by infectious agents from human and animal wastes led to cholera, dysentery, and typhoid epidemics. This concern about microbe-borne disease was largely confined to surface water—that is, water from rivers, lakes, and reservoirs. Water in the underground water table (which was retrieved through wells) tended to remain pure, since infectious agents were filtered out as the water seeped down through the earth. And with the advent of chlorination of water—first introduced in New Jersey in 1908—and improved general sanitation, epidemics of water-borne bacterial diseases became exceedingly rare in the United States. Thanks to chlorination, one of the most successful public health-control measures in all history, Americans could take the safety of their public water supplies for granted. Though reported problems with contamination are indeed increasing around the country, public-health and environmental experts say most American tap water is still safe.

Monitoring municipal water

Some chemical contaminants, such as arsenic and radon, have been found to occur naturally in water. But in recent decades, new sorts of potential contaminants—which are neither filtered out naturally nor eliminated by chlorination—have been discovered in some surface-water supplies and, more ominously, in previously secure groundwater reserves. Among the leading culprits are residues of pesticides, industrial wastes, discharges from sewage treatment plants, and toxic seepage from dumps. Still other contaminants come from materials used in supplying public water, notably lead from home plumbing. Unfortunately, water that may be hazardous to your health may look, taste, and smell fine.

In response, the Safe Drinking Water Act of 1974 and subsequent regulations, enforced by the Environmental Protection Agency (EPA), placed limits on the levels of more than eighty contaminants in drinking water; the agency's goal is to regulate an additional twenty-five contaminants by 1996. In addition, some states have placed more stringent limits on chemicals found in water. But these regulations apply only to municipal water supplies—if you get your water from a private well, you're on your own (see the following page).

Many public-health experts believe that the monitoring of safe-water regulations should be strengthened and further research carried out. One problem is that today there are hundreds of potential chemical contaminants of water. Little is known, for instance, about the health effects of compounds left behind when pesticides break down in the soil. It would be very costly to test for all potential contaminants, and probably unnecessary. In addition, experts don't agree on how to assess the risk, if any, posed by the minuscule levels of the various substances occasionally found in water (or in food). Is it worth spending millions of dollars to prevent one possible additional death from cancer per million people over a period of seventy years, as one scientific standard stipulates? Or should we allocate these funds to deal with the far greater known risks posed by lead and natural contaminants such as arsenic and radon?

Despite the debate, the consensus is that drinking water from municipal systems remains safe. That includes the water consumed by more than 80 percent of Americans. Public water companies are required to test their water periodically and make the analysis available to the public.

The average American uses anywhere from 50 to 150 gallons of water each day: 39 percent for bathing, dish washing, and laundry; 30 percent for swimming pools and lawn and garden watering; 29 percent for flushing the toilet; and only 1.5 percent for drinking and cooking. Per capita, Europeans and Japanese use about half as much water as Americans.

Testing water from a private well

Millions of other Americans, usually in rural areas, get their drinking water from private wells—and it's up to them to make sure their water is safe, since it's not tested by the municipality. A study from the University of Iowa in 1990 found that shallow wells (less than fifty feet deep) are the ones most likely to be contaminated with coliform bacteria, nitrate, and pesticides. If you get water from a private well, ask your local health department if there are groundwater problems. Depending on what you find out, have your well water tested periodically for bacteria, inorganic chemicals (such as arsenic), and radon. In agricultural areas, check for nitrate and pesticides. And if you live near a landfill, refinery, or chemical plant, test for organic chemicals. Also consider testing if you note a change in your water's color, taste, or smell.

Which test? There are different types of tests for different contaminants, so it's important to have some idea of what potential problems you may face. Prices can range from about twenty dollars for a simple lead test to several hundred dollars for tests for organic chemicals. Call your local or state health department for the name of a lab, or consult the Yellow Pages under "laboratories, testing." Rely on a private testing laboratory only if it is certified by the state or by the federal Environmental Protection Agency. Do not depend on tests by a company that sells water-treatment equipment. It's wise to consult a second lab before investing in expensive corrective action.

The following are widespread contaminants in well water:

Nitrate. Fertilizers and sewage are the main contributors of nitrate to water, so this tends to be a problem primarily in agricultural areas. Nitrate may pose an immediate threat to infants, since high levels can cause a rare form of anemia. It may also signal the presence of other contaminants.

Microorganisms. Coliform bacteria from human and animal wastes are still found on occasion in improperly treated drinking water. They are a sign of unsanitary conditions and may indicate the presence of more dangerous bacteria, viruses, or parasites. Giardia, an intestinal parasite, is a leading cause of water-borne outbreaks of diarrhea.

Organic chemicals. These include pesticides, benzene and other industrial solvents, gasoline, trihalomethanes (THMs, byproducts of chlorination), and most other pollutants regulated by the EPA.

Radon. This naturally occurring radioactive gas, which has been implicated as a cause of lung cancer, typically seeps from the earth through building foundations into household air. And if there's a high level of radon in your soil, there may also be radon in your water if it comes from a well on your property. Drinking radon-contaminated water is not considered a health risk. But the radon will be released from your running water, especially from hot water, and add to the radon in your household air. If tests have shown that the air in your house contains high levels of radon and you have a private well, test your water too. Some states or localities will test your water for you. Ventilating your bathroom and kitchen may help disperse radon released from water (see page 564 for more information on radon).

Water purifiers

If scientific testing reveals that your water supply is contaminated, your first reaction may be to buy a water-treatment device. The less you know about your water, the easier it is for a salesman to sell you unreliable equipment for a problem you may not even have. The water-purification business is rich in scams and hokum—always get an objective test and a second opinion before investing in a costly device. No single device can get rid of all contaminants: different contaminants call for different types of purifier. All purifiers need to be maintained properly, otherwise your water may end up even more contaminated. You may simply need a device to improve the water's look, taste, or smell.

Registration of a purifying device with the EPA is required on devices claiming to inhibit or kill microorganisms via chemically active ingredients. It does not imply EPA approval nor does it guarantee effectiveness. The following listing is based on a report in *Consumer Reports* in January, 1990:

Activated carbon (or charcoal) filters employ particles that attract certain contaminants. These may be attached to an individual faucets or installed under sink counters. There are also larger systems that filter all the water that enters a house. Small units, such as those attached to faucets or in pour-through pitchers, are virtually useless, since they quickly become ineffective and require frequent replacement. Carbon filters are best at removing bad tastes and odors, along with some organic chemicals such as pesticides. They generally don't remove lead (though some are designed to remove lead) and other metals, nitrate, dissolved minerals, or microbial contamination. The filters must be cleaned regularly: they eventually become clogged with sediment; bacteria build-up can occur in warm weather or periods of non-use.

Lead filter cartridges may be for you if lead is your only problem. They are relatively inexpensive and probably effective, provided you change them frequently.

Reverse osmosis filters employ a porous membrane that excludes most contaminants, along with a carbon filter. Consumer Reports found that they remove some lead and other toxic metals, nitrate, bacteria, and most inorganic and some organic chemicals. But if you have a serious problem with lead or bacterial contamination, you shouldn't rely on them. The devices waste lots of water—for every four gallons fed into the system, at least three go down the drain—and are usually expensive and difficult to maintain.

Distillers work via vaporization and condensation to remove lead and other heavy metals along with microorganisms, but not organic chemicals such as volatile pesticides. It can take more than five hours—plus considerable energy—to make a gallon of distilled water.

Water softeners filter out the calcium and magnesium found in hard water. These minerals limit sudsing and cause scaly deposits in bathtubs—but they are not a health problem. Softeners may add sodium and make the water more corrosive, thus increasing any leaching of lead from plumbing.

Bottled water that has a plastic taste may contain materials such as plasticizers—used to keep the bottle flexible—or compounds used in manufacturing to get the bottle out of its mold. If your bottled water tastes like plastic, you might be wise to either switch brands or go back to the tap.

How to choose the right system for you?

After appropriate testing, seek out a reliable dealer and ignore advertising claims. The National Sanitation Foundation (NSF) operates a voluntary certification program for water-treatment programs. A useful feature of the NSF label is its specification of the contaminants a device is qualified to remove. The Federal Trade Commission serves as watchdog for false claims, but applies no labeling standards. If a consumer complains, the FTC will have the offending device tested by the EPA or independent labs. You can also check with the Better Business Bureau.

Fluoridation

Fluoride in the water sometimes occurs naturally, as in Colorado Springs and other communities. And sometimes local governments, usually cities, add it to the water in controlled quantities. As medical science has known for decades, fluoride interacts with tooth enamel and hardens it, making it less susceptible to decay—50 to 70 percent less susceptible. In the generations born since the 1950s, when fluoridation came into wide use, toothaches and tooth extractions are almost an oddity.

Fluoridated water may also play a role in building strong bones, and warding off osteoporosis, a disease that decreases bone mass, weakens bones, and increases the likelihood of fractures, particularly among post-menopausal women. Studies have shown that women who live in areas with naturally fluoridated water suffer fewer osteoporotic fractures and have generally greater bone strength than those who drink nonfluoridated water.

Classified as a nutrient, fluoride occurs naturally in water and in soil. It is one of many elements that make up human tissue. As early as 1908, its properties as a tooth-decay preventive were deduced from observing dental health patterns in communities where the water supply was naturally fluoridated. According to a number of long-term studies, such communities have no greater incidence of cancer, heart disease, liver disease, or other ills than other places.

One well-known side effect of fluoride, however, is dental fluorosis, a light mottling of the tooth enamel that may be cosmetically unappealing. This condition occurs in some people in areas where the natural fluoride content is very high.

If you do install an NSF-approved water-treatment system, be sure you follow the manufacturer's maintenance instructions to the letter. But—we repeat—first have your water tested by a reputable lab.

Bottled water

Most people purchase bottled water not because their tap water is polluted, but because they like the taste or they feel bottled water confers health benefits. Supermarket shelves are packed with literally hundreds of brands of deluxe mineral waters, "bulk" waters, club sodas, seltzers, and flavored seltzers.

Bottled water, unfortunately, is not universally healthful, and there's no reason to believe it is purer than tap water from a municipal system. Some bottled waters come from sources high in sodium, for example. Three-quarters of the bottled water sold in the United States is simply processed tap water from local taps, with or without added carbonation. Some bottled waters are processed and bottled under conditions that actually give them higher bacteria counts than your own tap water (if bottled according to Food and Drug Administration (FDA) standards, however, bacteria must be very low). Some contain the same pollutants from pesticides and organic chemicals that your tap water may.

A report to Congress by the General Accounting Office concluded that bottled water "may contain levels of potentially harmful contaminants that are not allowed in public drinking water." The mineral content of any water is *not* nutritionally significant, except for the tooth-protecting fluoride that is either naturally present or added to the water supplies in most communities. Unfortunately, most bottled waters lack fluoride, and some are comparatively high in sodium.

On the plus side, bottled waters are not allowed to contain appreciable amounts of lead or any other heavy metal.

Price is another factor when selecting bottled water; an eight-ounce glass of mineral water can cost twenty-five to fifty cents, and even more in a restaurant.

The labels on bottled water generally provide little information about chemical content. Moreover, labeling terminology can be confusing. Here are some definitions and choices:

Distilled water is definitely the purest since it contains no solid matter of any kind and is essentially free of sodium. The water is first evaporated into steam, which leaves many impurities behind, and then is recondensed. However, it is the minerals that give water its satisfying taste: distilled water tastes flat and dead. In addition, distillation does not remove many of the suspect organic chemicals.

Mineral water is simply water that contains minerals—which is true of virtually all water except distilled water. "Natural mineral water" contains just the minerals present in the water as it comes from the ground. Simple "mineral water" may have been processed and had minerals added or removed. Most mineral water, whether or not it is identified as such, comes from a spring.

Seltzer is usually tap water that is filtered and carbonated, with no minerals or mineral salts added. Oddly enough, a few so-called "seltzers" contain sweeteners such as sucrose or corn syrup, giving them up to 100 calories per eight ounces. Diabetics and other people trying to avoid sugar should therefore always read the ingredients list of any seltzer. In contrast, flavored seltzer contains a minuscule amount, or "essence," of fruit juice, usually equal to one-tenth of one percent of total volume. It contains no calories, sugar, or mineral salts. You can, of course, make your own by squeezing a little fruit juice into plain seltzer.

Sparkling water is a generic term for any carbonated water. The carbonization can be "natural" (the gases are captured as they escape from water and later reinjected during bottling) or be added artificially. The results are the same. Most are relatively high in sodium.

Club soda is usually simple tap water, filtered and carbonated, to which a mix of minerals and mineral salts have been added to give it the distinctive taste associated with its brand. Many distributors, for instance, sell their special mineral mixes to local bottling companies, which then add the local water to the mix. Most are fairly high in sodium—30 to 65 milligrams per eight ounces. People on sodium-restricted diets should stick to seltzer.

Spring water is water that has risen naturally to the earth's surface. Water labeled "natural spring water" must not have been processed in any way before bottling, whereas simple "spring water" may or may not have been processed. As with any groundwater, spring water may be contaminated. The best choice is spring water that is bottled directly from a spring in a nonindustrial area where few pollutants can reach the water. Such water would be labeled something on the order of "natural spring water bottled directly from the source." It may or may not be called mineral water, and may or may not be carbonated.

Wood-Burning Stoves

More than a million wood-burning stoves are sold in the U. S. each year. Economical and cozy as such "natural" heating may be, it also entails certain risks. Besides the danger of a house fire, there's the problem of indoor and outdoor pollution.

Wood-burning stoves produce combustion by-products, notably gases such as carbon monoxide and nitrogen dioxide, along with particulates (the smoke and ash from incompletely burned wood). These stoves are far more polluting than other forms of heating; they can create significant air-quality problems in areas where they are used in large numbers. Inside your home, long-term exposure to these pollutants can contribute to respiratory problems (such as asthma and bronchitis) and have other adverse effects, especially in children, whose lungs are more susceptible.

The following steps will help ensure safer, cleaner, and more economical use of a wood stove:

• If you depend on a wood stove for heating, make sure it has been certified by the Environmental Protection Agency (EPA). If it's not EPA-certified, consider buying a new one—nearly all on the market today are certified. These new stoves are more efficient: some use catalytic converters to burn fuel more completely; others employ improvements such as baffles and secondary combustion chambers. They often consume only half as much wood as older models (and thus will save money in the long run), emit anywhere from 70 percent to 90 percent less particulate matter, and produce less of the creosote that can cause a fire in the chimney. As a general rule, stoves manufactured before July 1990 are less efficient (and thus emit more pollutants) than newer models. Avoid antique stoves.

• Before you buy a stove, check with your local fire marshall to see what local restrictions may apply to wood stoves. Have the stove installed by a professional. If you do it yourself, have the work checked by a fire or building inspector.

• Burn only dry, seasoned wood (less than 20 percent water content); this will improve combustion and thus cut down on pollutants. Hardwoods (such as maple, oak, or elm) burn more cleanly and evenly than softwoods (pine, spruce, or fir).

• Make small, hot fires rather than large smoky ones. This will burn the wood more thoroughly and reduce pollution. Attach a surface thermometer to the top of the stove—it should read between 300° and 500°F. If the temperature is lower, add more wood or open the air controls more.

• Look at the smoke coming out of the chimney. Smoke is unburned fuel: the darker it is, the more fuel (wood) it is wasting, and the more pollutants it is releasing. A properly burning fire should give off mostly white steam.

• Inspect the stove regularly for cracks and leaks; check that the doors fit tightly. To make sure your stove is airtight, make a fire and then shut off the air supply. The fire should go right out; if it continues to burn until the wood is gone, there's a leak that you should have repaired. Inexpensive devices that measure indoor carbon monoxide levels are available at many hardware stores.

• Have the chimney cleaned professionally at least once a year.

• Check the stovepipe periodically for corrosion.

• Never burn plastics, colored paper (such as magazines), treated or painted wood, or garbage in the stove. These produce harmful fumes, along with more smoke and other pollutants.

Outdoors

In addition to your home and workplace, your immediate environment also includes your yard, your community, and the places you travel to frequently. From barbecuing safely to preventing Lyme disease to ways you can help preserve the ozone layer, this chapter discusses some of the common environmental and safety concerns in the great outdoors.

Barbecues

Every summer about 10,000 Americans burn themselves at the backyard barbecue—by having the lighter fluid explode in their hands, being splashed by grease, or being caught by a flare-up from the fire. Here are some rules to help you avoid these hazards:

• Set up the grill away from the house and away from bushes or dry leaves. Never set it up in a tent, trailer, or garage or inside the house. In addition to the fire hazard, there is danger of carbon monoxide build-up.

• Don't wear clothes with hanging shirttails or frilly aprons.

• Pile the briquettes in a pyramid to start them. They'll light faster.

• Use only lighter fluid specifically designed for barbecues, never gasoline or kerosene. Let the fluid soak in before lighting it. Never add more liquid once the briquettes are lit or smoking. Better yet, use an electric starter or metal chimney starter that requires only a lit piece of newspaper to start the briquettes; these work quickly, are safe, and eliminate the chemical taste of fluids.

• Use long-handled utensils and gloves or mitts to avoid burns and spatters.

• Keep a spray bottle of water nearby so you can subdue flare-ups with a light mist of water. You might also keep a box of baking soda handy to sprinkle on a resistant grease fire. Also, a covered grill will minimize the chance of flare-ups.

• If you use a gas grill, reread the instructions the first time you use it each season in order to refresh your memory.

• Before each use and after a new gas tank is connected, apply soapy water around the connections and along the hose. If you see bubbles, you have a gas leak, which could lead to an explosion.

• Light gas grills with the lid open to prevent gas build-up and explosion.

Beach Pollution

By and large the public health danger of debris—even medical waste—washed up on the beaches has been blown out of proportion. While floating waste has been washing up on beaches for well over a century, the character of the waste has changed. Now there's more plastic and disposable waste, some of which is medical. This same waste is, of course, also turning up in municipal trash bins and landfills.

Most medical experts and health officials don't look on medical waste, however unattractive it may be, as a major public health threat. It's unlikely that anything in the ocean for any length of time could still be infectious. The chances of getting AIDS or any other illness by stepping on a used needle at a beach are virtually nil.

As for bacterial contamination, New Jersey's Department of Health looked into water quality for the summers of 1987 and 1988 and published figures concerning the incidence of illness reported by swimmers. Aside from one serious sewage spill, most water samplings were "excellent." Symptoms such as itchy eyes, sore throat, skin rash, stomach upset, and ear infections, the study concluded, are primarily the result of person-to-person transmission of viruses. Many people who get sick at the beach, the report implied, shouldn't necessarily blame pollution, but rather factors such as poor food handling at beach picnics or concessions.

Taking precautions

Pollution problems obviously vary from region to region. But wherever you are, the following commonsense measures can minimize any risks beach pollution may pose to your health:

•Check with local health officials about the condition of local waters—especially lakes and bays.

•Stay out of the water when warnings or closings are posted. In some areas, bacterial counts may rise after heavy rains because of raw sewage overflows and run-offs of storm waters.

•Avoid touching debris that looks like medical waste. Report it to lifeguards or other officials.

•Clean up your own act, if need be. Refrigerate picnic food; don't litter. Use public toilets instead of the ocean.

Lawn Mowers

About 32,000 people are injured by power lawn mowers each year. If you use a power mower, here are a few pointers to keep you safe:

•When mowing, wear close-fitting trousers and shoes that both protect your feet and give you traction. Sandals or cloth sneakers are not adequate. Avoid voluminous sleeves, dangling jewelry, or anything likely to get caught in the mower. Since a riding mower may hoist you up to tree branch level, safety goggles are a good idea.

•Clear the area of stones, large twigs, and other debris. These can break the blades—or can become high-speed missiles if the blades pick them up.

•Don't pull any mower backward. You may pull it too close to your feet.

•Store gasoline in an Underwriters Laboratories (UL)–labeled container. Fill the mower while the engine is cool, and always handle gasoline outdoors.

•Use an electric mower only on dry grass. Choose an extension cord with a UL seal that is intended for outdoor use.

•If it's a walk-behind mower, cut across slopes, not up and down them, to minimize the risk of the mower rolling back on you. But do the opposite with a riding mower to reduce the risk of tipping sideways.

•Keep children and pets out of the area where you are mowing, and don't offer

Sales of old-fashioned push mowers have risen in recent years. Not only are they less expensive and less likely to break down, but they don't pollute the air. (The typical walk-behind gas-powered mower produces as much air pollution in one hour as a new car does in more than eleven hours, according to the EPA.) Manual mowers also provide good exercise: pushing a manual mower burns between 420 and 480 calories an hour—as many calories as an hour of playing tennis.

rides on a riding mower. If children are outdoors while you are mowing, insist that they wear shoes.

• When buying a mower, look for the triangular emblem with the letters OPEI (Outdoor Power Equipment Institute). It's usually affixed to the mower near the discharge chute. This assures you that the mower meets minimum safety standards for machines with revolving parts and blades.

Lightning

At any moment there are about 1,800 lightning storms occurring on earth. Here is what happens: in a thunderstorm, air turbulence causes a negative charge to build up in the underside of a thundercloud, while positive charges build up on the earth below. Streamers of positive charges constantly flow up from the earth—from tips of trees, the edges of the eaves of houses, from poles, even from people as they walk through a large open space. Eventually the thundercloud sends a nearly invisible, negatively charged jagged streamer down toward the earth. As it approaches the ground, at least one positively charged streamer shoots up to meet it.

When the two streamers join, thus creating an ionized air channel between cloud and earth, a blinding positive stroke of lightning flashes *upward,* from the earth to the cloud. In four-tenths of a second, several strokes will rise up from the earth to create a bolt of lightning of as much as 30 million volts (compared to household current of 110 to 220 volts). The heat that such a bolt creates can run as high as 30,000 to 50,000° Fahrenheit. This causes an explosion of superheated air in the ionized channel, and thus a crack of thunder.

A direct hit by a lightning bolt is usually fatal. A sideflash—a bolt of lightning splashing off a tree or other object—can be fatal. Conducted current—a bolt of lightning sending its electrical charge through the telephone wire or the plumbing—can be fatal, or just stunning. Step voltage—the charge that radiation sends out into the ground around a struck tree—is often fatal to cattle or horses, but usually only jolts a person.

The most dangerous month for lightning is July. According to the National Weather Service, from 1959 to 1988, 29 percent of all lightning deaths occurred during this month.

Protecting lives and property

Not much will protect a house except a properly installed lightning rod. If you are in a house without a lightning rod, you will be safest if you stay away from metal objects, the telephone, plumbing, the fireplace, and open doors and windows during a thunderstorm.

Outside, stay away from lone trees, unprotected shelters, open fields, open boats, and wire fences. Anything that sticks up from the landscape can be the lightning rod from which a positive streamer rises to meet the negative streamer. In a grove of trees, stay out from under the taller trees. Get off your bike, horse, golf cart, or tractor. Don't swim. Look for a ravine or other low-lying spot, a small tree, or the underside of a cliff. If you are caught in the open, kneel down, bend low, and touch the ground only with your knees and feet.

If someone near you is struck, immediately perform cardiopulmonary resuscitation (CPR), even if the person appears to be dead. Although you may think a person has no chance of surviving a bolt of lightning, people do survive an indirect hit—even sometimes a direct hit.

Lyme Disease

By the end of 1993, a total of 57,206 cases of Lyme disease had been reported in the United States. Lyme disease poses a double bind for doctors and health officials: many people who have it don't know it, and many others are convinced they have it but don't. Although there's much debate about exactly how prevalent this tickborne disease is, more cases of it are reported each year. Yet despite the media hype and sensationalistic ads for tick repellents and testing kits, there is no reason to panic or, as some people are doing, avoid spending time outdoors. There is good reason, nonetheless, to take steps to protect yourself if you live in or visit an area where the disease is common, especially New York, Connecticut, Pennsylvania, and other Atlantic states, as well as northern California.

How Lyme disease spreads

The infection, caused by a corkscrew-shaped bacterium known as a spirochete (*Borrelia burgdorferi*), is transmitted primarily via certain species of deer ticks. These are smaller than the common dog tick, though it's often difficult to tell them apart. A deer tick, before it becomes engorged with blood, looks like a mole or blood blister. While the flat, eight-legged adults are less than one-tenth of an inch long, immature ticks (called nymphs) are about the size of a pinhead, and the larvae are nearly invisible. The male is black and the female is dark red and black. When filled with blood, the tick becomes gray and increases in size three- to five-fold.

Although deer can become infected, in the eastern United States, white-footed field mice serve as the main host for both the bacteria and the young ticks. The adult ticks usually feed and mate on deer, then drop off to lay eggs. These in turn hatch into minuscule larvae, which become infected by feeding on white-footed mice. The larvae molt and become infected nymphs. (In the West, the culprit is the closely related black-legged tick, also carried by wood rats.) Both nymphs and adult ticks feed on a variety of animals. *The nymphs are the chief threat to humans—about 70 to 90 percent of all cases are caused by nymph bites.* Adult ticks are generally less of a threat to humans because they're large enough to be seen and removed before they transfer the bacteria.

The nymphs and adults wait on low vegetation in wooded areas and adjacent grasslands and transfer themselves to whatever brushes by; they don't fly or jump. Dogs and cats can carry the ticks to your home and property.

Geographical distribution

Lyme disease was first identified as a form of arthritis in 1975 in the woodlands around Lyme, Connecticut (hence its name). Cases are known to have occurred in at least forty states. Those with the highest reported incidence in 1989 were, in descending order, Connecticut, Rhode Island, New York, Georgia, New Jersey, Wisconsin, and Pennsylvania. The ticks tend to thrive in those areas where suburban lawns meet woodlands. Deer, whose population has grown in the East in recent years, help spread infected ticks to new areas. Migratory birds have brought Lyme disease to the South.

Even city dwellers may be susceptible to Lyme disease. All it takes is a weekend excursion to the countryside for you—or your dog—to meet up with a tick.

Although this disease has received the most publicity in the United States, it has existed in Europe at least since the beginning of the century (though its assorted symptoms were often not attributed to a single disorder). Lyme disease is found today in all continents except Antarctica. While the peak periods may vary from region to region, this is primarily a summer disease. You're most likely to be bitten by a deer tick between May and September, when the nymphs are active. And that's also when people are outdoors most. The risk of being bitten is lower in April, October, and November, and lowest from December through March.

Even if you're certain you've been bitten by a deer tick and that the tick was infected, it's unlikely that you'll develop Lyme disease. In a study published in the *New England Journal of Medicine,* Yale researchers looked at 387 people who had been bitten by deer ticks; they found that the risk of infection after a deer-tick bite was only 1 percent, even in areas of Connecticut where Lyme disease is prevalent. A tick has to feed on a human for twenty-four to forty-eight hours before the disease can be transmitted.

Symptoms

Lyme disease is hard to diagnose because its symptoms can vary greatly from person to person. No single symptom appears in all cases, and there's no predictable time frame or sequence of symptoms. And the problem is complicated by the lack of a reliable test for the disease. So far the available blood tests for Lyme disease have been neither sensitive nor specific enough, yielding an unacceptable number of false positives and false negatives. The results of the tests vary from lab to lab, and the meaning of the results is not standardized. This greatly compounds the problems of diagnosis. In particular, during the first four weeks after someone becomes infected, the test is unlikely to detect the small amount of antibodies the body has produced in response to the bacteria. Even in the later stages of the disease, the current tests, as routinely performed, are so unreliable that they're virtually useless. (Newer, more reliable tests are in the experimental stage, but it will probably be several years before they are available for clinical use.) Still, three general phases have been identified:

Phase one. Most often, within thirty days of being bitten by an infected tick, you'll develop a small red bump at the site of the bite surrounded by a rash that gradually grows for several weeks and then fades. The rash may have a firm center area, feel warm to the touch, and disappear briefly only to reappear elsewhere on your body. At the same time, you may develop flulike symptoms: fatigue, chills, headache, muscle and joint aches, and a low fever. Remember, however, that you may not develop a rash but just the flulike symptoms—or you may have none of these early symptoms at all. In some people, Lyme disease doesn't progress beyond this early stage. But if it goes untreated, more severe symptoms may develop, sometimes many months later.

Phase two. About 20 percent of untreated people develop neurological or cardiac disorders weeks or months after the bite. These range from heart rhythm abnormalities to impaired motor coordination and even partial facial paralysis. These symptoms also usually disappear within a few weeks.

Phase three. About half of untreated people develop recurring or chronic arthritis after a latent period of up to two years. Thus the disease was first called "Lyme arthritis." The knees are almost always affected.

You don't need a special, costly tick repellent to ward off Lyme disease. Use insect repellents that contain the chemical deet; they will do the job just as well.

If in doubt, antibiotics?

Lyme disease is treatable and almost always curable, especially in its early stage. If you have—or had—the characteristic rash, your doctor will probably put you on antibiotics. Similarly, if you live in an area with a high incidence of the disease and find a tick on you, which your doctor or the local health department identifies as a deer tick,or a western black-legged tick if you life in California, you'll probably be put on antibiotics.

What if you have only the flulike symptoms, fatigue, or joint pain, but no memory of a tick bite? Some people may shop around till they find a physician who will treat them with antibiotics just in case. But overuse of antibiotics has a serious downside. All antibiotics can have adverse effects in sensitive individuals. Pregnant women, in particular, shouldn't be stampeded into unwarranted antibiotic treatment by overblown news reports of birth defects caused by Lyme disease. And the overuse of these drugs can also produce antibiotic-resistant organisms.

Preventing Lyme disease

To lessen the risks of contracting Lyme disease and free yourself from worry in the fields or woods, take these precautions:

•Wear a long-sleeved shirt with buttoned cuffs. Tuck the shirt into your pants and your pants into your socks or boots. Wear hard-finished, light-colored fabrics.

If you find a tick attached to you and engorged with blood, remove it (see page 314). If you think it may be a deer tick, save it in a small jar containing a little alcohol; label the jar with the date, the body location of the bite, and where you think the tick came from. This way you can show it to a doctor, if necessary. If you think the deer tick has been on you more than twenty-four hours, talk to your doctor, especially if you live in an area where Lyme disease is common.

A Tick-Free Yard

Ticks appear to be stubbornly embedded in our ecosystem, and there's not much we can do about it. Spraying the landscape with pesticides is apparently not an effective way to destroy them. Many ticks are underground in animal burrows, and others hide on the underside of leaves—either way, they may escape the spray.

Moreover, pesticide sprays are indiscriminate and endanger all insects and perhaps other creatures on your land as well. What about killing or removing the mice or deer that feed and transport the ticks? Even if this were desirable and feasible, it might not do much to prevent Lyme disease, since the ticks could find other host animals.

There may be a way, however. Scientists are intrigued by a product called Damminix, which was developed by researchers at Harvard's School of Public Health. These cardboard tubes filled with insecticide-impregnated cotton are "roach motels" with a twist. They don't attract the ticks themselves, but rather the mice that serve as host to both the young ticks and the Lyme disease bacteria in the eastern United States. The mice bring the cotton back to their burrows and thus become covered with the pesticide. The young ticks die when they come to feed on a treated mouse or when the mouse brings them back to its burrow.

Usage tips

Place the tubes at ten-yard intervals on your property wherever mice may be living; lawns don't need to be treated. Tests in infested areas have found that using Damminix can drastically reduce the number of infected ticks. It works in the northeast and upper midwest; tests are underway in California

Damminix is not cheap: a box of twenty-four tubes, a year's supply (two applications are recommended, one in spring and one in summer) for a typical half-acre property, costs about $70. The manufacturer points out that since ticks don't travel far and mice are territorial (that is, they tend to stay in a certain area), Damminix will work even if neighboring land isn't treated. Obviously, it would help if your neighbors treated their property, too.

Permethrin, the pesticide in Damminix, is also available in two aerosol sprays, Permanone and Duranon. Studies have found that permethrin may be an even more effective against ticks than deet. It is available in hardware stores in many states Make sure you use it only on clothing, not on your skin.

It's easier to spot ticks on white or tan trousers than on black ones.

- Use insect repellent on your pants, socks, and shoes.
- Try to stay near the center of trails in overgrown country.
- Check occasionally for ticks when you're in underbrush or wooded areas. Later do a thorough check of your entire body. Have someone look at your back and head if possible.

(For more information on ticks, see pages 313-315.)

Ozone Layer

The depletion of the earth's protective ozone layer is a health issue for all of us. While most of the measures needed to safeguard the ozone layer involve nations and industries, there are significant steps you can take—as an individual consumer and as a member of society.

There's good and bad ozone, depending on where it is, though both are chemically identical. Ozone is a gas formed when three atoms of oxygen, rather than the normal two, bind together. The ozone found at ground level, a by-product of car and factory pollution, is one of the more dangerous components of smog. But in the earth's stratosphere, about ten to twenty-five miles above us, ozone functions as a natural screen against the sun's most damaging ultraviolet (UV) rays. Unfortunately, the ozone that pollutes our air cannot reach the stratosphere's ozone layer.

Chlorofluorocarbons—the largest contributor

The stratospheric ozone layer is being destroyed in large part by manmade compounds called chlorofluorocarbons, or CFCs. These versatile chemicals, in liquid or gaseous form, have helped shape modern society. CFCs are used as coolants in our homes, cars, and refrigerators, as foaming agents (in foam insulation, mattresses, and food packaging), and as solvents that remove impurities from computer microchips and electronic equipment. The same properties that make CFCs efficient and safe for so many industrial uses also make them destructive to the environment. Their great stability ensures that when they are released into the air (during manufacturing processes, from leaky cooling systems, or upon disposal) CFCs eventually rise intact to the stratosphere, where intense radiation breaks them down into component atoms. One of these atoms, chlorine, has a devastating effect on ozone. Other compounds called halons, used in some fire extinguishers, are even more destructive of ozone.

Scientists predict that by allowing more UV radiation to reach the earth, the depletion of the ozone layer will lead to an increase in the number of cases of skin cancer (especially melanoma) and cataracts. In addition, they postulate that the increased UV radiation may damage crops, kill plankton that serve as a food source for marine life, and even have adverse effects on the human immune system. CFCs may also trap heat in the atmosphere and thus contribute to the global warming trend (greenhouse effect).

For all these reasons, an international agreement in Montreal in 1987 called for accelerating the phasing out of CFC and halon production. Reports by NASA that the ozone layer is being depleted even more rapidly than was previously projected, and the discovery of vast holes in the layer over Antarctica and the Arctic, have prompted scientists and environmental groups to call for a complete and rapid phase-out of CFCs. The Clean Air Act Amendments passed by Congress in 1990 require the EPA to phase out domestic production and imports of CFCs—along with several other substances that deplete the ozone layer—by 1996. To complement the phasing-out program, products containing or manufactured with ozone-depleting chemicals have to carry warning labels. The EPA also announced rules in 1993 that prohibit the release of CFCs into the atmosphere during the servicing and disposal of refrigerators and air conditioners in homes and businesses. The previous year, the agency ruled that service stations must recycle CFCs during the servicing of automobile air conditioners.

However, the impact of CFCs won't vanish overnight by virtue of these recent regulations. For one thing, companies can continue to sell existing inventories of products that use CFCs; they can also recycle CFCs. More importantly, even if we stopped using CFCs tomorrow, the damage to the ozone layer will continue, since those CFCs already released in the air will still be making their way to the stratosphere a decade from now and destroying ozone for up to a century.

Fortunately, many companies have already voluntarily eliminated ozone-depleting chemicals from their products. Substitutes have already been found for many uses of CFCs, from aerosol sprays to fire extinguishers. CFCs can also be modified so that they do much less damage to the ozone layer, or so that they break down quickly in the lower atmosphere. Industries are also seeking ways to recycle the chemicals so that they aren't released into the air. Du Pont, the world's largest manufacturer of CFCs, announced some years back that it would phase out production by the end of the century. The European Economic Community followed suit.

Seven ways you can help

The United States has been the leading producer and consumer of CFCs—though the recent EPA rulings should help dramatically reduce the American contribution to the destruction of the ozone layer: By following these steps, consumers can also contribute to this reduction:

1. Get auto air conditioners properly serviced. Before the new EPA regulations took effect, auto air conditioners were the single largest source of CFC emissions in the United States. If you have a leak, get it fixed; otherwise, the CFCs you add will end up in the atmosphere. By law, all service stations should be equipped to recycle the refrigerant used in car air conditioners. (The EPA has banned the sale of small cans of refrigerant, which allowed people to "top off" their air conditioners instead of repairing leaks.) Also, car air conditioners using less-harmful refrigerants are now available. (Home air conditioners, by and large, contain coolants that are far less ozone-depleting.)

2. Avoid products made of plastic foam (polystyrene), such as fast-food containers, egg cartons, Styrofoam cups, and foam trays for meats. Although many of these products are now made from less-damaging compounds, you may not be able to tell which are which, so limit your use of them.

3. Don't use foam plastic insulation in your home, unless it is made with ozone-safe agents. Instead use fiberglass, gypsum, fiberboard, or cellulose insulation.

4. Don't buy a halon fire extinguisher for home use. Halon extinguishers were no longer manufactured as of January, 1994, but some may still be available.

5. Check labels on aerosol cans and certain other products. Some VCR-head cleaners, boat horns, spray confetti, photo-negative cleaners, and drain plungers that contain the most dangerous CFCs may still be on the market, even after the 1996 ban on CFCs goes into effect.

6. When buying a new refrigerator, choose an energy-efficient model: it may contain as little as half the CFCs. To keep your fridge in the best working order, clean the coils regularly; that way it may last until models with CFC-free coolants and foam insulation, which are being developed, gradually come on the market. When disposing of an old refrigerator, you must ensure that CFCs are recovered so they don't escape into the air. The town you live in may take responsibility for this, or you may have to pay a refrigerator repair service to perform the task. (Although the insulating foam in refrigerators also contains CFCs, there is no law requiring them to be recovered.)

Pesticides

Developed in the late 1930s and introduced in 1945 as a heaven-sent boon to farmers, the pesticide DDT was outlawed twenty-seven years later in the United States as "environmentally persistent." Its toxic residues in food were found to be a threat to animal and human, as well as insect, life. Even now, however, the residues of scores of other insecticides remain on or in the food we eat, while their toxic effects remain in question.

The availability and variety of fruits and vegetables have increased tenfold in ten years—in large measure, due to pesticides and other agrichemicals that increase crop yield and ward off spoilage during storing and shipping. The residues of these compounds constitute a universal environmental and health hazard whose full scope remains to be determined. No one really knows how to address this problem at this time.

Apples have been found to contain the residues of as many as 43 of a total of 110 pesticides registered by the Environmental Protection Agency (EPA) for use on apples. Yet the Food and Drug Administration (FDA), which sets tolerance levels for such chemicals, tests only 1 percent of the fruits and vegetables (domestic and imported) marketed in the United States. Some experts feel that such skimpy testing provides an inadequate basis for predicting the long-term effects of pesticides on humans. Is consumption of fruits and vegetables—laden, after all, with vital nutrients as well as potentially dangerous agrichemicals—worth the risk, then? Some researchers imply that it is. In 1986, a report by researchers at the University of California at Berkeley, published in the *Annual Review of Public Health,* concluded: "With few exceptions, the delayed effects of pesticides on human health have been difficult to detect. Perhaps the health risks are sufficiently small that they are below the power of epidemiologic studies to detect."

While the Berkeley conclusions are correct, in 1988 the National Academy of Science, utilizing different assumptions, estimated the national risk of cancer from pesticide use at as many as 20,000 cases a year. The academy's report noted further: "some allowed levels [of pesticide residues in food] are being challenged by scientists as being too high." EPA-acceptable intake figures, for instance, are based on a diet that includes only 7.5 ounces of foods like cantaloupe, avocado, or squash a year. Most of us eat much more.

Although produce grown without pesticides may not look as appetizing— apples may have small blemishes or lettuce may have tiny holes in the leaves—it is not harmful. These fruits and vegetables are usually picked ripe and don't travel well, and may have more imperfections.

Despite the gaps in current research, there is enough evidence of toxicity to justify concern about the effects of these residues. Fortunately, there are a number of sensible protective measures you can adopt—some in the nature of short-term first aid, others with long-term aims in view. Abide by them, and what you eat may not only be safer, but better-tasting, too.

Eat a wide variety of foods. This helps minimize your exposure to any one pesticide.

Eat what's in season. Buy strawberries and cherries in June primarily, not December, and chances are you'll get more delicious fruit grown under optimum conditions. In the right season, there's less need for chemicals.

Eat local or at least domestic produce. Obviously, if you eat seasonal produce, it's more likely to be domestically grown. In this regard, FDA figures are significant; they show that 64 percent of imported produce contains pesticide residues, against 38 percent of domestic produce.

Wash carefully. Many water-soluble residues float away with thorough washing. Use a vegetable brush to scrub hard vegetables and fruits.

Don't use hanging pest strips, since these constantly release pesticide into the air you breathe. In addition, many of them contain DDVP (also called dichlorvos or Vapona), a carcinogen that the EPA has considered banning.

Mothballs

Several kinds of household insects feed on clothing—not just moths but several kinds of carpet beetles. Actually it's the larvae of all these creatures that can leave their mark on wool, silk, leather, cotton, as well as book bindings, depending on their tastes. Even synthetic fabrics are not always safe. What attracts the pests is not the fibers but spots of food, urine, or perspiration—often too small to be noticed by the human eye. Storage of clothing in unheated rooms slows down the life cycle of these insects, but sooner or later the hungry larvae emerge. For many years, people have fought them off with mothballs, but it may be wise to take another tack.

One hazardous aspect of mothballs is that children sometimes swallow them. Some mothballs, including camphor balls, contain naphthalene, which can be fatal to small children who eat them. Even a single mothball can make a child very sick. Cases of infant death have been reported when babies were exposed to clothing and blankets stored with naphthalene mothballs, and whole households have become ill from heavy exposure. Other mothballs contain paradichlorobenzene, which is less toxic if swallowed, but which may be a carcinogen.

These insecticides kill moth larvae and adults when their fumes reach a high enough concentration in a closet or chest. There are no studies of the effects of prolonged exposure of humans to these vapors, but wearing a sweater or sleeping under a blanket that has been stored in mothballs, or spending hours in a room where vapors are in the air, is unpleasant and a risk you don't need to run. Indeed, the manufacturers' labels always advise you to "avoid prolonged breathing of vapor or prolonged contact with the skin," but that's hard to do if clothing or indoor air is permeated with the fumes.

Storing clothes in a cedar chest or cedar closet is a traditional way of insect-proofing. While cedar oil can kill young larvae, it's probably the airtight construction that helps most. If you do use mothballs, be sure to air garments before wearing them. Seal closets with tape to keep vapors inside. And don't use paradichlorobenzene mothballs inside plastic bags—they can break the plastic down and make it stick to the fabric.

Pesticide-free alternatives

•Keep your clothing clean. Before storing, send woolens to the dry cleaner and wash the washables, then store them in a taped box or sealed bag.

• Vacuum often and thoroughly to keep down lint and dust balls, which are hiding places for fabric pests. Empty the vacuum bag frequently, since it may contain larvae or eggs. Keep the floors and walls of closets clean.

Trim vegetables and fruits. Based on federal and California state data, more celery samples contain toxic residues than any other of the twenty-six fruits and vegetables analyzed. But trimming celery tops and leaves gets rid of as much as 50 to 90 percent of some of these. Similarly, careful pruning of the outside layers of other leafy vegetables like lettuces and cabbages removes residues.

Peel anything that has a wax coating. Some nutrients may be tossed out with your apple or cucumber peelings, but so are the surface residues. The wax coating, harmless in itself, not only fends off the hard knocks of shipping and storage but seals in residues, including those left by fungicides.

In states where the term means anything, you may wish to buy "organic" foods. Buying produce raised without chemicals isn't easy to do in many cities or states, and "organically grown" doesn't always mean "pesticide-free." A certification plan is in force in many states to ensure that foods labeled "organic" must not have been raised with pesticides.

Even big grocery chains are beginning to stock organically grown produce. Since you'll probably have to pay a 10 to 20 percent premium for organic fruits and vegetables, try to be sure they really are grown without the aid of chemical fertilizers or pesticides, although this can be difficult to ascertain. You can ask your supermarket produce manager, but be aware that while he may reassure you, he may not really know.

The home garden—no longer a chemical battlefield

Most gardeners are now aware that chemical pesticides can endanger human health as well as kill insects. The trend in gardening is away from chemical use and back to safer and more pleasant alternatives.

According to experts at the University of California, Berkeley, the rationale for using pesticides in home gardens is so weak that you should probably not use them at all. You can adopt gardening methods that will reduce the number of insects and thus the need for pesticides. Spring is the time to begin—but what you do in the fall is important, too.

•Choose a garden site in a well-drained area, and don't overwater. Practice crop rotation. Even in a small garden, this will help keep down specific pests.

•Use a high-quality fertilizer. Healthy plants are more likely to resist diseases and insects. Pull weeds regularly.

•Plant garlic, nasturtiums, onions, or chives around the garden border. They help repel some insects.

•Buy insect- and disease-resistant seedlings when possible.

•If you buy a pesticide, be just as wary of so-called "botanicals," "biologicals," or "natural pesticides" as of manmade chemicals. Whether it occurs in nature or not, a pesticide is a pesticide and can be harmful to people and animals. Pyrethrum and rotenone, for example, classified as natural, are both toxic and not very selective. Be wary of nonselective pesticides and herbicides—the ones that kill a broad spectrum of organisms.

•Neatness counts. Harvest produce as soon as it is ripe. After you finish harvesting, promptly dispose of all crop residues—vines, roots, stems, and leaves. If you have fruit trees, dispose of shriveled fruit on the ground or on branches. Be sure the garden area is free of boards, boxes, stones, and other potential hiding places for insect eggs. Deep tilling in spring and fall will kill many residual pests.

Snakebites

Compared with other risks, such as injuries on the highway, getting bitten by a snake is a pretty remote possibility, unless you handle snakes regularly or camp out for long periods. The bite of a poisonous snake can be painful or even fatal, and requires hospitalization and treatment. Out of about 45,000 snakebites reported every year in the United States, only about 8,000 are venomous. Fewer than twenty people die each year. The great majority of venomous bites occur in the Southern states and the Southwest, including California. Rattlesnakes are responsible for two-thirds of the bites and almost all the deaths. Copperheads, cottonmouths, imported snakes (kept by collectors), and the occasional coral snake account for the rest of the bites. Lore about snakes and snakebites, of course, is richly embroidered.

Here is a small sampling of snakebite myths:
- A snake can't strike more than once.
- A snakebite always consists of two fang marks.
- A venomous snake always injects venom when it bites.
- If you're bitten, it's essential to cut across the fang marks with a razor and suction or suck the venom from the wound.
- If you're bitten, it's essential to cut off all blood flow with a tourniquet. Then ice the wound.

None of these statements is correct or sound advice. Snakes can bite twice in rapid succession, and the wound may consist of tooth marks only, one or more fang marks, or both tooth and fang marks. The wound may be deep or superficial. Even if you're bitten by a viper, you may be lucky: a snake doesn't always inject its venom. Surprisingly, the amount of poison it injects may vary—from none up to a potentially lethal dose. Venoms consist of many proteins and enzymes that can affect blood coagulation, as well as damage the lungs, other organs, and central nervous system. Cutting the wound and sucking the venom should only be done in the most extreme circumstances, when no other help is available. And a tourniquet is not recommended because it can do permanent damage.

Snakebite first aid

If you are certain the snake that bit you was nonvenomous, the bite can be treated like any other wound (including, possibly, a tetanus shot). If you've been bitten by a poisonous snake, or if you're not sure what kind it was, it's important to get medical help at once. Get to the nearest emergency room, preferably with a companion, since you may quickly begin to experience pain and weakness if the snake did inject you with venom. Never try to capture or kill the snake and take it along. That only wastes valuable time and puts you at risk of being bitten again. It's also important to try to immobilize the bitten body part and keep it below heart level. If your foot or leg has been bitten, it's a good idea to be carried, if there's any way to arrange this. Try not to panic—antivenins are available and effective.

If the bite is on the hand or arm, remove rings and other constricting items, since most snakebite wounds will cause swelling. If possible, cleanse the wound with soap and water and cover it with sterile gauze or other clean dressing. If you're caring for a snakebite victim, keep him warm and try to keep him calm. Remember that the most important task is finding medical assistance.

Do not apply ice: this can actually drive the venom deeper, as well as damage tissue if left in place too long. Nor should you apply a tourniquet that shuts off the flow of arterial blood, as this can result in loss of the limb. In very special circumstances—if medical help is more than half an hour away, and if not more than five minutes has elapsed since the bite—use a constricting band around a bitten arm or leg. Apply it two to three inches above the bite and tighten it so that you can still slip two fingers under the band. Check for a pulse below the band to make sure the blood is still circulating, and keep checking periodically. (Pulse points can be felt in the wrist and on the top of the foot above the instep.)

Cutting a wound and sucking out the poison, once thought essential, should be considered only in extreme situations (if you're hours away from medical care, for example), and then only if you have a suction cup, can start treatment within five minutes, and have had some training in the procedure.

And no matter what old-timers do in the movies, don't give a snakebite victim a shot of whiskey or alcohol in any form.

The best treatment: prevention

• If you or an acquaintance keeps snakes as pets, don't handle them until you've had proper training. Never tease or hurt a snake.

• If you see a snake outdoors, stay away from it. Snakes try to avoid people.

• If you're out in the wilderness, wear long pants and footgear that covers your ankles. Thick gloves are practical, too, if you're gathering firewood.

• Be cautious when turning over a rock or a fallen branch. Don't reach or step into dark places, such as heavy underbrush. Make sure you can see what you're getting into. Don't put your hand into rocky crevices while climbing.

• Camp in an open space, and never gather firewood at night.

Tornadoes

According to meteorologists, clashing air masses fueled by warm, moist air from the Gulf of Mexico cause tornadoes in the United States. Tornadoes most commonly strike west Texas, Oklahoma, Arkansas, Missouri, and Kansas. But other areas have also experienced serious tornado outbreaks—Ohio, Illinois, Michigan, Pennsylvania, New York, New England, the Carolinas, the Gulf states, and even parts of Canada. Tornadoes are almost unknown west of the Rockies. An average of 773 tornadoes occur in the United States each year, killing about eighty people and injuring 200 more—one of the highest tolls of all natural disasters. April, May, and June are the prime times with May the peak. But tornadoes occasionally strike in summer or fall and out of their customary area.

Unlike hurricanes, tornadoes often arrive with little warning—the first sign being high winds, flying debris, or the roar of the approaching funnel. A study of a series of tornadoes that killed ninety-one people in the northeastern United States and Canada in 1985 found that only a third of the injured (in one Pennsylvania locality) had known a tornado was on the way. Among survivors interviewed in Ontario, fewer than 10 percent had as much as a five-minute warning that a twister was coming. Most of these people had telephones, television sets, and radios, but because of a power failure, local stations were unable to issue warnings.

However, these and other studies have revealed that people caught in a tornado or violent windstorm can take protective action, if they know in advance what to do.

The right shelter

The main danger in a tornado is being picked up by the wind or hit by flying objects. Thus a basement or cellar is the safest place. Stay away from windows, and if there is no basement or cellar available, go to an interior room on the lowest level of the building you're in. Crouch down and try to protect your head: dragging a mattress over you is a good idea. A closet is a good place to hide, and people have survived by seeking shelter in the bathtub. If you're caught on the street, go to the interior of the nearest building. Staying in a car or truck is not safe. Get out and use whatever time you have to run for cover indoors. If no shelter is in sight, lie flat in a nearby ditch or ravine. Cover your head with your hands. You're better off on the ground than in a vehicle, which might become airborne.

Mobile homes and other poorly anchored houses are the most dangerous locales in severe storms. Government authorities have urged local agencies in tornado-prone states to provide residents of mobile home parks with accessible tornado shelters. If you live in the tornado belt in a mobile home or a house that might easily be pulled off its moorings, find out where the nearest shelter would be—perhaps an office building or nearby school. Ask the local health or police department what tornado safety provisions have been made.

If there's hail or a bad thunderstorm, find out if the weather bureau has declared a tornado watch (the first stage) or issued a tornado warning. Keep a small battery radio in the house; you shouldn't turn on the TV if there's heavy lightning. If you live in a trailer, go to a shelter when warnings are issued—never try to wait it out. If there's no better solution, leave the trailer and lie in the nearest ditch.

A tornado can travel up to seventy miles an hour, and not even the best of meteorologists can predict the course of its winding path.

Transportation

You may think that you have no control over your safety when traveling by car, plane, or boat. But there is a lot you can do to prevent accidents or to lessen your chance of injury should an accident occur. For example, simply by wearing a seat belt every time you get into a car, you can reduce your risk of being injured or killed in an automobile accident by more than half. This chapter begins with a discussion of how to protect yourself in airplanes and boats, and ends with an in-depth look at driving safety.

Airplane Safety

Despite sensational headlines, few people are killed in airplane accidents, and in many cases lives might have been saved if the victims had been ready for an emergency. Unfortunately, many experienced travelers may turn a deaf ear to safety instructions or take a fatalistic attitude toward crashes. You are as safe or safer in a plane than on the highway, yet accidents do happen—usually on takeoff or landing. (In the United States, an air accident is defined as any incident that damages a plane or seriously injures an occupant.)

According to statistics collected by the National Transportation Safety Board, passengers who think ahead systematically about their safety are more likely to emerge from an accident alive and uninjured. As with any emergency, the best advice is to be as well informed as possible and to stay calm. Use the first few minutes on a plane to avail yourself of all safety instructions, make a plan, and commit it to memory. The following steps will keep you prepared for an emergency:

•After you take your seat, find the nearest exit and mentally rehearse the path you would take to get there. Count the number of rows to the exit so you could find it if the lights were out. According to the National Transportation Safety Board, fifty people who died in a post-crash fire in a DC-10 at Malaga, Spain, in 1982 were sitting in the back of the plane and had failed to move up the aisle to the nearest available exit.

•When you sit down, fasten your seat belt as tight as tolerable around your hips. Make sure that you can unfasten it easily. Remember that a loose seat belt will not keep you from lunging forward during an abrupt stop. Instead, the belt may slide over your stomach and cause internal injuries. As the pilot may remind you, it pays to keep your belt fastened throughout the flight. A National Transportation Safety Board study showed that in thirty-five turbulence accidents from 1977 to 1983, no injuries occurred to those who were snugly buckled in.

•Although it may not be exciting reading, study the seat-pocket card. No matter how many times you've heard them before, listen to the flight attendant's instructions. Different airplanes may have different safety procedures.

•If you are traveling with a small child, airlines are required to allow you to bring a regulation car safety seat on board. To exercise this option, you may have to purchase a ticket for a child under two years of age (who otherwise may be able to fly for free). Check with the airline to see if a ticket is necessary. Also check the labels on your car seat; since 1985, seats providing acceptable protection carry labels stating that they meet Federal motor vehicle safety standards and that they are certified for use on aircraft.

•If possible, wear comfortable clothing, including shoes that you can easily walk or run in. High heels reduce your stability in the aisles, even on an uneventful flight, and could seriously hamper a quick getaway via the exit door and chute.

•If your oxygen mask drops during the flight, don't wait to be told to use it. If cabin pressure is dropping at 40,000 feet, you'll have only about fifteen seconds to put on the mask before the reduced pressure will begin to affect you. You must pull the tube to start the flow of oxygen. If traveling with children, put your own mask on before you assist them with theirs.

•In any kind of airplane accident, the greatest danger is fire. Don't stop to gather your belongings. Proceed toward the exit door as quickly as possible and, since smoke rises, keep your head low.

•In an emergency landing, brace yourself against impact. If the seats are close together, cross your arms on the top of the seat in front of you and put your head on your arms; if the seats are well apart, place your head on your knees and wrap your arms around your legs. In both cases keep your feet flat on the floor, slightly ahead of the seat edge.

Driving a boat when you're drunk is just as dangerous as driving a car while intoxicated, and will often incur the same penalty. Many states consider a boating DWI (driving while intoxicated) conviction to be the same as a DWI motor vehicle offense.

Boating Safety

Careless handling, oversized motors, overloading, hazardous water conditions, and alcohol consumption can all turn a boating outing into an accident. The National Safe Boating Council estimates that alcohol is involved in more than half of all boating accidents. In most cases in which a boating accident results in death, the victim could have been saved by a life preserver. Federal law requires life preservers—personal flotation devices—on all recreational boats. Unfortunately, too many people don't have the proper flotation devices or don't use them.

There are two basic types of life preservers: wearable models and models designed for throwing and grasping. The law requires that boats sixteen feet long and over must carry one wearable for each passenger, and at least one throwable per boat. Boats less than sixteen feet long are not required to carry wearable models—but they should, since nearly half of the fatalities involve smaller boats.

Test the buoyancy of your life preserver in shallow water before setting out; it should keep your head above the surface. On board, wear it at all times. And follow these other tips to avoid falling overboard: cross other boats' wakes at a right angle; crouch, don't stand up when changing position; don't hang over the sides or ends of a boat. Above all, limit your alcohol intake.

Driving Safety

Driving really is safer than it used to be. The experts know more than they did twenty years ago about safe driving— highway and automotive research has paid

The Low-Risk Driver

According to statistics, driving is on average about ten times more dangerous than traveling by plane or train. But that's average: if you are a low-risk driver, according to General Motors researchers, you are more than 1,000 times less likely to die in a car crash than a high-risk driver. Thus automobile travel for a low-risk driver may be no more risky than travel by plane or train.

Who is a low-risk driver? The researchers defined him or her as a forty-year-old who is sober when driving and wears a seat belt. Travel on rural interstate highways in a heavy car lowers the risk even more, though these factors are less important than, for instance, age, sobriety, or wearing a seat belt.

The high-risk driver, in contrast, was defined as an eighteen-year-old, intoxicated male traveling on average roads in a light-weight car without wearing a seat belt. Of course, luck is always involved: anyone could be hit by a car driven by a drunk teenager. Even then, though, you would be more likely to survive if you take care of the factors that are in your control, such as wearing a seat belt and driving only when sober.

Be extra careful driving during the first half hour of a rainfall. A little water plus the oil and dirt on the road form a slick film. This film is eventually washed away in a heavy rain.

dividends, and much of the new knowledge has been put to practical use. Cars are better engineered than ever, and safety has become a more important issue for car makers and buyers. Seat belts are standard equipment, and 90 percent of new 1994 cars now have at least one air bag. Better roads, better laws and law enforcement, and education programs, as well as increases in the legal drinking age, have also played their role. Thus fatalities on American roads have declined. In 1992 and 1993 they numbered about 40,000—the lowest since 1961 (and there are more than twice as many vehicles on the road now).

Still, the driver is the most important key to traffic safety. Driving an automobile, or even riding in one, may be the most dangerous thing you do on a regular basis. At some point in their lives, according to the National Traffic Safety Institute, half of all Americans will be involved in a serious car crash, or will have an immediate family member involved in one.

When you hear the words "car crash," you probably picture a car smashing head-on into something, perhaps a telephone pole. But side-impact crashes—usually one in which a car runs a traffic light or stop sign at an intersection and barrels into another auto—are also common, especially in drivers over age fifty. Such side-impact crashes cause nearly half of all serious or fatal automobile injuries, and account for some 8,000 deaths in the United States each year. Side-impact and frontal crashes are very different. Knowing which kind you're most likely to be in may help you be on your guard and take precautions.

Side-impact crashes. About 76 percent of these involve drivers over the age of fifty, and 28 percent of the drivers are over seventy. Two reasons that may account for the higher risk in older drivers are age-related vision and reflex changes and unfamiliarity with traffic safety rules. Side crashes most often occur during the day and infrequently involve alcohol or drug use. In 69 percent of the crashes, the driver of the struck car was at fault because of a driving error; in 17 percent of the cases, this driver committed a traffic violation. Slightly more than half of the resulting injuries involve the chest and abdomen.

Frontal crashes (single vehicle). These generally involve young drivers; only 26 percent of the resulting fatalities occur in people over age fifty, and only 8 percent in those over age seventy. Most of these crashes are alcohol or drug related. The majority occur at night, and often involve head injuries.

How to handle troublesome situations

Driving defensively means that you avoid putting yourself in dangerous situations, and you know how to react intelligently in a crisis, should one develop. Learning to drive defensively could be one of the most important actions you could take. Think of it this way: the safest driver of all may well be the professional racer. Although he's going well over 150 miles per hour, he's wearing several seat belts, the chassis in his vehicle is a cage of steel tubing, and most importantly, he's trained to react to danger up ahead. We can't all be race-car drivers; yet we could be better drivers than we are. Below are some common situations that routinely give people trouble:

Braking. The safest way to brake is to do so as far in advance as possible. A basic principle of defensive driving is never to get into a situation that calls for slamming on the brakes. This can throw you into a skid (see below) that may injure you and your passengers. Good breaking technique is to pump the brakes repeatedly until you come to a full stop. If you are forced to brake fast, "threshold" braking is the best technique: push the brake just short of locking and hold it there.

Antilock brakes can make braking quickly safer. These brakes detect potential skids and react accordingly, pulsing the brake power and bringing the vehicle to a faster, safer stop than conventional brakes, especially in hazardous road conditions such as ice and snow. Antilocks are now standard equipment in many car models and an option in others, at a cost of $700 to $1,000. About half of the new cars on American roads have this feature.

But antilock brakes do not mean you needn't worry about skids, nor do they shorten braking time in all situations. If any wheel is about to lose traction and lock, thus potentially throwing the car into a skid, the control unit reduces brake pressure very briefly so that the tire regains traction, and you stay in control. When you are braking on wet or icy pavement, this can be the crucial factor in preventing a skid. But if you are driving fast on a slick road, antilocks are not magic. And on a dry surface, where wheels are less likely to lock, your car will stop as fast without antilock brakes as with them.

You may assume that on a slick road you should brake gently or pump your brakes to prevent a skid, just as you would without antilocks, but in fact you need continuous brake pressure to activate the system. Pumping the brake is what antilocks do for you. If you do the pumping, the system won't work.

Skidding. To avoid skidding, be aware of dangerous situations such as a wet or icy highway, leaves on the road, or a sharp curve ahead. Keep your speed reasonable for

---

Avoiding Animals

Each year more than 10,000 Americans are injured and 120 are killed in collisions with animals. In many states across the country, deer have become a special problem because their population has risen in recent years—not just in rural areas but in many suburban areas as well.

If you're coming up on an animal in the road, don't assume that it will get out of your way. The American Automobile Association recommends that you tap lightly on the horn well in advance when approaching a large animal. And, if traveling at night, flick your lights from bright to dim, since animals are attracted to—and often become immobilized by—headlights. Slamming on the brakes and swerving to avoid the animal is especially dangerous at night and on a wet or icy road; you may crash into another car or a tree. Under these conditions, travel at low speeds so that you can safely steer clear of the animal if need be.

road conditions. Avoid sudden braking, accelerating, or shifting to a lower gear. Smooth and precise driving will help you avoid skids. Try to avoid getting in a situation where you need to slam on the brakes. If you have antilock brakes and have to make an emergency stop, don't pump the brakes. The antilock system will pump them for you. If you don't have antilocks, do pump. But skids can happen to even the most careful driver.

•If you do skid, try to stay calm. Take your foot off the brake and the accelerator. Shift to neutral. Look and steer in the direction you want the front of the car to go. As soon as the wheels grip the road again, return to driving gear and slowly accelerate.

Tailgating. Following the car in front of you at a safe distance gives you room to stop in case of an unforeseen emergency. (One of the riskiest things a driver can do is to tailgate.) To be sure you're following at a safe distance, pick out some definite marker (a driveway, a bridge abutment, a sign) on the road ahead, and when the car in front of you passes it, start counting seconds, "one thousand and one, one thousand and two." Two seconds should elapse before your own car reaches the marker. In bad weather, when it's harder to stop, make it four seconds. That gives you a safety cushion of space.

Instead of tailgating, develop the habit of allowing more space between you and the car ahead. If you are following a car that signals a turn, you can actually gain time by allowing a wide gap between your car and his, since you won't have to reduce your speed as much or brake as hard. When the turn is completed, you'll still be traveling faster than the turning car. You can easily come back up to speed, and you'll have saved both time and fuel.

If someone is tailgating you and the car in front of you is at a safe distance away, tap the brakes and start to slow down—gradually, keeping an eye on the rearview mirror. If the tailgater is daydreaming, tapping your brakes (and activating the brake lights) should wake him up. If he's being aggressive, you've politely signaled him to let up. If he doesn't stop tailgating, pull over as soon as you can and let him pass.

Highway driving. Contrary to popular opinion, statistics show that six-lane highways are safer than smaller roads. Many people find highways intimidating simply because they use them infrequently. Gaining experience will boost your confidence. Ask an experienced highway driver to accompany you and advise you about any weak points in your driving skills.

Changing lanes. When preparing to change lanes on a multilane highway, you should turn on your directional signal, check your mirrors, be aware of the traffic in front of you, and take your eyes off the road momentarily to glance over your shoulder at the lane you're planning to move into. Many people forget this last step, but it's essential. You always have a blind spot (about a car length behind you on either side) and may not be able to see an overtaking vehicle in either mirror.

Older drivers often fail to look to the rear when changing lanes because of stiffness in the neck or upper body. If you have problems looking behind you, it may be wise to invest in a large, wide-angle rearview mirror and a right-side exterior mirror. Flexibility exercises may also help relieve stiffness.

Inclement weather. At least one out of every ten automobile accidents can be attributed to adverse weather conditions. Many of these accidents occur because drivers fail to prepare their cars for winter driving or are unfamiliar with winter

Air pressure in tires

An underinflated tire is more likely to overheat and possibly blow out at high speeds, and is more likely to skid on a wet surface. Underinflation also decreases fuel efficiency. According to a 1991 report from the American Automobile Association almost 40 percent of cars tested at a diagnostic center had underinflated tires. Look in your owner's manual for recommended pressures. A tire can look perfectly okay and still be underinflated. Overinflation is undesirable, too, since it makes for a hard ride and wears the tire out faster.

Check pressure with a gauge once a month—and don't forget to check the spare.

Myth: Drunk drivers don't get hurt in car crashes.

Fact: Drunk drivers aren't only more apt to be in a car crash, they are more likely to be hurt or killed in one.

Many people think that alcohol somehow "limbers up" a person and protects him from serious harm, but according to one study that examined over a million accidents involving one or two vehicles, the opposite is true. When all other factors were equal, drinking drivers were injured or killed more often than nondrinking drivers, and their injuries were likely to be more severe. Head injuries were more likely to be fatal to drinkers because alcohol makes brain tissue swell.

Surprisingly, drinkers tended to sustain severe injuries even in low speed, low damage crashes, which suggests that alcohol in the blood enhances the degree of any injury that occurs. Although the study didn't compare the fate of intoxicated and sober passengers, the researchers theorized that drinkers, even when not driving, would be more susceptible to injury.

driving techniques. It doesn't have to snow for the road to be slippery—rain can create treacherous conditions, especially on heavily used roads. The main precautions you can take involve your driving skills. Adjust your speed according to the road conditions. Even if the speed limit is fifty-five, drive at forty-five or even slower if conditions are bad. The best rule is to not do anything suddenly. That includes changing lanes, slamming on the brakes, and jackrabbit starts. In slippery conditions, avoid braking on a curve. When you have to slow down, shift to a lower gear instead of braking. When you must use the brakes on a slippery surface, depress and release the brake pedal repeatedly and gently. In fog or snow, don't use high beams; the light just reflects back at you. You'll see farther with low beams.

In addition, take these precautions:

Use snow tires. Radial tires are not snow tires. You can get away with so-called "all-weather radials" only if you live in an area that doesn't get much snow. If there's a heavy snowfall, you need snow tires. It's best to put them on all four wheels, but you must put them at least on the drive wheels. Check tire pressure periodically. Air contracts in cold weather and tires lose about one pound of pressure for every drop of ten degrees, so you may have to add air in very cold weather to maintain the right pressure. Some people let a little air out of their tires, thinking mistakenly that this improves traction because more tire surface will come in contact with the road. It's the worst thing you can do. (This goes for very hot weather as well.) Keep tires at the recommended maximum air pressure, and check them weekly.

Clean off snow. If it snows, clear off the car completely, including all lights and windows, the hood, and roof, so that blowing snow will not obscure your vision. If your car has recessed wipers, make sure they are not frozen in place. You can burn out the wiper motor or blow a fuse if you turn on the wipers when they're frozen.

Driving and alcohol and drugs

Most people are aware of the dangers of driving after drinking alcohol. But they may not know how alcohol affects your driving abilities, or how other drugs—such as marijuana, cocaine, and even some prescription and over-the-counter drugs, such as cold preparations—can significantly decrease driving performance.

Alcohol. Alcohol does not affect your abilities equally. Simple perception— seeing and hearing—is affected least of all, at least at low levels of alcohol consumption. But your ability to process the information you receive and to perform complex tasks based on that information begins to be impaired at blood alcohol levels slightly above 0.05 percent (more than one drink per hour for a 160-pound man). At slightly higher levels, up to 0.10 percent (two or three drinks an hour), your vigilance and accuracy are reduced, your reaction time is significantly lengthened, and your short-term memory is impaired. While alcohol may not immediately affect your simple skills, it quite quickly and insidiously impairs your ability to make quick decisions.

Alcohol affects different parts of your body at different rates because of variations in the way alcohol is distributed by the blood. Blood-rich organs, such as the brain and lungs, get the highest dose earliest, and the central nervous system is affected faster than the muscles and skeleton. If you think of your brain as a computer, alcohol doesn't shut the whole mechanism down until you've drunk a lot, but simply short-circuits it—usually without your being aware of what's happening to you.

Don't drive if you've gotten drunk—not even the next morning. One study found that driving ability is still impaired the following day. Performance results of a driving test declined 20 percent even after participants had a chance to sleep it off. Even those who said they didn't have a hangover performed as poorly as those who said they felt awful.

Planning Trips

The following tips will help keep long car trips safe and enjoyable:

Give your car a complete physical. Check your tires for tread depth and keep them inflated to the required tire pressure. Don't forget to check the spare tire, too. Make sure your windshield wipers are in good condition and that you have plenty of wiper fluid. Clean your car windows inside and out—dirty windows greatly impair your vision. Have a mechanic give your car a good once-over, paying special attention to the braking system. In cold weather, keep at least a half tank of gas in your car at all times. If the gas tank is less full, the gas line can freeze.

Take along emergency provisions. In winter, pack a blanket, first-aid supplies, a flashlight, an ice scraper, some crackers, chocolate bars, or other high-energy foods, and some bottled water in case bad weather strikes and you have to stay in your car. Keep these items in your back seat—you may not be able to reach your trunk in a storm. In your trunk, you may want to have the following on hand: a shovel, emergency flares, sand or tracking mats, and jumper cables.

Make sure you are well rested. Get enough sleep the night before you drive. Stop every two or three hours to stretch your muscles. Trying to cover too much distance in one day causes tension and fatigue. The National Safety Council recommends that you drive no more than seven or eight hours a day.

Avoid taking any over-the-counter cold remedies when driving. These medications often contain antihistamines, which can cause drowsiness. Indeed, any medication may affect your driving skills. If you're taking a new medication, avoid driving until you know how it will affect you.

Keep the car properly ventilated. Carbon monoxide from the car's exhaust can cause drowsiness. Even on the coldest days, leave your car windows open a crack. Fresh air will help keep you awake.

Stay alert. "Highway hypnosis"—the trancelike state caused by the monotony of driving over miles of roadway—impairs your judgment and cuts down on your reaction time. Avoid continuously staring at the road ahead—look in your rearview and sideview mirrors frequently. Listen to the radio, sing, or carry on a conversation with others in the car. Be aware of your surroundings.

Avoid arguing with your car mates. Anger and frustration can temporarily impair your driving ability and may cause you to take risks you normally would not take. If heavy traffic is getting to you, pull off the highway and take a breather.

Thus you may not be the best judge of whether or not you are able to drive safely.

Just as alcohol affects your brain and body at different rates, the level in your blood is not entirely predictable. Factors such as body size, alcohol concentration per drink, other drugs used, how well you feel, how tired you are, if you ate while you drank, and how fast you drank are all important, too. People with the same blood alcohol level will behave differently. And remember, any level of alcohol in your blood will lead to some deterioration of your driving ability.

If you think you may have to drive after drinking, follow these rules:

•Don't drink on an empty stomach. Milk and cheese, or any large or especially fatty meal, can lengthen the time the alcohol takes to get into the blood.

•Don't consume more than one drink per hour. Intersperse the alcohol with something nonalcoholic.

•Don't depend on caffeine to counteract the effects of alcohol. It won't.

•Don't mix alcohol with marijuana or other drugs.

Even if you've followed the four rules above, you should still wait at least an hour after your last drink before driving. Be honest: if you don't succeed in following this plan, don't drive. Best plan of all: if you're driving, drink no alcohol at all.

Marijuana. The effect of marijuana on the smoker's ability to drive or operate machinery is harder to gauge than that of alcohol. The principal mind-altering ingredient in marijuana, known as THC (tetrahydrocannabinol), passes rapidly from the bloodstream into the brain and fatty tissue. But unlike alcohol, which is flushed out of the system fairly quickly, THC may linger for days or even weeks. Studies have shown that intoxication can return—for no apparent reason—even when a person has not recently smoked.

Marijuana definitely decreases performance, but not in any consistent relationship to THC blood levels. Unlike testing for blood alcohol levels, there's no simple way to tell if someone has been using marijuana. The marijuana user won't have a telltale breath or slurred speech. Rather than disturbing the simple motor skills involved in driving, marijuana seems to interfere with perception and attention processes. In combination with alcohol, it can be extremely deleterious to judgment and performance.

Thus, though the effects of marijuana on driver performance are hard to measure precisely, they can certainly endanger human life. And these effects may even be delayed and unpredictable. Anyone who has recently smoked marijuana—let alone a habitual user—should not drive.

Legal medications. Some prescription drugs—such as some blood pressure medications and sleeping pills (even one taken the night before) and many over-the-counter drugs, such as cold, sinus, or hay fever preparations—can cause drowsiness and greatly reduce your driving ability. If you take any medication, even occasionally, discuss the possible effects on your driving with your physician or pharmacist.

Staying awake and alert

Falling asleep while driving is a leading cause of car crashes and, after alcohol, the second most common cause of vehicle fatalities. It's thought that drowsy drivers cause 600,000 crashes a year and 12,000 highway deaths.

Fatigue, the monotony of the road, the drone of the engine, an uncomfortably warm or stuffy environment, an alcoholic drink (even one you might have had many hours before driving), lack of sleep, and some medications can all produce

One defensive driving tip comes from a course for individuals over age fifty sponsored by the American Association for Retired Persons: it is safer to drive a white, beige, or yellow car because it is easier for other drivers to see it.

drowsiness. Some drivers believe that using the cruise control makes them drowsy, though there's no scientific evidence for this. Anybody who is deprived of sleep, feeling under par, or taking tranquilizers or other medications that affect alertness—or who has been driving too long and finds his eyes drooping. Sleep disorders or chronic insomnia can contribute, but fatigue is usually the main cause.

Your first reaction to feeling drowsy should be to pull safely over to the roadside and take stock. Obviously, if you have a passenger who's also a qualified driver, change drivers. If not, consider stopping for the night. Or find a secure place (a roadside rest area, for example, but not the shoulder of an expressway) and take a nap in the locked car. When you wake up, take a walk if possible, or do some stretching or other simple exercises in the car. Have something to eat and drink (nonalcoholic) as soon as you can. Music can be helpful if you play it loudly and sing along, and so can opening the window and letting fresh air hit your face.

Generally speaking, it's good policy not to drive long hours after dark, or to leave for a long drive Friday night after work. If you do plan to drive long distances, don't drink alcohol—even the day before. Don't drive at all if you're taking medications that induce drowsiness. Don't rely on any kind of drug to keep you awake; if you're really tired, even caffeine won't keep you from falling asleep. Whether you feel sleepy or not, it's always wise to break up a long drive with rest stops, occasional snacks, and some stretching or walking outside the car.

Check your night vision

Few people realize that even though they may have 20/20 vision in daytime, their nighttime vision will have considerably lessened by the time they turn forty, and this is something that the motor vehicle department seldom tests. According to the latest figures from the National Safety Council, nighttime accidents account for about 25 percent more fatalities than daytime accidents. Although factors such as exhaustion and alcohol play a role in this, no driver can see as well at night as in the day. One study has shown that 87 percent of all drivers who hit a pedestrian at night said they didn't see the person in time—while only 11 percent of daytime drivers made the same claim.

The speed with which the eye accommodates itself to darkness starts decreasing in young adulthood. In daytime, the retina resolves visual data primarily by means of a specialized set of cells called cones, but at nighttime, it relies chiefly on another, more sensitive set called rods. The older you are, the longer it may take to make the switch, which could make driving more difficult along a road where light conditions are changing rapidly. Along with a decline in the eye's ability to accommodate itself to darkness comes a drop in visual acuity in early adulthood, and night vision deteriorates faster than daytime vision. It is possible your ability to perceive a pedestrian or some potential hazard in the darkness up ahead on a country road may start to decline when you are in your twenties. It will be greatly reduced by the time you are fifty or so. Most people become aware of this at about age forty.

This need not be a disaster, however, for driver awareness of reduced night vision is thought to be the best protection of all. Research shows that drivers who realize they have poor night vision voluntarily reduce night driving trips or eliminate them completely.

If you must drive at night, drive more slowly and carefully. Even under ideal

It's not true that you are safer being thrown clear of a car rather than being strapped into it by a seat belt. You are twenty-five times more likely to be fatally injured if ejected than if you stay inside and are buckled up.

conditions no one can spot a pedestrian at night much farther away than 300 feet—and if you are driving 55 miles per hour, it will take more than 300 feet to bring your car to a stop. Unless there is an approaching car, use your high beams—but remember that your headlights may temporarily blind a pedestrian. And keep your dashboard lights low so that your eyes are not constantly readjusting from light to darkness.

Protecting yourself in a crash

Even the best driver in the world needs to protect himself in case of a car crash; your driving skills may be first rate, but you cannot always avoid a driver who isn't in your league. Other drivers may not pay attention to the road, ignore traffic signals, loose control of their car, or drive while intoxicated. The two best ways to prevent injury and protect your life are wearing a seat belt and driving a car with an airbag.

Seat belts

There is no doubt: if you are in a car crash, a properly worn seat belt can reduce the severity of injury and indeed may save your life. According to the National Highway Traffic Safety Administration, in the event of a crash, wearing a lap-shoulder belt reduces your chances of being injured or killed by 57 percent. If everyone wore a seat belt every time they drove or rode in a car, about 17,000 lives would be saved every year.

And yet, despite the overwhelming evidence in their favor, many people still do not wear seat belts. Even in states with mandatory seat belt laws, front seat belts are used only about half the time.

Despite the benefits of seat belts, however, they must be worn properly to be effective. The following tips will help ensure correct seat belt use:

• Wear the seat belt low across the pelvis, not the abdomen. In a crash, the belt can exert a pressure equal to twenty to fifty times your body weight, and only the pelvis can withstand this load. If the belt is worn higher (across the abdomen) and the car stops suddenly, the belt can cause serious injury to internal organs.

• Sit upright. If you slump, the belt can slide up the pelvis onto the soft abdominal wall.

• Keep the belt tight. Some people wear belts loosely just to comply with seat belt laws. A loose belt offers little protection and may, in fact, compound injuries in a crash. An occupant can be thrown forcefully against the belt itself, or can slide forward under the loose belt and suffer head or neck injuries from the shoulder strap.

• Never wear the shoulder strap under your arm or across your neck. Some people complain about neck, shoulder, or breast irritation because of the shoulder strap and find that they can avoid this by wearing the strap under the arm instead of over the shoulder. However, in a crash, wearing the strap under the arm can concentrate pressure on the abdomen, diaphragm, and lungs. In many cases in which fatal injuries were caused by underarm positioning of shoulder straps, the victims probably would have survived had they worn the straps correctly.

When properly worn, the strap rests on the middle of the collarbone and the upper chest, both of which are better suited to absorb the strap's pressure. It must never cross at the neck. It's essential for short people to have the shoulder portion

It is impossible to hold a child in your arms in the event of a collision. For example, the momentum of a crash or even a sudden stop can launch a twenty-pound baby forward with a force equivalent to 400 pounds. And if you're not wearing a seat belt, your body could crush the child against the dashboard.

Seat Belts: Special Concerns

Pregnant women

Use of a seat belt is imperative for the safety of both the woman and her fetus. There's no evidence that a seat belt increases the risk of injury to the fetus or uterus, even in an accident, according to the American College of Obstetricians and Gynecologists. The fetus is well protected in a fluid-filled sac in a very elastic uterus, which is cushioned by surrounding organs, muscle, and bones. In a crash the fetus may be squeezed by the seat belt for a short time, but it almost always recovers quickly.

The fetus is at much greater risk when the mother doesn't wear a seat belt. *The leading cause of fetal death or injury in a crash is death or injury of the mother.* Since a seat belt ensures the safety of the mother, doctors strongly recommend wearing one during the entire pregnancy—including the ride to the hospital for the birth.

For maximum protection, wear the belt under your abdomen—across your upper thighs and as low on your hips as possible—and wear the shoulder strap across your shoulder and chest. Never wear the lap belt above your abdomen or too loosely, which may injure your ribs or abdomen. Place the strap between your breasts; there should be less than three inches of slack between the strap and chest.

Children

Automobile accidents are the leading cause of death and serious injury for children over six months old. All states now require children to ride buckled up—yet surveys show that many children travel without any restraints at all.

Children over age four who have outgrown infant or toddler safety seats pose a special problem. As with adults, the complete protection provided by lap-shoulder straps is better than lap-only belts, but shoulder straps tend to cross over young children's necks or faces. In any case, few cars have rear-seat shoulder straps. The solution is to put a child (four to eight years old, forty to sixty-five pounds) in a restraining device called a "booster seat," such as the two below.

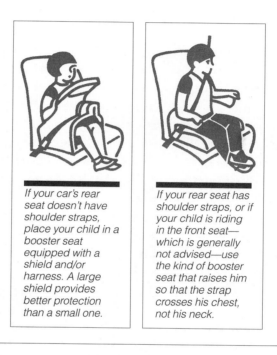

If your car's rear seat doesn't have shoulder straps, place your child in a booster seat equipped with a shield and/or harness. A large shield provides better protection than a small one.

If your rear seat has shoulder straps, or if your child is riding in the front seat—which is generally not advised—use the kind of booster seat that raises him so that the strap crosses his chest, not his neck.

Seventy-five percent of all car crashes involving injury or death occur within twenty-five miles of home. More than half occur at speeds under forty miles per hour.

of the three-point strap lowered so that it doesn't choke them. This can easily be done by the dealer who sold you your car.

If the shoulder strap causes irritation, try keeping a little slack in it—no more than two inches of slack, however—just enough to allow you to place your fist between the strap and your chest. Or place a piece of foam rubber under the strap where it's bothering you.

Rear seat belts. Controversy has continued about the safety of using seat belts without shoulder straps in the rear seat, ever since the National Transportation Safety Board reported that lap-only belts can cause severe and fatal injuries in serious head-on collisions. No one doubts that combination lap-shoulder straps are safer than lap-only belts, and therefore the major auto makers are planning to phase in rear-seat shoulder harnesses as standard equipment. Some auto companies now offer to refit cars with shoulder strap units. However, these units aren't available for all makes and models, and some dealers don't stock them. In the meantime, most evidence suggests that you're better off wearing lap-only belts than wearing no belt at all. Using the belt properly, as described on page 596, should minimize the risk of belt-induced injury.

Airbags

The experts know that the death and serious injury rate from head-on automobile crashes could be halved if all motorists used three-point lap-shoulder belts in combination with an airbag that inflates automatically in head-on collisions. Indeed, if everyone used seat belts and all cars were equipped with airbags, it would save an estimated 9,000 lives and prevent 150,000 serious injuries each year. Currently, more than 90 percent of all new 1994 cars have at least one airbag.

At a speed of only thirty miles per hour, a 150-pound passenger involved in a car crash will hit the dashboard or steering wheel with a force of 4,500 pounds. A combination lap-shoulder belt does something to soften the blow, but an airbag can do more. An airbag is a tough cloth bag usually concealed in the steering wheel. Activated by a crash sensor, the bag inflates automatically with harmless nitrogen gas to cushion the driver on impact. Some people imagine that the bag would pin them against the seat, but deflation occurs within a second.

Another worry has been that the bags might inflate unpredictably, or be triggered by a quick stop or low-speed accident. But there's almost no chance that this would happen. Airbag-equipped Mercedes-Benz cars, according to a company report, have logged some five billion miles with no inadvertent deployments. Even if an airbag inflated for no apparent reason, tests have shown that it would not cause you to lose control of your car.

But remember, airbags protect only in head-on collisions—your seat belt is still your first line of defense. With a seat belt you'll be 42 percent safer in a crash than without one; in a head-on crash or one from a front angle, an air bag adds another 5 percent to that equation. If you have an air bag but don't buckle up, you're settling for just an 18 percent increase in safety. An air bag is designed to inflate only in frontal crashes. It won't protect you the way a seat belt does. People who have

Can airbags cause injury?

Injuries caused by inflating airbags are rare, and the great majority of those reported have been minor bruises or abrasions. In addition, those who were injured were often not wearing seat belts. Besides buckling up, you can protect yourself against any possible air bag injury by positioning your seat as far back from the steering wheel as is comfortable. If you're short, adjust the seat upward, or sit on a cushion so that an inflating air bag would not hit you in the face. Seat belts and air bags do not guarantee, of course, that you won't be hurt in a very severe crash. Indeed, preliminary data indicate that leg or internal injuries may occur in the kind of crash that would have been fatal without a seat belt and air bag.

No child in a safety seat should ride in the front, particularly if you have a passenger-side air bag. Inflating air bags can injure an infant.

Are Big Cars Safer?

Fatality statistics clearly show that large heavy cars are safer than small lightweight ones. Indeed the American Automobile Association recommends a larger car for older drivers, not only on grounds of safety, but also for ease in getting in and out. But because so many variables affect car safety, the data are hard to interpret. True, all things being equal, a heavier car will be safer than a lighter one, since it's a law of physics that the heavy car will be better able to absorb the force of impact than the small one. But in the real world all things seldom are equal.

The size of the car (wheel base) or interior volume, for instance, may be just as important as its weight; for one thing, large cars have more "crush space" to absorb the forces of a crash, and are less likely to roll over in a crash than narrow cars. Complicating matters is the fact that different makes and kinds of cars are driven by different kinds of people. Young men, who are the riskiest drivers by far, tend to choose small cars, especially sporty high-performance models, while older, cautious drivers select big cars. Thus certain models have lower rates of seat-belt use and higher rates of drunk driving. So the accident statistics may say as much about the personality and driving patterns of people who buy a particular make as about the safety of the car itself.

When all is said and done, the weight of your car is only one factor in determining your overall risk while driving. How you drive is almost always more important than what you drive.

been in crashes where their air bags deployed usually love them: 96 percent of a group surveyed said they'd definitely want an air bag in their next car.

Think of air bags as additional protection in a kind of crash that's unlikely to happen anyway.

Older drivers

There is no set age at which an older person should stop driving. Today there are 30 million licensed drivers over sixty-five in the United States, and some of them drive safely into their eighties. When all accident and injury rates are taken into consideration, older drivers are about as bad as those under twenty-four. While teenage drivers have the highest rate of traffic injuries (mile for mile), drivers age seventy-five and over have the highest fatality rate. And those over sixty-five are involved in a third more driving fatalities than forty-year-olds. That's why insurance companies may raise rates steadily for older customers or cancel policies after the slightest fender-bender. Still, a recent Canadian study showed that while seniors' crash records were worse than those in their forties, their poor performance was largely attributable to drivers over seventy-five. But though the crash and fatality rates may be high among seniors, the number of crashes and deaths are relatively low because such older drivers usually limit the time they spend on the road.

Reduced vision and reduced reaction times that come with aging are common problems in older drivers. So are decreased head and neck mobility. If you're wondering whether to continue driving, or are trying to make this decision for someone in the family, the driver's state of health is important. You may need a physician's advice. Use of prescription drugs (especially tranquilizers) may seriously affect driving abilities, and older drivers on medication should always ask how it might affect driving skills and should read package inserts as well. (Those starting new medications should inquire particularly about possible drug interactions.)

A study done for the American Automobile Association at West Virginia University found that while older drivers were generally less proficient than younger ones at handling vehicles, older drivers who rated high on cardiovascular fitness (that is, people who exercised as opposed to the sedentary) were better drivers than others the same age. Drivers in this study improved after following an exercise program designed to improve flexibility and observational skills, and to reduce the emotional stress that often plagues older drivers.

Glossary

Words in italics in the definition of a term are defined elsewhere in the glossary.

A

Abduction. Movement of limbs away from the midline of the body.

Achilles tendinitis. Inflammation of the Achilles *tendon,* which connects the calf muscles to the bones of the foot. This stress injury is most often due to tight calf muscles and is common among runners.

Acquired immune deficiency syndrome (AIDS). A fatal, incurable disease caused by a blood-borne virus (called *HIV* or human immunodeficiency virus) that attacks and eventually destroys the body's immune system. AIDS is transmitted via bodily fluids primarily through sexual relations and also by contaminated hypodermic needles and syringes, and blood transfusions if donated blood is contaminated. In addition, it can be contracted in utero or during birth.

Acute mountain sickness (AMS). A condition, characterized by shortness of breath, fatigue, headaches, nausea, and other flu-like symptoms, that occurs at high altitudes due to a lack of oxygen. Most people don't experience symptoms until they reach heights well above five thousand feet.

Adduction. Movement of limbs toward the midline of the body.

Adipose cells. Specialized cells in the body that store *fat.*

Aerobic exercise. Continuous rhythmic exercise using the large muscles of the body over an extended period of time. Aerobic exercise increases the body's demand for oxygen, thereby adding to the workload of the heart and lungs, and elevating the heart rate. Among its many benefits, it strengthens the *cardiovascular* system and allows the body to burn *fat* for energy. Aerobic activities include brisk walking, running, swimming, cycling, and cross-country skiing.

Aflatoxin. A toxin produced by several species of fungus that grow on some crops, especially peanuts, but also on wheat, corn, beans, and rice. It is known to injure the liver and may be a factor in liver *cancer* if ingested in large quantities.

Amino acids. Building blocks of *protein* molecules that are necessary for every bodily function. There are twenty different types of amino acids, which come in two forms: nonessential, which the body can produce; and essential, which the body must extract from foods.

Anaerobic exercise. Exercise in which energy is released without the use of oxygen. *Glycogen* is the primary fuel. Activities that require short bursts of energy, such as weight lifting, sprinting, and *calisthenics,* are anaerobic.

Anaphylactic shock. An overreaction of the immune system that occurs in some people in response to a substance that the person has been previously sensitized to, such as an insect sting from a bee or wasp or drugs like penicillin. This overreaction causes nausea, flushing, depressed blood pressure, irregular heartbeat, vomiting, and difficult breathing, and may lead to coma or death.

Anemia. A condition characterized by a decreased amount of *hemoglobin* circulating in the cells. The most common type is iron-deficiency anemia (usually due to a diet low in iron) in which red blood cells are reduced in size and number, and *hemoglobin* levels are low.

Angina. Chest pain resulting from lack of blood (and therefore oxygen) to the heart muscle. The correct medical term is angina pectoris.

Antioxidants. Chemical compounds that neutralize cell-damaging *free radicals* created when oxygen is utilized inside the body's cells. In combating free radicals, antioxidants appear to protect against *cancer* and possibly other diseases. The principal antioxidant nutrients are *beta carotene,* the *mineral* selenium, and *vitamins* C and E.

Arthritis. A term that encompasses a number of joint diseases, the most common of which is osteoarthritis, characterized by a gradual loss of *cartilage* and often an overgrowth of bone at the joints. Osteoarthritis is usually associated with aging and is divided into two forms:

primary, in which there is no apparent cause, and secondary, which is the result of injury, disease, or metabolic disorder. Another more serious type is rheumatoid arthritis, which is due to chronic inflammation of joint linings, leading to the deterioration of joints.

Astigmatism. A defect of the *cornea* or lens of the eye that leads to variable blurred vision.

Atherosclerosis. A condition characterized by the accumulation of *plaque* within the arterial walls. This results in a narrowing of the arteries, which reduces blood and oxygen flow to the heart and brain as well as to other parts of the body and can lead to a heart attack, *stroke*, or loss of function or gangrene of other tissues.

ATP (adenosine triphosphate). An energy-storing compound found in the cells which releases energy when needed by the body. The body produces ATP from food.

Axons. Finger-like projections of nerve cells, or *neurons,* that serve as transmitters of information between neighboring neurons.

B

Ballistic stretching. A potentially injurious type of stretching in which one performs quick, bouncing stretches, forcing a muscle to lengthen. The muscles react by reflexively contracting or shortening, increasing the likelihood of muscle tears and soreness.

Basal cell carcinoma. The most common form of skin *cancer.* Basal cell carcinoma usually grows slowly and rarely spreads, and therefore is easily treated.

Beta carotene. A *nutrient* that the body converts to *vitamin* A. One of a family of nutrients called carotenoids, it is found in orange and yellow fruits and vegetables such as cantaloupe and carrots and in green leafy vegetables such as broccoli and spinach. Acting as an *antioxidant,* beta carotene may protect against some forms of *cancer.* It does not have the *toxicity* of vitamin A.

Biofeedback. A relaxation technique. An individual is provided read-outs of physiological functions that are commonly considered involuntary—*systolic blood pressure,* finger temperature or moisture, the tension of the muscles in the forehead, or any combination of these. These measurements are communicated to the individual, who is told to lower them but without any instructions on how to do this.

Blood chemistry tests. Blood tests that measure the levels of naturally occurring circulating chemicals or ingested drugs in the blood, including *glucose,* urea nitrogen, creatinine, and electrolytes such as potassium and sodium.

Blood pressure. The force of the blood against the walls of the arteries. It is measured in two ways; *systolic pressure* and *diastolic pressure.*

Botulism. A form of food poisoning caused by the bacterium Clostridium botulinum, which is commonly found in soil. Potential sources of botulism include improperly canned foods and any food contaminated by soil and subsequently mishandled. Botulism affects the nervous system, causing weakness; blurred vision; difficulty in breathing, swallowing, and speaking; and can be fatal if not diagnosed in time.

Brachialis. A muscle in the upper arm that flexes the elbow and rotates the forearm.

Brachioradialis. A muscle in the upper arm that helps to stabilize and bend the elbow.

C

Calcaneus. The heel bone.

Calisthenics. Systematic and rhythmic exercises, such as sit-ups, that are usually performed without equipment. Calisthenics are designed to tone and strengthen muscles.

Calorie. A measure of the energy released when a food is digested, more accurately called a *kilocalorie.*

Cancer. A group of diseases characterized by the uncontrolled growth of abnormal cells which can occur in any organ or tissue of the body.

Carbo-loading. An eating regimen followed by some athletes that involves consuming large quantities of *carbohydrates* several days before an endurance event or long distance competition in order to enhance performance and prevent early exhaustion. There is no evidence that carbo-loading has any benefit for anyone other than highly trained athletes.

Carbohydrates. The sugars and starches in food. Sugars are called simple carbohydrates and found in such foods as fruit and table sugar *(sucrose).* Complex carbohydrates (starches) are composed of large numbers of sugar molecules joined together, and are found in grains, legumes, and vegetables like potatoes, squash, and corn.

Carcinogen. Any substance capable of causing *cancer.*

Cardiovascular. Pertaining to the heart and blood vessels.

Cartilage. Specialized fibrous connective tissue that forms the skeleton of an embryo and much of the skeleton in an infant. As the child grows, the cartilage becomes bone. In adults, cartilage is present in and around joints and makes up the primary skeletal structure in some parts of the body, such as the ears and the tip of the nose.

Cerebellum. The part of the brain—located in the back of the head—that coordinates movement and balance.

Cerebral cortex. The outer layer of the brain containing three control areas: motor areas, which control voluntary and certain types of involuntary movement; sensory areas, which receive incoming information from the sense organs (such as the ears and eyes); and association areas, which are responsible for thought, learning, language, and personality, and may store memories.

Cerebrovascular. Pertaining to the brain and the blood vessels supplying it.

Cholesterol. A waxy, fat-like substance manufactured in the liver and found in all tissues. In foods, only animal products contain cholesterol. An excess of cholesterol in the bloodstream can contribute to the development of *atherosclerosis.*

Circuit training. A form of weight training designed for *aerobic* benefit as well as strength building. Circuit training requires the use of weight machines set up in a circuit of "stations;" the aerobic benefit comes from moving quickly from station to station between sets of exercises.

Coenzymes. Small molecules composed of nonprotein substances—often *vitamins*—that assist *enzymes* in their functions.

Collagen. The main supportive and connective tissue in the body. It forms the basic structure for *tendons, ligaments,* skin, and *cartilage.*

Complete blood count. A test that measures the composition of the blood. It includes *hemoglobin* concentration, red blood cell count, hematocrit, and white blood cell count.

Contract-relax stretching. A way of stretching muscles that allows for a reflex relaxation of the muscle. It involves contracting a muscle against resistance—usually another person—then relaxing into a static extension of the muscle while the partner pushes the muscle into a stretch that extends it farther than before.

Cornea. The transparent layer that covers the iris and pupil of the eye.

Coronary artery disease (CAD). Narrowing or blockage of the coronary arteries, which reduces the supply of blood, and therefore of oxygen, to the heart muscle.

CPR (Cardiopulmonary resuscitation). A combination of chest compression and mouth-to-mouth breathing, used to help restore breathing and heartbeat until more sophisticated cardiac life support can be used.

Cross training. Regularly performing more than one *aerobic* activity to exercise different muscle groups and provide variety. Interchanging jogging with bicycling and swimming is an example of cross training.

D

Dehydration. A depletion of body fluids that can hinder the body's ability to regulate its own temperature. During exercise, one can become dehydrated if the fluids lost through perspiration are not replaced by drinking water.

Delayed-onset muscle soreness (DOMS). Discomfort believed to be a possible symptom of microscopic injury to muscle tissue. DOMS typically affects those who only exercise occasionally or perform exercise to which they are not accustomed, and usually sets in one to two days after the workout.

Dendrites. Finger-like projections of nerve cells or *neurons* that serve as receivers of information between neighboring neurons.

Dental plaque. A gummy film made up of *polysaccharides* that adheres to teeth and seals in bacteria, especially along the gum line. Other material, such as calcium and saliva, can become entrapped in it. It can lead to cavities and *periodontal disease.*

Dermatitis. A general term used to refer to eruptions or rashes on the skin. There are many causes of dermatitis—for example, contact dermatitis is skin irritation caused by contact with an irritating substance such as the *urushiol* in poison ivy.

Dextrose. A simple sugar containing one sugar unit; also another name for *glucose.*

Diabetes. A condition characterized by the body's inability to produce enough *insulin* or to use it properly. Diabetes is found in two forms. In insulin-dependent diabetes (IDDM), also known as type I or juvenile-onset, the pancreas makes little or no insulin, so the diabetic must receive insulin injections every day. More common is noninsulin-dependent diabetes (NIDDM), also known as type II or adult-onset, in which the pancreas makes insulin but either the amount is insufficiently released or the body cannot properly utilize what is available. This type of diabetes can often be controlled without insulin injections through diet, weight management, and other types of medications.

Diastolic blood pressure. The lowest pressure in the arteries, which occurs when the heart is relaxed between beats. It is represented by the bottom number in the fraction of a blood pressure reading.

Disaccharides. Sugars consisting of two-sugar units. For example, when *fructose* and *glucose,* two single sugars, are combined, they form the disaccharide *sucrose.*

Disc (intervertebral disc). A ring of *cartilage* and fibrous tissue with a pulpy or gel-like center located between the vertebrae in the spine. Discs act as shock absorbers and contribute to the spine's flexibility.

Diuretic. A substance that increases fluid output through urination. Caffeine, alcohol, and a number of medications act as diuretics, and can cause the excretion of important *vitamins* and *minerals.*

Diverticulitis. A condition where diverticula (tiny pouches in the colon wall) become blocked with feces, resulting in infection and inflammation. This may cause abdominal pain, diarrhea, and fever.

Diverticulosis. A condition where tiny pouches (called diverticula) form in the wall of the colon. This condition is usually harmless and without symptoms; however, when the pouches are infected or inflamed, it can turn into *diverticulitis.*

Dysmenorrhea. The medical term for menstrual pain.

Dysplasia. A disturbance in the usual organization or appearance of cells, which may indicate a precancerous condition.

E

Edema. An abnormal accumulation of fluid in the body's tissues that can produce swelling or inflammation.

Electrocardiogram (ECG). A recording of the electroconductivity of the heart. Also referred to as an EKG. Probably the most useful test of heart function, it can detect and determine the cause of irregular heartbeats and, at times, damage to the heart muscle. It also can determine enlargement of the heart's chambers, mineral imbalances in the blood and whether someone has had or is having a heart attack. ECGs are usually performed while the subject is at rest; an exercising ECG (also called a stress test) can provide more information on how the heart responds under stress.

Endometrium. The lining of the uterus. Each month, if pregnancy does not occur, part of the endometrium sloughs off during *menstruation.*

Endorphins. Chemical substances produced by the central nervous system that suppress pain.

Enzymes. Proteins produced by the cells that are crucial in chemical reactions and in building up or synthesizing most compounds in the body. Each enzyme has a specific function; for example, the digestive enzyme amylase acts on *carbohydrates* in foods to break them down.

Epinephrine. A *hormone* secreted by the adrenal medulla gland in response to threatening situations. Also known as adrenaline, it causes elevated *blood pressure,* increased heart rate, and the rerouting of blood to those areas called upon in threatening situations, such as the brain, heart, and muscles.

Estrogen. One of the female sex *hormones* produced by the ovaries.

Extension. A straightening out of a joint. Kicking your knee outward from a sitting position is an example of extension.

Extensor digitorum. A slender muscle that runs along the back of the forearm and works with two smaller muscles to extend the hand and fingers.

F

Fats. The body's most concentrated source of energy, technically termed *lipids.* All fats are made up of carbon, hydrogen, and oxygen atoms arranged in combinations of glycerol and *fatty acids.* (Some fats contain other substances as their organic basis.) Fats found in foods are either in solid or liquid (oil) form. In the body, fat is part of all cell membranes, where it serves as a stored form of energy, helps cushion organs, and helps create certain *hormones.*

Fatty acids. Chemical chains of carbon, hydrogen, and oxygen atoms that are part of a *fat (lipid)* and are the major component of *triglycerides.* Depending on the number and arrangement of these atoms, fatty acids are classified as either *saturated,* polyunsaturated, or monounsaturated. (See also *unsaturated fatty acid.*)

FDA (Food and Drug Administration). The government agency that regulates and monitors food and drug safety; its many responsibilities include regulating the labeling on packaged foods, establishing safe limits of food additives, and ruling on the safety of new drugs before they are made available to the public.

Femur. The thigh bone; the largest bone in the body.

Fiber. The indigestible part of plants. Nutritionists have divided fiber into two basic types—*insoluble* and *soluble*—and have identified five major forms of fiber: cellulose, hemicellulose, lignin, pectin, and gums. Fiber is resistant to human digestive *enzymes* and therefore passes through much of the digestive tract virtually unaltered, absorbing water and helping to speed elimination. Some types of fiber are broken down by microorganisms in the large bowel into substances that can be absorbed by the body. These substances produce various physiological effects, such as inhibiting the production of *cholesterol.*

Fibula. The smaller of the two bones in the lower leg.

Flexion. The bending of a joint. Curling your fingers inward toward your palm is an example of flexion.

Free radicals. Unstable molecules, usually containing oxygen, created by normal chemical processes in the body as well as by radiation (especially X-rays) and other environmental influences. The interaction of free radicals with DNA and other macromolecules leads to impaired functioning of the cells. Free radicals are most likely an important factor in *cancer* development.

Fructose. A *monosaccharide,* sometimes known as fruit sugar. This form of sugar is sweeter than other sugars.

G

Gamma globulin. A *protein* formed in the blood that contains antibodies to all of the diseases to which an individual is immune. It can be extracted from donated blood and is used in the prevention and treatment of certain diseases, such as hepatitis A and Rh factor disorders. It is often given as an injection to individuals who may come into contact with a disease, but who are not immune to it.

Gastrocnemius. The calf muscle.

Glaucoma. A disease characterized by increased pressure in the eyeball, which can ultimately damage the optic nerve and lead to blindness. The most common form—called open-angle glaucoma—usually has no symptoms the patient can observe.

Glucose. A sugar that is the simplest form of *carbohydrate.* It is commonly referred to as blood sugar. The body breaks down carbohydrates in foods into glucose, which serves as the primary fuel for the muscles and the brain. Excess glucose is either converted by the liver to *glycogen* or turned into body fat. In foods, glucose is formed in plants via the process of photosynthesis.

Gluteus maximus. The large powerful muscle—more commonly called the buttocks—that helps to maintain the trunk's erect posture and extends, abducts, and externally rotates the hip.

Glycogen. A compound produced by the liver from *glucose* and stored in the liver and muscles. It acts as an energy source for muscles, and releases glucose from the liver to maintain blood sugar.

Gram. The metric unit of weight measurement equivalent to 1/1000 of a *kilogram.* One ounce is equal to 28.35 grams. A paper clip weighs about a gram.

GRAS (Generally recognized as safe). A list established by the *Food and Drug Administration* of food additives in long-term use and considered safe. The list is subject to revision as new facts become known.

H

Hamstrings. A group of three muscles that run along the back of the thigh.

HDL (High-density lipoprotein). A molecular package that picks up *cholesterol* from the tissues and delivers it to the liver for reprocessing or excretion. Because it clears cholesterol out of the cardiovascular system, HDL has been called the "good" cholesterol. There are several types of HDL.

Heme iron. The type of iron that makes up about 40 percent of the iron in meats. It is the type most easily absorbed by the body.

Hemoglobin. The oxygen-carrying *protein* of the blood found in red blood cells.

Hemorrhoid. A swollen blood vessel in the anus. Cushions of blood vessels, muscle, and connective tissue are normally present in the anus. When one of the veins becomes swollen and tender as a result of constipation, pregnancy, or *obesity,* it is called a hemorrhoid.

Hepatitis. An inflammatory disease of the liver most commonly caused by viruses, but also by alcohol, drugs, or overexposure to toxic chemicals. The viruses that cause hepatitis are spread in different ways. Hepatitis A, the most common type, is transmitted orally via food, water, or other objects that have been contaminated with feces. Hepatitis B, or serum hepatitis, is transmitted primarily through direct blood contact, as in blood transfusions or contaminated needles or syringes. Hepatitis B can also be transmitted through sexual intercourse. Hepatitis C is also transmitted through direct blood contact, primarily from intravenous drug use. It is not clear whether hepatitis C can be transmitted sexually.

High altitude pulmonary edema (HAPE). A serious, potentially life-threatening condition due to the accumulation of fluid in the lungs that may occur in individuals who ascend to heights greater than eight thousand feet.

Hippocampus. A part of the brain that screens sensory data for discard or storage.

HIV (Human immunodeficiency virus). The virus that causes *AIDS.*

Hormones. Chemical substances secreted by a variety of body organs that are carried by the bloodstream and usually influence cells some distance from the source of production. Hormones signal certain *enzymes* to perform their functions. In this way, hormones regulate such body functions as blood sugar levels, *insulin* levels, the menstrual cycle, and growth.

Humerus. The bone of the upper arm.

Hydrogenation. The process of adding hydrogen atoms to an unsaturated *fat* to make it more saturated, more solid, and more resistant to chemical change. Manufacturers often hydrogenate fats to give them a longer shelf life.

Hyperglycemia. A condition characterized by an abnormally high blood *glucose* level; it occurs in people with untreated or inadequately controlled *diabetes.*

Hyperhydrosis. A condition characterized by very heavy perspiring not related to exercise. Most probably a genetic condition, it usually affects the armpits, palms, or soles of the feet.

Hypertension. High *blood pressure.* A persistent elevation of blood pressure above 140/90 millimeters of mercury (mm Hg.). Hypertension increases the risk of heart attack, *stroke,* and kidney failure because it adds to the workload of the heart, causing it to enlarge and, over time, to weaken; in addition, it may damage the walls of the arteries.

Hypoglycemia. A condition characterized by an abnormally low blood *glucose* level. Severe hypoglycemia is rare and dangerous. It can be caused by medications such as *insulin* (diabetics are prone to hypoglycemia), severe physical exhaustion, and some illnesses. The significance of reactive hypoglycemia—a lowering of blood sugar levels after meals in some people—is uncertain, but the symptoms reported, such as lightheadedness, weakness, and rapid heart beat, usually do not correlate with blood sugar levels.

Hypothalamus. A small part of the brain that controls many unconscious functions. It regulates food intake and the release of several *hormones,* helps to main fluid balance and body temperature, and influences sexual behavior and the emotional aspects of sensory input.

Hypothermia. A condition in which body temperature drops to a dangerous level. This is most likely to occur from being outdoors in very cold weather for extended periods, particularly if one does not engage in enough physical activity to keep warm, or is wet or injured.

I

Iliotibial band. A *tendon* running along the outside of the thigh that helps to stabilize the knee joint.

Immunization. A procedure in which a dead or inactive bacteria, virus, or toxin is given orally or by injection to trigger the production of antibodies to that specific disease so that the individual is then immune to it.

Impotence. The inability to achieve and maintain an erection.

Insoluble fiber. A type of dietary *fiber* that absorbs many times its weight in water and swells up in the intestine. Found primarily in whole grains as well as in vegetables, in the peels of fruits, and on the outside of seeds and legumes, it includes cellulose, some hemicellulose, and lignin. By increasing stool bulk, insoluble fiber plays a significant role in promoting efficient waste elimination from the colon, and there is evidence that it may help prevent colon *cancer.*

Insomnia. Difficulty in falling or staying asleep.

Insulin. A *hormone* secreted by the pancreas in response to elevated blood glucose levels. Insulin stimulates the liver, muscles, and fat cells to remove glucose from the blood for use or storage.

Interval training. A method of exercising that alternates spurts of intense exertion with lower-intensity periods in one exercise session.

Irritable bowel syndrome. A condition that occurs when the regular rhythmic contractions that normally propel waste through the intestines become irregular, resulting in constipation or diarrhea and other abdominal disorders.

Isokinetic exercise. Muscle-developing exercise performed on weight machines that provides maximal resistance through a full range of movement at a constant speed.

Isometric exercise. Strengthening exercise in which a muscle group is contracted without moving the joint to which the muscles are attached, such as pressing the hands together at the chest.

Isotonic exercise. Strength training that usually involves raising and lowering a maximal amount of weight.

K

Keratin. A *protein* found in the hair, nails, and outer layer of the skin.

Kilocalorie. The amount of heat necessary to raise the temperature of a liter of water one degree Celsius. What is usually referred to as a food *"calorie"* is more accurately a kilocalorie.

Kilogram. A metric unit of weight measurement equivalent to 2.2 pounds.

Kyphosis. Progressive rounding of the upper back.

L

Lactic acid. A byproduct of the breakdown of *glycogen* during *anaerobic* metabolism. An excess buildup of lactic acid is associated with muscle fatigue and certain forms of muscle soreness.

Lactose. The sugar found in milk. Lactose is a *disaccharide* composed of *glucose* and galactose.

LDL (Low-density lipoprotein). A carrier of *cholesterol* in the bloodstream, LDL delivers cholesterol to tissues and has been implicated in the accumulation of *plaque* within the arteries. Often referred to as "bad" cholesterol.

Ligaments. Bands of connective tissue that join bones together.

Lipids. The technical term for *fats,* waxes, and fatty compounds.

Lipoproteins. Packages of proteins, *cholesterol,* and *triglycerides* assembled by the intestine and liver and circulating in the bloodstream. One of the chief functions is to carry cholesterol.

Lordosis. Exaggerated forward curvature of the lower back; sway-back.

Lumbar region. The five vertebrae in the lower spine that form the largest natural curve in the back.

Lyme disease. An infectious disease caused by bacteria spread primarily via certain species of deer ticks. Symptoms are varied, but include a rash at the site of the tick bite, chills, fever, headache, muscle and joint aches, and low fever. Several months later, more severe symptoms—such as cardiac abnormalities, neurological disorders, and recurring or chronic *arthritis*—may occur in untreated individuals.

M

Macronutrients. A category of *nutrients*—including *carbohydrates, proteins,* and *fats*—that are present in foods in large quantities.

Mammogram. A low-dose X-ray that can detect abnormalities of the breast and therefore can spot any sign of breast *cancer* at the earliest possible stage.

Maximum heart rate (MHR). The highest heart rate you can achieve during your greatest effort exercising. MHR decreases with age, and is determined by subtracting your age from 220. MHR is used to compute your *target heart rate.*

Megadose. A quantity of a *vitamin* or *mineral* that far exceeds the *RDA,* or Recommended Dietary Allowance. In some cases, megadoses can be toxic and cause severe side effects.

Melanin. A dark pigment produced in the skin. Dark-skinned individuals produce more melanin, and melanin production increases in response to sunlight, causing the skin to become darker.

Melanoma. A malignant form of skin *cancer* that usually arises from a mole and can invade other parts of the body if not caught early.

Menopause. The state resulting in the cessation of *menstruation* that usually occurs when a woman reaches her late forties or early fifties. During menopause, *estrogen* production declines and ovulation ceases.

Menstruation. The monthly shedding of blood and the *endometrium* in a premenopausal woman who is not pregnant.

Metabolism. The sum total of the chemical reactions in the body that are necessary to sustain life. All metabolic processes are driven by energy derived from the major *nutrients* in foods.

Metatarsals. The arching bones between the ankles and the toes that form the top of your foot.

Microminerals. The *minerals* present in the body in small amounts (less than five grams). Also known as trace minerals, these include chromium, cobalt, copper, fluorine, iodine, iron, manganese, molybdenum, nickel, selenium, silicon, tin, vanadium, and zinc. The body must replenish these from foods.

Micronutrients. The *nutrients* that are present in foods in small amounts, such as *vitamins* and *minerals*.

Migraine. A severely painful type of headache caused by constriction of the blood vessels in the head. Migraines usually affect one side of the head and may be accompanied by distorted vision, nausea, and numbness or tingling in the limbs.

Milligram. The metric unit of weight measurement that is equivalent to 1/1000 of a *gram*.

Millimole. A chemical measure—one-thousandth of a mole—that is based on the molecular weight of a substance. It is part of the International System, which is used in Canada and many other countries.

Minerals. Inorganic substances that are basic components of the earth's crust; they are also found in the human body. Humans constantly replenish their mineral supply with food and water. Minerals are crucial in a wide variety of bodily functions, including *enzyme* synthesis, regulation of the heart rhythm, bone formation, and digestion.

Monosaccharides. Sugars consisting of a single sugar molecule, such as *glucose, fructose,* and galactose.

Muscular endurance. The ability to perform repeated muscular contractions in rapid succession, such as repeatedly lifting a weight or doing a series of sit-ups.

Muscular strength. The force a muscle produces in one effort, such as a single lift or jump.

Myoglobin. An oxygen-carrying muscle *protein* that makes oxygen available to the muscles for contraction.

N

Neurons. Active cells of the nervous system that transmit and receive messages.

Neurotransmitters. Chemicals in the brain that aid in the transmission of nerve impulses. Various neurotransmitters are responsible for different functions including controlling mood and muscle movement and inhibiting or causing the sensation of pain.

Non-REM sleep. The deepest stages of sleep characterized by general absence of body movement and slow, regular brain activity.

Nonheme iron. The type of iron that makes up all of the iron in eggs, dairy products, vegetables, fruits, grains, and enriched flours and cereals and makes up about 60 percent of the iron in animal tissue. Nonheme iron is not as well absorbed by the body as *heme iron.*

Nonoxynol-9. A spermicide used in many contraceptive foams and jellies.

Norepinephrine. A *hormone* secreted by the adrenal medulla gland in conjunction with *epinephrine* in response to threatening situations.

Nutrients. Components necessary for virtually all bodily functions that must be obtained from foods (or in some cases supplements), since the body cannot manufacture them. Nutrients include *protein, fat, carbohydrates, vitamins, minerals,* and water.

O

Obesity. A medical term that refers to the storage of excess *fat* in the body. A person is usually considered obese when his or her weight is 20 percent greater than the appropriate weight as determined by conventional height-weight tables.

Occult blood test. A diagnostic test performed on a stool sample for the presence of hidden (occult) blood, which may indicate colon *cancer.*

Omega-3 fatty acids. A unique group of poly-unsaturated *fatty acids* found in fish oil and some seeds (such as in linseed oil). Omega-3s in fish oil significantly reduce blood clotting. They make platelets less likely to stick together and to blood vessels, thus lessening the chance of a heart attack or *stroke.*

Opiates. Narcotic pain relievers, such as morphine.

Orthoses. Foot supports that fit in shoes to correct for abnormal foot motion and alignment. Orthoses should be custom designed by a podiatrist or orthopedist.

Osteoporosis. A disease in which bone tissue becomes porous and brittle. The disease primarily affects postmenopausal women.

Ovulation. The monthly process in which a mature ovum (egg) is released from the ovary.

Oxalic acid. A substance that, when joined with calcium in the body, forms insoluble salts and hinders iron absorption from food. It is found in such vegetables as spinach, chard, and rhubarb.

P

PABA (para-aminobenzoic acid). A chemical compound that is one of the most commonly used ingredients in sunscreens. The derivatives made from it—such as Padimate O—effectively screen out the ultraviolet rays responsible for sunburn, but don't offer protection against the full spectrum of ultraviolet rays, including those that may play a role in causing skin *cancer.*

Pap smear. A diagnostic test for detecting cervical *cancer* in which a sample of cervical cells is examined for cellular changes. Among women who have regular Pap smears, the death rate from cervical cancer is almost zero.

Patella. The kneecap, which protects the front of the knee joint.

Periodontal disease. Inflammation or destruction of the supporting structures—the gums and bone—around the teeth. Periodontal disease—which is reversible in its earliest stages—is the most common cause of tooth loss in adults.

Placebo. A medication, most frequently used in medical research, that contains no active ingredients. Because people may feel better after taking medication simply because they expect to, placebos are commonly used ·in tests of new drugs to check whether the drug is actually having an effect.

Plantar fascia. A thick, pad-like band of tissue along the bottom of the foot. Undue stress to this area from running or jumping can cause *plantar fascitis.*

Plantar fascitis. A pain or discomfort in the heel that often travels up the sole of the foot; it is caused by a partial or full tear in the *ligament* in the arch of the foot.

Plaque (arterial). Deposits of fatty substances, such as *cholesterol,* in the inner lining of the artery walls. The buildup of these deposits can lead to *atherosclerosis.*

Polysaccharides. *Carbohydrates* that consist of many simple sugars linked together. Starch, *glycogen,* and cellulose are polysaccharides.

Premenstrual syndrome (PMS). Disruptive emotional and physical symptoms that appear to precede *menstruation* and may last two weeks or more. Though PMS has been widely publicized, physicians have yet to agree on either its cause or a reliable treatment.

Presbycusis. A common age-related degeneration of the inner ear that results in some degree of hearing loss in both ears.

Presbyopia. An eye condition due to aging in which the lens becomes less able to focus on close objects. This condition occurs to some degree in everyone over the age of forty. It can often be corrected with reading glasses.

Progesterone. A female sex *hormone* secreted by the ovaries. Progesterone and *estrogen* regulate changes that occur during the menstrual cycle.

Progressive muscle relaxation. A tension-reducing technique in which muscle groups from head to toe are each tensed for a few seconds and then relaxed in sequence.

Protein. Compounds composed of hydrogen, oxygen, and nitrogen present in the body and in foods that form complex combinations of *amino acids.* Protein is essential for life. Foods that supply the body with protein include meats, dairy products, eggs, and seafood as well as grains, legumes, and vegetables.

Pruritus. The medical term for itching.

PSA. A test that measures blood levels of the prostate-specific antigen, a protein produced by the prostate gland that may be elevated when cancer is present. The test has come into wide use as a routine screening device, especially for men over fifty.

Q

Quadriceps. A group of four muscles that extend down the front of the thigh and join in a single *tendon* at the kneecap. They extend or straighten the lower leg.

R

RDA (Recommended Dietary Allowances). The estimated amount of *nutrients* needed daily to maintain good health. These estimates differ for various conditions and ages, such as women, men, children, the elderly, and pregnant and lactating women. Developed by the Food and Nutrition Board of the National Research Council, the RDAs are not minimum amounts required, but amounts recommended for optimal health.

Relaxation response. A set of changes in bodily functions that take place as a result of meditating or practicing other relaxation techniques. First described by Herbert Benson of the Harvard Medical School, the response includes a slowing of heart rate and respiration, and an increase in the brain waves associated with relaxation.

REM sleep. A phase of sleep during which the sleeper's eyes move quickly (REM stands for "rapid eye movement"), heartbeat and *metabolism* speed up, and toes and fingers twitch. Dreaming takes place during REM sleep.

Resting heart rate (RHR). The number of heartbeats per minute while the body is at rest. It is most accurately measured by taking your pulse before rising in the morning.

Resting metabolic rate (RMR). The total amount of energy your body uses in a given period of time when at rest. RMR depends on body size, body composition, age, and other factors, and can be temporarily affected by activity level and diet.

Retrovirus. A virus that has the ability to take over certain cells and interrupt their normal genetic function.

Rhinoviruses. One of the main groups of viruses that cause colds.

RICE. An acronym for a recommended method of alleviating exercise-related injuries, both acute and overuse. RICE stands for: REST the injured body part; apply ICE; apply COMPRESSION; and ELEVATE the injured extremity above heart level.

Rotator cuff. Four small muscles and their tendons that stabilize the upper arm in the shoulder socket and allow the shoulder its range of motion.

Runner's knee. A condition brought on by repeated stress to the knee, which is usually signaled by dull pain at the kneecap. It most commonly affects those who run, ski, cycle, or do high-impact aerobics.

S

Salmonella. A group of bacteria that causes intestinal infection. A frequent contaminator of foods, salmonella is probably the most common cause of food poisoning.

Saturated fatty acids. *Fats* containing all the hydrogen atoms they can carry. Such fats, which are solid at room temperature, come chiefly from animal sources (such as beef, butter, whole-milk dairy products, dark meat poultry, and poultry skin) as well as tropical vegetable oils (coconut, palm, and palm kernel). Saturated fatty acids in the diet are the chief contributors to elevated blood *cholesterol* levels.

Sciatica. A severe pain along the sciatic nerve, which runs from the lower back into the leg. Strain to the lower back or a slipped disc are common causes, though often no cause can be identified.

Scoliosis. A sideways curvature of the spine.

Serotonin. A compound made from the *amino acid* tryptophan that serves as one of the brain's principal *neurotransmitters*. When a person eats a meal, the level of serotonin is raised or lowered—depending on the amounts of *proteins, carbohydrates,* and other substances consumed—and this level may affect mood.

Shin splint. A term that applies to a variety of overuse injuries that cause inflammation of muscles and *tendons* in the lower leg.

Sigmoidoscopy. A screening procedure to detect colon cancer and other abnormalities of the lower portion of the large intestine and of the rectum. The test is done by viewing the area with a long thin tube that is inserted into the rectum.

Sleep apnea. A potentially dangerous condition in which breathing stops temporarily during sleep. It is often associated with deep snoring when breathing resumes.

Solanine. A toxic substance that in large amounts is a powerful inhibitor of nerve impulses. It is found in the skin of potatoes that are damaged, old, soft, sprouted, or greenish as well as in potato sprouts.

Soleus. A flat muscle that extends along the back of the calf underneath the *gastrocnemius.*

Soluble fiber. A type of dietary *fiber* which includes pectins, some hemicellulose, and gums, found in fruits, vegetables, seeds, brown rice, oats, and oat bran. When ingested, soluble fiber can promote a softer stool and works chemically to prevent or reduce the absorption of certain substances into the bloodstream. It appears to lower blood *cholesterol* levels and may help regulate blood sugar.

Spasm. A prolonged, painful, involuntary muscular contraction.

SPF (Sun protection factor). A number on sunscreen products that indicates the relative length of time that the sunscreen will protect you against sunburn as compared to using no sunscreen. A product with an SPF of 15, for example, would allow you to stay in the sun without burning fifteen times longer, on average, than if you didn't apply sunscreen.

Sprain. An injury that damages a *ligament* or ligaments, as well as joint capsules. Ranging from small tears to serious ruptures, sprains are often the result of a sudden forceful movement.

Strain. The injury to a muscle that occurs from an excessive effort, such as lifting a heavy weight or sudden overextension of a muscle, as when you stretch to catch a baseball. When this occurs, small tears are usually present in the muscle. The thigh, groin, and shoulder are the most common sites for strains.

Stress fracture. A microscopic break in a bone caused by repeated impact. Stress fractures are common among aerobic dancers and long distance runners, and usually affect the foot, shin, or thigh.

Stress injury. An exercise-related injury—usually referring to an overuse or chronic injury—that results from the wear-and-tear of performing a repetitive activity such as cycling, running, playing tennis, or even swimming.

Stroke. A hemorrhage or a blockage in a blood vessel that supplies the brain, resulting in insufficient blood (and therefore oxygen) to a portion of the brain. The most common manifestation is some degree of paralysis, but small strokes may occur without symptoms. If recurrent, strokes can lead to mental deterioration.

Sucrose. White table sugar made from cane or beets. A combination of *fructose* and *glucose* bonded together, it also occurs naturally in many vegetables and fruits.

Swimmer's ear. A painful, itchy infection of the external ear canal that can develop after long periods of swimming or bathing. Water gets trapped in the ear canal and breaks down the skin lining, allowing bacteria or fungi to breed.

Synapses. The connections between *neurons*.

Systolic blood pressure. The maximum pressure in the arteries when the heart is contracting. It is represented by the top number in the fraction of a *blood pressure* reading.

T

Talus. The ankle bone.

Tannins. Soluble astringent substances found in some plants that may reduce iron and trace *mineral* absorption.

Tartar. Another name for dental plaque.

Temperomandibular joint syndrome (TMJ). Painful grinding, clicking, and soreness of the jawbone muscles when chewing.

Tendinitis. A condition characterized by an inflammation of the *tendons* that usually occurs from overuse, especially in those who perform one sport or movement regularly and intensely.

Tendons. The cords of connective tissue that anchor muscles to bones.

Tennis elbow. A form of *tendinitis* that is caused by forceful, repetitive movements of the arm muscle, such as in tennis, raking, and working with heavy tools. It is characterized by pain that can range from the shoulder to the wrist.

Testosterone. The principal male sex *hormone* that induces and maintains the changes that occur in males at puberty. In men, the testicles continue to produce testosterone throughout life, though there is some decline with age.

Tibia. The larger of two bones in the lower leg.

Tibialis anterior. A long muscle in front of the calf that raises the foot.

Tinnitus. Persistent or recurring ringing or other noises in the ears. When it occurs, episodes of tinnitus usually appear intermittently in middle age, then may become chronic as a person grows older.

Toxicity. The potential ability of a substance to harm a living organism. Almost any substance in food, air, and water can become toxic if taken in a high enough concentration.

Target heart rate (THR). A level of exercise intensity that enables one to gain the maximum training benefits from an *aerobic* workout. Also called training heart rate, THR is computed by taking 60 per-cent and 90 percent of your *maximum heart rate (MHR)*. During aerobic exercise, the number of heartbeats per minute should fall between these two figures.

Trans fatty acids. *Fatty acids* that have undergone *hydrogenation,* making them more saturated and changing their structure in other subtle ways. Studies have shown that trans fats act more like saturated fats, raising levels of total and *LDL* ("bad") *cholesterol.*

Trichinosis. An illness caused by eating raw or undercooked pork infested with worms called trichinae. The disease is usually characterized by muscular pain, fever, and tissue swelling.

Triglyceride. The main form of *fat* found in foods and the human body. Containing three *fatty acids* and one unit of glycerol, triglycerides are stored in *adipose cells* in the body, which, when broken down, release fatty acids into the blood.

Tubal ligation. A surgical procedure for birth control in which a woman's fallopian tubes are tied off so that fertilization of the ovum cannot take place. Tubal ligation is safe, convenient, and permanent, but it is also extremely difficult to reverse.

U

U.S. RDA. A condensed version of the *RDA* figures used by the *Food and Drug Administration* for legal regulation of food labeling. The values are based on RDAs and are used for all persons over the age of four. On food labels, they are expressed in percentages.

Unsaturated fatty acids. In foods, *fats* missing hydrogen atoms in specific places on the *fatty acid* molecule; depending on the number of missing atoms, these fats are classified as either monounsaturated or polyunsaturated. Main dietary sources are plants and fish. These fats are generally liquid at room temperature.

Urinalysis. The laboratory examination of a urine specimen. This routine examination is generally performed with a specially coated strip of paper that can reveal the presence of various substances and chemicals. Usually the sample is also inspected under a microscope for bacteria and other visible signs of urinary tract disorders.

Urushiol. The toxic material secreted by poison ivy and poison oak that causes itching, burning, and a blistery rash in those who are exposed and sensitive.

V

Vasectomy. A permanent method of birth control for men that involves cutting the vas deferens—the tube through which sperm cells pass from the testicles to the penis. The procedure is safe and effective, though irreversible to a great degree.

Vegetarian. An individual who eats a diet that omits meat. The basic categories of vegetarians include semi-vegetarians, who omit red meat; lacto-ovo vegetarians, who omit all animal foods except milk, milk products, and eggs; and vegans, who omit all animal products from their diets.

Vitamins. Organic substances (excluding the essential amino acids) that the body requires to help regulate metabolic functions. Vitamins must be ingested; the body cannot manufacture them.

W

Weight-bearing exercise. An exercise in which the legs support the body, such as in running, walking, and jumping rope.

Wisdom teeth. The last molars (in a full set of teeth) on each side of the upper and lower jaw. Because wisdom teeth may cause trouble when they grow in, which usually occurs in late adolescence, they commonly are removed.

Z

Zinc oxide ointment. A blend of zinc oxide powder and ointment that functions as a skin protector and a sunblock. Unlike chemical sunscreens—such as *PABA*—zinc oxide prevents any ultraviolet light from reaching the skin.

Index

A

Acclimatization to altitude, 481
Acesulfame-K, 100
Acetaminophen:
    and muscular pain, 410
    as cold remedy, 342
    compared to other pain relievers, 519
    for exercise injuries, 424
    for headache relief, 471
    side effects of, 519
Acetic acid, 154
Achilles tendinitis, 412
Achilles tendon, 413, 448
    exercises for, 414
Acids, in art materials, 529-530
Acne, 297-298
Acquired Immune Deficiency
    Syndrome, *see* AIDS
Acupuncture, 521
Acute Mountain Sickness, 481
Acyclovir, 390
Addiction:
    to analgesics, 517
    to smoking, 63. *See also* Smoking
Addictive behavior:
    and addictive personalities, 72
    and sugar, 99
    and weight control, 45
Adipose cells, 107. *See also* Fat
Adolescent diet:
    calcium requirements for, 137
    iron requirements for, 141
    nutritional needs of, 80
Adrenaline, 313, 458
Aerobic exercise, 232-236, 248
    and anxiety reduction, 454
    and cholesterol levels, 47
    and neurological functioning in
        elderly, 28
    and weight reduction, 42
    as therapy for arthritis, 426-427
    effects on aging process, 234
    in postmenopausal women, 28
    psychological benefits of, 233
Aerobic movement, 249-252
    high-impact, 238, 250
    low-impact, 238, 250
Aerobics shoes, 242
Aerosol cans, environmental effects of,
    528
Aerosol sprays:
    adverse effects of, 528-529
    and contact lenses, 330
Aflatoxin, 153, 222
African Americans
    and genetic predisposition to
        overweight, 33
    and sun exposure, 301
    hypertension in, 56
    risk of glaucoma in, 339
Aging:
    and aerobic capacity, 28
    and benefits of aerobic exercise,
        28, 234

and hearing loss, 347-350
and memory changes, 465-466
and sexuality, 406-407
and sleep patterns, 474-476
and susceptibility to colds, 341
and vitamin D deficiency, 24
effects on skin, 304-306
AIDS (Acquired Immune Deficiency
    Syndrome), 392-399
    and AIDS-related complex (ARC),
        394
    and blood donation, 396
    and blood transfusions, 396, 494
    and children, 395
    and treatment with AZT, 393, 397
    groups at high risk for, 393
    in health care workers, 396
    mandatory screening for, 398
    myths concerning, 393-397
    risk of in dental care, 397
    spread by insects, 395-396
    testing for, 397-399
    transmission through casual
        contact, 393
Air, indoor, 550-553
    controlling allergens in, 553
    eliminating pollutants in, 552-553
    quality of, and houseplants, 551
Airbags, automobile, 598
Air conditioners:
    and allergens, 552
    and hay fever, 344
    car:
    and allergies, 552
    and chlorofluorocarbons (CFCs),
        579
Air freshener, alternatives to, 548
Airplanes:
    cabin environment of, 480-481
    safety, 587-588
Air purifiers, household, 551-552
Al-Anon, 75
Alcohol, concentration in blood, 70
Alcohol abuse treatment, 75
Alcohol consumption, 68-75
    and atherosclerosis, 72
    and boating accidents, 588
    and breast cancer, 14, 72
    and cholesterol levels, 72
    and driving, 592-594
    and hangovers, 73
    and headaches, 470
    and healthy diet, 78
    and heart disease, 73
    and highway fatalities, 69
    and hypertension, 73
    and impotence, 407-408
    and longevity, 22
    and osteoporosis, 430
    and pregnancy, 72
    and premature death, 69
    and smoking and oral cancer, 15
    diuretic effect of, 71, 240
    effects of heavy consumption,
        72-74

effects of moderate consumption,
    71-72
effect on brain, 72
effect on cardiovascular system, 73
effect on central nervous system, 71
effect on gastrointestinal tract, 72
effect on liver, 73
effect on sleep, 479
ineffective as cold remedy, 343
on airplanes, 481
reducing, 71
relationship to other health risks, 15
short-term effects of, 71
Alcohol-free beverages, 71
Alcoholics Anonymous, 75
Alcoholism, 74-75
    and acetaminophen, 342
Alcohol, rubbing, as treatment for cuts
    and scrapes, 309
Allergens, 291, 345, 553
Allergic reactions:
    to antiperspirants, 308
    to cosmetics, 295
    to ear piercing, 294
    to eye drops, 332
    to insect stings, 313
Aloe vera, 25, 308
Almonds, 221
Alopecia areata, 323
Alpha waves, 459
Altitude, adjustment to, 481
Aluminum chlorohydrate, 308
Alzheimer's disease, 466
Amaranth, 188-189
American College of Obstetricians and
    Gynecologists (ACOG), 506
American College of Sports Medicine
    (ACSM), 233, 248
American Heart Association, 117
American Medical Association (AMA)
    Directory of Physicians, 491
Amino acids, 119
Ammonia, alternatives to, 548
Amniocentesis, 401
Anal fissure, 374
Analgesics, 517-519
Anal intercourse, risk of AIDS from, 393,
    395
Anal itching, 373-374
Anaphylactic shock, 313
Anemia, iron-deficiency, 140, 143, 499
Anesthesiologists, 490
Anger, managing, 456-457
Angiotensin, 133
Ankles, 413-415
    footwear to support, 414
    injuries to, 412, 413-414
Ankle weights, 251
ANSI (American National Standards
    Institute), 332
Antacids, 367
Antibiotic ointments, 309-310
Antibiotics:
    and Lyme disease, 578
    in animal feed, 378

Antihistamines:
    as cold remedy, 342
    effect on driving ability, 593
Antilock brakes, 591
Antioxidant nutrients, 22, 24
    and vitamins, 125
    potential benefits of, 23, 125
    recommended intakes, 126
Antiperspirants and deodorants, 307-308
Apnea, sleep, 477
Appetite:
    effect of coffee on, 145
    effect of exercise on, 42-44
Apples, 156
Apricots, 156
Arrhythmias and caffeine consumption, 145
Arsenic, in drinking water, 568
Arthritis, 425-427
    and Lyme disease, 577
    exercises for, 426
Artichokes, 165, 166
Artificial colors and flavors in foods, 153, 154, 155
Artificial fingernails, safety of, 325-326
Artificial sweeteners, 100
Art supplies and safety, 529-531
    for children, 530
Arugula, 173
Asbestos, 531-532, 547
Asian cuisine, 93
Asparagus, 165
Aspartame, 100
Aspirin:
    and muscular pain, 410
    and vitamin C metabolism, 127
    as cold remedy, 342
    compared to other pain relievers, 519
    for exercise injuries, 424
    for headache relief, 471
    side effects of, 519
Astigmatism, 327
Atherosclerosis:
    and electrocardiograms, 500
    and cholesterol, 47
    and hypertension, 56
    and smoking, 61
Athlete's cramps, 410-411
Athlete's foot, 446
ATP (adenosine triphosphate), 79
Autologous transfusions, 494
Automobile crashes, alcohol-related, 69
Automobile safety, see Driving safety
Automotive supplies, safe disposal of, 547
Avocados, 165
Axons, 465
AZT, 393, 397

B

Babesiasis, 313
Babies, swimming instruction for, 271
Back care, 431-443
Back-care products, 441-442
Back exercises, 434
Back pain
    and sports, 435
    and stress, 442
    bed rest as therapy for, 432
    causes of, 431-432
    medical care for, 433
    preventing, 437

    treatment, 432-433
Back schools, 441
Bad breath, 356
Bagels, 194
Bags under eyes, 305
Baldness, 321
Ballistic stretching, 2137-238, 282-283
Ballroom dancing, 251
Banana bread, health claims for, 223
Bananas, 157
Bandages, 310-311
Barbecues, 573
Barbiturates, 478
Barley, 189
Basal cell carcinoma, 299, 300. See also Skin cancer
Batteries, safe disposal of, 548
Beach pollution, 573-574
Beans, 165
    as protein source, 120
    canned, high sodium content of, 198
    dried, 197-199
Beef, 199-203
    and hormones, 202
    cooking tips for, 199
    ground, 201
    nutritional content of, 200
    USDA grades of, 201
Beer, nonalcoholic, 71
Beer, poor as exercise drink, 239
Beet greens, 173
Beets, 168
Benadryl, 482
Benzocaine, 294
Benzophenones, 302
Benzoyl peroxide and acne, 298
Bereavement and stress, 456
Beta carotene
    food sources of, 22
    in fruits and juices, 156, 159
    in vegetables, 165
    role in cancer prevention, 22
Beta carotene, as an antioxidant, 125-126
    in fruits and vegetables, 177
    in juices, 159
BHA (butylated hydroxyanisole), 153, 154
BHT (butylated hydroxytoluene), 153, 154
Bibb lettuce, 173
Bicycles, getting a proper fit, 256
Bicycling, see Cycling
Bifocals, 333
Biker's knee, 256
Biofeedback:
    and pain relief, 522
    and stress reduction, 461
    as remedy for tinnitus, 351
    for hypertension, 59
Biotin, 124
Birth control, 381-388. See also Oral contraceptives
    methods compared, 382
    safety and effectiveness, 382
Bites:
    dog, 311
    insect, 312-316
Black beans, 197
Black-eyed peas, 197
Blackstrap molasses, 97, 142
Bladder cancer:
    and coffee drinking, 146

    and smoking, 60-61
Blisters, 447
Blood chemistry tests, 497-499
    blood urea nitrogen (BUN), 499
    creatinine, 499
    electrolytes, 499
    glucose, 498
Blood clotting and fish oils, 116, 209
Blood donation and risk of AIDS infection, 396
Blood pressure. See also Hypertension
    defined, 54
    diastolic, 54
    effect of meditation on, 459
    effect of weight lifting on, 56
    measuring, 54
    monitoring, 57
    systolic, 54
Blood transfusions, 494
Blueberries, 157
Blue light, protecting eyes from, 335-336
Boating safety, 588
Body fat, 32-33
    and energy, 79
Body shape and risk of heart disease, 32
Bok choy, 166
Bones and teeth, role of calcium in building, 136-137
Boron, 137
Boston lettuce, 173
Bottled water, 570-571
Botulism, 376, 378-380
Bowel movements, 104, 364
Bowling, effect on back, 435
Braking, proper technique for, 590
Bran, as source of fiber, 105
Bran muffins, health claims for, 223
Brazil nuts, 221
Bread, 120, 193-195
    nutritional content of, 194
Breakfast, 82-84
Breakfast cereals, 190-193
Breakfast foods, 83
Breast cancer:
    and alcohol consumption, 14-15, 22, 72
    and body fat distribution, 32
    and fat consumption, 117
    and obesity, 26, 32
    and oral contraceptives, 384
    risks for, 14
    self-exam for, 502
Bridges, dental, 357-358
Broccoli, 21, 22, 24, 168
Bronchitis, and effects of smoking, 62
Brown rice, 189
Brussels sprouts, 24, 168
Buckwheat, 189
Buffalo meat, 208
Bunions, 447-448
Burns, 308
Bursitis, prevention and treatment tips, 427-428
Butter, 218
Butterhead lettuce, 173
Buttermilk, 180

C

Cabbage, 24, 168
Cactus spines, removing from skin, 313
Cadence, in cycling, 255-257
Caffeine, 144-148

Ectopic heartbeats, 500
Egg noodles, 187-188
Eggplant, 171-172
Eggs, 186-188
    and egg substitutes, nutritional content of, 186
    safe cooking and storage of, 377
    safety measures, 187-188
EKG, see Electrocardiogram
Elbow brace for tennis elbow, 420
Elderly:
    nutritional needs of, 80
    vitamin supplements for, 127
Elective surgery, 493-494
Electrical fields, 539-540
Electrical nerve stimulation, 520
Electric blankets, safe use of, 540
Electric toothbrushes, 354
Electrocardiogram (EKG or ECG), 500, 511-512
    for travel abroad, 483
Electronic-digital blood pressure equipment, 57
Electrostatic filters, for indoor air, 551
Electrostatic precipitators and hay fever, 345
ELISA (enzyme-linked immuno-absorbent assay), 394, 397. *See also* AIDS
Emergency medicine specialists, 490
Emergency rooms, 492
Emollients, 293-294
Emphysema and smoking, 62
Emulsifiers, 154
Endometrium, 21
Endorphins, 520
English muffins, 194
Enriched bread, 194
Enriched foods, 150 *See also* Food labeling
Entoptic phenomena, 334
Environmental Protection Agency (EPA):
    and noise levels, 348, 559
    regulation of lead, 554
    regulation of pesticides, 567, 581
Epicondylitis (tennis elbow), 412, 419-420
Epidemiology, 13
Epinephrine (adrenaline), 313
Escarole, 173
    Eskimos, health effects of fish oil consumption by, 110
Essential amino acids, 119
Essential hypertension, 55, 133
Estrogen, 383, 384
Estrogen replacement therapy (ERT), 404-405
Evaporated milk, 180
Exercise:
    aerobic, 213-215, 232-235
    anaerobic, 213
    and appetite, 44
    and blood cholesterol reduction, 51
    and hypertension, 57-58
    and reducing cancer risk, 24
    and regression of atherosclerosis, 26
    and risk of heart disease, 26
    and stress reduction, 451
    and weight reduction, 42-44
    dehydration during, 239-240
    effect on blood cholesterol tests, 53
    for abdominals, 277-279

    for back pain, 434
    for flexibility, 232, 282-283, 286-287
    for preventing sports injuries, 413-422
    for strength, 232, 276, 280-282, 284-285
    for stress relief, 454
    general guidelines for, 234, 237-239, 248
    in polluted air, 247
    in the cold, 243-245
    in the heat, 243
Exercise bicycles, 259
Exercise machines vs. free weights, 281
Exercise performance:
    and blood sugar, 99
    and carbohydrates, 96
    and protein consumption, 121
Exercise programs:
    and aging, 241
    convenience in, 238
    guidelines for, 238
    recording progress, 238
    setting goals, 238
    variety in, 238
Exercise shoes, 242
Exertion headaches, 471
Exotic fruits, 160
Exotic vegetables, 166
Expiration date, of medications, 524
Eye care, 327-339
    checkup timetable, 328
    specialists for, 328
Eye drops, 332
    nonprescription, 526
Eyeglasses, 327, 332, 334-337
Eye makeup:
    and preventing eye infection, 333
    choosing and applying, 333
Eye problem chart, 329
Eye protection, for racquet sports, 264
Eyestrain, 337-338, 471, 539
Eyewashes, 332

F

Family exercise activities, 241
Family practitioners, 488
Farsightedness, 327
Fast food, 88
Fasting, as method of weight reduction, 34
Fat, 107-118
    as energy source, 79
    calculating daily needs, 42
    content of foods, 111-115
    in common foods, 41
    in processed foods, 108
Fat cells, function and development, 32-33
Fat consumption:
    and cancer, 117
    and heart disease, 109-110
    and longevity, 20-21
    and overweight, 41
    reduction of, 77
Fat deposits and risk of heart disease, 32
Fat-soluble vitamins, 107, 124
Fatty acids, saturated vs. unsaturated, 107
Fatty fish and blood cholesterol levels, 47
Feet, care of, 444-449
Fennel, 166

Fetus:
    development of fat cells, 33
    effects of mother's alcohol consumption on, 72
    risk of contracting AIDS from mother, 398
Fiber, 102-106
    and blood cholesterol reduction, 51-52
    and calcium binding, 105
    and cancer prevention, 22
    and colon cancer, 104
    and constipation, 104
    and flatulence, 366
    and heart disease, 104
    and intestinal disorders, 102-104
    benefits of, 103-105
    content of foods, 103
    effect on mineral absorption, 105
    in cranberries, 157
    increasing intake of, 105
    insoluble, 102, 104
    soluble, 102-103, 104
    supplements, 106
    vegetables high in, 167
Fig bars, fiber content of, 105
"Fight or flight" response to stress, 458
Fingernails, 324-326
    artificial, safety of, 325-326
Finger stretches, 426
Fire extinguishers, 543-544
Fireplace safety, 542
Fish, 209-216
    cooked, nutritional content of, 211
    cooking tips, 210
    fat content of, 209
    raw, hazards of, 211
    safety guidelines, 210-211
Fish oils, 110, 116-117
    supplements, 110
Fish tapeworm and roundworm, 210
Fitness, 232-236
    aerobic, 232
    and aging, 27-28
Flatulence, 366
Flexibility, 282-283. *See also* Stretching
    exercises for drivers, 593, 595
Floaters, 334
Flooring, asbestos-containing, 531
Floss, dental, 353
Fluid replacement, 239-240
Fluorescent lights, 539
Fluoridation (of drinking water), 570
Fluoride, 137, 354, 570
Fluorine, 129
Flu vaccine, 514
Flying, coping with, 480-481
Foam plastic insulation and destruction of ozone layer, 583
Folacin, 124-126
    and pregnancy, 400
    benefits of, 125
    in fruits and vegetables, 177
    recommended intake, 126
Follicles, hair, 319
Folliculitis, 422
Food, on airplanes, 482
Food additives, 152-155
Food and Drug Administration (FDA):
    and antiperspirants, 307
    and hair dyes, 323
    and prescription medications, 523
    and Retin-A regulation, 304
    condom reliability, 386

Lightning, 575
Light sensitivity and prescription drugs, 335-336
Lignin, 102. *See also* Fiber
Liniments, effectiveness of, 410
Linoleic acid, 116
Linolenic acid, 107
Lip protection, from sun, 301
Lipid profile, and cholesterol testing, 53
Lipid Research Clinics (LRC), 53
Lipids, *see* Fats
Lipstick and sun protection, 301
Listerial bacteria, in raw milk, 180
Liver, effects of alcohol on, 73
Liver cancer and aflatoxin, 222
Liver spots, 292
Lordosis, 432
Lovastatin, 52
Low blood sugar, 98-99
Low-calorie foods, 150. *See also* Food labeling
Lower-back pain, stretching to relieve, 434
Lower leg, injuries to, 417
Low-fat diet, and longevity, 21
Low-fat milk, 180
Low-fat substitutes, 116
Low-impact exercise, 248, 250, 268
L-tryptophan, 122, 478
Lunch, 84-89
Lung cancer, and smoking, 62
Lychee, 160
Lye (sodium hydroxide), hazards of, 560
Lyme disease, 313-315, 576-579
Lysine, 119

M

Macadamia nuts, 221
Macrobiotic diet, 25
Macrominerals, 128
Macronutrients, 79
Magnesium, 129
    and bone formation, 137
    and hypertension, 58-59
    function in body, 128-129
Magnetic fields, health effects of, 539-540
Magnetic resonance imaging (MRI), 513
Mail-order food, precautions, 379
Malaria, preventing, 483-484
Male pattern baldness, 321
Malignant melanoma, 299, 300-301. *See also* Skin cancer
Maltose, 97
Mammogram, 501, 504
Manganese, 128, 129, 137
Mango, 160
Maple syrup, 97
Margarine, 218-219
Marijuana use and driving, 594
Marquis *Directory of Medical Specialists,* 491
Mascara, 333
Massage:
    as headache treatment, 472
    for pain relief, 522-523
Masters and Johnson Institute, 408
Maximum heart rate, 241
Mayonnaise, 229, 378
Measles immunization, 516
Medications, 523-526
    as hazard to children, 562-563
    for pain, 424, 517
    prescription, and driving ability, 594

safe disposal of, 549
    safe storage and handling of, 563
Medicine cabinet safety, 524
Meditation, 59, 461-462
Megadoses:
    of niacin for cholesterol reduction, 52
    of vitamin C for colds, 342
    of vitamins, 127
Melanin, 301
Melanoma, 299-301. *See also* Skin cancer
Melons, 162
Memory, 464-468
Menopause, 402-406
    alternative treatments for, 404
    and arthritis risk, 429-430
    and effects of aerobic exercise, 28
    and hormone replacement therapy, 405
Menstruation, 399-402
    and headaches, 470
    and iron intake, 140
    cramps, 399
Mental performance and caffeine, 144
Mercury, in dental fillings, 357
Metal polish, safe substitutes for, 548
Metatarsals, 444
Methionine, 119
Methylene chloride, 148. *See also* Decaffeinated coffee
Methyl methacrylate, in artificial fingernails, 325-326
Microminerals, 128
Micronutrients, 79
Microwave ovens, 536-537
    and food safety, 375
Microwave popcorn, 116
Midwives, 495-496
Migraines, 470
Milk, 179-182
    consumption trends in the United States, 136
    hormones in, 181
    nutritional content of, 180
    raw, 179-180
    vitamin D-fortified, 24
Milk sugar, 101
Millet, 189
Mineral imbalance, and leg cramps, 410-411
Minerals, 128-130
    as part of healthy diet, 78
    chelated, 130
    effect of fiber on absorption of, 105-106
    in vegetarian diets, 87
    trace, 128
Mineral water, 494
Minoxidil and baldness, 322
Mirrored lenses, in sunglasses, 336
Miscarriage, and computer use, 534, 535
Mobile homes, formaldehyde gas levels in, 545
Moisturizers, 293-294
Molasses, 97
Molds:
    and hay fever, 344
    in automobile air conditioners, 552
    in humidifiers, 549
Moles and malignant melanoma, 300-301
Mollusks, 212

Molybdenum, 129
Monocytes, 500
Monounsaturated fats, 108
Morphine, 517
Motion sickness, 482
Mourning, dealing with, 456
Mouth cancer
    and alcohol consumption, 22
    and smoking, 60-61
MSG (monosodium glutamate):
    as food additive, 154
    in cold cuts, 205
    in egg substitutes, 187
    sodium content of, 131
Multiple-choice tests, 465
Mumps, 516
Mung beans, 197
Muscles:
    injuries, 409-425
    pulls, 411
    soreness, 237, 409-410
    spasms, 410
Muscular endurance, defined, 232
    strength, defined, 232
Mushrooms, 174
Mustard, 230
Myoglobin, 140

N

Nail care, 324-326
Naloxone, 520
Napping, 474
Narcotics, as headache remedy, 471
Nasal sprays, nonprescription, 526
National Aeronautics and Space Administration (NASA), 579
National Cancer Institute (NCI), 105
National Heart, Lung and Blood Institute, 48
National Institute for Occupational Safety and Health (NIOSH), 538
National Library of Medicine, 16
National Transportation Safety Board (NTSB), 587
Natural cosmetics, 295
Natural foods, 151. *See also* Food labeling
Navy beans, 197
Nearsightedness, 327
    surgery for, 334
Neck stretches, 443
Nectarines, 162
Nervous system, lead damage to, 554
Neurologists, 490
Neurons, 465
Neurosurgeons, 490
Newborn, risk of contracting AIDS from mother, 398
Niacin, 124
Nickel allergies, 294
Nicotine:
    and quitting smoking, 63
    as stimulant, 60
    effect on sleep, 479
Night, exercising during, 246
Night blindness, 124
Night driving safety, 590, 595-596
Nightmares, 476
Nitrate, in water, 568
Nitrites and nitrates, and cancer risk, 22
Nitrosamines, 22
Noise pollution, 559-560
Nonalcoholic beverages, 71